U. S. DEPARTMENT OF AGRICULTURE,
BUREAU OF ANIMAL INDUSTRY.
J. R. MOHLER, Chief of Bureau.

SPECIAL REPORT

ON

DISEASES OF THE HORSE.

BY

Drs. PEARSON, MICHENER, LAW, HARBAUGH, TRUMBOWER, LIAUTARD,
HOLCOMBE, HUIDEKOPER, MOHLER, EICHHORN,
HALL, AND ADAMS.

REVISED EDITION, 1923.

WASHINGTON:
GOVERNMENT PRINTING OFFICE.
1923.

[Extract from "An act making appropriations for the Department of Agriculture for the fiscal year ending June 30, 1924, and for other purposes," approved February 26, 1923. Public—No. 446.]

For printing, binding, and distribution of the publications entitled " Diseases of the Horse" and "Diseases of Cattle," $200,000: *Provided*, That said publications shall be deposited one-third in the folding room of the Senate and two-thirds in the folding room of the House of Representatives, and said documents shall be distributed by Members of the Senate and House of Representatives.

2

CONTENTS.

3

ILLUSTRATIONS.

SPECIAL REPORT

ON

DISEASES OF THE HORSE.

THE EXAMINATION OF A SICK HORSE.

By LEONARD PEARSON, B. S., V. M. D.

In the examination of a sick horse it is important to have a method or system. If a definite plan of examination is followed one may feel reasonably sure, when the examination is finished, that no important point has been overlooked and that the examiner is in a position to arrive at an opinion that is as accurate as is possible for him. Of course, an experienced eye can see, and a trained hand can feel, slight alterations or variations from the normal that are not perceptible to the unskilled observer. A thorough knowledge of the conditions that exist in health is of the highest importance, because it is only by a knowledge of what is right that one can surely detect a wrong condition. A knowledge of anatomy, or of the structure of the body, and of physiology, or the functions and activities of the body, lie at the bottom of accuracy of diagnosis. It is important to remember that animals of different races or families deport themselves differently under the influence of the same disease or pathological process. The sensitive and highly organized thoroughbred resists cerebral depression more than does the lymphatic draft horse. Hence a degree of fever that does not produce marked dullness in a thoroughbred may cause the most abject dejection in a coarsely bred, heavy draft horse. This and similar facts are of vast importance in the diagnosis of disease and in the recognition of its significance.

The order of examination, as given hereafter, is one that has proved to be comparatively easy of application and sufficiently thorough for the purpose of the readers of this work, and is recommended by several writers.

7

HISTORY.

It is important to know, first of all, something of the origin and development of the disease; therefore the cause should be looked for. The cause of a disease is important, not only in connection with diagnosis, but also in connection with treatment. The character of feed that the horse has had, the use to which he has been put, and the kind of care he has received should all be closely inquired into. It may be found by this investigation that the horse has been fed on damaged feed, such as brewers' grains or moldy silage, and this may be sufficient to explain the profound depression and weakness that are characteristic of forage poisoning. If it is learned that the horse has been kept in the stable without exercise for several days and upon full rations, and that he became suddenly lame in his back and hind legs, and finally fell to the ground from what appeared to be partial paralysis, this knowledge, taken in connection with a few evident symptoms, will be enough to establish a diagnosis of azoturia (excess of nitrogen in the urine). If it is learned that the horse has been recently shipped in the cars or has been through a dealer's stable, we have knowledge of significance in connection with the causation of a possible febrile disease, which is, under these conditions, likely to prove to be influenza, or edematous pneumonia.

It is also important to know whether the particular horse under examination is the only one in the stable, or on the premises, that is similarly afflicted. If it is found that several horses are afflicted much in the same way, we have evidence of a common cause of disease which may prove to be of an infectious nature.

Another item of importance in connection with the history of the case relates to the treatment that the horse may have had before he is examined. It sometimes happens that medicine given in excessive quantities produces symptoms resembling those of disease, so it is important that the examiner be fully informed as to the medication that has been employed.

ATTITUDE AND GENERAL CONDITION.

Before beginning the special examination, attention should be paid to the attitude and general condition of the animal. Sometimes horses assume positions that are characteristic of a certain disease. For example, in tetanus (lockjaw) the muscles of the face, neck, and shoulders are stiff and rigid, as well as the muscles of the jaw. This condition produces a peculiar attitude, that once seen is subsequently recognized as rather characteristic of the disease. A horse with tetanus stands with his muscles tense and his legs in a somewhat bracing position, as though he were gathered to repel a shock. The neck is stiff and hard. the head is slightly extended upon it, and the face is drawn, and the nostrils are dilated. The tail is usually held up a little, and when pressed down against the thighs it springs back to its previous position. In inflammation of the throat, as in pharyngolaryngitis, the head is extended upon the neck and the angle between the jaw and the lower border of the neck is opened as far as possible to relieve the pressure that otherwise would fall upon the throat. In dumminess, or immobility, the hanging position of the head and the stupid expression are rather characteristic. In pleurisy, peritonitis, and some other painful diseases of the internal organs, the rigid position of the body denotes an effort of the animal to avoid pressure upon and to protect the inflamed sensitive region.

The horse may be down in the stall and unable to rise. This condition may result from paraplegia (paralysis), from azoturia, from forage poisoning, from tetanus, or from painful conditions of the bones or feet, such as osteoporosis or founder. Lying down at unusual times or in unusual positions may indicate disease. The first symptom of colic may be a desire on the part of the horse to lie down at an unusual or inappropriate time or place. Sometimes disinclination to lie down is an indication of disease. When there is difficulty in breathing, the horse knows that he can manage himself better upon his feet than upon his breast or his side. It happens, therefore, that in nearly all serious diseases of the respiratory tract he stands persistently, day and night, until recovery has commenced and breathing is easier, or until the animal falls from sheer exhaustion. If there is stiffness and soreness of the muscles, as in rheumatism, inflammation of the muscles from overwork, or of the bones in osteoporosis, or of the feet in founder, or if the muscles are stiff and beyond control of the animal, as in tetanus, a standing position is maintained, because the horse seems to realize that when he lies down he will be unable to rise.

Abnormal attitudes are assumed in painful diseases of the digestive organs (colic). A horse with colic may sit upon his haunches, like a dog, or may stand upon his hind feet and rest upon his knees in front, or he may endeavor to balance himself upon his back, with all four feet in the air. These positions are assumed because they give relief from pain by lessening pressure or tension upon the sensitive structures.

Under the general condition of the animal it is necessary to observe the condition or state of nutrition, the conformation, so far as it may indicate the constitution, and the temperament. By observing the condition of nutrition one may be able to determine to a certain extent the effect that the disease has already had upon the animal and to estimate the amount of strength that remains and that will be available for the repair of the diseased tissues. A good condition of nutrition is shown by the rotundity of the body, the pliability and softness of the skin, and the tone of the hair. If the subcutaneous fat has disappeared and the muscles are wasted, allowing the bony prominences to stand out; if the skin is tight and inelastic and the coat dry and harsh, we have evidence of a low state of nutrition. This may have resulted from a severe and long-continued disease or from lack of proper feed and care. When an animal is emaciated—that is, becomes thin—there is first a loss of fat and later the muscles shrink. By observing the amount of shrinkage in the muscles one has some indication as to the duration of the unfavorable conditions under which the animal has lived.

By constitution we understand the innate ability of the animal to withstand disease or unfavorable conditions of life. The constitution depends largely upon the conformation. The type of construction that usually accompanies the best constitution is deep, broad chest, allowing plenty of room for the lungs and heart, indicating that these vital organs are well developed; capacious abdomen, allowing sufficient space for well-developed organs of digestion; the loins should be short—that is, the space should be short between the last rib and the point of the hip; the head and neck should be well molded, without superfluous or useless tissue; this gives a clear-cut throat. The ears, eyes, and face should have an expression of alertness and good breeding. The muscular development should be good; the shoulders, forearms, croup, and thighs must have the appearance of strength. The withers are sharp, which means that they are not loaded with useless, superfluous tissue; the legs are straight and their axes are parallel; the knees and hocks are low, which means that the forearms and thighs are long and the cannons relatively short. The cannons are broad from in front to behind and relatively thin from side to side. This means that the bony and tendinous structures of the legs are well developed and well placed. The hoofs are compact, tense, firm structures, and their soles are concave and frogs large. Such a horse is likely to have a good constitution and to be able to resist hard work, fatigue, and disease to a maximum degree. On the other hand, a poor constitution is indicated by a shallow, narrow chest, small bones, long loins, coarse neck and head, with thick throat, small, bony, and muscular development, short thighs and forearms, small joints, long, round cannons, and hoofs of open texture with flat soles.

The temperament is indicated by the manner in which the horse responds to external stimuli. When the horse is spoken to, or when he sees or feels anything that stimulates or gives alarm, if he responds actively, quickly, and intelligently, he is said to be of lively, or nervous, temperament. On the other hand, if he responds in a slow, sluggish manner, he is said to have a sluggish, or lymphatic, temperament. The temperament is indicated by the gait, by the expression of the face, and by the carriage of the head and ears. The nature of the temperament should be taken into consideration in an endeavor to ascertain the severity of a given case of illness, because the general expression of an animal in disease as well as in health depends to a large extent on the temperament.

THE SKIN AND THE VISIBLE MUCOUS MEMBRANES.

The condition of the skin is a fair index to the condition of the animal. The effect of disease and emaciation upon the pliability of the skin have been referred to above. There is no part of the body that loses its elasticity and tone as a result of disease sooner than the skin. The practical herdsman or flockmaster can gain a great deal of information as to the condition of an animal merely by grasping the coat and looking at and feeling the skin. Similarly, the condition of the animal is shown to a certain extent by the appearance of the mucous membranes. For example, when the horse is anemic as a result of disease or of inappropriate feed the mucous membranes become pale. This change in the mucous membranes can be seen most readily in the lining of the eyelids and in the lining of the nostril. For convenience of examination the eyelids can readily be everted. Paleness means weak circulation or poor blood. Increased redness occurs physiologically in painful conditions, excitement, and following severe exertion. Under such conditions the increase of circulation is transitory. In fevers there is an increased redness in the mucous membrane, and this continues so long as the fever lasts. In some diseases red spots or streaks form in the mucous membrane. This usually indicates an infectious disease of considerable severity, and occurs in blood poisoning, purpura hemorrhagica, hemorrhagic septicemia, and in urticaria. When the liver is deranged and does not operate, or when the red-blood corpuscles are broken down, as in serious cases of influenza, there is a yellowish discoloration of the mucous membrane. The mucous membranes become bluish or blue when the blood is imperfectly oxidized and contains an excess of carbon dioxid. This condition exists in any serious disease of the respiratory tract, as pneumonia, and in heart failure.

The temperature of the skin varies with the temperature of the body. If there is fever the temperature of the skin is likely to be increased. Sometimes, however, as a result of poor circulation and irregular distribution of the blood, the body may be warmer than normal, while the extremities (the legs and ears) may be cold. Where the general surface of the body becomes cold it is evident that the small blood vessels in the skin have contracted and are keeping the blood away, as during a chill, or that the heart is weak and is unable to pump the blood to the surface, and that the animal is on the verge of collapse.

The skin is moist, to a certain degree, at all times in a healthy horse. This moisture is not in the form of a perceptible sweat, but it is enough to keep the skin pliable and to cause the hair to have a soft, healthy feel. In some chronic diseased conditions and in fever, the skin becomes dry. In this case the hair has a harsh feel that is quite different from the condition observed in health, and from the fact of its being so dry the individual hairs do not adhere to one another, they stand apart, and the animal has what is known as "a staring coat." When, during a fever, sweating occurs, it is usually an indication that the crisis is passed. Sometimes sweating is an indication of pain. A horse with tetanus or azoturia sweats profusely. Horses sweat freely when there is a serious impediment to respiration; they sweat under excitement, and, of course, from the well-known physiological causes of heat and work. Local sweating, or sweating of a restricted area of the body, denotes some kind of nerve interference.

Swellings of the skin usually come from wounds or other external causes and have no special connection with the diagnosis of internal diseases. There are, however, a number of conditions in which the swelling of the skin is a symptom of a derangement of some other part of the body. For example, there is the well-known "stocking," or swelling of the legs about the fetlock joints, in influenza. There is the soft swelling of the hind legs that occurs so often in draft horses when standing still and that comes from previous inflammation (lymphangitis) or from insufficient heart power. Dropsy, or edema of the skin, may occur beneath the chest or abdomen from heart insufficiency or from chronic collection of fluid in the chest or abdomen (hydrothorax, ascites, or anemia). In anasarca or purpura hemorrhagica large soft swellings appear on any part of the skin, but usually on the legs, side of the body, and about the head.

Gas collects under the skin in some instances. This comes from a local inoculation with an organism which produces a fermentation beneath the skin and causes the liberation of gas which inflates the skin, or the gas may be air that enters through a wound penetrating some air-containing organ, as the lungs. The condition here described is known as emphysema. Emphysema may follow the fracture of a rib when the end of a bone is forced inward and caused to penetrate the lung, or it may occur when, as a result of an ulcerating process, an organ containing air is perforated. This accident is more common in cattle than it is in horses. Emphysema is recognized by the fact that the swelling that it causes is not hot or sensitive on pressure. It emits a peculiar crackling sound when it is stroked or pressed upon.

Wounds of the skin may be of importance in the diagnosis of internal disease. Wounds over the bony prominence, as the point of the hip, the point of the shoulder, and the greatest convexity of the ribs, occur when a horse is unable to stand for a long time and, through continually lying upon his side, has shut off the circulation to the portion of the skin that covers parts of the body that carry the greatest weight, and in this way has caused them to mortify. Little, round, soft, doughlike swellings occur on the skin and may be scattered freely over the surface of the body when the horse is afflicted with urticaria. Similar eruptions, but distributed less generally, about the size of a silver dollar, may occur as a symptom of dourine, or colt distemper. Hard lumps, from which radiate weltlike swellings of the lymphatics, occur in glanders, and blisterlike eruptions occur around the mouth and pasterns in horsepox.

THE ORGANS OF CIRCULATION.

The first item in this portion of the examination consists in taking the pulse. The pulse may be counted and its character may be determined at any point where a large artery occupies a situation close to the skin and above a hard tissue, such as a bone, cartilage, or tendon. The most convenient place for taking the pulse of the horse is at the jaw. The external maxillary artery runs from between the jaws, around the lower border of the jawbone, and up on the outside of the jawbone to the face. It is located immediately in front of the heavy muscles of the cheek. Its throb can be felt most distinctly just before it turns around the lower border of the jawbone. The balls of the first and second or of the second and third fingers should be pressed lightly on the skin over this artery when its pulsations are to be studied.

The normal pulse of the healthy horse varies in frequency as follows:

Stallion	28 to 32 beats per minute.
Gelding	33 to 38 beats per minute.
Mare	34 to 40 beats per minute.
Foal 2 to 3 years old	40 to 50 beats per minute.
Foal 6 to 12 months old	45 to 60 beats per minute.
Foal 2 to 4 weeks old	70 to 90 beats per minute.

The pulse is accelerated by the digestion of rich food, by hot weather, exercise, excitement, and alarm. It is slightly more rapid in the evening than it is in the morning. Well-bred horses have a slightly more rapid pulse than sluggish, cold-blooded horses. The pulse should be regular; that is, the separate beats should follow each other after intervals of equal length, and the beats should be of equal fullness, or volume.

In disease, the pulse may become slower or more rapid than in health. Slowing of the pulse may be caused by old age, great exhaustion, or excessive cold. It may be due to depression of the central nervous system, as in dumminess, or be the result of the administration of drugs, such as digitalis or strophanthus. A rapid pulse is almost always found in fever, and the more severe the infection and the weaker the heart the more rapid is the pulse. Under these conditions, the beats may rise to 80, 90, or even 120 per minute. When the pulse is above 100 per minute the outlook for recovery is not promising, and especially if this symptom accompanies high temperature or occurs late in an infectious disease. In nearly all of the diseases of the heart and in anemia the pulse becomes rapid.

The pulse is irregular in diseases of the heart, and especially where the valves are affected. The irregularity may consist in varying intervals between the beats or the dropping of one or more beats at regular or irregular intervals. The latter condition sometimes occurs in chronic diseases of the brain. The pulse is said to be weak, or soft, when the beats are indistinct, because little blood is forced through the artery by each contraction of the heart. This condition occurs when there is a constriction of the vessels leading from the heart and it occurs in certain infectious and febrile diseases, and is an indication of heart weakness.

In examining the heart itself it is necessary to recall that it lies in the anterior portion of the chest slightly to the left of the median line and that it extends from the third to the sixth rib. It extends almost to the breastbone, and a little more than half of the distance between the breastbone and the backbone. In contracting, it rotates slightly on its axis, so that the point of the heart, which lies below, is pressed against the left chest wall at a place immediately above the point of the elbow. The heart has in it four chambers—two in the left and two in the right side. The upper chamber of the left side (left auricle) receives the blood as it comes from the lungs, passes it to the lower chamber of the left side (left ventricle), and from here it is sent with great force (for this chamber has very strong, thick walls) through the aorta and its branches (the arteries) to all parts of the body. The blood returns through the veins to the upper chamber of the right side (right auricle), passes then to the lower chamber of the right side (right ventricle), and from this chamber is forced into the lungs to be oxidized. The openings between the chambers of each side and into the aorta are guarded by valves.

If the horse is not too fat, one may feel the impact of the apex of the heart against the chest wall with each contraction of the heart by placing the hand on the left side back of the fifth rib and above the point of the elbow. The thinner and the better bred the horse is the more distinctly this impact is felt. If the animal is excited, or if he has just been exercised, the impact is stronger than when the horse is at rest. If the horse is weak, the impact is reduced in force.

The examination of the heart with the ear is an important matter in this connection. Certain sounds are produced by each contraction of the normal heart. It is customary to divide these into two, and to call them the first and second sounds. These two sounds are heard during each pulsation, and any deviation of the normal indicates some alteration in the structure or the functions of the heart. In making this examination, one may apply the left ear over the heavy muscles of the shoulder back of the shoulder joint, and just above the point of the elbow, or, if the sounds are not heard distinctly, the left fore leg may be drawn forward by an assistant and the right ear placed against the lower portion of the chest wall that is exposed in this manner.

The first sound of the heart occurs while the heart muscle is contracting and while the blood is being forced from the heart and the valves are rendered taut to prevent the return of the blood from the lower to the upper chambers. The second sound follows quickly after the first and occurs during rebound of blood in the arteries, causing pressure in the aorta and tensions of the valves guarding its opening into the left ventricle. The first sound is of a high pitch and is longer and more distinct than the second. Under the influence of disease these sounds may be altered in various ways. It is not profitable, in a work such as this, to describe the details of these alterations. Those who are interested will find this subject fully discussed in the veterinary textbooks.

TEMPERATURE.

The temperature of the horse is determined roughly by placing the fingers in the mouth or between the thighs or by allowing the horse to exhale against the cheek or back of the hand. In accurate examination, however, these means of determining temperature are not relied upon, but recourse is had to the use of the thermometer. The thermometer used for taking the temperature of a horse is a self-registering clinical thermometer, similar to that used by physicians, but larger, being from 5 to 6 inches long. The temperature of the animal is measured in the rectum.

The normal temperature of the horse varies somewhat under different conditions. It is higher in the young animal than in the old, and is higher in hot weather than in cold. The weather and exercise decidedly influence the temperature physiologically. The normal temperature varies from 99.5° to 101° F. If the temperature rises to 102.5° the horse is said to have a low fever; if the temperature reaches 104° the fever is moderate; if it reaches 106° it is high, and above this point it is regarded as very high. In some diseases, such as tetanus or sunstroke, the temperature goes as high as 108° or 110°. In the ordinary infectious diseases it does not often exceed 106°. A temperature of 107.5° and above is very dangerous and must be reduced promptly if the horse is to be saved.

THE ORGANS OF RESPIRATION.

In examining this system of organs and their functions it is customary to begin by noting the frequency of the respiratory movements. This point can be determined by observing the motions of the nostrils or of the flanks; on a cold day one can see the condensation of the moisture of the warm air as it comes from the lungs. The normal rate of respiration for a healthy horse at rest is from 8 to 16 per minute. The rate is faster in young animals than in old, and is increased by work, hot weather, overfilling of the stomach, pregnancy, lying upon the side, etc. Acceleration of the respiratory rate where no physiological cause operates is due to a variety of conditions. Among these is fever; restricted area of active lung tissue, from filling of portions of the lungs with inflammatory exudate, as in pneumonia; compression of the lungs or loss of elasticity; pain in the muscles controlling the respiratory movements; excess of carbon dioxid in the blood; and constriction of the air passages leading to the lungs.

Difficult or labored respiration is known as dyspnea. It occurs when it is difficult, for any reason, for the animal to obtain the amount of oxygen that it requires. This may be due to filling of the lungs, as in pneumonia; to painful movements of the chest, as in rheumatism or pleurisy; to tumors of the nose and paralysis of the throat, swellings of the throat, foreign bodies, or weakness of the respiratory passages, fluid in the chest cavity, adhesions between the lungs and chest walls, loss of elasticity of the lungs, etc. Where the difficulty is great the accessory muscles of respiration are brought into play. In great dyspnea the horse stands with his front feet apart, with his neck straight out, and his head extended upon his neck. The nostrils are widely dilated, the face has an anxious expression, the eyeballs protrude, the up-and-down motion of the larnyx is aggravated, the amplitude of the movement of the chest walls increased, and the flanks heave.

The expired air is of about the temperature of the body. It contains considerable moisture, and it should come with equal force from each nostril and should not have an unpleasant odor. If the stream of air from one nostril is stronger than from the other, there is an indication of an obstruction in a nasal chamber. If the air possesses a bad odor, it is usually an indication of putrefaction of a tissue or secretion in some part of the respiratory tract. A bad odor is found where there is necrosis of the bone in the nasal passages or in chronic catarrh. An ulcerating tumor of the nose or throat may cause the breath to have an offensive odor. The most offensive breath occurs where there is necrosis, or gangrene, of the lungs.

In some diseases there is a discharge from the nose. In order to determine the significance of the discharge it should be examined closely. One should ascertain whether it comes from one or both nostrils. If but from one nostril, it probably originates in the head. The color should be noted. A thin, watery discharge may be composed of serum, and it occurs in the earlier stages of coryza, or nasal catarrh. An opalescent, slightly tinted discharge is composed of mucus and indicates a little more severe irritation. If the discharge is sticky and puslike, a deeper difficulty or more advanced irritation is indicated. If the discharge contains flakes and clumps of more or less dried, agglutinated particles, it is probable that it originates within a cavity of the head, as the sinuses or guttural pouches. The discharge of glanders is of a peculiar sticky nature and adheres tenaciously to the wings of the nostrils. The discharge of pneumonia is of a somewhat red or reddish brown color and, on this account, has been described as a prune-juice discharge. The discharge may contain blood. If the blood appears as clots or as streaks in the discharge, it probably originates at some point in the upper part of the respiratory tract. If the blood is in the form of a fine froth, it comes from the lungs.

In examining the interior of the nasal passage one should remember that the normal color of the mucous membrane is a rosy pink and that its surface is smooth. If ulcers, nodules, swellings, or tumors are found, these indicate disease. The ulcer that is characteristic of glanders is described fully in connection with the discussion of that disease.

Between the lower jaws there are several clusters of lymphatic glands. These glands are so small and so soft that it is difficult to find them by feeling through the skin, but when a suppurative disease exists in the upper part of the respiratory tract these glands become swollen and easy to feel. They may become soft and break down and discharge as abscesses; this is seen constantly in strangles. On the other hand, they may become indurated and hard from the proliferation of connective tissue and attach themselves to the jawbone, to the tongue, or to the skin. This is seen in chronic glanders. If the glands are swollen and tender to pressure, it indicates that the disease causing the enlargement is acute; if they are hard and insensitive, the disease causing the enlargement is chronic.

54763°—23——2

The manner in which the horse coughs is of importance in diagnosis. The cough is a forced expiration, following immediately upon a
forcible separation of the vocal cords. The purpose of the cough is
to remove some irritant substance from the respiratory passages, and
it occurs when irritant gases, such as smoke, ammonia, sulphur vapor,
or dust, have been inhaled. It occurs from inhalation of cold air if
the respiratory passages are sensitive from disease. In laryngitis,
bronchitis, and pneumonia, cough is very easily excited and occurs
merely from accumulation of mucus and inflammatory product upon
the irritated respiratory mucous membrane. If one wishes to determine the character of the cough, it can easily be excited by pressing
upon the larynx with the thumb and finger. The larynx should be
pressed from side to side and the pressure removed the moment the
horse commences to cough. A painful cough occurs in pleurisy, also
in laryngitis, bronchitis, and bronchial pneumonia. Pain is shown
by the effort the animal exerts to repress the cough. The cough is
not painful, as a rule, in the chronic diseases of the respiratory tract.
The force of the cough is considerable when it is not especially painful and when the lungs are not seriously involved. When the lungs
are so diseased that they can not be filled with a large volume of air,
and in heaves, the cough is weak, as it is also in weak, debilitated
animals. If mucus or pus is coughed out, or if the cough is accompanied by a gurgling sound, it is said to be moist; it is dry when
these characteristics are not present—that is, when the air in passing
out passes over surface not loaded with secretion.

In the examination of the chest we resort to percussion and auscultation. When a cask or other structure containing air is tapped
upon, or percussed, a hollow sound is given forth. If the cask contains fluid, the sound is of a dull and of quite a different character.
Similarly, the amount of air contained in the lungs can be estimated
by tapping upon, or percussing, the walls of the chest. Percussion is
practiced with the fingers alone or with the aid of a special percussion hammer and an object to strike upon known as a pleximeter.
If the fingers are used, the middle finger of the left hand should be
pressed firmly against the side of the horse and should be struck with
the ends of the fingers of the right hand bent at a right angle so as to
form a hammer. The percussion hammer sold by instrument makers
is made of rubber or has a rubber tip, so that when the pleximeter,
which is placed against the side, is struck the impact will not be
accompanied by a noise. After experience in this method of examination one can determine with a considerable degree of accuracy
whether the lung contains a normal amount of air or not. If, as in
pneumonia, air has been displaced by inflammatory product occupying the air space, or if fluid collects in the lower part of the chest, the
percussion sound becomes dull. If, as in emphysema, or in pneu-

mothorax, there is an excess of air in the chest cavity, the percussion sound becomes abnormally loud and clear.

Auscultation consists in the examination of the lungs with the ear applied closely to the chest wall. As the air goes in and out of the lungs a certain soft sound is made which can be heard distinctly, especially upon inspiration. This sound is intensified by anything that accelerates the rate of respiration, such as exercise. This soft, rustling sound is known as vesicular murmur, and wherever it is heard it signifies that the lung contains air and is functionally active. The vesicular murmur is weakened when there is an inflammatory infiltration of the lung tissue or when the lungs are compressed by fluid in the chest cavity. The vesicular murmur disappears when air is excluded by the accumulation of inflammatory product, as in pneumonia, and when the lungs are compressed by fluid in the chest cavity. The vesicular murmur becomes rough and harsh in the early stages of inflammation of the lungs, and this is often the first sign of the beginning of pneumonia.

By applying the ear over the lower part of the windpipe in front of the breastbone a somewhat harsh, blowing sound may be heard. This is known as the bronchial murmur and is heard in normal conditions near the lower part of the trachea and to a limited extent in the anterior portions of the lungs after sharp exercise. When the bronchial murmur is heard over other portions of the lungs, it may signify that the lungs are more or less solidified by disease and the blowing bronchial murmur is transmitted through this solid lung to the ear from a distant part of the chest. The bronchial murmur in an abnormal place signifies that there exists pneumonia or that the lungs are compressed by fluid in the chest cavity.

Additional sounds are heard in the lungs in some diseased conditions. For example, when fluid collects in the air passages and the air is forced through it or is caused to pass through tubes containing secretions or pus. Such sounds are of a gurgling or bubbling nature and are known as mucous râles. Mucous râles are spoken of as being large or small as they are distinct or indistinct, depending upon the quantity of fluid that is present and the size of the tube in which this sound is produced. Mucous râles occur in pneumonia after the solidified parts begin to break down at the end of the disease. They occur in bronchitis and in tuberculosis, where there is an excess of secretion.

Sometimes a shrill sound is heard, like the note of a whistle, fife, or flute. This is due to a dry constriction of the bronchial tubes and it is heard in chronic bronchitis and in tuberculosis.

A friction sound is heard in pleurisy. This is due to the rubbing together of roughened surfaces, and the sound produced is similar to a dry rubbing sound that is caused by rubbing the hands together or by rubbing upon each other two dry, rough pieces of leather.

THE EXAMINATION OF THE DIGESTIVE TRACT.

The first point in connection with the examination of the organs of digestion is the appetite and the manner of taking food and drink. A healthy animal has a good appetite. Loss of appetite does not point to a special diseased condition, but comes from a variety of causes. Some of these causes, indeed, may be looked upon as being physiological. Excitement, strange surroundings, fatigue, and hot weather may all cause loss of appetite. Where there is cerebral depression, fever, profound weakness, disorder of the stomach, or mechanical difficulty in chewing or swallowing, the appetite is diminished or destroyed. Sometimes there is an appetite or desire to eat abnormal things, such as dirty bedding, roots of grass, soil, etc. This desire usually comes from a chronic disturbance of nutrition.

Thirst is diminished in a good many mild diseases unaccompanied by distinct fever. It is seen where there is great exhaustion or depression or profound brain disturbance. Thirst is increased after profuse sweating, in diabetes, diarrhea, in fever, at the crises of infectious diseases, and when the mouth is dry and hot.

Some diseases of the mouth or throat make it difficult for the horse to chew or swallow his feed. Where difficulty in this respect is experienced, the following-named conditions should be borne in mind and carefully looked for: Diseases of the teeth, consisting in decay, fracture, abscess formation, or overgrowth; inflammatory conditions, or wounds or tumors of the tongue, cheeks, or lips; paralysis of the muscles of chewing or swallowing; foreign bodies in upper part of the mouth between the molar teeth; inflammation of throat. Difficulty in swallowing is sometimes shown by the symptom known as " quidding." Quidding consists in dropping from the mouth well-chewed and insalivated boluses of feed. A mouthful of hay, for example, after being ground and masticated, is carried to the back part of the mouth. The horse then finds that from tenderness of the throat, or from some other cause, swallowing is difficult or painful, and the bolus is then dropped from the mouth. Another quantity of hay is similarly prepared, only to be dropped in turn. Sometimes quidding is due to a painful tooth, the bolus being dropped from the mouth when the tooth is struck and during the pang that follows. Quidding may be practiced so persistently that a considerable pile of boluses of feed accumulate in the manger or on the floor of the stall. In pharyngitis one of the symptoms is a return through the nose of fluid that the horse attempts to swallow.

In some brain diseases, and particularly in chronic internal hydrocephalus, the horse has a most peculiar manner of swallowing and of taking feed. A similar condition is seen in hyperemia of the brain. In eating the horse will sink his muzzle into the grain in the feed box and eat for a while without raising the head. Long pauses are made while the feed is in the mouth. Sometimes the horse will eat very rapidly for a little while and then slowly; the jaws may be brought together so forcibly that the teeth gnash. In eating hay the horse will stop at times with hay protruding from the mouth and stand stupidly, as though he has forgotten what he was about.

In examining the mouth one should first look for swellings or for evidence of abnormal conditions upon the exterior; that is, the front and sides of the face, the jaws, and about the muzzle. By this means wounds, fractures, tumors, abscesses, and disease accompanied by eruptions about the muzzle may be detected. The interior of the mouth is examined by holding the head up and inserting the fingers through the interdental space in such a way as to cause the mouth to open. The mucous membrane should be clean and of a light-pink color, excepting on the back of the tongue, where the color is a yellowish gray. As abnormalities of this region, the chief are diffuse inflammation, characterized by redness and catarrhal discharge; local inflammation, as from eruptions, ulcers, or wounds; necrosis of the lower jawbone in front of the first back tooth; and swellings. Foreign bodies are sometimes found embedded in the mucous membrane lining of the mouth or lodged between the teeth.

The examination of the pharynx and of the esophagus is made chiefly by pressing upon the skin covering these organs in the region of the throat and along the left side of the neck in the jugular gutter. Sometimes, when a more careful examination is necessary, an esophageal tube or probang is passed through the nose or mouth down the esophagus to the stomach.

Vomiting is an act consisting in the expulsion of all or part of the contents of the stomach through the mouth or nose. This act is more difficult for the horse than for most of the other domestic animals, because the stomach of the horse is small and does not lie on the floor of the abdominal cavity, so that the abdominal walls in contracting do not bring pressure to bear upon it so directly and forcibly, as is the case in many other animals. Beside this, there is a loose fold of mucous membrane at the point where the esophagus enters the stomach, and this forms a sort of valve which does not interfere with the passage of food into the stomach, but does interfere with the exit of food through the esophageal opening. Still, vomiting is a symptom that is occasionally seen in the horse. It occurs when the stomach is very much distended with food or with gas. Distention stretches the mucous membrane and eradicates the valvular fold referred to, and also makes it possible for more pressure to be exerted upon the stomach through the contraction of the abdominal muscles. Since the distention to permit vomiting must be extreme, it not infrequently happens that it leads to rupture of the stomach walls. This has caused the impression in the minds of some that vomiting can not occur in the horse without rupture of the stomach, but this is incorrect, since many horses vomit and afterwards become entirely sound. After rupture of the stomach has occurred vomiting is impossible.

In examination of the abdomen one should remember that its size depends largely upon the breed, sex, and conformation of the animal, and also upon the manner in which the animal has been fed and the use to which it has been put. A pendulous abdomen may be the result of an abdominal tumor or of an accumulation of fluid in the abdominal cavity; or, on the other hand, it may merely be an indication of pregnancy, or of the fact that the horse has been fed for a long time on bulky and innutritious food. Pendulous abdomen occurring in a work horse kept on a concentrated diet is an abnormal condition. The abdomen may increase suddenly in volume from accumulation of gas in tympanic colic. The abdomen becomes small and the horse is said to be "tucked up" from long-continued poor appetite, as in diseases of the digestive tract and in fever. This condition also occurs in tetanus from the contraction of the abdominal walls and in diarrhea from emptiness.

In applying the ear to the flank, on either the right or left side, certain bubbling sounds may be heard that are known as peristaltic sounds, because they are produced by peristalsis, or wormlike contraction of the intestines. These sounds are a little louder on the right side than on the left on account of the fact that the large intestines lie in the right flank. Absence of peristaltic sounds is always an indication of disease, and suggests exhaustion or paralysis of the intestines. This may occur in certain kinds of colic and is an unfavorable symptom. Increased sounds are heard where the intestines are contracted more violently than in health, as in spasmodic colic, and also where there is an excess of fluid or gas in the intestinal canal.

The feces show, to a certain extent, the thoroughness of digestion. They should show that the feed has been well ground, and should, in the horse, be free from offensive odor or coatings of mucus. A coating of mucus shows intestinal catarrh. Blood on the feces indicates severe inflammation. Very light color and bad odor may come from inactive liver. Parasites are sometimes in the dung.

Rectal examination consists in examination of the organs of the pelvic cavity and posterior portion of the abdominal cavity by the hand inserted into the rectum. This examination should be attempted by a veterinarian only, and is useless except to one who has a good knowledge of the anatomy of the parts concerned.

THE EXAMINATION OF THE NERVOUS SYSTEM.

The great brain, or cerebrum, is the seat of intelligence, and it contains the centers that control motion in many parts of the body. The front portion of the brain is believed to be the region that is most important in governing the intelligence. The central and posterior portions of the cerebrum contain the centers for the voluntary motions of the face and of the front and hind legs. The growth of a tumor or an inflammatory change in the region of a center governing the motion of a certain part of the body has the effect of disturbing motion in that part by causing excessive contraction known as cramps, or inability of the muscles to contract, constituting the condition known as paralysis. The nerve paths from the cerebrum, and hence from these centers to the spinal cord and thence to the muscles, pass beneath the small brain, or the cerebellum, and through the medulla oblongata to the spinal cord. Interference with these paths has the effect of disturbing motion of the parts reached by them. If all of the paths on one side are interfered with, the result is paralysis of one side of the body.

The small brain, or cerebellum, governs the regularity, or coordination, of movements. Disturbances of the cerebellum cause a tottering, uncertain gait. In the medulla oblongata, which lies between the spinal cord and the cerebellum, are the centers governing the circulation and breathing.

The spinal cord carries sensory messages to the brain and motor impressions from the brain. The anterior portions of the cord contain the motor paths, and the posterior portions of the cord contain the sensory paths.

Paralysis of a single member or a single group of muscles is known as monoplegia and results from injury to the motor center or to a nerve trunk leading to the part that is involved. Paralysis of one-half of the body is known as hemiplegia and results from destruction or severe disturbances of the cerebral hemisphere of the opposite side of the body or from interference with nerve paths between the cerebellum, or small brain, and the spinal cord. Paralysis of the posterior half of the body is known as paraplegia and results from derangement of the spinal cord. If the cord is pressed upon, cut, or injured, messages can not be transmitted beyond that point, and so the posterior part becomes paralyzed. This is seen when the back is fractured.

Abnormal mental excitement may be due to congestion of the brain or to inflammation. The animal so afflicted becomes vicious, pays no attention to commands, cries, runs about in a circle, stamps with the feet, strikes, kicks, etc. This condition is usually followed by a dull, stupid state, in which the animal stands with his head down, dull and irresponsive to external stimuli. Cerebral depression also occurs in the severe febrile infectious diseases, in chronic hydrocephalus, in chronic diseases of the liver, in poisoning with a narcotic substance, and with chronic catarrh of the stomach and intestines.

Fainting is a symptom that is not often seen in horses. When it occurs it is shown by unsteadiness of gait, tottering, and, finally, inability to stand. The cause usually lies in a defect of the small brain, or cerebellum. This defect may be merely in respect of the blood supply, to congestion, or to anemia, and in this case it is likely to pass away and may never return, or it may be due to some permanent cause, as a tumor or an abscess, or it may result from a hemorrhage, from a defect of the valves of the heart, or from poisoning.

Loss of consciousness is known as coma. It is caused by hemorrhage in the brain, by profound exhaustion, or may result from a saturation of the system with the poison of some disease. Coma may follow upon cerebral depression, which occurs as a secondary state of inflammation of the brain.

Where the sensibility of a part is increased the condition is known as hyperesthesia, and where it is lost—that is, where there is no feeling or knowledge of pain—the condition is known as anesthesia. The former usually accompanies some chronic disease of the spinal cord or the earlier stages of irritation of a nerve trunk. Hyperesthesia is difficult to detect in a nervous, irritable animal, and sometimes even in a horse of less sensitive temperament. An irritable, sensitive spot may be found surrounded by skin that is not sensitive to pressure. This is sometimes a symptom of beginning of inflammation of the brain. Anesthesia occurs in connection with cerebral and spinal paralysis, section of a nerve trunk leading to a part, in severe mental depression, and in narcotic poisoning.

URINARY AND SEXUAL ORGANS.

In considering the examination of the urinary and sexual organs we may consider, at the beginning, a false impression that prevails to an astonishing extent. Many horsemen are in the habit of pressing upon the back of a horse over the loins or of sliding the ends of the fingers along on either side of the median line of this region. If the horse depresses his back it is at once said "his kidneys are weak." Nothing could be more absurd or further from the truth. Any healthy horse—any horse with normal sensation and with a normally flexible back—will cause it to sink when manipulated in this way. If the kidneys are inflamed and sensitive, the back is held more rigidly and is not depressed under this pressure.

To examine the kidneys by pressure the pressure should be brought to bear over these organs. The kidneys lie beneath the ends of the transverse processes of the vertebræ of the loins and beneath the hindmost ribs. If the kidneys are actually inflamed and especially sensitive, pressure or light blows applied here may cause the horse to shrink.

The physical examination of the sexual and generative organs is made in large part through the rectum, and this portion of the examination should be carried out by a veterinarian only. By this means it is possible to discover or locate cysts of the kidneys, urinary calculi in the ureters, bladder, or upper urethra, malformations, and acute inflammations accompanied by pain. The external genital organs are swollen, discolored, or show a discharge as a result of local disease or from disease higher in the tract.

The manner of urinating is sometimes of considerable diagnostic importance. Painful urination is shown by frequent attempts, during which but a small quantity of urine is passed; by groaning, by constrained attitude, etc. This condition comes from inflammation of the bladder or urethra, urinary calculi (stones of the bladder or urethra), hemorrhage, tumors, bruises, etc. The urine is retained from spasms of the muscle at the neck of the bladder, from calculi, inflammatory growths, tumors, and paralysis of the bladder.

The urine dribbles without control when the neck of the bladder is weakened or paralyzed. This condition is seen after the bladder is weakened from long-continued retention and where there is a partial paralysis of the hind quarters.

Horses usually void urine five to seven times a day, and pass from 4 to 7 quarts. Disease may be shown by increase in the number of voidings or of the quantity. Frequent urination indicates an irritable or painful condition of the bladder or urethra or that the quantity is excessive. In one form of chronic inflammation of the kidneys (interstitial nephritis) and in polyuria the quantity may be increased to 20 or 30 quarts daily. Diminution in the quantity of urine comes from profuse sweating, diarrhea, high fever, weak heart, diseased and nonsecreting kidneys, or an obstruction to the flow.

The urine of the healthy horse is a pale or at times a slightly reddish yellow. The color is less intense when the quantity is large, and is more intense when the quantity is diminished. Dark-brown urine is seen in azoturia and in severe acute muscular rheumatism. A brownish-green color is seen in jaundice. Red color indicates admixture of blood from a bleeding point at some part of the urinary tract, usually in the kidneys.

The urine of the healthy horse is not clear and transparent. It contains mucus, which causes it to be slightly thick and stringy, and a certain amount of undissolved carbonates, causing it to be cloudy, A sediment collects when the urine is allowed to stand. The urine of the horse is normally alkaline. If it becomes acid the bodies in suspension are dissolved and the urine is made clear. The urine may be unusually cloudy from the addition of abnormal constituents, but to determine their character a chemical or microscopic examination is necessary. Red or reddish flakes or clumps in the urine are always abnormal, and denote a hemorrhage or suppuration in the urinary tract.

The normal specific gravity of the urine of the horse is about 1.040. It is increased when the urine is scanty and decreased when the quantity is excessive.

Acid reaction of the urine occurs in chronic intestinal catarrh, in high fever, and during starvation. Chemical and microscopic tests and examinations are often of great importance in diagnosis, but require special apparatus and skill.

Other points in the examination of a sick horse require more discussion than can be afforded in this connection, and require special training on the part of the examiner. Among such points may be mentioned the examination of the organs of special sense, the examination of the blood, the microscopic examination of the secretions and excretions, bacteriological examinations of the secretions, excretions, and tissues, specific reaction tests, and diagnostic inoculation.

FUNDAMENTAL PRINCIPLES OF DISEASE.

By Rush Shippen Huidekoper, M. D., Vet.

[Revised by Leonard Pearson, B. S., V. M. D.]

ANIMAL TISSUES.

The nonprofessional reader may regard the animal tissues, which are subject to inflammation, as excessively simple structures, as similar, simple, and fixed in their organization as the joists and boards which frame a house, the bricks and iron coils of pipe which build a furnace, or the stones and mortar which make the support of a great railroad bridge. Yet while the principles of structure are thus simple, for the general understanding by the student who begins their study the complete appreciation of the shades of variation, which differentiate one tissue from another, which define a sound tendon or a ligament from a fibrous band—the result of disease filling in an old lesion and tying one organ with another—is as complicated as the nicest jointing of Chinese woodwork, the building of a furnace for the most difficult chemical analysis, or the construction of a bridge which will stand for ages and resist any force or weight.

All tissues are composed of certain fundamental and similar elements which are governed by the same rules of life, though at first glance they may appear to be widely different. These are (a) amorphous substances, (b) fibers, and (c) cells.

(a) Amorphous substances may be in liquid form, as in the fluid of the blood, which holds a vast amount of salts and nutritive matter in solution; or they may be in a semiliquid condition, as the plasma which infiltrates the loose meshes of connective tissue and lubricates the surface of some membranes; or they may be in the form of a glue or cement, fastening one structure to another, as a tendon or muscle end to a bone; or, again, they hold similar elements firmly together, as in bone, where they form a stiff matrix which becomes impregnated with lime salts. Amorphous substances, again, form the protoplasm or nutritive element of cells or the elements of life.

(b) Fibers are formed of elements of organic matter which have only a passive function. They can be assimilated to little strings, or cords, tangled one with another like a mass of waste yarn, woven regularly like a cloth, or bound together like a rope. They are of two

27

kinds—white connective tissue fibers, only slightly extensible, pliable, and very strong, and yellow elastic fibers, elastic, curly, ramified, and very dense. These fibers once created require the constant presence of fluids around them in order to retain their functional condition, as a piece of harness leather demands continual oiling to keep its strength, but they undergo no change or alteration in their form until destroyed by death.

(c) Cells, which may even be regarded as low forms of life, are masses of protoplasm or amorphous living matter, with a nucleus and frequently a nucleolus, which are capable of assimilating nutriment or food, propagating themselves either into others of the same form or into fixed cells of another outward appearance and different function but of the same constitution. It is simply in the mode of the grouping of these elements that we have the variation in tissues, as (1) loose connective tissue, (2) aponeurosis and tendons, (3) muscles, (4) cartilage, (5) bones, (6) epithelia and endothelia, (7) nerves.

(1) Loose connective tissue forms the great framework, or scaffolding, of the body, and is found under the skin, between the muscles surrounding the bones and blood vessels, and entering into the structures of almost all the organs. In this the fibers are loosely meshed together like a sponge, leaving spaces in which the nutrient fluid and cells are irregularly distributed. This tissue we find in the skin, in the spaces between the organs of the body where fat accumulates, and as the framework of all glands.

(2) Aponeurosis and tendons are structures which serve for the termination of muscles and for their contention, and for the attachment of bones together. In these the fibers are more frequent and dense, and are arranged with regularity, either crossing each other or lying parallel, and here the cells are found in minimum quantity.

(3) In the muscles the cells lie end to end, forming long fibers which have the power of contraction, and the connective tissue is in small quantity, serving the passive purpose of a band around the contractile elements.

(4) In cartilage a mass of firm amorphous substance, with no vascularity and little vitality, forms the bed for the chondroplasts, or cells of this tissue.

(5) Bone differs from the above in having the amorphous matter impregnated with lime salts, which gives it its rigidity and firmness.

(6) Epithelia and endothelia, or the membranes which cover the body and line all its cavities and glands, are made up of single or stratified and multiple layers of cells bound together by a glue of amorphous substance and resting on a layer composed of fibers.

When the membrane serves for secreting or excreting purposes, as in the salivary glands or the kidneys, it is usually simple; when it serves the mechanical purpose of protecting a part, as over the tongue or skin, it is invariably multiple and stratified, the surface wearing away while new cells replace it from beneath.

(7) In nerves, stellate cells are connected by their rays to each other, or to fibers which conduct the nerve impressions, or they act as receptacles, storehouses, and transmitters for them, as the switch-board of a telephone system serves to connect the various wires.

All these tissues are supplied with blood in greater or less quantity. The vascularity depends upon the function which the tissue is called upon to perform. If this is great, as in the tongue, the lungs, or the sensitive part of the hoof, a large quantity of blood is required; if the labor is a passive one, as in cartilage, the membrane over the withers, or the tendons of the legs, the vessels only reach the periphery, and nutrition is furnished by imbibition of the fluids brought to their surface by the blood vessels.

Blood is brought to the tissues by arterioles, or the small terminations of the arteries, and is carried off from them by the veinlets, or the commencement of the veins. Between these two systems are small, delicate networks of vessels called capillaries, which subdivide into a veritable lacework so as to reach the neighborhood of every element.

In health the blood passes through these capillaries with a regular current, the red cells or corpuscles floating rapidly in the fluid in the center of the channel, while the white or ameboid cells are attracted to the walls of the vessels and move very slowly. The supply of blood is regulated by the condition of repose or activity of the tissue, and under normal conditions the outflow exactly compensates the supply. The caliber of the blood vessels, and consequently the quantity of blood which they carry, is governed by nerves of the sympathetic system in a healthy body with unerring regularity, but in a diseased organ the flow may cease or be greatly augmented. In health a tissue or organ receives its proper quantity of blood; the nutritive elements are extracted for the support of the tissue and for the product, which the function of the organ forms. The force required in the achievement of this is furnished by combustion of the hydrocarbons and oxygen brought by the arterial blood, then by the veins this same fluid passes off, less its oxygen, loaded with the waste products, which are the result of the worn-out and disintegrated tissues, and of those which have undergone combustion. The foregoing brief outline indicates the process of nutrition of the tissues.

Hypernutrition, or excessive nutrition of a tissue, may be normal or morbid. If the latter, the tissue becomes congested or inflamed.

CONGESTION.

Congestion is an unnatural accumulation of blood in a part. Excessive accumulation of blood may be normal, as in blushing or in the red face which temporarily follows a violent muscular effort, or, as in the stomach or liver during digestion, or in the lungs after severe work, from which, in the latter case, it is shortly relieved by a little rapid breathing. The term congestion, however, usually indicates a morbid condition, with more or less lasting effects. Congestion is active or passive. The former is produced by an increased supply of blood to the part, the latter by an obstacle preventing the escape of blood from the tissue. In either case there is an increased supply of blood, and as a result increased combustion and augmented nutrition.

ACTIVE CONGESTION.

Active congestion is caused by—

(1) *Functional activity.*—Any organ which is constantly or excessively used is habituated to hold an unusual quantity of blood; the vessels become dilated; if overstrained the walls become weakened, lose their elasticity, and any sudden additional quantity of blood engorges the tissues so that they can not contract, and congestion results. Example: The lungs of a race horse, after an unusual burst of speed or severe work, in damp weather.

(2) *Irritants.*—Heat and cold, chemical or mechanical. Any of these, by threatening the vitality of a tissue, induce immediately an augmented flow of blood to the part to furnish the means of repair—a hot iron, frostbites, acids, or a blow.

(3) *Nerve influence.*—This may produce congestion either by acting on the part reflexly or as the result of some central nerve disturbance affecting the branch which supplies a given organ.

(4) *Plethora and sanguinary temperament.*—Full-blooded animals are much more predisposed to congestive diseases than those of a lymphatic character or those in an anemic condition. The circulation in them is forced to all parts with much greater force and in large quantities. A well-bred, full-blooded horse is much more subject to congestive diseases than a common, coarse, or old, worn-out animal.

(5) *Fevers.*—In fever the heart works more actively and forces the current of blood more rapidly; the tissues are weakened, and it requires but a slight local cause at any part to congest the structures already overloaded with blood. Again, in certain fevers, we find alteration of the blood itself, rendering it less or more fluid, which interferes with its free passage through the vessels and induces a local predisposition to congestion.

(6) *Warm climate and summer heat.*—Warmth of the atmosphere relaxes the tissues; it demands of the animals less blood to keep up their own body temperature, and the extra quantity accumulates in the blood-vessel system. It causes sluggishness in the performance of the organic functions, and in this way it induces congestion, especially of the internal organs. So we find founders, congestive colics, and staggers more frequent in summer than in winter.

(7) *Previous congestion.*—Whether the previous congestion of any organ has been a continuous normal one—that is, a repeated functional activity—or has been a morbid temporary overloading, it always leaves the walls of the vessels weakened and more predisposed to recurrent attacks from accidental causes than are perfectly healthy tissues. Thus a horse which has had a congestion of the lungs from a severe drive is liable to have another attack from even a lesser cause.

The alterations of congestion are distention of the blood vessels, accumulation of the cellular elements of the blood in them, and effusion of a portion of the liquid of the blood into the fibrous tissues which surround the vessels. When the changes produced by congestion are visible, as in the eye, the nostril, the mouth, the genital organs, and on the surface of the body in white or unpigmented animals, the part appears red from the increase of blood; it becomes swollen from the effusion of liquid into the spongelike connective tissues; it is at times more or less hot from the increased combustion; the part is frequently painful to the animal from pressure of the effusion on the nerves, and the function of the tissue is interfered with. The secretion or excretion of glands may be augmented or diminished. Muscles may be affected with spasms or may be unable to contract. The eyes and ears may be affected with imaginary sights and sounds.

PASSIVE CONGESTION.

Passive congestion is caused by interference with the return of the current of blood from a part.

Old age and debility weaken the tissues and the force of the circulation, especially in the veins, and retard the movement of the blood. We then see horses of this class with stocked legs, swelling of the sheath of the penis or of the milk glands, and of the under surface of the belly. We find them also with effusions of the liquid parts of the blood into the lymph spaces of the posterior extremities and organs of the pelvic cavity.

Tumors or other mechanical obstructions, by pressing on the veins, retard the flow of blood and cause it to back up in distal parts of the body causing passive congestion.

The alterations of passive congestion, as in active congestion, consist of an increased quantity of blood in the vessels and an exudation

PLATE II.

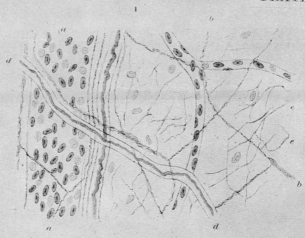

1-*Non-inflamed mesentery of the frog, 400 diameters, reduced ½: a, a, Venule with red and white corpuscles; b, b, Gelatinous nerve fibre; c, Capillary; d, d, Dark-bordered nerve fibre; e, e, Connective tissue with connective tissue corpuscles and leucocytes scattered sparsely through it.*

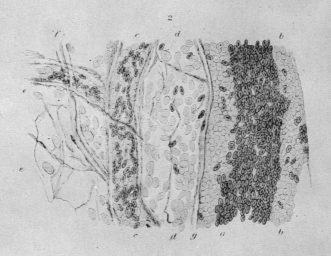

2-*Inflamed mesentery or the frog, 400 diameters, reduced ½: a, b, Venule filled with red and white corpuscles; the red in the centre and the white crowding along the walls; c, c, Capillary distended with red and white corpuscles; number of the white much decreased; d, d, Connective tissue between venule and capillary filled with migrated leucocytes; e, e, Connective tissue with less infiltration; f, Dark-bordered nerve fibre; g, Number of nuclei in sheaths increased.*

Haines, del. after Agnew.

INFLAMMATION.

spavins, ringbones, inflammation of the glands of the less vascular skin of the extremities, greasy heels, thrush, etc.

Young horses have inflammation of the membranes lining the air passages and digestive tract, while older animals are more subject to troubles in the closed serous sacs and in the bones.

The work to which a horse is put (saddle or harness, speed or draft) will influence the predisposition of an animal to inflammatory diseases. As in congestion, the functional activity of a part is an important factor in localizing this form of disease. Given a group of horses exposed to the same draft of cold air or other exciting cause of inflammation, the one which has just been eating will be attacked with an inflammation of the bowels; the one that has just been working so as to increase its respiration will have an inflammation of the throat, bronchi, or lungs; the one that has just been using its feet excessively will have a founder or inflammation of the laminæ of the feet.

The direct cause of inflammation is usually an irritant of some form. This may be a pathogenic organism—a disease germ—or it may be mechanical or chemical, external or internal. Cuts, bruises, injuries of any kind, parasites, acids, blisters, heat, cold, secretions, such as an excess of tears over the cheek or urine on the legs, all cause inflammation by direct injury to the part. Strains or wrenches of joints, ligaments, and tendons cause trouble by laceration of the tissue.

Inflammations of the internal organs are caused by irritants as above, and by sudden cooling of the surface of the animal, which drives the blood to that organ which at the moment is most actively supplied with blood. This is called repercussion. A horse which has been worked at speed and is breathing rapidly is liable to have pneumonia if suddenly chilled, while an animal which has just been fed is more liable to have a congestive colic if exposed to the same influence, the blood in this case being driven from the exterior to the intestines, while in the former it was driven to the lungs.

Symptoms.—The symptoms of inflammation are, as in congestion, change of color, due to an increased supply of blood; swelling, from the same cause, with the addition of an effusion into the surrounding tissues; heat, owing to the increased combustion in the part; pain, due to pressure on the nerves, and altered function. This latter may be augmented or diminished, or first one and then the other. In addition to the local symptoms, inflammation always produces more or less constitutional disturbance or fever. A splint or small spavin will cause so little fever that it is not appreciable, while a severe spavin, an inflamed joint, or a pneumonia may give rise to a marked fever.

54763°—23——3

The alterations in an inflamed tissue are first those of congestion, distention of the blood vessels, and exudation of the fluid of the blood into the surrounding fibers, with, however, a more nearly complete stagnation of the blood; fibrin, or lymph, a plastic substance, is thrown out as well, and the cells, which we have seen to be living organisms in themselves, no longer carried in the current of the blood, migrate from the vessels and, finding proper nutriment, proliferate or multiply with greater or lesser rapidity. The cells which lie dormant in the meshes of the surrounding fibers are awakened into activity by the nutritious lymph which surrounds them, and they also multiply.

Whether the cell in an inflamed part is the white ameboid cell of the blood or the fixed connective tissue embedded in the fibers, it multiplies in the same way. The nucleus in the center is divided into two, and then each again into two, ad infinitum. If the process is slow, each new cell may assimilate nourishment and become, like its ancestor, an aid in the formation of new tissues; if, however, the changing takes place rapidly, the brood of young cells have not time to grow or use up the surrounding nourishment, and, but half developed, they die, and we then have destruction of tissue, and pus or matter is formed, a material made up of the imperfect dead elements and the broken-down tissue. Between the two there is an intermediate form, where we have imperfectly formed tissues, as in "proud flesh," large, soft splints; fungous growths, greasy heels, and thrush.

Whether the inflamed tissue is one like the skin, lungs, or intestines, very loose in their texture, or a tendon or bone, dense in structure, and comparatively poor in blood vessels, the principle of the process is the same. The effects, however, and the appearance may be widely different. After a cut on the face or an exudation into the lungs, the loose tissues and multiple vessels allow the proliferating cells to obtain rich nourishment; absorption can take place readily, and the part regains its normal condition entirely, while a bruise at the heel or at the withers finds a dense, inextensible tissue where the multiplying elements and exuded fluids choke up all communication, and the parts die (necrose) from want of blood and cause a serious quittor, or fistula.

This effect of structure of a part on the same process shows the importance of a perfect knowledge in the study of a local trouble, and the indispensable part which such knowledge plays in judging of the gravity of an inflammatory disease, and in formulating a prognosis or opinion of the final termination of it. It is this which allows the veterinarian, through his knowledge of the intimate structure of a part and the relations of its elements, to judge of the severity of a disease, and to prescribe different modes of treatment in two animals for troubles which, to the less experienced observer, appear to be absolutely identical.

Termination of inflammation.—Like congestion, inflammation may terminate by resolution. In this case the exuded lymph undergoes chemical change, and the products are absorbed and carried off by the blood vessels and lymphatics, to be thrown out of the body by the kidneys, liver, the glands of the skin, and the other excretory organs. The cells, which have wandered into the neighboring tissues from the blood vessels, gradually disappear or become transformed into fixed cells. Those which are the result of the tissue cells, wakened into active life, follow the same course. The vessels themselves contract, and, having resumed their normal caliber, the part apparently reassumes its normal condition; but it is always weakened, and a new inflammation is more liable to reappear in a previously inflamed part than in a sound one. The alternate termination is necrosis, or mortification. If the necrosis, or death of a part, is gradual, by small stages, each cell losing its vitality after the other in more or less rapid succession, it takes the name of ulceration. If it occurs in a considerable part at once, it is called gangrene. If this death of the tissues occurs deep in the organism, and the destroyed elements and proliferated and dead cells are inclosed in a cavity, the result of the process is called an abscess. When it occurs on a surface, it is an ulcer, and an abscess by breaking on the exterior becomes then also an ulcer. Proliferating and dying cells, and the fluid which exudes from an ulcerating surface and the débris of broken-down tissue is known as pus, and the process by which this is formed is known as suppuration. A mass of dead tissue in a soft part is termed a slough, while the same in bone is called a sequestrum. Such changes are especially liable to occur when the part becomes infected with microorganisms that have the property of destroying tissue and thus causing the production of pus. These are known as pyogenic microorganisms. There are also bacilli that are capable of multiplying in tissues and so irritating them as to cause them to die (necrose) without forming pus.

Treatment of inflammation.—The study of the causes and pathological alterations of inflammation has shown the process to be one of hypernutrition, attended by excessive blood supply, so this study will indicate the primary factor to be employed in the treatment of it. Any agent which will reduce the blood supply and prevent the excessive nutrition of the elements of the part will serve as a remedy. The means employed may be used locally to the part, or they may be constitutional remedies, which act indirectly.

Local treatment.—Removal of the cause will frequently allow the part to heal at once. Among causes of inflammation may be mentioned a stone in the frog, causing a traumatic thrush; a badly fitting harness or saddle, causing ulcers of the skin; decomposing manure and urine in a stable, which, by their vapors, irritate the air tubes and lungs and cause a cough.

Motion stimulates the action of the blood, and thus feeds an inflamed tissue. This is alike applicable to a diseased point irritated by movement to an inflamed pair of lungs surcharged with blood by the use demanded of them in a working animal, or to an inflamed eye exposed to light, or an inflamed stomach and intestines still further fatigued by feed. Rest, absolute quiet, a dark stable, and small quantities of easily digested feed will often cure serious inflammatory troubles without further treatment.

The application of ice bags or cold water by bandages, douching with a hose, or irrigation with dripping water, contracts the blood vessels, acts as a sedative to the nerves, and lessens the vitality of a part; it consequently prevents the tissue change which inflammation produces.

Either dry or moist heat acts as a derivative. It quickens the circulation and renders the chemical changes more active in the surrounding parts; it softens the tissues and attracts the current of blood from the inflamed organ; it also promotes the absorption of the effusion and hastens the elimination of the waste products in the part. Heat may be applied by hand rubbing or active friction and the application of warm coverings (bandages) or by cloths wrung out of warm water; or steaming with warm, moist vapor, medicated or not, will answer the same purpose. The latter is especially applicable to inflammatory troubles in the air passages.

Local bleeding frequently affords immediate relief by carrying off the excessive blood and draining the effusion which has already occurred. It affords direct mechanical relief, and, by a stimulation of the part, promotes the chemical changes necessary for bringing the diseased tissues to a healthy condition. Local blood-letting can be done by scarifying, or making small punctures into the inflamed part, as in the eyelid of an inflamed eye, or into the sheath of the penis, or into the skin of the latter organ when congested, or the leg when acutely swelled.

Counterirritants are used for deep inflammations. They act by bringing the blood to the surface and consequently lessening the blood pressure within. The derivation of the blood to the exterior diminishes the amount in the internal organs and is often very rapid in its action in relieving a congested lung or liver. The most common counterirritant is mustard flour. It is applied as a soft paste mixed with warm water to the under surface of the belly and to the sides, where the skin is comparatively soft and vascular. Colds in the throat or inflammations at any point demand the treatment applied in the same manner to the belly and sides and not to the throat or on the legs, as so often used. Blisters, iodin, and many other irritants are used in a similar way.

Constitutional treatment in inflammation is designed to reduce the current of blood, which is the fuel for the inflammation in the diseased part, to quiet the patient, and to combat the fever or general effects of the trouble in the system, and to favor the neutralization or elimination of the products of the inflammation.

Reduction of blood is obtained in various ways. The diminution of the quantity of the blood lessens the amount of pressure on the vessels, and, as a sequel, the volume of it which is carried to the point of inflammation; it diminishes the body temperature or fever; it numbs the nervous system, which plays an important part as a conductor of irritation in diseases.

Blood-letting is the most rapid means, and frequently acts like a charm in relieving a commencing inflammatory trouble. One must remember, however, that the strength of the body and repair depend on the blood; hence blood-letting should be practiced only in full-blooded, well-nourished animals and in the early stages of the disease.

Cathartics act by drawing off a large quantity of fluid from the blood through the intestines, and have the advantage over the last remedy of removing only the watery and not the formed elements from the circulation. The blood cells remain, leaving the blood as rich as it was before. Again, the glands of the intestines are stimulated to excrete much waste matter and other deleterious material which may be acting as a poison in the blood.

Diuretics operate through the kidneys in the same way.

Diaphoretics aid depletion of the blood by pouring water in the form of sweat from the surface of the skin and stimulating the discharge of waste material out of its glands, which has the same effect on the blood pressure.

Antipyretics are remedies to reduce the temperature. This may be accomplished by depressing the center in the brain that controls heat production. Some coal-tar products are very effective in this way, but they have the disadvantage of depressing the heart, which should always be kept as strong as possible. If they are used it must be with knowledge of this fact, and it is well to give heart tonics or stimulants with them. The temperature of the body may be lowered by cold packs or by showering with cold water. This is a most useful procedure in many diseases.

Depressants are drugs which act on the heart. They slow or weaken the action of this organ and reduce the quantity and force of the current of the blood which is carried to the point of local disease; they lessen the vitality of the animal, and for this reason are now used much less than formerly.

Anodynes quiet the nervous system. Pain in the horse, as in the man, is one of the important factors in the production of fever, and the dulling of the former often prevents, or at least reduces, the latter. Anodynes produce sleep, so as to rest the patient and allow recuperation for the succeeding struggle of the vitality of the animal against the exhausting drain of the disease.

The diet of an animal suffering from acute inflammation is a factor of the greatest importance. An overloaded circulation can be starved to a reduced quantity and to a less rich quality of blood by reducing the quantity of feed given to the patient. Feeds of easy digestion do not tire the already fatigued organs of an animal with a torpid digestive system. Nourishment will be taken by a suffering brute in the form of slops and cooling drinks when it would be totally refused if offered in its ordinary form, as hard oats or dry hay, requiring the labor of grinding between the teeth and swallowing by the weakened muscles of the jaws and throat.

Tonics and stimulants are remedies which are used to meet special indications, as in the case of a feeble heart, and which enter into the after treatment of inflammatory troubles as well as into the acute stages of them. They brace up weakened and torpid glands; they stimulate the secretion of the necessary fluids of the body, and hasten the excretion of the waste material produced by the inflammatory process; they regulate the action of a weakened heart; they promote healthy vitality of diseased parts, and aid the chemical changes needed for returning the altered tissues to their normal condition.

FEVERS.

Fever is a general condition of the animal body in which there is an elevation of the animal body temperature, which may be only a degree or two or may be 10° F. The elevation of the body temperature, which represents tissue change or combustion, is accompanied with an acceleration of the heart's action, a quickening of the respiration, and an aberration in the functional activity of the various organs of the body. These organs may be stimulated to the performance of excessive work, or they may be incapacitated from carrying out their allotted tasks, or, in the course of a fever, the two conditions may both exist, the one succeeding the other. Fever as a disease is usually preceded by chills as an essential symptom.

Fevers are divided into essential fevers and symptomatic fevers. In symptomatic fever some local disease, usually of an inflammatory character, develops first, and the constitutional febrile phenomena are the result of the primary point of combustion irritating the whole body, either through the nervous system or directly by means of the waste material which is carried into the circulation and through the blood vessels, and is distributed to distal parts. Essential fevers are those in which there is from the outset a general disturbance of the whole economy. This may consist of an elementary alteration in the blood or a general change in the constitution of the tissues. Fevers of the latter class are usually due to some infecting agent and belong, therefore, to the class of infectious diseases.

Essential fevers are subdivided into ephemeral fevers, which last but a short time and terminate by critical phenomena; intermittent fevers, in which there are alterations of exacerbations of the febrile symptoms and remissions, in which the body returns to its normal condition or sometimes to a depressed condition, in which the functions of life are but badly performed; and continued fevers, which include contagious diseases, such as glanders, influenza, etc., the septic diseases, such as pyemia, septicemia, etc., and the eruptive fevers, such as variola, etc.

Whether the cause of the fever has been an injury to the tissues, such as a severe bruise, a broken bone, an inflamed lung, or excessive work, which has surcharged the blood with the waste products of the combustion of the tissues, which were destroyed to produce force, or the toxins of influenza in the blood, or the presence of irritating material, either in the form of living organisms or of their products, as in glanders or tuberculosis—the general train of symptoms are much the same, varying as the amount of the irritant differs in quantity, or when some special quality in them has a specific action on one or another tissue.

There is in fever at first a relaxation of the small blood vessels, which may have been preceded by a contraction of the same if there was a chill, and as a consequence there is an acceleration of the current of the blood. There is, then, an elevation of the peripheral temperature, followed by a lowering of tension in the arteries and an acceleration in the movement of the heart. These conditions may be produced by a primary irritation of the nerve centers of the brain from the effects of heat, as is seen in thermic fever, or sunstroke, or by the entrance into the blood stream of disease-producing organisms or their chemical products, as in anthrax, rinderpest, influenza, etc.

There are times when it is difficult to distinguish between the existence of fever as a disease and a temporary feverish condition which is the result of excessive work. Like the condition of congestion of the lungs, which is normal up to a certain degree in the lungs of a race horse after a severe race, and morbid when it produces more than temporary phenomena or when it causes distinct lesions, the temperature may rise from physiological causes as much as four degrees, so fever, or, as it is better termed, a feverish condition, may follow any work or other employment of energy in which excessive tissue change has taken place; but if the consequences are ephemeral, and no recognizable lesion is apparent, it is not considered morbid. This condition, however, may predispose to severe organic disturbance and local inflammations which will cause disease, as an animal in this condition is liable to take cold and develop lung fever or a severe enteritis, if chilled or otherwise exposed.

Fever in all animals is characterized by the same general phenomena, but we find the intensity of the symptoms modified by the species of animals affected, by the races which subdivide the species, by the families which form groups of the races, and by certain conditions in individuals themselves. For example, a pricked foot in a Thoroughbred may cause intense fever, while the same injury in the foot of a Clydesdale may scarcely cause a visible general symptom. In the horse, fever produces the following symptoms:

The normal body temperature, which varies from 99° to 100° F., is elevated from 1° to 9°. A temperature of 102° or 103° F. is moderate fever, 104° to 105° F. is high, and 106° F. and over is excessive. The temperature is accurately measured by means of a clinical thermometer inserted in the rectum.

This elevation of temperature can readily be felt by the hand placed in the mouth of the animal, or in the rectum, and in the cleft between the hind legs. It is usually appreciable at any point over the surface of the body and in the expired air emitted from the nostrils. The ears and cannons are often as hot as the rest of the body, but are sometimes cold, which denotes a debility in the circulation and irregular distribution of the blood. The pulse, which in a healthy horse is felt beating about 42 to 48 times in the minute, is increased to 60, 70, 90, or even 100. The respirations are increased from 14 or 16 to 24, 30, 36, or even more. With the commencement of a fever the horse usually has diminished appetite, or it may have total loss of appetite if the fever is excessive. There is, however, a vast difference among horses in this regard. With the same degree of elevation of temperature one horse may lose its appetite entirely, while another, usually of the more common sort, will eat at hay throughout the course of the fever, and will even continue to eat oats or other grains. Thirst is usually increased, but the animal desires only a small quantity of water at a time, and in most cases of fever a bucket of water should be kept standing before the patient, which may be allowed to drink ad libitum. The skin becomes dry and the hairs stand on end. Sweating is almost unknown in the early stage of fevers, but frequently occurs later in their course, when an outbreak of warm sweat is often a most favorable symptom. The mucous membranes, which are most easily examined in the conjunctivæ of the eyes and inside of the mouth, change color if the fever is an acute one; without alteration of blood the mucous membranes become of a rosy or deep-red color at the outset; if the fever is attended with distinct alteration of the blood, as in influenza, and at the end of two or three days in severe cases of pneumonia or other extensive inflammatory troubles the mucous membranes are tinged with yellow, which may even become a deep ocher in color, the result of the decomposition of the blood corpuscles and the freeing of their coloring matter, which acts as a stain. At the outset of a fever the various glands are checked in their secretions, the salivary glands fail to secrete the saliva, and we find the surface of the tongue and inside of the cheeks dry and covered with a brownish, bad-smelling deposit. The excretion from the liver and intestinal glands is diminished and produces an inactivity of the digestive organs which causes a constipation. If this is not remedied at an early period, the undigested material acts as an irritant, and later we may have it followed by an inflammatory process, producing a severe diarrhea.

The excretion from the kidneys is sometimes at first entirely suppressed. It is always considerably diminished, and what urine is passed is dark in color, undergoes ammoniacal change rapidly, and deposits quantities of salts. At a later period the diminished excretion may be replaced by an excessive excretion, which aids in carrying off waste products and usually indicates an amelioration of the fever.

While the ears, cannons, and hoofs of a horse suffering from fever are usually found hot, they may frequently alternate from hot to cold, or be much cooler than they normally are. This latter condition usually indicates great weakness on the part of the circulatory system.

It is of the greatest importance, as an aid in diagnosing the gravity of an attack of fever and as an indication in the selection of its mode of treatment, to recognize the exact cause of a febrile condition in the horse. In certain cases, in very nervous animals, in which fever is the result of nerve influence, a simple anodyne, or even only quiet with continued care and nursing, will sometimes be sufficient to diminish it. When fever is the result of local injury, the cure of the cause produces a cessation in the constitutional symptoms. When it is the result of a pneumonia or other severe parenchymatous inflammation, it usually lasts for a definite time, and subsides with the first improvement of the local trouble, but in these cases we constantly have exacerbations of fever due to secondary inflammatory processes, such as the formation of small abscesses, the development of secondary bronchitis, or the death of a limited quantity of tissue (gangrene).

In specific cases, such as influenza, strangles, and septicemia, there is a definite poison in the blood-vessel system and carried to the heart and to the nervous system, which produces a peculiar irritation, usually lasting for a specific period, during which the temperature can be but slightly diminished by any remedy.

In cases attended with complications, the diagnosis at times becomes still more difficult, as at the end of a case of influenza which becomes complicated with pneumonia. The high temperature of the simple inflammatory disease may be grafted on that of the specific trouble, and the determination of the cause of the fever, as between the two, is therefore frequently a difficult matter but an important one, as upon it depends the mode of treatment.

Any animal suffering from fever, whatever the cause, is much more susceptible to attacks of local inflammation, which become complications of the original disease, than are animals in sound health. In fever we have the tissues and the walls of the blood vessels weakened, we have an increased current of more or less altered blood flowing through the vessels and stagnating in the capillaries, which need but an exciting cause to transform the passive congestion of fever into an active congestion and acute inflammation. These conditions become still more distinct when the fever is accompanied with a decided deterioration in the blood itself, as is seen in influenza, septicemia, and at the termination of severe pneumonias.

Fever, with its symptoms of increased temperature, acceleration of the pulse, acceleration of respiration, dry skin, diminished secretions, etc., must be considered as an indication of organic disturbance. This organic disturbance may be the result of local inflammation or other irritants acting through the nerves on nerve centers, alterations of the blood, in which a poison is carried to the nerve centers, or direct irritants to the nerve centers themselves, as in cases of heat stroke, injury to the brain, etc.

The treatment of fever depends upon its cause. One of the important factors in treatment is absolute quiet. This may be obtained by placing a sick horse in a box stall, away from other animals and extraneous noises and sheltered from excessive light and drafts of air. Anodynes, belladonna, hyoscyamus, and opium act as antipyretics simply by quieting the nervous system. As an irritant exists in the blood in most cases of fever, any remedy which will favor the excretion of foreign elements from it will diminish this cause. We therefore use diaphoretics to stimulate the sweat and excretions from the skin; diuretics to favor the elimination of matter by the kidneys; cholagogues and laxatives to increase the action of the liver and intestines, and to drain from these important organs all the waste material which is aiding to choke up and congest their rich plexuses of blood vessels. The heart becomes stimulated to increased action at the outset of a fever, but this does not indicate increased strength; on the contrary, it indicates the action of an irritant to the heart that will soon weaken it. It is, therefore, irrational further to depress the heart by the use of such drugs as aconite. It is better to strengthen it and to favor the elimination of the substance that is irritating it. The increased blood pressure throughout the body may be diminished by lessening the quantity of blood. This is obtained in some cases with advantage when the disease is but starting and the animal is plethoric by direct abstraction of blood, as in bleeding from the jugular or other veins; or by derivatives, such as mustard, turpentine, or blisters applied to the skin; or by setons, which draw to the surface the fluid of the blood, thereby lessening its volume without having the disadvantage of impoverishing the elements of the blood found in bleeding. In many cases antipyretics given by the mouth and cold applied to the skin are most useful.

When the irritation which is the cause of fever is a specific one, either in the form of bacteria (living organisms), as in glanders, tuberculosis, influenza, septicemia, etc., or in the form of a foreign element, as in rheumatism, gout, hemaglobinuria, and other so-called diseases of nutrition, we employ remedies which have been found to have a direct specific action on them. Among the specific remedies for various diseases are counted quinin, carbolic acid, salicylic acid, antipyrene, mercury, iodin, the empyreumatic oils, tars, resins, aromatics, sulphur, and a host of other drugs, some of which are of known effect and others of which are theoretical in action. Certain remedies, like simple aromatic teas, vegetable acids, such as vinegar, lemon juice, etc., alkalines in the form of salts, sweet spirits of niter, etc., which are household remedies, are always useful, because they act on the excreting organs and ameliorate the effects of fever. Other remedies, which are to be used to influence the cause of fever, must be selected with judgment and from a thorough knowledge of the nature of the disease.

METHODS OF ADMINISTERING MEDICINES.

By CH. B. MICHENER, V. S.

[Revised by Leonard Pearson, B. S., V. M. D.]

Medicine may enter the body through any of the following designated channels: First, by the mouth; second, by the air passages; third, by the skin; fourth, by the tissue beneath the skin (hypodermic methods); fifth, by the rectum; sixth, by the genito-urinary passages; and, seventh, by the blood (intravenous injections).

BY THE MOUTH.—Medicines can be given by the mouth in the form of solids, as powders or pills; liquids, and pastes, or electuaries.

Powders.—Solids administered as powders should be as finely pulverized as possible, in order to obtain rapid solution and absorption. Their action is in this way facilitated and intensified. Powders must be free from any irritant or caustic action upon the mouth. Those that are without any disagreeable taste or smell are readily eaten with the feed or taken in the drinking water. When placed with the feed they should first be dissolved or suspended in water and thus sprinkled on the feed. If mixed dry the horse will often leave the medicine in the bottom of his manger. Nonirritant powders may be given in capsules, as balls are given.

Pills, or " balls," when properly made, are cylindrical in shape, 2 inches in length and about three-fourths of an inch in diameter. They should be fresh, but if necessary to keep them some time they should be made up with glycerin, or some such agent, to prevent their becoming too hard. Very old, hard balls are sometimes passed whole with the manure without being acted upon at all. Paper is sometimes wrapped around balls when given, if they are so sticky as to adhere to the fingers or the balling gun. Paper used for this purpose should be thin but firm, as the tougher tissue papers. Balls are preferred to drenches when the medicine is extremely disagreeable or nauseating; when the dose is not too large; when the horse is difficult to drench; or when the medicine is intended to act slowly. Certain medicines can not or should not be made into balls, as medicines requiring to be given in large doses, oils, caustic substances, unless in small dose and diluted and thoroughly mixed with the vehicle, deliquescent, or efflorescent salts. Substances suitable for balls can be made up by the addition of honey, sirup, soap, etc., when required for immediate use. Gelatin capsules of different sizes are now obtainable and are a convenient means of giving medicines in ball form.

44

When balls are to be given we should observe the following directions: In shape they should be cylindrical, of the size above mentioned, and soft enough to be easily compressed by the fingers. If made round or egg-shaped, if too long or too hard, they are liable to become fixed in the gullet and cause choking. Balls may be given with the "balling gun" (obtainable at any veterinary instrument maker's) or by the hand. If given by the hand a mouth speculum or gag may be used to prevent the animal from biting the hand or crushing the ball. Always loosen the horse before attempting to give a ball; if tied he may break his halter and injure himself or the one giving the ball. With a little practice it is much easier to give a ball without the mouth gag, as the horse always fights more or less against having his mouth forced open. The tongue must be firmly grasped with the left hand and gently pulled forward; the ball, slightly moistened, is then to be placed with the tips of the fingers of the right hand as far back into the mouth as possible; as the tongue is loosened it is drawn back into the mouth and carries the ball backward with it. The mouth should be kept closed for a minute or two. We should always have a pail of water at hand to offer the horse after balling. This precaution will often prevent him from coughing out the ball or its becoming lodged in the gullet.

Pastes or electuaries are medicines mixed with licorice-root powder, ground flaxseed, molasses, or sirup to the consistency of honey, or a "soft solid." They are intended, chiefly, to act locally upon the mouth and throat. They are given by being spread upon the tongue, gums, or teeth with a wooden paddle or strong, long-handled spoon.

Liquids.—It is, very often, impossible to get balls properly made, or to induce owners or attendants to attempt to give them, and for these reasons medicines by the mouth are mostly given in the form of liquids. Liquids may be given as drenches when the dose is large, or they may, when but a small quantity is administered, be injected into the mouth with a hard-rubber syringe or be poured upon the tongue from a small vial.

When medicine is to be given as a drench we must be careful to use water or oil enough to dissolve or dilute it thoroughly; more than this makes the drench bulky and is unnecessary. Insoluble medicines, if not irritant or corrosive, may be given simply suspended in water, the bottle to be well shaken immediately before giving the drench. The bottle used for drenching purposes should be clean, strong, and smooth about its neck; it should be without shoulders, tapering, and of a size to suit the amount to be given. A horn or tin bottle may be better, because it is not so easily broken by the teeth. If the dose is a small one the horse's head may be held up by the left hand, while the medicine is poured into the mouth by the right. The left thumb is to be placed in the angle of the lower jaw, and the fingers spread out in such manner as to support the lower lip. Should the dose be large, the horse ugly, or the attendant unable to support the head as directed above, the head is then to be held up by running the tines of a long-handled wooden fork under the noseband of the halter or the halter strap or a rope may be fastened to the noseband and thrown over a limb, beam, or through a pulley suspended from the ceiling. Another way of supporting the head is to place a loop in the end of a rope, and introduce this loop into the mouth just behind the upper front teeth or tusks of the upper jaw, the free end to be run through a pulley, as before described, and held by an assistant. It is never to be fastened, as the horse might in that case do himself serious injury. The head is to be elevated just enough to prevent the horse from throwing the liquid out of his mouth. The line of the face should be horizontal, or only the least bit higher. If the head is drawn too high the animal can not swallow with ease or even with safety. (If this is doubted, just fill your mouth with water, throw back the head as far as possible, and then try to swallow.) The person giving the drench should stand on some object in order to reach the horse's mouth—on a level, or a little above it. The bottle or horn is then to be introduced at the side of the mouth, in front of the molar teeth, in an upward direction. This will cause the horse to open his mouth, when the base of the bottle is to be elevated, and about 4 ounces of the liquid allowed to escape on the tongue as far back as possible, care being taken not to get the neck of the bottle between the back teeth. The bottle is to be immediately removed, and if the horse does not swallow this can be encouraged by rubbing the fingers or neck of the bottle against the roof of the mouth, occasionally removing them. As soon as this is swallowed repeat the operation until he has taken all the drench. If coughing occurs, or if, by any mishap, the bottle should be crushed in the mouth, lower the head immediately.

Do not rub, pinch, or pound the throat nor draw out the tongue when giving a drench. These processes in no way aid the horse to swallow and oftener do harm than good. In drenching, swallowing may be hastened by pouring into the nose of the horse, while the head is high, a few teaspoonfuls of clean water, but *drenches must never be given through the nose*. Large quantities of medicine given by pouring into the nose are liable to strangle the animal, or, if the medicine is irritating, it sets up an inflammation of the nose, fauces, windpipe, and sometimes the lungs.

BY THE AIR PASSAGES.—Medicines are administered to the lungs and upper air passages by insufflation, inhalation, injection, and nasal douche.

Insufflation consists in blowing an impalpable powder directly into the nose. It is but rarely resorted to.

Inhalation.—Gaseous and volatile medicines are given by inhalation, as is also medicated steam or vapor. Of the gases used there may be mentioned, as the chief ones, sulphurous acid gas and, occasionally, chlorin. The animal or animals are to be placed in a tight room, where these gases are generated until the atmosphere is sufficiently impregnated with them. Volatile medicines—as the anesthetics (ether, chloroform, etc.)—are to be given by the attending surgeon only. Medicated vapors are to be inhaled by placing a bucket containing hot water, vinegar and water, scalded hay or bran, to which carbolic acid, iodin, compound tincture of benzoin, or other medicines have been added, in the bottom of a long grain bag. The horse's nose is to be inserted into the top of the bag, and he thus inhales the "medicated steam." Care must be taken not to have it hot enough to scald the animal. The vapor from scalding bran or hay is often thus inhaled to favor discharges in sore throat or "distemper."

Injections are made into the trachea by means of a hypodermic syringe. This method of medication is used for the purpose of treating local diseases of the trachea and upper bronchial tubes. It has also been used as a mode of administering remedies for their constitutional effect, but is now rarely used for this purpose.

The nasal douche is employed by the veterinarian in treating some local diseases of the nasal chambers. Special appliances and professional knowledge are necessary when using liquid medicines by this method. It is not often resorted to, even by veterinary surgeons, since, as a rule, the horse objects very strongly to this mode of medication.

BY THE SKIN.—Medicines are often administered to our hair-covered animals by the skin, yet care must be taken in applying some medicines—as tobacco water, carbolic-acid solutions, strong creolin solutions, mercurial ointment, etc.—over the entire body, as poisoning and death follow in some instances from absorption through the skin. For the same reasons care must also be exercised and poisonous medicines not applied over very large raw or abraded surfaces. With domestic animals medicines are only to be applied by the skin to allay local pain or cure local disease.

BY THE TISSUE BENEATH THE SKIN (HYPODERMATIC METHOD).—Medicines are frequently given by the hypodermic syringe under the skin. It is not safe for any but medical or veterinary practitioners to use this form of medication, since the medicines thus given are powerful poisons. There are many precautions to be observed, and a knowledge of anatomy is indispensable. One of the chief precautions has to do with the sterilization of the syringe. If it is not sterile an abscess may be produced.

BY THE RECTUM.—Medicines may be given by the rectum when they can not be given by the mouth, or when they are not retained in

DISEASES OF THE DIGESTIVE ORGANS.

By CH. B. MICHENER, V. S.

[Revised by John R. Mohler, V. M. D.]

It is not an easy task to write "a plain account of the common diseases, with directions for preventive measures, hygienic care, and the simpler forms of medical treatment," of the digestive organs of the horse. Being limited as to space, the endeavor has been made to give simply an outline—to state the most important facts—leaving many gaps, and continually checking the disposition to write anything like a full description as to cause, prevention, and modes of treatment of diseases.

WATER.

It is generally held, at least in practice, that any water that stock can be induced to drink is sufficiently pure for their use. This practice occasions losses that would startle us if statistics were at hand. Water that is impure from the presence of decomposing organic matter, such as is found in wells and ponds in close proximity to manure heaps and cesspools, is frequently the cause of diarrhea, dysentery, and many other diseases of stock, while water that is impregnated with different poisons and contaminated in very many instances with specific media of contagion produces death.

Considering first the quantity of water required by the horse, it may be stated that when our animals have access to water continually they never drink to excess. Were the horse subjected to ship voyages or any other circumstances where he must depend upon his attendant for the supply of water, it may be roughly stated that he requires a daily average of about 8 gallons of water. This varies somewhat upon the character of his feed; if upon green feed, less water will be needed than when fed upon dry hay and grain.

The time of giving water should be carefully studied. At rest, the horse should receive it at least three times a day; when at work, more frequently. The rule should be to give it in small quantities and often. There is a popular fallacy that if a horse is warm he should not be allowed to drink, many asserting that the first swallow of water "founders" the animal or produces colic. This is erroneous. No matter how warm a horse may be, it is always entirely safe to allow him from six to ten swallows of water. If this is given on

49

going into the stable, he should have at once a pound or two of hay and allowed to rest about an hour before feeding. If water is now offered him it will in many cases be refused, or at least he will drink but sparingly. The danger, then, is not in the "first swallow" of water, but is due to the excessive quantity that the animal will take when warm if he is not restrained.

Ice-cold water should never be given to horses. It may not be necessary to add hot water, but we should be careful in placing water troughs about our barns to have them in such position that the sun may shine upon the water during the winter mornings. Water, even though it is thus cold, seldom produces serious trouble if the horse has not been deprived for a too great length of time.

In reference to the purity of water, Smith, in his "Veterinary Hygiene," classes spring water, deep-well water, and upland surface water as wholesome; stored rain water and surface water from cultivated land as suspicious; river water to which sewage gains access and shallow-well water as dangerous. The water that is used so largely for drinking purposes for stock throughout some States can not but be impure. I refer to those sections where there is an impervious clay subsoil. It is the custom to scoop, or hollow out, a large basin in the pastures. During rains these basins become filled with water. The clay subsoil, being almost impervious, acts as a jug, and there is no escape for the water except by evaporation. Such water is stagnant, but would be kept comparatively fresh by subsequent rains were it not for the fact that much organic matter is carried into it by surface drainage during each succeeding storm. This organic matter soon undergoes decomposition, and, as the result, we find diseases of different kinds much more prevalent where this water is drunk than where the water supply is wholesome. Again, it must not be lost sight of that stagnant surface water is much more certainly contaminated than is running water by one diseased animal of the herd, thus endangering the remainder.

The chief impurities of water may be classified as organic and inorganic. The organic impurities are either animal or vegetable substances. The salts of the metals are the inorganic impurities. Lime causes hardness of water, and occasion will be taken to speak of this when describing intestinal concretions. Salts of lead, iron, and copper are also frequently found in water; they also will be referred to.

About the only examination of water that can be made by the average stock raiser is to observe its taste, color, smell, and clearness. Pure water is clear and is without taste or smell.

Chemical and microscopic examination will frequently be necessary in order to detect the presence of certain poisons, bacteria, etc., and can, of course, be conducted by experts only.

FEEDS AND FEEDING.

In this place one can not attempt anything like a comprehensive discussion of the subject of feeds and feeding, and I must content myself with merely giving a few facts as to the different kinds of feed, preparation, digestibility, proper time of feeding, quality, and quantity. Improper feeding and watering will doubtless account for more than one-half the digestive disorders met with in the horse, and hence the reader can not fail to see how very important it is to have some proper ideas concerning these subjects.

KINDS OF FEED.

In this country horses are fed chiefly upon hay, grass, corn fodder, roots, oats, corn, wheat, and rye. Many think that they could be fed on nothing else. Stewart, in "The Stable Book," gives the following extract from Loudon's Encyclopedia of Agriculture, which is of interest at this point:

In some sterile countries they [horses] are forced to subsist on dried fish, and even on vegetable mold; in Arabia, on milk, flesh balls, eggs, broth. In India horses are variously fed. The native grasses are judged very nutritious. Few, perhaps no, oats are grown; barley is rare, and not commonly given to horses. In Bengal a vetch, something like the tare, is used. On the western side of India a sort of pigeon pea, called gram (*Cicer arietinum*), forms the ordinary food, with grass while in season, and hay all the year round. Indian corn or rice is seldom given. In the West Indies maize, guinea corn, sugar-corn tops, and sometimes molasses are given. In the Mahratta country salt, pepper, and other spices are made into balls, with flour and butter, and these are supposed to produce animation and to fine the coat. Broth made from sheep's head is sometimes given. In France, Spain, and Italy, besides the grasses, the leaves of limes, vines, the tops of acacia, and the seeds of the carob tree are given to horses.

We can not, however, leave aside entirely here a consideration of the digestibility of feeds; and by this we mean the readiness with which they undergo those changes in the digestive canal that fit them for absorption and deposition as integral parts of the animal economy.

The age and health of the animal will, of course, modify the digestibility of feeds, as will also the manner and time of harvesting, preserving, and preparing.

In the horse digestion takes place principally in the intestines, and here, as in all other animals and with all feeds, it is found that a certain part only of the provender is digested; another portion is undigested. This proportion of digested and undigested feed must claim passing notice at least, for if the horse receives too much feed, or bulky feed containing much indigestible waste, a large portion of it must pass out unused, entailing not only the loss of this unused feed, but also calling for an unnecessary expenditure of vital force on the part of the digestive organs of the horse. It is thus that, in fact, too much feed may make an animal poor.

In selecting feed for the horse we should remember the anatomical arrangement of the digestive organs, as well as the physiological functions performed by each one of them. Feeds must be wholesome, clean, and sweet, the hours of feeding regular, the mode of preparation found by practical experience to be the best must be adhered to, and cleanliness in preparation and administration must be observed.

The length of time occupied by stomach digestion in the horse varies with the different feeds. Hay and straw pass out of the stomach more rapidly than oats. It would seem to follow, then, that oats should be given after hay, for if reversed the hay would cause the oats to be sent onward into the intestines before being fully acted upon by the stomach, and as a result produce indigestion. Experience confirms this. There is another good reason why hay should be given first, particularly if the horse is very hungry or if exhausted from overwork, namely, it requires more time in mastication (insuring proper admixture of saliva) and can not be bolted, as are the grains. In either instance water must not be given soon after feeding, as it washes or sluices the feed from the stomach before it is fitted for intestinal digestion.

The stomach begins to empty itself very soon after the commencement of feeding, and continues rapidly while eating. Afterwards the passage is slower, and several hours are required before the stomach is entirely empty. The nature of the work required of the horse must guide us in the selection of his feed. Rapid or severe labor can not be performed on a full stomach. For such labor feed must be given in small quantity and about two hours before going to work. Even horses intended for slow work must never be engorged with bulky, innutritious feed immediately before going to labor. The small stomach of the horse would seem to lead us to the conclusion that he should be fed in small quantities and often, which, in reality, should be done. The disproportion between the size of the stomach and the quantity of water drunk tells us plainly that the horse should always be watered before feeding. One of the common errors of feeding, and the one that produces more digestive disorders than any other, is *to feed too soon after a hard day's work*. This must never be done. If a horse is completely jaded, it will be found beneficial to give him an alcoholic stimulant on going into the stable. A small quantity of hay may then be given, but his grain should be withheld for one or two hours. These same remarks will apply with equal force to the horse that for any reason has been fasting for a long time. After a fast, feed less than the horse would eat, for if allowed too much the stomach becomes engorged, its walls paralyzed, and "colic" is almost sure to follow. The horse should be fed three or four times a day. It will not do to feed him entirely upon concentrated feed. Bulky feed must be given to detain the grains in their passage through the intestinal tract; bulk also favors distention, and thus mechanically aids absorption. For horses that do slow work the greater part of the time, chopped or cut hay fed with crushed oats, ground corn, etc., is the best manner of feeding, as it gives the required bulk, saves time, and half the labor of feeding.

Sudden changes of diet are always dangerous. When desirous of changing, do so very gradually. If a horse is accustomed to oats, a sudden change to a full meal of corn will almost always sicken him. If we merely intend to increase the quantity of the *usual* feed, this also must be done gradually. The quantity of feed given must always be in proportion to the amount of labor to be performed. If a horse is to do a small amount of work, or rest entirely from work for a few days, he should receive a proportionate quantity of feed. If this should be observed even on Saturday night and Sunday, there would be fewer cases of "Monday morning sickness," such as colics and lymphangitis.

Feeds should also be of a more laxative nature when the horse is to stand for several days.

Musty or moldy feeds.—Above all things, avoid feeding musty or moldy feeds. They are very frequent causes of disease of different kinds. Lung trouble, such as bronchitis and "heaves," often follows their use. The digestive organs always suffer from moldy or musty feeds. Musty hay is generally considered to produce disorder of the kidneys, and all know of the danger from feeding pregnant animals upon ergotized grasses or grains. It has often been said to produce that peculiar disease known variously as cerebrospinal meningitis, putrid sore throat, or choking distemper.

Hay.—The best hay for horses is timothy. It should be about one year old, of a greenish color, crisp, clean, fresh, and possessing a sweet, pleasant aroma. Even this good hay, if kept too long, loses part of its nourishment, and, while it may not be positively injurious, it is hard, dry, and indigestible. New hay is difficult to digest, produces much salivation (slobbering), and occasional purging and irritation of the skin. If fed at all it should be mixed with old hay.

Second crop, or aftermath.—This is not considered good hay for horses, but it is prized by some farmers as good for milch cows, the claim being made that it increases the flow of milk. The value of hay depends upon the time of cutting, as well as care in the curing. Hay should be cut when in full flower, but before the seeds fall; if left longer it becomes dry, woody, and lacks in nutrition.

An essential point in making hay is that when the crop is cut it should remain in the field as short a time as possible. If left too long in the sun it loses color, flavor, and dries or wastes. Smith asserts that one hour more than is necessary in the sun causes a loss of 15 to 20 per cent in the feeding value of hay. It is impossible to state any fixed time that hay must have to cure, this depending, of course, upon the weather, thickness of the crop, and many other circumstances; but it is well known that in order to preserve the color and aroma of hay it should be turned or tedded frequently and cured as quickly as possible. On the other hand, hay spoils in the mow if harvested too green or when not sufficiently dried. Mow-burnt hay produces disorder of the kidneys and bowels and causes the horse to fall off in condition.

The average horse on grain should be allowed from 10 to 12 pounds of good hay a day. It is a mistake of many to think that horses at light work can be kept entirely on hay. Such horses soon become pot-bellied, fall off in flesh, and do not thrive. The same is true of colts; unless the latter are fed with some grain they grow up to be long, lean, gawky creatures, and never make so good horses as those accustomed to grain with, or in addition to, their hay.

STRAW.—The straws are not extensively fed in this country, and when used at all they should be cut and mixed with hay and ground or crushed grain. Wheat, rye, and oat straw are the ones most used; of these, oat straw is most easily digested and contains the most nourishment. Pea and bean straw are occasionally fed to horses, the pea being preferable, according to most writers.

CHAFF.—Wheat and rye chaff should never be used as a feed for horses. The beards frequently become lodged in the mouth or throat and are productive of more or less serious trouble. In the stomach and intestines they often serve as the nucleus of the "soft concretions," which are to be described when treating of obstructions of the digestive tract.

Oat chaff, if fed in small quantities and mixed with cut hay or corn fodder, is very much relished by horses. It is not to be given in large quantities, as I have repeatedly witnessed a troublesome and sometimes fatal diarrhea following the practice of allowing horses or cattle free access to a pile of oat chaff.

GRAINS.—Oats take precedence of all grains as a feed for horses, as the ingredients necessary for the complete nutrition of the body exist in them in the best proportions. Oats are, besides, more easily digested and a larger proportion absorbed and converted into the various tissues of the body. Care must be taken in selecting oats. According to Stewart, the best oats are one year old, plump, short, hard, clean, bright, and sweet. New oats are indigestible. Kiln-dried oats are to be refused, as a rule, for even though originally good this drying process injures them. Oats that have sprouted or fermented are injurious and should never be fed. Oats are to be given either whole or crushed—whole in the majority of instances; crushed to old horses and those having defective teeth. Horses that bolt their feed are also best fed upon crushed oats and out of a manger large enough to permit of spreading the grain in a thin layer.

In addition to the allowance of hay above mentioned, the average horse requires about 12 quarts of good oats daily. The best oats are those cut about one week before they are fully ripe. Not only is the grain richer in nutritive materials at this time, but there is also less waste from "scattering" than if left to become dead ripe. Moldy oats, like hay and straw, not only produce serious digestive disorders but have been the undoubted cause of outbreaks of that dread disease in horses, already referred to, characterized by inability to eat or drink, sudden paralysis, and death.

WHEAT AND RYE.—These grains are not to be used for horses except in small quantities, bruised or crushed, and fed mixed with other grains or hay. If fed alone, in any considerable quantities, they are almost certain to produce digestive disorders, laminitis (founder), and similar troubles. They should never constitute more than one-fourth the grain allowance, and should always be ground or crushed.

BRAN.—The bran of wheat is the one most used, and its value as a feeding stuff is variously estimated. It is not to be depended upon if given alone, but may be fed with other grains. It serves to keep the bowels open. Sour bran is not to be given, for it disorders the stomach and intestines and may even produce serious results.

MAIZE (CORN).—This grain is not suitable as an exclusive feed for young horses, as it is deficient in salts. It is fed whole or ground. Corn on the cob is commonly used for horses affected with "lampas." If the corn is old and is to be fed in this manner it should be soaked in pure, clean water for 10 or 12 hours. Corn is better given ground, and fed in quantities of from 1 to 2 quarts at a meal, mixed with crushed oats or wheat bran. Great care should be taken in giving corn to a horse that is not accustomed to its use. It must be commenced in small quantities and very gradually increased. I know of no grain more liable to produce what is called acute indigestion than corn if these directions are not observed.

LINSEED.—Ground linseed is occasionally fed with other feeds to keep the bowels open and to improve the condition of the skin. It is of particular service during convalescence, when the bowels are sluggish in their action. Linseed tea is very often given in irritable or inflamed conditions of the digestive organs.

POTATOES.—These are used as an article of feed for the horse in many sections. If fed raw and in large quantities they often produce indigestion. Their digestibility is increased by steaming or boiling. They possess, in common with other roots, slight laxative properties.

BEETS.—These are not much used as feed for horses.

CARROTS.—These make a most excellent feed, particularly during sickness. They improve the appetite and slightly increase the action of the bowels and kidneys. They possess also certain alterative properties, making the coat smooth and glossy. Some veterinary writers assert that chronic cough is cured by giving carrots for some time. The roots may be considered, then, as an adjunct to the regular regimen, and if fed in small quantities are highly beneficial.

GRASSES.—Grass is the natural food of horses. It is composed of a great variety of plants, differing widely as to the amount of nourishment contained, some being almost entirely without value and only eaten when nothing else is obtainable, while others are positively injurious, or even poisonous. None of the grasses are sufficient to keep the horse in condition for work. Horses thus fed are "soft," sweat easily, purge, and soon tire on the road or when at hard work. Grass is indispensable to growing stock, and there is little or no doubt that it acts as an alterative when given to horses accustomed to grain and hay. It must be given to such horses in small quantities at first. The stomach and intestines undergo rest, and recuperate if the horse is turned to grass for a time each year. It is also certain that during febrile diseases grass acts almost as a medicine, lessening the fever and favoring recovery. Wounds heal more rapidly than when the horse is on grain, and some chronic disorders (chronic cough, for instance) disappear entirely when at grass. In my experience, grass does more good when the horse crops it himself. This may be due to the sense of freedom he enjoys at pasture, to the rest to his feet and limbs, and for many other similar reasons. When cut for him it should be fed fresh or when but slightly wilted.

SILAGE.—Regarding silage as a feed for horses, Rommel in Farmers' Bulletin 578 writes as follows:

Silage has not been generally fed to horses, partly on account of a certain amount of danger which attends its use for this purpose, but still more, perhaps, on account of prejudice. In many cases horses have been killed by eating moldy silage, and the careless person who fed it at once blamed the silage itself, rather than his own carelessness and the mold which really was the cause of the trouble. Horses are peculiarly susceptible to the effects of molds, and under certain conditions certain molds grow on silage which are deadly poisons to both horses and mules. Molds must have air to grow, and therefore silage which is packed air-tight and fed out rapidly will not become moldy. If the feeder watches the silage carefully as the weather warms up he can soon detect the presence of mold. When mold appears, feeding to horses or mules should stop immediately.

It is also unsafe to feed horses frozen silage on account of the danger of colic. * * *

To summarize, silage is safe to feed to horses and mules only when it is made from fairly mature corn, properly stored in the silo. When it is properly stored and is not allowed to mold, no feed exceeds it as a cheap winter ration. It is most valuable for horses and mules which are not at heavy work, such as brood mares and work horses during the slack season. With plenty of grain on the cornstalks, horses will keep in good condition on a ration of 20 pounds of silage and 10 pounds of hay for each 1,000 pounds of live weight.

PREPARATION OF FEEDS.

Feed is prepared for any of the following reasons: To render it more easily eaten; to make it more digestible; to economize in amount; to give it some new property; and to preserve it. We have already spoken of the preparation of drying, and need not revert to this again, as it only serves to preserve the different feeds. Drying does, however, change some of the properties of feed, *i. e.*, removes the laxative tendency of most of them.

The different grains are more easily eaten when ground, crushed, or even boiled. Rye or wheat should never be given whole, and even of corn it is found that there is less waste when ground, and, in common with all other grains, it is more easily digested than when fed whole.

Hay and fodder are economized when cut in short pieces. Not only will the horse eat the necessary quantity in a shorter time, but it will be found that there is less waste, and the mastication of the grains (whole or crushed) fed with them is insured.

Reference has already been made to those horses that bolt their feed, and we need only remark here that the consequences of such ravenous eating may be prevented if the grains are fed with cut hay, straw, or fodder. Long or uncut hay should also be fed, even though a certain quantity of hay or straw is cut and fed mixed with grain.

One objection to feeding cut hay mixed with ground or crushed grains, and wetted, must not be overlooked during the hot months. Such feed is liable to undergo fermentation if not fed directly after it is mixed; even the mixing trough, unless frequently scalded and cleaned, becomes sour and enough of its scrapings are given with the feed to produce flatulent (wind) colic. A small quantity of salt should always be mixed with such feed. Bad hay should never be cut simply because it insures a greater consumption of it; bad feeds are dear at any price, and should never be fed.

The advantage of boiling roots has been mentioned. Not only does this render them less liable to produce digestive disorders, but it also makes them clean. Boiling or steaming grains is to be recommended when the teeth are poor, or when the digestive organs are weak.

DISEASES OF THE TEETH.

Dentition.—This covers the period during which the young horse is cutting his teeth—from birth to the age of 5 years. With the horse more difficulty is experienced in cutting the second or permanent teeth than with the first or milk teeth. There is a tendency among farmers and many veterinarians to pay too little attention to the teeth of young horses. Percivall relates an instance illustrative of this that is best told in his own words:

I was requested to give my opinion concerning a horse, then in his fifth year, who had fed so sparingly for the last fortnight, and so rapidly declined in condition in consequence, that his owner, a veterinary surgeon, was under no light apprehensions about his life. He had himself examined his mouth without having discovered any defect or disease, though another veterinary surgeon was of opinion that the difficulty or inability manifested in mastication, and the consequent cudding, arose from preternatural bluntness of the surfaces of the molar teeth, which were, in consequence, filed, but without beneficial result. It was after this that I saw the horse, and I confess I was, at my first examination, quite as much at a loss to offer any satisfactory interpretation as others had been. While meditating, however, after my inspection, on the apparently extraordinary nature of the case, it struck me that I had not seen the tusks. I went back into the stable and discovered two little tumors, red and hard, in the situation of the inferior tusks, which, when pressed, gave the animal insufferable pain. I instantly took out my pocketknife and made crucial incisions through them both, down to the coming teeth, from which moment the horse recovered his appetite and, by degrees, his wonted condition.

The mouths of young horses should be examined from time to time to see whether one or more of the milk teeth are not remaining too long, causing the second teeth to grow in crooked, in which case the first teeth should be removed with the forceps.

Irregularities of teeth.—There is a fashion of late years, especially in large cities, to have horses' teeth regularly "floated," or "rasped," by "veterinary dentists." In some instances this is very beneficial, while in most cases it is entirely unnecessary. From the character of the feed, the rubbing, or grinding, surface of the horse's teeth should be rough. Still, we must remember that the upper jaw is somewhat wider than the lower, and that, from the fact of the teeth not being perfectly apposed, a sharp ridge is left unworn on the inside of the lower molars and on the outside of the upper, which may excoriate the tongue or cheeks to a considerable extent. This condition may readily be felt by the hand, and these sharp ridges when found should be rasped down by a guarded rasp. In some instances the first or last molar tooth is unnaturally long, owing to the fact that its fellow in the opposite jaw has been lost or does not close perfectly against it. Should it be the last molar that is thus elongated,

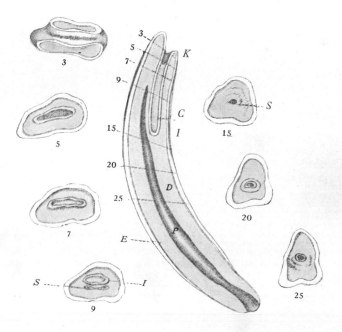

AGE OF HORSES AS INDICATED BY TEETH.

Longitudinal section of left central lower incisor and cross sections of same tooth showing table surfaces as they appear at the ages of 3, 5, 7, 9, 15, 20 and 25 years. C, Cement; D, Dentine; E, Enamel; I, Infundibulum; K, Cup; P, Pulp Cavity; S, Star.

it will require the aid of the veterinary surgeon, who has the necessary forceps or chisel for cutting it. The front molar may be rasped down, if much patience is taken. In decay of the teeth it is quite common to find the tooth corresponding to the decayed one on the opposite jaw very much elongated, sometimes to such an extent that the mouth can not be perfectly closed. Such teeth must also be shortened by the tooth forceps, chisel, tooth saw, or rasp. In all instances in which horses " quid " their feed, if they are slobbering, or evince pain in mastication, shown by holding the head to one side while chewing, the teeth should be carefully examined. Horses whose teeth have unduly sharp edges are liable to drive badly; they pull to one side, do not bear on the bit, or bear on too hard and " big," toss the head, and start suddenly when a tender spot is touched. If, as is mostly the case, all the symptoms are referable to sharp corners or projections, these must be removed by the rasp. If decayed teeth are found, or other serious difficulty detected, or if the cause of the annoying symptoms is not discovered, an expert should be called.

Toothache.—This is rare in the horse and is mostly witnessed when there is decay of a tooth or inflammation about its root. Toothache is to be discovered in the horse by the pain expressed by him while feeding or drinking cold water. I have seen horses, affected with toothache, that would suddenly stop chewing, throw the head to one side, and slightly open the mouth. They behave as though some sharp body had punctured the mouth. If upon examination no foreign body is found, we must then carefully examine each tooth. If this can not be done with the hand in the mouth, we can, in most instances, discover the aching tooth by pressing each tooth from without. By tapping the teeth in succession with a hard object, such as a small hammer, the one that is tender may be identified. The horse will flinch when the sore tooth is pressed or tapped upon. In most cases there is nothing to be done but extract the decayed tooth, and this, of course, is to be attempted by the veterinarian only.

Deformity.—There is a deformity, known as parrot-mouth, that interferes with prehension, mastication, and, indirectly, with digestion. The upper incisors project in front of and beyond the lower ones. The teeth of both jaws become unusually long, as they are not worn down by friction. Such horses experience much difficulty in grazing. Little can be done except to examine the teeth occasionally, and if those of the lower jaw become so long that they bruise the " bars " of the upper jaw, they must be shortened by the rasp or saw. Horses with this deformity should never be left entirely at pasture.

The method of determining the age of a horse by the teeth is illustrated in Plate IV.

DISEASES OF THE MOUTH.

LAMPAS.

Lampas is the name given to a swelling of the mucous membrane covering the hard palate and projecting in a more or less prominent ridge immediately behind the upper incisors. The hard palate is composed of spongy tissue that fills with blood when the horse is feeding, which causes the ridges to become prominent, and they then help to keep feed from dropping from the mouth. This swelling is entirely natural and occurs in every healthy horse. Where there is some irritation in the mouth, as in stomatitis or during teething, the prominence of the hard palate may persist, owing to the increased blood supply. In such cases the cause of the irritation should be sought for and removed. By way of direct treatment, slight scarification is the most that will be required. Burning the lampas is barbarous and injurious, and it should never be tolerated.

It is a quite common opinion among owners of horses and stablemen that lampas is a disease that very frequently exists. In fact whenever a horse fails to eat, and if he does not exhibit very marked symptoms of a severe illness, they say at once " he has the lampas." It is almost impossible to convince them to the contrary; yet it is not the case. It may be put down, then, as an affliction of the stableman's imagination rather than of the horse's mouth.

STOMATITIS.

Stomatitis is an inflammation of the mucous membrane lining the mouth and is produced by irritating medicines, feeds, or other substances. The symptoms are swelling of the mouth, which is also hot and painful to the touch; there is a copious discharge of saliva; the mucous membrane is reddened, and in some cases vesicles or ulcers in the mouth are observed. The treatment is simple, soft feed alone often being all that is necessary. A bucket of fresh, cold water should be kept constantly in the manger so that the horse may drink or rinse his mouth at will. In some instances, it may be advisable to use a wash of chlorate of potash, borax, or alum, about one-half ounce to a pint of water. Hay, straw, or oats should not be fed unless steamed or boiled. A form of contagious stomatitis, characterized by the formation within the mouth of small vesicles, or blisters, sometimes occurs. In this disease the horse should be isolated from other horses, and his stall, especially the feed box, and his bit should be disinfected.

GLOSSITIS (INFLAMMATION OF THE TONGUE).

Glossitis, or inflammation of the tongue, is very similar to stomatitis, and mostly exists with it and is due to the same causes. Injuries to the tongue may produce this simple inflammation of its covering membrane, or, if severe, may produce lesions much more extensive, such as lacerations, abscesses, etc. These latter would require surgical treatment, but for the simpler forms of inflammation of the tongue the treatment recommended for stomatitis should be followed.

SALIVATION (PTYALISM).

Ptyalism, or salivation, consists in an abnormal and excessive secretion of saliva. This is often seen as a symptom of irregular teeth; inflammation of the mouth or tongue, or of the use of such medicines as lobelia, mercury, and many others. Some feeds, such as clover, and particularly second crop, produce it; foreign bodies, such as nails, wheat chaff, and corncobs becoming lodged in the mouth, also are causes. If the cause is removed no further attention is necessary, as a rule. Astringent washes may be applied to the mouth as a gargle or by means of a sponge.

PHARYNGITIS.

Pharyngitis is an inflammation of the mucous membrane lining of the pharynx or throat. It rarely exists unless accompanied with stomatitis or laryngitis, especially the latter. In those rare instances in which the inflammation is mostly confined to the pharynx are noticed febrile symptoms—difficulty of swallowing either liquids or solids; there is but little cough except when trying to swallow; there is no soreness on pressure over larynx (head of the windpipe). Increased flow of saliva, difficulty of swallowing liquids in particular, and cough only when attempting to swallow, are the symptoms best marked in pharyngitis. In some cases the throat becomes gangrenous and the disease ends in death. For treatment a wet sheet should be wrapped around the throat and covered with rubber sheeting and a warm blanket. This should be changed three times daily; or the region of the throat may be rubbed with mercurial ointment twice daily until the skin becomes irritated, but no longer; chlorate of potash may be given in 2-dram doses four times daily, mixed with flaxseed meal or licorice-root powder and honey, as an electuary. Soft feeds should be given, and fresh water should be constantly before the horse.

PARALYSIS OF THE PHARYNX.

Paralysis of the pharynx, or, as it is commonly called, "paralysis of the throat," is a rare but very serious disease. The symptoms are as follows: The horse will constantly try to eat or drink, but will be unable to do so; if water is offered him from a pail he will apparently drink with avidity, but the quantity of water in the pail will remain about the same; he will continue by the hour to try to drink; if he can get any fluid into the back part of the mouth it will come out at once through the nose. Feeds also return through the nose, or are dropped from the mouth, quidded. An examination of the mouth by inserting the hand fails to find any obstruction or any abnormal condition. These cases go on from bad to worse; the horse constantly and rapidly loses in condition, becomes very much emaciated, the eyes are hollow and lusterless, and death occurs from inanition.

Treatment is very unsatisfactory. A severe blister should be applied behind and under the jaw; the mouth is to be frequently swabbed out with alum or chlorate of potash, 1 ounce to a pint of water, by means of a sponge fastened to the end of a stick. Strychnia may be given in 1-grain doses two or three times a day.

This disease may be mistaken at times for foreign bodies in the mouth or for the so-called cerebrospinal meningitis. It is to be distinguished from the former, upon a careful examination of the mouth, by the absence of any offending body and by the flabby feel of the mouth, and from the latter by the animal appearing in perfect health in every particular except this inability to eat or drink.

ABSCESSES.

Abscesses sometimes form back of the pharynx and give rise to symptoms resembling those of laryngitis or distemper. Interference with breathing that is of recent origin and progression, without any observable swelling or soreness about the throat, will make one suspect the formation of an abscess in this location. But little can be done in the way of treatment, save to hurry the ripening of the abscess and its discharge by steaming with hops, hay, or similar substances and by poulticing the throat. The operation for opening an abscess in this region necessitates an intimate knowledge of the complex anatomy of the throat region.

DISEASES OF THE ESOPHAGUS OR GULLET.

It is rare to find diseases of this organ, except as a result of the introduction of foreign bodies too large to pass or to the administering of irritating medicines. In the administration of irritant or caustic medicines great care should be taken that they be thoroughly diluted. If this is not done, erosions and ulcerations of the throat ensue, and this again is prone to be followed by constriction (narrowing) of the gullet.

CHOKING.

The mechanical trouble of choking is quite common. It may occur when the animal is suddenly startled while eating apples or roots, and we should be careful never to approach suddenly or put a dog after horses or cows that are feeding upon such substances. If left alone these animals very rarely attempt to swallow the object until it is sufficiently masticated.

Choking also arises from feeding oats in a deep, narrow manger to such horses as eat very greedily or bolt their feed. Wheat chaff is also a frequent cause of choke. This accident may result from the attempts to force eggs down without breaking or from giving balls that are too large or not of the proper shape.

Whatever object causes the choking, it may lodge in the upper part of the esophagus, at its middle portion, or close to the stomach, giving rise to the designations of pharyngeal, cervical, and thoracic choke. In some cases where the original obstruction is low we find all that part of the gullet above it to be distended with feed.

Symptoms.—The symptoms vary somewhat according to the position of the body causing choke. In pharyngeal choke the object is lodged in the upper portion of the esophagus. The horse will present symptoms of great distress, hurried breathing, frequent cough, excessive flow of saliva, sweating, trembling, or stamping with the fore feet. The abdomen rapidly distends with gas. The diagnosis is completed by manipulating the upper part of the throat from without and by the introduction of the hand into the back part of the mouth, finding the body lodged here. In cervical choke (where the obstruction is situated at any point between the throatlatch and the shoulder) the protrusion caused by the object can be seen and the object can be felt. The symptoms here are not so severe; the horse will be seen occasionally to draw himself up, arch his neck, and make retching movements as though he wished to vomit. The abdomen may be tympanitic. Should there be any question as to the trouble, a conclusion may be reached by pouring water into the throat from a bottle. If the obstruction is complete, by standing on the left side of the horse and watching the course of the esophagus, you can see the gullet, just above the windpipe, become distended with each bottle of water. This is not always a sure test, as the obstruction may be an angular body, in which case liquids would pass it. Solids taken would show in these cases; solids should not, however, be given, as they serve to increase the trouble by rendering the removal of the body more difficult.

In thoracic choke the symptoms are less severe. Feed or water may be ejected through the nose or mouth after the animal has taken a few swallows. There will be some symptoms of distress, fullness of the abdomen, cough, and occasionally retching movements. Sometimes a choking horse is heard to emit groans. The facial expression always denotes great anxiety and the eyes are bloodshot. The diagnosis is complete if, upon passing the probang (a flexible tube made for this purpose), an obstruction is encountered.

Treatment.—If the choke is at the beginning of the gullet (pharyngeal) an effort must be made to remove the obstacle through the mouth. A mouthgag, or speculum, is to be introduced into the mouth to protect the hand and arm of the operator. Then, while an assistant, with his hands grasped tightly *behind* the object, presses it upward and forward with all his force, the operator must pass his hand into the mouth until he can seize the obstruction and draw it outward. This mode of procedure must not be abandoned with the first failure, as by continued efforts we may get the obstacle farther toward the mouth. If we fail with the hand, forceps may be introduced through the mouth and the object seized when it is just beyond the reach of the fingers. Should our efforts entirely fail, we must then endeavor to force the obstruction downward by means of the probang. This instrument, which is of such signal service in removing choke in cattle, is decidedly more dangerous to use for the horse, and I can not pass this point without a word of caution to those who have been known to introduce into the horse's throat such objects as whipstalks, shovel handles, etc. These are always dangerous, and more than one horse has been killed by such barbarous treatment.

In cervical as well as in thoracic choke we must first of all endeavor to soften or lubricate the obstruction by pouring oil or mucilaginous drinks down the gullet. After this has been done endeavor to move the object by gentle manipulations with the hands. If choked with oats or chaff (and these are the objects that most frequently produce choke in the horse), begin by gently squeezing the lower portion of the impacted mass and endeavor to work it loose a little at a time. This is greatly favored at times if we apply hot fomentations immediately about the obstruction. Persist in these efforts for at least an hour before deciding to resort to other and more dangerous modes of treatment. If unsuccessful, however, the probang may be used. In the absence of the regular instrument, a piece of inch hose 6 feet long or a piece of new three-quarter-inch manila rope well wrapped at the end with cotton twine and thoroughly greased with tallow should be used. The mouth is to be kept open by a gag of wood or iron and the head slightly raised and extended. The probang is then to be carefully guided by the hand into the upper part of the gullet and gently forced downward until the obstruction is reached. Pressure must then be gradual and firm. At first too much force should not be used, or the esophagus will be ruptured. Firm, gentle pressure should be kept up until the object is felt to move, after which it should be followed rapidly to the stomach. If this mode of treatment is unsuccessful, a veterinarian or a physician should be called, who can remove the object by cutting down upon it. This should scarcely be attempted by a novice, as a knowledge of the anatomy of the parts is essential to avoid cutting the large artery, vein, and nerve that are closely related to the esophagus in its cervical portion.

Thoracic choke can be treated only by means of the introduction of oils and mucilaginous drinks and the careful use of the probang.

STRICTURE OF THE ESOPHAGUS.

This is due to corrosive medicines, previous choking (accompanied with lacerations, which, in healing, narrow the passage), or pressure on the gullet by tumors. In the majority of cases of stricture, dilatation of the gullet in front of the constricted portion soon occurs. This dilatation is the result of the frequent accumulation of solid feed above the constriction. Little can be done in either of these instances except to give sloppy or liquid feed.

SACULAR DILATATION OF THE ESOPHAGUS.

This follows choking, and is due to stretching or rupture of the muscular coat of the gullet, allowing the internal, or mucous, coat to protrude through the lacerated muscular walls. Such a dilatation, or pouch, may gradually enlarge from the frequent imprisonment of feed. When liquids are taken, the solid materials are partially washed out of the pouch.

The symptoms are as follows: The horse is able to swallow a few mouthfuls without apparent difficulty; then he will stop feeding, paw, contract the muscles of his neck, and eject a portion of the feed through his nose or mouth, or it will gradually work down to the stomach. As the dilatation thus empties itself the symptoms gradually subside, only to reappear when he has again taken solid feed. Liquids pass without any, or but little, inconvenience. Should this dilatation exist in the cervical region, surgical interference may sometimes prove effectual; if in the thoracic portion, nothing can be done, and the patient rapidly passes from hand to hand by "swapping," until, at no distant date, the contents of the sac become too firm to be dislodged as heretofore, and the animal succumbs.

DISEASES OF THE STOMACH AND INTESTINES.

As a rule it is most difficult to distinguish between diseases of the stomach and of the intestines of the horse. The reason for this is that the stomach is relatively small. It lies away from the abdominal wall, and so pressure from without can not be brought to bear upon it to reveal sensitiveness or pain. Nor does enlargement, or distention, of the stomach produce visible alteration in the form of the abdomen of the horse. Moreover, it is a rule to which there are few exceptions, that an irritant or cause of disease of the stomach acts likewise upon the intestines, so that it is customary to find them similarly deranged. For these reasons it is logical to discuss together the diseases of the stomach and intestines and to point out such localizations in one organ or another as are of importance in recognizing and treating the diseases of the digestive organs of the horse.

It should be understood that gastritis signifies an inflammation of the stomach and enteritis an inflammation of the intestines. The two terms may be used together to signify a disease of the stomach and intestines, as gastroenteritis.

COLIC.

The disease of the horse that is most frequently met with is what is termed "colic," and many are the remedies that are reputed to be "sure cures" for this disease. Let us discover, then, what the word "colic" means. This term is applied loosely to almost all diseases of the organs of the abdomen that are accompanied with pain. If the horse evinces abdominal pain, he probably will be considered as suffering with colic, no matter whether the difficulty is a cramp of the bowel, an internal hernia, overloading of the stomach, or a painful disease of the bladder or liver. Since these conditions differ so much in their causation and their nature, it is manifestly absurd to treat them alike and to expect the same drugs or procedures to relieve them all. Therefore, it is important that, so far as possible, the various diseased states that are so roughly classed together as colic shall be separated and individualized in order that appropriate treatments may be prescribed. With this object in view, colics will be considered under the following headings: (1) Engorgement colic, (2) obstruction colic, (3) flatulent or tympanitic colic, (4) spasmodic colic. Worm colic is discussed under the heading "Gastrointestinal parasites," page 90.

The general symptoms of abdominal pain, and therefore of colic, are restlessness, cessation of whatever the horse is about, lying down, looking around toward the flank, kicking with the hind feet upward and forward toward the belly, jerky switching of the tail, stretching as though to urinate, frequent change of position, and groaning. In the more intense forms the horse plunges about, throws himself, rolls, assumes unnatural positions, as sitting on the haunches, and grunts loudly. Usually the pain is not constant, and during the intermissions the horse may eat and appear normal. During the period of pain sweat is poured out freely. Sometimes the horse moves constantly in a circle. The respirations are accelerated, and usually there is no fever.

ENGORGEMENT COLIC.—This form of colic consists in an overloading of the stomach with feed. The horse may have been overfed or the feed may have collected in the stomach through failure of this organ to digest it and pass it backward into the intestines. Even a normal quantity of feed that the horse is unaccustomed to may cause disease. Hence a sudden change of feed may produce engorgement colic. Continued full rations while the horse is resting for a day or two or working too soon after feeding may serve as a cause. New oats, corn, or hay, damaged feed, or that which is difficult of digestion, such as barley or beans, may incite engorgement colic. This disease may result from having fed the horse twice by error or from its having escaped and taken an unrestricted meal from the grain bin. Ground feeds that pack together, making a sort of dough, may cause engorgement colic if they are not mixed with cut hay. Greedy eaters are predisposed to this disease.

Symptoms.—The horse shows the general signs of abdominal pain, which may be long continued or of short duration. Retching or vomiting movements are made; these are shown by labored breathing, upturned upper lip, contraction of the flank, active motion at the throat, and drawing in of the nose toward the breast, causing high arching of the neck. The horse may assume a sitting position like a dog. At times the pain is very great and the horse makes the most violent movements, as though mad. At other times there is profound mental depression, the horse standing in a sleepy, or dazed, way, with the head down, the eyes closed, and leaning his head against the manger or wall. There is, during the struggles, profuse perspiration. Following retching, gas may escape from the mouth, and this may be followed by a sour froth and some stomach contents. The horse can not vomit except when the stomach is violently stretched, and, if the accumulation of feed or gas is great enough to stretch the stomach so that vomiting is possible, it may be great enough to rupture that organ. So it happens not infrequently that a horse dies from ruptured stomach after vomiting. After the stomach ruptures, however, vomiting is impossible. The death rate in this form of colic is high.

Treatment.—The bowels should be stimulated to contraction by the use of clysters of large quantities of water and of glycerin. Veterinarians use hypodermic injections of eserin or arecolin or intravenous injections of barium chlorid, but they must be employed with great caution. It is not profitable to give remedies by the stomach, for they can not be absorbed. But small doses of morphin (5 grains) or of the fluid extract of Indian hemp (2 drams) may be placed in the mouth and are absorbed in part, at least, without passing to the stomach. These drugs lessen pain and thus help to overcome the violent movements that are dangerous, because they may be the means of causing rupture of the diaphragm or stomach. If facilities are available, relief may be afforded by passing an esophageal tube through which some of the gaseous and liquid contents of the stomach may escape.

Rupture of the stomach.—This mostly occurs as a result of engorged or tympanitic stomach (engorgement colic) and from the horse violently throwing himself when so affected. It may result from disease of the coats of the stomach, gastritis, stones (calculi), tumors, or anything that closes the opening of the stomach into the intestines, and very violent pulling or jumping immediately after the animal has eaten heartily of bulky feed. These or similar causes may lead to this accident.

The symptoms of rupture of the stomach are not constant or always reliable. Always make inquiry as to what and how much the horse has been fed at the last meal. Vomiting may precede rupture of this organ, as stated above. This accident appears to be most liable to occur in heavy draft horses. A prominent symptom observed (though it may also occur in diaphragmatic hernia) is when the horse, if possible, gets the front feet on higher ground than the hind ones or sits on his haunches, like a dog. This position affords relief to some extent, and it will be maintained for several minutes; it is also quickly regained when the horse has changed it for some other. Colicky symptoms, of course, are present, which vary much and present no diagnostic value. As the case progresses the horse will often stretch forward the fore legs, lean backward and downward until the belly nearly touches the ground, and then rise up again with a groan, after which the fluid from his nostrils is issued in increased quantity. The pulse is fast and weak, breathing hurried, body bathed in a clammy sweat, limbs tremble violently, the horse reels or staggers from side to side, and death quickly ends the scene.

In the absence of any pathognomonic symptom we must consider the history of the case; the symptoms of colic that cease suddenly and are succeeded by cold sweats and tremors; the pulse quick and small and thready, growing weak and more frequent, and at length running down and becoming altogether imperceptible; looking back at the flank and groaning; sometimes crouching with the hind quarters; with or without eructation and vomiting.

There is no treatment that can be of any use whatever. Could we be sure of our diagnosis it would be better to destroy the animal at once. Since, however, there is always the possibility of a mistake in diagonsis, we may give powdered opium in 1-dram doses every two or three hours, with the object of keeping the stomach as quiet as possible.

OBSTRUCTION COLIC.—The stomach or bowels may be obstructed by accumulations of partly digested feed (fecal matter), by foreign bodies, by displacements, by paralysis, or by abnormal growths.

Impaction of the large intestines.—This is a very common bowel trouble and one which, if not promptly recognized and properly treated, results in death. It is caused by overfeeding, especially of bulky feed containing an excess of indigestible residue; old, dry, hard hay, or stalks when largely fed; deficiency of secretions of the intestinal tracts; lack of water; want of exercise, medicines, etc.

Impaction of the large bowels is to be diagnosed by a slight abdominal pain, which may disappear for a day or two to reappear with more violence. The feces are passed somewhat more frequently, but in smaller quantities and drier; the abdomen is full, but not distended with gas; the horse at first is noticed to paw and soon begins to look back at his sides. Probably one of the most characteristic symptoms is the position assumed when down. He lies flat on his side, head and legs extended, occasionally raising his head to look toward his flank; he remains on his side for from five to fifteen minutes at a time. Evidently this position is the one giving the most freedom from pain. He rises at times, walks about the stall, paws, looks at his sides, backs up against the stall, which he presses with his tail, and soon lies down again, assuming his favored position. The intestinal sounds, as heard by applying the ear to the flank, are diminished, or there is no sound, indicating absence of motion of the bowels. The bowels may cease entirely to move. The pressure of the distended intestine upon the bladder may cause the horse to make frequent attempts to urinate. The pulse is but little changed at first, being full and sluggish; later, if this condition is not overcome, it becomes rapid and feeble. Horses may suffer from impaction of the bowels for a week, yet eventually recover, and cases extending two or even three weeks have ended favorably. As a rule, however, they seldom last more than four or five days, many, in fact, dying sooner than this.

The treatment consists of efforts to produce movement of the bowels and to prevent inflammation of the same from arising. A large cathartic is to be given as early as possible. Either of the following is recommended: Powdered Barbados aloes 1 ounce, calomel 2 drams, and powdered nux vomica 1 dram; or linseed oil 1 pint and croton oil 15 drops; or from 1 pint to 1 quart of castor oil may be given. Some favor the administration of Epsom or Glauber's salt, 1 pound, with one-quarter pound of common salt, claiming that this causes the horse to drink largely of water, thus mechanically softening the impacted mass and favoring its expulsion. Whichever physic is selected, it is essential that a full dose be given. This is much better than small and repeated doses. It must be borne in mind that horses require about twenty-four hours in which to respond to a physic, and under no circumstances is it to be repeated sooner. If aloes has been given and has failed to operate at the proper time, oil or some different cathartic should then be administered. Allow the horse all the water he will drink. Calomel may be administered in half-dram doses, the powder being placed on the tongue, one dose every two hours until four doses are given.

Enemas of glycerin, 2 to 4 ounces, are often beneficial. Rubbing or kneading of the abdominal walls and the application of stimulating liniments or strong mustard water also, at times, favor the expulsion of this mass. Walking exercise must occasionally be given. If this treatment is faithfully carried out from the start the majority of cases will terminate favorably. When relief is not obtained inflammation of the bowels may ensue and cause death.

Constipation, or costiveness.—This is often witnessed in the horse, and particularly in the foal. Many colts die every year from failure on the part of the attendant to note the condition of the bowels soon after birth. Whenever the foal fails to pass any feces, and in particular if it presents any signs of colicky pains—straining, etc.—immediate attention must be given it. As a rule, it will be necessary only to give a few injections of soapy water in the rectum and to introduce the finger through the anus to break down any hardened mass of dung found there. If this is not effective a purgative must be given. Oils are the best for these young animals, and preferably castor oil, giving from 2 to 4 ounces. The foal should always get the first of the mother's milk, which, for a few days, possesses decidedly laxative properties. If a mare, while suckling, is taking laudanum, morphin, atropia, or similar medicines, the foal during this time should be fed by hand and the mare milked upon the ground. Constipation in adult horses is often the result of long feeding on dry, innutritious feed, deficiency of intestinal secretions, scanty water supply, or lack of exercise. If the case is not complicated with colicky symptoms a change to light, sloppy diet, linseed gruel or tea, with plenty of exercise, is all that is required. If colic exists a cathartic is needed. In very many instances the constipated condition of the bowels is due to lack of intestinal secretions, and when so caused may be treated by giving fluid extract of belladonna in 2-dram doses three times a day and handful doses of Epsom salt daily in the feed. It is always best, when possible, to overcome this trouble by a change of diet rather than by the use of medicines. For the relief of constipation such succulent feeds as roots, grass, or green forage are recommended. Silage, however, should be fed sparingly, and not at all unless it is in the very best condition. Moldy silage may cause fatal disease.

Foreign bodies (calculi, stones) in the stomach.—There are probably but few symptoms exhibited by the horse that will lead one to suspect the presence of gastric calculi, and possibly none by which we can unmistakably assert their presence. They have been found most frequently in millers' horses fed sweepings from the mills. A depraved and capricious appetite is common in horses that have a stone forming in the stomachs. There is a disposition to eat the wood-work of the stable, earth, and, in fact, almost any substance within their reach. This symptom must not, however, be considered as pathognomonic, since it is observed when calculi are not present. Occasional colics may result from these " stomach stones," and when the latter lodge at the outlet of the stomach they may give rise to symptoms of engorged stomach, already described. There is, of course, no treatment that will prove effective. Remedies to move the bowels, to relieve pain, and to combat inflammation should be given.

Intestinal concretions (calculi or stones in the intestines).—These concretions are usually found in the large bowels, though they are occasionally seen in the small intestines. They are of various sizes, weighing from 1 ounce to 25 pounds; they may be single or multiple, and differ in composition and appearance, some being soft (com-posed mostly of animal or vegetable matter), while others are porous, or honeycombed (consisting of animal and mineral matter), and others are entirely hard and stonelike. The hair balls, so common to the stomach and intestines of cattle, are very rare in horses. Intestinal calculi form around some foreign body, as a rule—a nail or piece of wood—whose shape they may assume to a certain extent. Layers are arranged concentrically around such nucleus until the sizes above spoken of are attained. These stones are also often found in millers' horses, as well also as in horses in limestone dis-tricts, where the water is hard. When the calculi attain a sufficient size and become lodged or blocked in some part of the intestines, they cause obstruction, inflammation of the bowels, colicky symp-toms, and death. There are no certain signs or symptoms that re-veal them. Recurring colics of the type of impaction colic, but more severe, may lead one to suspect the existence of this condition. Examination through the rectum may reveal the calculus.

The symptoms will be those of obstruction of the bowels. Upon post-mortem examinations these stones will be discovered mostly in the large bowels; the intestines will be inflamed or gangrenous about the point of obstruction. Sometimes calculi have been expelled by the action of a physic, or they may be removed by the hand when found to occupy the rectum.

As in concretions of the stomach, but little can be done in the way of treatment more than to overcome spasm (if any exists), and to give physics with the hope of dislodging the stone or stones and carrying them on and outward.

Intussusception, or invagination.—This is the slipping of a portion of the intestine into another portion immediately adjoining, like a partially turned glove finger. This may occur at any part of the bowels, but is most frequent in the small guts. The invaginated portion may be slight—2 or 3 inches only—or extensive, measuring as many feet. In intussusception, the inturned bowel is in the direction of the anus. There are adhesions of the intestines at this point, congestion, inflammation, or even gangrene. This accident is most liable to occur in horses that are suffering from spasm of the bowel, or in those in which a small portion of the gut is paralyzed. The natural wormlike or ringlike contraction of the gut favors the passage of the contracted or paralyzed portion into that immediately behind it. It may occur during the existence of almost any abdominal trouble, as diarrhea, inflammation of the bowels, or from injuries, exposure to cold, etc. A fall or leaping may give the initial maldirection. Foals are most likely to be thus afflicted.

Unless the invaginated portion of the gut becomes strangulated, probably no symptoms except constipation will be appreciable. Strangulation of the bowel may take place suddenly, and the horse die within 24 hours, or it may occur after several days—a week even—and death then follow. There are no symptoms positively diagnostic. Colicky pains, more or less severe and continuous, are observed, and at first there may be diarrhea, followed by constipation. Severe straining occurs in some instances of intussusception, and when this occurs it should receive due credit. As death approaches, the horse sweats profusely, sighs, presents an anxious countenance, the legs and ears become cold, and there is often freedom from pain immediately before death. In some rare instances he recovers, even though the invaginated portion of the gut has become strangulated. In this case the imprisoned portion sloughs away so gradually that a union has taken place between the intestines at the point where one portion has slipped into that behind it. The piece sloughing off is found passed with the manure. Such cases are exceedingly rare. Nonirritating laxatives, such as castor oil, sweet oil, or calomel in small doses, should be given. Soft feed and mucilaginous and nourishing drinks should be given during these attacks. E. Mayhew Michener has operated successfully on a foal with intussusception by opening the abdomen and releasing the imprisoned gut.

Volvulus, gut tie, or twisting of the bowels.—These are the terms applied to the bowels when twisted or knotted. This accident is rather a common one, and frequently results from the violent manner in which a horse throws himself about when attacked by spasmodic colic. The symptoms are the same as those of intussusception and obstructions of the bowels; the same directions as to treatment are therefore to be observed.

Paralysis of the intestine.—This occurs in old, debilitated animals that have been fed on coarse, innutritious fodder. This produces a condition of dilatation so pronounced as to make it impossible for the intestine to advance its contents, and so obstruction results. The symptoms are as in other forms of obstruction colic. The history of the case is of much service in diagnosing the trouble. The treatment consists in the administration of laxatives. One may give 1 quart of raw linseed oil and follow it the next day with 1 pound of Glauber's salt dissolved in a quart of warm water. Strychnia may be given in doses of 1 grain two or three times daily. If the stagnant mass of feces is in the rectum, it must be removed with the hand.

Abnormal growths, such as tumors or fibrous tissue, producing contraction or stricture, may be causes of obstruction. The colic caused by these conditions is chronic. The attacks occur at gradually shortening intervals and become progressively more severe. Relief is afforded by the use of purgatives that render the feces soft and thin and thus enable them to pass the obstruction, but in time the contracted place is liable to close so far that passage is impossible and the horse will die.

FLATULENT COLIC (TYMPANITIC COLIC, WIND COLIC, OR BLOAT).— Among the most frequent causes of this form of colic are to be mentioned sudden changes of feed, too long fasting and feed then given while the animal is exhausted, new hay or grain, large quantities of feed that is green or that has lain in the manger for some time and become sour, indigestible feed, irregular teeth, crib biting, and, in fact, anything that produces indigestion may produce flatulent colic.

Symptoms.—The symptoms of wind colic are not so suddenly developed nor so severe as those of cramp colic. At first the horse is noticed to be dull, paws slightly, and may or may not lie down. The pains from the start are continuous. The belly enlarges, and by striking it in front of the haunches a drumlike sound results. If not soon relieved the above symptoms are aggravated, and in addition difficult breathing, bloodshot eyes, and red mucous membranes, loud tumultuous heart beat, profuse perspiration, trembling of front legs, sighing respiration, staggering from side to side are noticed, and, finally, plunging forward dead. The diagnostic symptom of flatulent colic is the distention of the bowels with gas, detected by the bloated appearance and resonance on percussion.

Treatment.—The treatment for wind colic differs very greatly from that of cramp colic. Absorbents are of some service, and charcoal may be given in any quantity. Relaxants and antispasmodics are also beneficial in this form of colic. Chloral hydrate not only possesses these qualities, but it also is an antiferment and a pain reliever. It is, then, particularly well adapted to the treatment of wind colic, and should be given in the same-sized doses and in the manner directed for spasmodic colic. Aromatic spirits of ammonia in 1-ounce doses may be given at short intervals.

A physic should always be given as early as possible in flatulent colic, the best being Barbados aloes in the dose already mentioned. Injections, per rectum, of turpentine 1 to 2 ounces, linseed oil 8 ounces, may be given frequently to stimulate the peristaltic motion of the bowels and to favor the escape of wind. Blankets wrung out of hot water do much to afford relief; they should be renewed every 5 or 10 minutes and covered with a dry woolen blanket. This form of colic is much more fatal than cramp colic, and requires prompt and persistent treatment. It is entirely unsafe to predict the result, some apparently mild attacks going on to speedy death, while others that at the onset appear to be very severe yielding rapidly to treatment. No efforts should be spared until the animal is known to be dead. In these severe cases puncturing of the bowels in the most prominent (distended) part by means of a small trocar and cannula or with a needle of a hypodermic syringe, thus allowing the escape of gas, has often saved life, and such punctures, if made with a clean, sharp instrument that is not allowed to remain in the horse too long, are accompanied with little danger and do more to relieve the patient quickly than any other treatment.

SPASMODIC OR CRAMP COLIC.—This is the name given to that form of colic produced by contraction, or spasm, of a portion of the small intestines. It is produced by indigestible feed; large drinks of cold water when the animal is warm; driving a heated horse through deep streams; cold rains; drafts of cold air, etc. Unequal distribution of or interference with the nervous supply here produces cramp of the bowels, the same as external cramps are produced. Spasmodic colic is much more frequently met with in high-bred, nervous horses than in coarse, lymphatic ones.

Symptoms.—These should be carefully studied in order to diagnose this from other forms of colic requiring quite different treatment. Spasmodic colic always begins suddenly. If feeding, the horse is seen to stop abruptly, stamp impatiently, and probably look back. He soon evinces more acute pain, shown by pawing, suddenly lying down, rolling, and getting up. During the period of pain the intestinal sounds, as heard by applying the ear over the flank, are louder than in health. There is then an interval of ease; he will resume feeding and appear to be entirely well. In a little while, however, the pains return and are increased in severity, only to pass off again for a time. As the attack progresses these intervals of ease become shorter and shorter, and pain may be continuous, though even then there are exacerbations of pain. Animals suffering from this form of colic evince the most intense pain; they throw themselves, roll over and over, jump up, whirl about, drop down again, paw, or strike rather, with the front feet, steam and sweat, and make frequent attempts to pass their urine. Only a small quantity of water is passed at a time; this is due to the bladder being so frequently emptied. These attempts to urinate are often regarded by horsemen as symptoms of trouble of the kidneys or bladder. In reality they are only one of the many ways in which the horse expresses the presence of pain. As a matter of fact, diseases of the bladder or kidneys of the horse are exceedingly rare.

To recapitulate the symptoms of spasmodic colic: The history of the case, the type of horse, the suddenness of the attack, the increased intestinal sounds, the intervals of ease (which become of shorter duration as the case progresses), the violent pain, the normal temperature and pulse during the intervals of ease, the frequent attempts to urinate, etc., should be kept in mind, and there is then but little danger of confounding this with other forms of colic.

Treatment.—Since the pain is due to spasm or cramp of the bowels, medicines that overcome spasms—antispasmodics—are the ones indicated. Chloral hydrate may be used. This is to be given in a dose of 1 ounce in a pint of water as a drench. As this drug is irritant to the throat and stomach, it has to be well diluted. A common and good remedy is sulphuric ether and laudanum, of each 2 ounces, in a half pint of linseed oil. Another drench may be composed of 2 ounces each of sulphuric ether and alcohol in 8 ounces of water. Jamaica ginger is useful. If relief is not obtained in one hour from any of the above doses, they may then be repeated. The body should be warmly clothed and perspiration induced. Blankets dipped in very hot water to which a small quantity of turpentine has been added should be placed around the belly and covered with dry blankets, or the abdomen may be rubbed with stimulating liniments or mustard water. The difficulty, however, of applying hot blankets and keeping them in place forces us in most instances to dispense with them. If the cramp is due to irritants in the bowels, a cure is not complete until a cathartic of 1 ounce of aloes or 1 pint of linseed oil is given. Injections of warm, soapy water or salt and water into the rectum aid the cure.

Rectal injections, clysters, or enemas as a rule should be lukewarm, and from 3 to 6 quarts are to be given at a time. They may be repeated every half hour if necessary. Great care is to be taken not to injure the rectum in giving such injections. A large syringe or a piece of rubber hose 4 or 5 feet long, with a funnel attached at one end, affords the best means by which to give them. The pipe of the syringe or the hose introduced into the rectum must be blunt, rounded, and smooth; it is to be thoroughly oiled and then carefully pushed through the anus in a slightly upward direction. Much force must be avoided, for the rectum may be lacerated and serious complications or even death result. Exercise will aid the action of the bowels in this and similar colicky troubles, but severe galloping or trotting is to be avoided. If the horse can have a loose box or paddock, it is the best, as he will then take what exercise he wants. If the patient is extremely violent, it is often wise to restrain him by leading him with a halter, since rupture of the stomach or displacement of the bowels may result and complicate the trouble.

INDIGESTION OR GASTROINTESTINAL CATARRH.

From the facts that they merge insensibly into each other and usually occur simultaneously, there is ample reason for considering these conditions together. This condition may be acute—that is, of sudden onset—or it may be chronic. The changes of structure produced by this disease occur in the mucous membrane lining of the stomach and intestines. This membrane becomes red from increased blood supply or from hemorrhage into it, is swollen, and is covered by a coating of slimy mucus. In some especially severe cases the membrane is destroyed in spots, causing the appearance of ulcers or of erosions.

The causes of indigestion are numerous, but nearly all are the result of errors in feeding.

Some horses are naturally endowed with weak digestive organs, and such are predisposed to this condition. Anything that irritates the stomach or intestines may cause this disease. Feeds that the animal is unaccustomed to, sudden changes of diet, imperfectly cured, unripe, or damaged feeds are all fruitful causes, and so are worms. In suckling foals this condition may come from some disease of the dam that renders her milk indigestible, or from overexertion or overheating of the mare. Another prolific cause is bad teeth, making mastication imperfect, and thus causing the horse to swallow his feed in a condition unfit for the action of the digestive juices. Working a horse too soon or too hard after feeding may cause either colic or indigestion. Any condition that reduces the vitality, such as disease, overwork, poor feed, or lack of care, may directly bring on indigestion by weakening the digestive organs.

Symptoms.—Indigestion is characterized by irregular appetite; refusing all feed at times, and at others eating ravenously; the appetite is not only irregular, but is often depraved; there is a disposition on the part of the horse to eat unusual substances, such as wood, soiled bedding, or even his own feces; the bowels are irregular to-day, loose and bad smelling, to-morrow bound; whole grain is often passed in the feces, and the hay passed in balls or impacted masses, undergoing but little change; the horse frequently passes considerable quantities of sour-smelling wind. The animal loses flesh, the skin presents a hard, dry appearance and seems very tight (hide-bound). If the stomach is very seriously involved, the horse may yawn by stretching the head forward and upward and by turning the upper lip outward. There may be more or less colicky pain. In the chronic cases there is mental depression; the horse is sluggish and dull. The abdomen gradually becomes small, giving a "tucked up" appearance, or, on the other hand, it becomes flaccid and pendulous.

Treatment.—One should commence with the feed—its quality, quantity, and time of feeding; examine the water supply, and see, besides, that it is given before feeding; then carefully observe the condition of the mouth and teeth; and, continuing the observations as best we may, endeavor to find the seat of the trouble. If the teeth are sharp or irregular they must be rasped down; if any are decayed they must be extracted; if indigestion is due to ravenous eating or bolting, the feed must then be given from a large manger where the grain can be spread and the horse thus compelled to eat slowly.

Any irritation, such as worms, undigested feed, etc., that is operating as a cause is to be removed by appropriate treatment, as advised elsewhere. If there is a tendency to distention of the stomach and bowels, with gas, during indigestion, the following may be used: Baking soda, powdered ginger, and powdered gentian, equal parts. These are to be thoroughly mixed and given in heaping tablespoonful doses, twice a day, before feeding. This powder is best given by dissolving the above-named quantity in a half pint of water and given as a drench.

As a digestive tonic the following is good: Glauber's salt, 2 pounds; common salt, 1 pound; baking soda, one-half pound. Of this a heaping tablespoonful may be given in each feed. If diarrhea exists, the treatment advised below may be used.

DIARRHEA.

Diarrhea is due to indigestion or intestinal catarrh or to irritation of the bowels from eating moldy or musty feed, drinking stagnant water, diseased condition of the teeth, eating irritating substances, to being kept on low, marshy pastures, and to exposure during cold nights, or in low, damp stables. Some horses are predisposed to scour and are called "washy" by horsemen; they are those with long bodies, long legs, and narrow, flat sides. Horses of this build are almost sure to scour if fed or watered immediately before being put to work. Fast or road work, of course, aggravates this trouble. Diarrhea may exist as a complication of other diseases, as pneumonia and influenza, for instance, and again during the diseases of the liver.

The symptoms are the frequent evacuations of liquid stools, with or without pronounced abdominal pain, loss of appetite, emaciation, etc.

Treatment is at times very simple, but requires the utmost care and judgment. If due to faulty feed or water it is sufficient to change these. If it results from some irritant in the intestines this is best gotten rid of by the administration of an oleaginous purge, for which nothing is better than castor oil, although raw linseed oil may be used if the case is not severe. The diarrhea often disappears with the cessation of the operation of the medicine. If, however, purging continues it may be checked by giving wheat flour in water, starch water, white-oak bark tea, chalk, opium, or half-dram doses of sulphuric acid in one-half pint of water twice or thrice daily. Good results follow the use of powdered opium 2 drams and subnitrate of bismuth 1 ounce, repeated three times a day. In all cases it should be remembered to look to the water and feed the horse is receiving. If either of these is at fault it is at once to be discontinued. We should feed sparingly of good, easily digested feeds. With that peculiar build of nervous horses that scour on the road but little can be done as a rule. They should be watered and fed as long as possible before going on a drive. If there is much flatulency accompanying diarrhea baking soda or other alkaline medicines may effect a cure, while if the discharges have a very disagreeable odor it may be corrected by 1 ounce of sulphite of soda or dram doses of creolin in water, repeated twice a day. Be slow to resort to either the vegetable or mineral astringents, since the majority of cases will yield to change of feed and water or the administration of oils. Afterwards feed upon wheat-flour gruel or other light feeds. The body should be warmly clothed.

SUPERPURGATION.—This is the designation of that diarrhea, or flux from the bowels, that, at times, is induced by and follows the action of a physic. It is accompanied with much irritation or even inflammation of the bowels and is always of a serious character. Although in rare instances it follows from a usual dose of physic and where every precaution has been taken, it is most likely to result under the following circumstances: Too large a dose of physic; giving physics to horses suffering from pneumonia, influenza, or other debilitating diseases; riding or driving a horse when purging; exposure or drafts of cold air; or giving large quantities of cold water while the physic is operating. There is always danger of superpurgation if a physic is given to a horse suffering from diseases of the respiratory organs. Small and often-repeated physics are also to be avoided, as they produce debility and great depression of the system and predispose to this disorder. When a physic is to be given one should rest the horse and give him sloppy feed until the medicine begins to operate; clothe the body with a warm blanket; keep out of drafts; give only warm water in small quantities. After a horse has purged from twelve to twenty-four hours it can mostly be stopped, or " set," as horsemen say, by feeding on dry oats and hay. Should the purging continue, however, it is best treated by giving demulcent drinks—linseed tea and oatmeal or wheat-flour gruel. After this the astringents spoken of for diarrhea may be given. Besides this the horse is to receive brandy in doses of from 2 to 4 ounces, with milk and eggs, four or five times a day.

Laminitis ("founder") is a frequent sequel of superpurgation and is to be guarded against by removing the shoes and standing the horse on moist sawdust or some similar bedding.

DYSENTERY.

This disease, sometimes called "bloody flux," is an intestinal disease attended with fever, occasional abdominal pains, and fluid discharges mingled with blood. Discharges in dysentery are coffee colored or bloody, liquid, and very offensive in odor, and passed with much straining. It is rare in the horse, but is sometimes quite prevalent among foals.

Causes.—Probably the most common cause is keeping young horses in particular for a long time on low, wet, marshy pastures, without other feed (a diarrhea of long standing sometimes terminates in dysentery) ; exposure during cold, wet weather; decomposed feeds; stagnant water that contains large quantities of decomposing vegetable matter; low, damp, and dark stables, particularly if crowded; the existence of some disease, as tuberculosis of the abdominal form. In suckling foals it may come from feeding the dam on irritant feeds or from disease of the udder. In other foals it may be produced by exposure to cold and damp, to irritant feed, or to worms.

Symptoms.—The initial symptom is a chill, which probably escapes notice in the majority of instances. The discharges are offensive and for the most part liquid, although it is common to find lumps of solid fecal matter floating in this liquid portion; shreds of mucous membrane and blood may be passed or the evacuations may be muco-purulent; there is much straining, and, rarely, symptoms of abdominal pain; the subject lies down a great deal; the pulse is quickened and the temperature elevated. Thirst is a prominent symptom. In the adult, death rarely follows under two to three weeks, but in foals the disease may end in death after a few days.

Treatment.—This is most unsatisfactory, and I am inclined to place more dependence upon the care and feed than any medication that may be adopted. First of all the horse must be placed in a dry, warm, yet well-ventilated stable; the skin is to receive attention by frequent rubbings of the surface of the body, with blankets, and bandages to the legs. The water must be pure and given in small quantities; the feed, that which is light and easily digested. Medicinally, give at first a light dose of castor oil, about one-half pint, to which has been added 2 ounces of laudanum. The vegetable or mineral astringents are also to be given. Starch injections containing laudanum often afford great relief. The strength must be kept up by milk punches, eggs, beef tea, oatmeal gruel, etc. In spite of the best care and treatment, however, dysentery is likely to prove fatal. In the case of nurslings, the dam should be placed in a healthy condition or, failing in this, milk should be had from another mare or from a cow.

GASTROENTERITIS.

This condition consists in an inflammation of the stomach and intestines. Instead of being confined to the mucous, or lining, membrane, as in gastrointestinal catarrh, the inflammatory process extends deeper and may even involve the entire thickness of the wall of the organ.

This disease may be caused by irritant feed, hot drinks, sudden chilling, moldy or decayed feeds, foul water, parasites, or by chemical poisons. It may also complicate some general diseases, especially infectious diseases, as anthrax, influenza, rabies, or petechial fever. Long-continued obstruction of the bowels or displacement resulting in death are preceded by enteritis.

Symptoms.—The symptoms differ somewhat with the cause and depend also, to some extent, upon the chief location of the inflammation. In general the animal stops eating or eats but little; it shows colicky pain; fever develops; the pulse and respiration become rapid; the mucous membrane becomes red; the mouth is hot and dry. Pressure upon the abdomen may cause pain. Intestinal sounds can not be heard at the flank. There is constipation in the earlier stages that is followed later by diarrhea. The extremities become cold. Sometimes the feces are coated with or contain shreds of fibrin, looking like scraps of dead membrane, and they have an evil, putrid odor. If the disease is caused by moldy or damaged feed there may be great muscular weakness, with partial paralysis of the throat, as shown by inability to swallow. If chemical poisons are the cause, this fact may be shown by the sudden onset of the disease, the history of the administration of a poison or the entire absence of known cause, the rapid development of threatening symptoms, the involvement of a series of animals in the absence of a contagious disease, and the special symptoms and alterations known to be produced by certain poisons. To make this chain of evidence complete, the poison may be discovered in the organs of the horse by chemical analysis. In nearly all cases of gastroenteritis there is nervous depression.

The poisons that are most irritant to the digestive tract are arsenic, corrosive sublimate, sugar of lead, sulphate of copper, sulphate or chlorid of zinc, lye, or other strong alkalies, mineral acids, and, among the vegetable poisons, tobacco, lobelia, and water hemlock.

Treatment.—The treatment will depend upon the cause, but if this can not be detected, certain general indications may be observed. In all cases feed should be given in small amounts and should be of the most soothing description, as oatmeal gruel, flaxseed tea, hay tea, fresh grass, or rice water. The skin should be well rubbed with alcohol and wisps of straw, to equalize the distribution of the blood; the legs, after being rubbed until warm, should be bandaged in raw cotton or with woolen bandages. The horse should be warmly blanketed. It is well to apply to the abdomen blankets wrung out of hot water and frequently changed; or mustard paste may be rubbed on the skin of the belly. Internally, opium is of service to allay pain, check secretion, and soothe the inflamed membrane. The dose is from 1 to 2 drams, given every three of four hours. If there is constipation, the opium should be mixed with 30 grains of calomel. Subnitrate of bismuth may be given with the opium or separately in 2-dram doses. Stimulants, such as aromatic spirits of ammonia or camphor, may be given in 2-ounce doses, mixed with warm water to make a drench.

If putrid feed has been consumed, creolin may be administered in doses of 2 drams, mixed with 1 pint of warm water or milk. If there is obstinate constipation and if a laxative must be employed, it should be sweet or castor oil, from 1 pint to 1 quart.

Antidotes for poisons.—For the various poisons the remedies are as follows:

Arsenic: Oxyhydrate of iron solution, 1 pint to 1 quart; or calcined magnesia, one-half ounce in 1 pint of water.

Corrosive sublimate (bichlorid of mercury): The whites of a dozen eggs, or 2 ounces of flowers of sulphur.

Sugar of lead: Glauber's salt, 1 pound in 1 quart of warm water; to be followed with iodid of potash, 3 drams at a dose, in water, three times daily for five days.

Sulphate of copper: Milk, the whites of eggs, or reduced iron.

Sulphate or chlorid of zinc: Milk, the whites of eggs, or calcined magnesia.

Lye or alkalies, as caustic potash or soda: Vinegar, dilute sulphuric acid, and linseed tea, with opium, 3 drams.

Mineral acids: Chalk, or calcined magnesia, or baking soda; later give linseed tea and opium.

HEMORRHOIDS, OR PILES.

These are rare, comparatively, in horses. They are diagnosed by the appearance of bright-red irregular tumors after defecation, which may remain visible at all times or be seen only when the horse is down or after passing his manure. They are mostly due to constipation, irritation, or injuries, or follow from the severe straining during dysentery. I have observed them to follow from severe labor pains in the mare.

54763°—23——6

Treatment.—Attention must be paid to the condition of the bowels; they should be soft, but purging is to be avoided. The tumors should be washed in warm water and thoroughly cleansed, after which scarify them and gently but firmly squeeze out the liquid that will be seen to follow the shallow incisions. After thus squeezing these tumors and before replacing through the anus, bathe the parts with some anodyn wash. For this purpose the glycerite of tannin and laudanum in equal parts is good. Mucilaginous injections into the rectum may be of service for a few days.

HERNIA, OR RUPTURE.

There are several kinds or hernias that require notice, not all of which, however, produce serious symptoms or results. Abdominal hernias, or ruptures, are divided into reducible, irreducible, and strangulated, according to condition; and into inguinal, scrotal, ventral, umbilical, and diaphragmatic, according to their situation. A hernia is reducible when the displaced organ can be returned to its natural location. It consists of a soft swelling, without heat, pain, or any uneasiness, generally larger on full feed, and decreases in size as the bowels become empty. An irreducible hernia is one that can not be returned into the abdomen, and yet does not cause any pain or uneasiness. Strangulated hernia is one in which the contents of the sac are greatly distended, or when from pressure upon the blood vessels of the imprisoned portion the venous circulation is checked or stopped, thereby causing congestion, swelling, inflammation, and, if not relieved, gangrene of the part and death of the animal. According to the time or mode of origin, hernias may be congenital or acquired.

CONGENITAL SCROTAL HERNIA.—Not a few foals are noticed from birth to have an enlarged scrotum, which gradually increases in size until about the sixth month, sometimes longer. Sometimes the scrotum of a six-months-old colt is as large as that of an adult stallion, and operative treatment is considered. This is unnecessary in the great majority of cases, as the enlargement often disappears by the time the colt has reached his second year. Any interference, medicinal or surgical, is worse than useless. If the intestine contained within the scrotum should at any time become strangulated, it must then be treated the same as in an adult horse.

SCROTAL HERNIA is caused by dilatation of the sheath of the testicle, combined with relaxation of the fibrous tissues surrounding the inguinal ring, thus allowing the intestine to descend to the scrotum. At first this is intermittent, appearing during work and returning when the horse is at rest. For a long time this form of hernia may not cause the least uneasiness or distress. In course of time, however, the imprisoned gut becomes filled with feces, its return into the abdominal cavity is prevented, and it becomes strangulated. While the gut is thus filling the horse often appears dull, is disinclined to move, appetite is impaired, and there is rumbling and obstruction of the bowels. Colicky symptoms now supervene. Strangulation and its consequent train of symptoms do not always follow in scrotal hernia, for often horses have this condition for years without suffering inconvenience.

INGUINAL HERNIA is but an incomplete scrotal hernia, and, like the latter, may exist and cause no signs of distress, or, again, it may become strangulated and cause death. Inguinal hernia is seen mostly in stallions, next in geldings, and very rarely in the mare. Bearing in mind that scrotal hernia is seen only in entire horses, we may proceed to detail the symptoms of strangulated, inguinal, and scrotal hernia at the same time. When, during the existence of colicky symptoms, we find a horse kicking with his hind feet while standing or lying upon his back, we should look to the inguinal region and scrotum. If scrotal hernia exists, the scrotum will be enlarged and lobulated; by pressure we may force a portion of the contents of the gut back into the abdomen, eliciting a gurgling sound. If we take a gentle but firm hold upon the enlarged scrotum and then have an assistant cause the horse to cough, the swelling will be felt to expand and as quickly contract again.

The history of these cases will materially aid us, as the owner can often assure us of preceding attacks of "colic," more or less severe, that have been instantaneously relieved in some (to him) unaccountable manner. The colicky symptoms of these hernias are not diagnostic, but, probably, more closely resemble those of enteritis than any other bowel diseases. In many cases the diagnosis can be made only by a veterinarian, when he has recourse to a rectal examination; the bowels can here be felt entering the internal abdominal ring.

Treatment of inguinal hernia.—If the reader is sure of the existence of hernia, he should secure the horse upon its back, and, with a hand in the rectum, endeavor to catch hold of the wandering bowel and pull it gently back into the cavity of the abdomen. Pressure should be made upon the scrotum during this time. If this fails, a veterinarian must be called to reduce the hernia by means of incising the inguinal ring, replacing the intestines, and to castrate, using clamps and performing the "covered operation."

VENTRAL HERNIA.—In this form of hernia the protrusion is through some accidental opening or rupture of the abdominal wall. It may occur at any part of the belly except at the umbilicus, and is caused by kicks, blows, hooks, severe jumping or pulling, etc. Ventral hernia is most common in pregnant mares, and is here due to the weight of the fetus or to some degenerative changes taking place in the abdominal coats. It is recognized by the appearance of a swelling, at the base of which can be felt the opening or rent in the abdominal tunics, and from the fact that the swelling containing the intestines can be made to disappear when the animal is placed in a favorable position.

Treatment of ventral hernia.—In many instances there is no occasion for treatment, and again, where the hernial sac is extensive, treatment is of no avail. If the hernia is small, a cure may be attempted by the methods to be described in treating of umbilical hernia. If one is fortunate enough to be present when the hernia occurs, and particularly if it is not too large, he may, by the proper application of a pad and broad bandage, effect a perfect cure.

UMBILICAL HERNIA is the passing of any portion of the bowel or omentum ("caul") through the navel, forming a "tumor" at this point. This is often congenital in our animals, and is due to the imperfect closure of the umbilicus and to the position of the body. Many cases of umbilical hernia, like inguinal and scrotal of the congenital kind, disappear entirely by the time the animal reaches its second or third year. Advancing age favors cure in these cases from the fact that the omentum (swinging support of the bowels) is proportionally shorter in adults than in foals, thus lifting the intestines out of the hernial sac and allowing the opening in the walls to close. Probably one of the most frequent causes of umbilical hernia in foals is the practice of keeping them too long from their dams, causing them to fret and worry, and to neigh, or cry, by the hour. The contraction of the abdominal muscles and pressure of the intestines during neighing seem to open the umbilicus and induce hernia. Accidents may cause umbilical hernia in adults in the same manner as ventral hernia is produced, though this is very rare.

Treatment of umbilical hernia.—In the treatment of umbilical hernia it should be remembered that congenital hernias are often removed with age, but probably congenital *umbilical hernias* less frequently than others. Among the many plans of treatment are to be mentioned the application of a pad over the tumor, the pad being held in place by a broad, tight bandage placed around the animal's body. The chief objection to this is the difficulty in keeping the pad in its place. Blisters are often applied over the swelling, and, as the skin hardens and contracts by the formation of scabs, an artificial bandage or pressure is produced that at times is successful. Another treatment that has gained considerable repute of late years consists in first clipping off the hair over the swelling. Nitric acid is then applied with a small brush, using only enough to moisten the skin.

This sets up a deep-seated, adhesive inflammation, which, in very many cases, closes the opening in the navel. Still another plan is to inject a solution of common salt by means of the hypodermic syringe at three or four points about the base of the swelling. This acts in the same manner as the preceding, but may cause serious injury if the syringe or solution is not sterile.

Others, again, after keeping the animal fasting for a few hours, cast and secure it upon its back; the bowel is then carefully returned into the abdomen. The skin over the opening is pinched up and one or two skewers are run through the skin from side to side as close as possible to the umbilical opening. These skewers are kept in place by passing a cord around the skin between them and the abdomen and securely tying it. Great care must be taken not to draw these cords too tight, as this would cause a speedy slough of the skin, the intestines would extrude, and death result. If properly applied, an adhesion is established between the skin and the umbilicus, which effectually closes the orifice. Special clamps are provided for taking up the fold of the skin covering the hernial sac and holding it until the adhesion is formed.

DIAPHRAGMATIC HERNIA.—This consists of the passage of any of the abdominal viscera through a rent in the diaphragm (midriff) into the cavity of the thorax. It is a rather rare accident, and one often impossible to diagnose during life. Colicky symptoms, accompanied with great difficulty in breathing, and the peculiar position so often assumed (that of sitting upon the haunches), are somewhat characteristic of this trouble, though these symptoms, as we have already seen, may be present during diseases of the stomach or anterior portion of the bowels. Even could we diagnose with certainty this form of hernia, there is little or nothing that can be done. Leading the horse up a very steep gangway or causing him to rear up may possibly cause the hernial portion to return to its natural position. This is not enough, however; it must be kept there.

PERITONITIS.

Peritonitis is an inflammation of the serous membrane lining the cavity of and covering the viscera contained within the abdomen. It is very rare to see a case of primary peritonitis. It is, however, somewhat common as a secondary disease from extension of the inflammatory action involving organs covered by the peritoneum. Peritonitis is often caused by injuries, as punctured wounds of the abdomen, severe blows or kicks, or, as is still more common, following the operation of castration. It follows strangulated hernia, invagination, or rupture of the stomach, intestines, liver, or womb.

Symptoms.—Peritonitis is mostly preceded by a chill; the horse is not disposed to move, and, if compelled to do so, moves with a stiff or sore gait; he paws with the front feet and may strike at his belly with the hind ones; lies down very carefully; as the pain is increased while down, he maintains the standing position during most of the time; he walks uneasily about the stall. Constipation is usually present. Pressure on the belly causes acute pain, and the horse will bite, strike, or kick if so disturbed; the abdomen is tucked up; the extremities are fine and cold. The temperature is higher than normal, reaching from 102° to 104° F. The pulse in peritonitis is rather characteristic; it is quickened, beating from 70 to 90 beats a minute, and is hard and wiry. This peculiarity of the pulse occurs in inflammation of the serous membrane, and if accompanied with colicky symptoms, and, in particular, if following any injuries, accidental or surgical, of the peritoneum, there is reason to think that peritonitis is present. Peritonitis in the horse is mostly fatal when it is at all extensive. If death does not occur in a short time, the inflammation assumes a chronic form, in which there is an extensive effusion of water in the cavity of the belly, constituting what is known as ascites, and which, as a rule, results in death.

Treatment.—The treatment of peritonitis is somewhat like that of enteritis. Opium in powder, 1 to 2 drams, with calomel, one-half dram, is to be given every two, three, or four hours, and constitutes the main dependence in this disease. Extensive counterirritants over the belly, consisting of mustard plasters, applications of mercurial ointment, turpentine stupes, or even mild blisters, are recommended. Purgatives must never be given during this complaint. Should we desire to move the bowels, it can be done by gentle enemas, though it is seldom necessary to resort even to this.

ASCITES, OR DROPSY OF THE ABDOMEN.

This is seen as a result of subacute or chronic peritonitis, but may be due to diseases of the liver, kidneys, heart, or lungs. There will be found, on opening the cavity of the belly, a large collection of yellowish or reddish liquid; from a few quarts to several gallons may be present. It may be clear in color, though generally it is yellowish or of a red tint, and contains numerous loose flakes of coagulable lymph.

Symptoms.—There is slight tenderness on pressure; awkward gait of the hind legs; the horse is dull, and may have occasional very slight colicky pains, shown by looking back and striking at the belly with the hind feet. Oftener, however, these colicky symptoms are absent. Diarrhea often precedes death, but during the progress of the disease the bowels are alternately constipated and loose. On percussing the abdominal walls we find that dullness exists to the same height on both sides of the belly; by suddenly pushing or striking the abdomen we can hear the rushing or flooding of water. If the case is an advanced one, the horse is potbellied in the extreme, and dropsical swellings are seen under the belly and upon the legs.

Treatment is, as a rule, unsatisfactory. Saline cathartics, as Epsom or Glauber's salt, and diuretics, ounce doses of saltpeter, may be given. If a veterinarian is at hand he will withdraw the accumulation of water by tapping and then endeavor to prevent its recurrence (though this is almost sure to follow) by giving three times a day saltpeter 1 ounce and iodid of potash 1 dram, and by the application of mustard or blisters over the abdominal walls. Tonics, mineral and vegetable, are also indicated. Probably the best tonic is one consisting of powdered sulphate of iron, gentian, and ginger in equal parts; a heaping tablespoonful of the mixture is given as a drench or mixed with the feed, twice a day. Good nutritious feeds and gentle exercise complete the treatment.

DISEASES OF THE LIVER.

In the United States the liver of the horse is but rarely the seat of disease, and when we consider how frequently the liver of man is affected this can not but appear strange. The absence of the gall bladder may account to a certain extent for his freedom from liver diseases, as overdistention of this and the presence in it of calculi (stones) in man is a frequent source of trouble. In domestic animals, as in man, hot climates tend to produce diseases of the liver, just as in cold climates lung diseases prevail. Not only are diseases of the liver rare in horses in temperate climates, but they are also very obscure, and in many cases pass totally unobserved until after death. There are some symptoms, however, which, when present, should make us examine the liver as carefully as possible. These are jaundice (yellowness of the mucous membranes of the mouth, nose, and eyes) and the condition of the dung, it being light in color and pasty in appearance.

HEPATITIS, OR INFLAMMATION OF THE LIVER.

This disease may be general or local, and may assume an acute or chronic form.

Symptoms.—The symptoms of acute hepatitis are: Dullness; the horse is suffering from some internal pain, but not of a severe type; constipated and clay-colored dung balls; scanty and high-colored urine; and general febrile symptoms. If lying down, he is mostly found on the left side; looks occasionally toward the right side, which, upon close inspection, may be found to be slightly enlarged over the posterior ribs, where pain upon pressure is also evinced. Obscure lameness in front, of the right leg mostly, may be a symptom of hepatitis. The horse, toward the last, reels or staggers in his gait and falls backward in a fainting fit, during one of which he finally succumbs. Death is sometimes due to rupture of the enveloping coat of the liver or of some of its blood vessels.

Causes.—Among the causes that lead to this disease we must mention first the stimulating effect of overfeeding, particularly during hot weather. Horses that are well fed and receive but little exercise are the best subjects for diseases of this organ. We must add to these causes the more mechanical ones, as injuries on the right side over the liver, worms in the liver, gallstones in the biliary ducts, foreign bodies—as needles or nails that have been swallowed and in their wanderings have entered the liver—and, lastly, in some instances, the extension of inflammation from neighboring parts, thus involving this organ. Acute hepatitis may terminate in chronic inflammation, abscesses, rupture of the liver, or may disappear, leaving behind no trace of disease whatever.

Treatment.—This should consist, at first, of the administration of 1 ounce of Barbados aloes or other physic. General blood-letting, if had recourse to early, must prove of much benefit in acute inflammation of the liver. The vein in the neck (jugular) must be opened, and from 4 to 6 quarts of blood may be drawn. Saline medicines, as Glauber's salt or the artificial Carlsbad salt, are indicated. These may be given with the feed in tablespoonful doses. The horse is to be fed sparingly on soft feed, bran mashes chiefly. If treatment proves successful and recovery takes place, see to it that the horse afterwards gets regular exercise and that his feed is not of a too highly nutritious character and not excessive.

JAUNDICE, ICTERUS, OR THE YELLOWS.

This is a condition caused by the retention and absorption of bile into the blood. It was formerly considered to be a disease of itself, but is now regarded as a symptom of disorder of the liver. "The yellows" is observed by looking at the eyes, nose, and mouth, when it will be seen that these parts are yellowish instead of the pale-pink color of health. In white or light-colored horses the skin even may show this yellow tint. The urine is saffron colored, the dung is of a dirty-gray color, and constipation is usually present. Jaundice may be present as a symptom of almost any inflammatory disease. We know that when an animal has fever the secretions are checked, the bile may be retained and absorbed throughout the system, and yellowness of the mucous membranes follows. Jaundice may also exist during the presence of simple constipation, hepatitis, biliary calculi, abscesses, hardening of the liver, etc.

Treatment.—When jaundice exists we must endeavor to rid the system of the excess of bile, and this is best accomplished by giving purgatives that act upon the liver. Calomel, 2 drams, with aloes, 7 drams, should be given. Glauber's salt in handful doses once or twice a day for a week is also effective. May apple, rhubarb, castor oil, and other cathartics that act upon the first or small bowels may be selected. We must be careful to see that the bowels are kept open by avoiding hard, dry, bulky feeds.

RUPTURE OF THE LIVER.

This is known to occur at times in the horse, most frequently in old, fat horses and those that get but little exercise. Horses that have suffered from chronic liver disease for years eventually present symptoms of colic and die quite suddenly. Upon post-mortem examination we discover that the liver has ruptured. The cicatrices, or scars, that are often found upon the liver indicate that this organ may suffer *small* rupture and yet the horse may recover from it. This can not be the result, however, if the rent or tear is extensive, since in such cases death must quickly follow from hemorrhage, or, later, from peritonitis. Enlarged liver is particularly liable to rupture.

The immediate causes of rupture appear to be excessive muscular exertion, as leaping a fence, a fall, a blow from a collision, a kick from a horse, or sudden distention of the abdomen with gas.

The symptoms of rupture of the liver will depend upon the extent of the laceration. If slight, there will be simply the symptoms of abdominal pain, looking back to the sides, lying down, etc.; if extensive, the horse is dull and dejected, has no appetite, breathing becomes short and catching, he sighs or sobs, visible mucous membranes are pale, extremities cold, pulse fast, small, and weak or running down. Countenance now shows much distress, he sweats profusely, totters in his gait, props his legs wide apart, reels, staggers, and falls. He may get up again, but soon falls dead. The rapid running-down pulse, paleness of the eyes, nose, and mouth, sighing, stertorous breathing, tottering gait, etc., are symptoms by which we know that the animal is dying from internal hemorrhage.

Treatment.—But little can be done in the way of treatment. Opium in powder, in doses of 2 drams every two or three hours, may be given, with the idea of preventing as much as possible all movements of internal organs. If there is reason to suspect internal bleeding, we should give large and frequent doses of white-oak bark tea, dram doses of tannic or gallic acid, or the same quantity of sugar of lead, every half hour or hour. Fluid extract of ergot or tincture of the chlorid of iron, in ounce doses, may be selected. Cold water dashed upon the right side or injected into the rectum is highly spoken of as a means of checking the hemorrhage.

BILIARY CALCULI, OR GALLSTONES.

These are rarely found in the horse, but may occupy the hepatic ducts, giving rise to jaundice and to colicky pains. There are no absolutely diagnostic symptoms, but should one find a horse that suffers from repeated attacks of colic, accompanied with symptoms of violent pain, and that during or following these attacks the animal is jaundiced, it is possible that gallstones are present. There is little or nothing to be done except to give medicines to overcome pain, trusting that these concretions may pass on to the bowels, where, from their small size, they will not occasion any inconvenience.

DISEASES OF THE PANCREAS AND SPLEEN.

Diseases of the pancreas and spleen are so rare, or their symptoms so little understood, that it is impossible to write anything concerning either of these organs and their simple diseases that will convey to the reader information of practical value.

GASTROINTESTINAL PARASITES.

[By Maurice C. Hall, Ph. D., D. V. M.]

Horses are subject to infestation by a number of species of worms, these worms being especially numerous at certain points in the alimentary canal.

The tapeworms of the horse are relatively unimportant and not very common. There are three species, the smallest about two inches long and the largest about eight inches long. These two occur in the small intestine; a form intermediate in size may also be found in the cecum and colon. These are flat, segmented worms with the head at the smaller end.

Flukes occur in horses elsewhere, but have apparently never been reported in the United States.

Roundworms, or nematodes, constitute the most important group of parasitic worms in the horse. The more important of these are as follows:

ROUNDWORM (*Ascaris equorum*).—This is the common large, yellowish roundworm (Pl. V, fig. 5), about the size of a lead pencil or larger, which may be found in horses almost anywhere in the

United States. It occurs in the intestine and probably occasions little damage as a rule, except when present in large numbers, in which case it will probably be found in the droppings. The symptoms occasioned by it are rather obscure and are such as might arise from a number of other causes, namely, colicky pains, depraved appetite, diarrhea or constipation, and general unthriftiness. In a general way, the presence of parasites may be suspected when an animal shows no fever but is unthrifty, debilitated, and shows disordered bowel movements in cases where there is no evident explanation in the way of feed, care, and surroundings.

Treatment for the removal of this worm consists in the use of anthelmintics such as tartar emetic, turpentine, and carbon bisulphid, but as these remedies are essentially poisons intended to kill the worm, and as their use by persons unused to determining conditions unfavorable for their use is dangerous and likely to result in the death of the animal or in permanent injury to the kidneys or other organs, it is advisable to call in a veterinarian in such cases.

PINWORM (*Oxyuris equi*).—This is a rather large worm (Pl. V, fig. 1), somewhat smaller than the foregoing and readily distinguishable from it by the presence of a long, slender tail. It also occurs generally throughout the United States, and except when present in large numbers probably does very little damage. It inhabits the large intestine and hence is difficult to reach with medicines administered by the mouth. The use of a half ounce of gentian on the feed night and morning for a week has been recommended, but the use of rectal enemas will give more prompt and perhaps more certain results. These enemas may be made up with one or two tablespoonfuls of salt to the pint, or infusions of quassia chips, a half pound to the gallon of water, and injected into the rectum once or twice a day.

STOMACH WORMS OF THE HORSE (*Habronema* spp.).—These worms (Pl. V, fig. 4) occur in nodules in the mucous lining of the horse's stomach and are credited with doing more or less damage. Their presence is not likely to be diagnosed in the present state of our knowledge, but in case their presence is determined or suspected in connection with the summer sores noted later, tartar emetic is recommended. At least one of these worms has an intermediate stage in the ordinary housefly, the fly becoming infested while it is a larva developing in horse manure. Obviously, therefore, any measures looking toward the eradication of the fly or the proper disposal of manure will aid in the control and eradication of this worm. The United States Bureau of Entomology has shown that fly maggots travel downward through a manure pile as it comes time for the maggot to enter the ground and pupate, and an excellent maggot trap, consisting of an exposed manure platform raised on posts which are set in a concrete basin extending under the platform and filled with three or four inches of water, has been devised. As maggots work down they come to the platform and escape through the spaces between the boards, left open for the purpose, to the water in the concrete basin, where they are drowned. In this way the exposed manure pile serves to attract flies with a deceptive proffer of a breeding place.

Apparently it is the young forms of these stomach worms which develop at times on the skin, causing a cutaneous habronemiasis known as summer sores. This is discussed under diseases of the skin.

STRONGYLES (*Strongylus* spp. and *Cylicostomum* spp.).—These worms (Pl. V, figs. 2 and 3) live in the large intestines of the horse as adult worms and are often present in enormous numbers. Many of them are very small, and the largest are less than two inches long. The adult worms do considerable damage, but the immature or larval worms do even more.

The larva of *Strongylus vulgaris* enters the blood vessels of the intestinal wall and finally attaches in the great mesenteric artery, where it causes aneurisms; here it transforms to an adult without sexual organs, which passes to the walls of the cecum and encysts, giving rise to small cysts or abscesses; these cysts finally discharge to the interior of the cecum, setting the worms, now mature, at liberty in the lumen of the intestines.

The larvæ of *Strongylus equinus* are found principally in the liver, lungs, and pancreas.

The larvæ of *Strongylus edentatus* may be met with almost anywhere, especially under the serous membranes, the pleura and peritoneum.

The embryos and larvæ of species of *Cylicostomum* are found in the mucosa of the large intestine.

Aneurisms impede the circulation of the blood, and may give rise to intermittent lameness. The aneurism may rupture, since it constitutes a weak place in the wall of the blood vessel, and the horse die of the resulting hemorrhage. Particles of blood clots in the aneurisms may break off and plug a blood vessel at the point where they lodge, thereby causing the death of the part from which the blood is shut off and occasioning a type of colic which often terminates fatally. The larvæ of *Cylicostomum* form cysts in the walls of the large intestine, and when these open they give rise to small sores; when they are numerous they cause a thickening and hardening which impair the proper functioning of the intestine. Abscesses sometimes perforate, causing death. The adult worm attacks the intestinal wall, causing bleeding which results in anemia. The

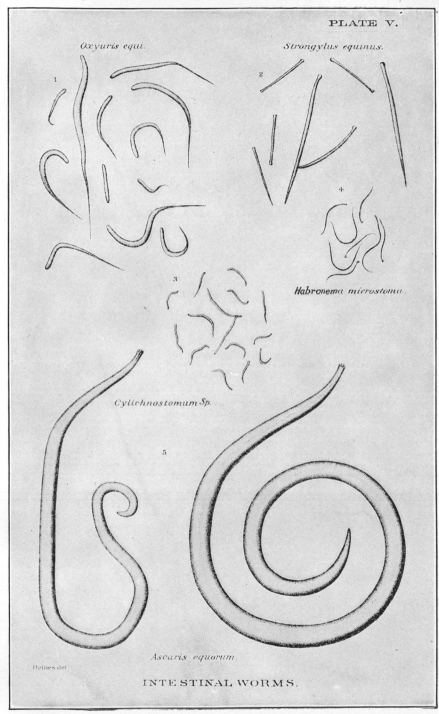

INTESTINAL WORMS.

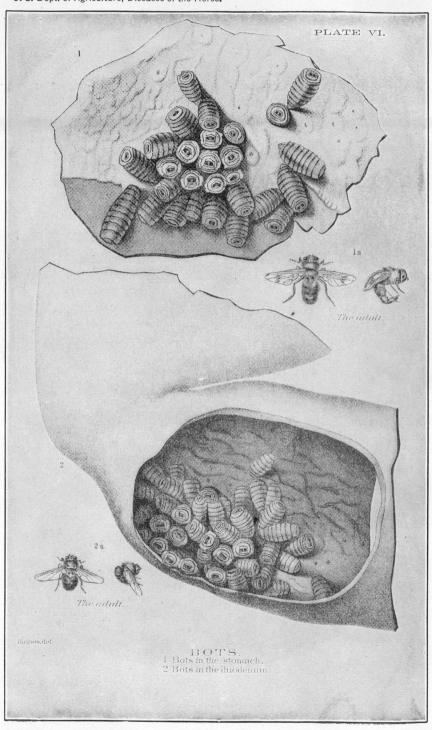

PLATE VI.

The adult.

The adult.

Hanes del.

BOTS.
1 Bots in the stomach.
2 Bots in the duodenum.

numerous small sores thus caused allow bacteria to get into the circulation, sometimes resulting in localized abscesses or in septic arthritis or joint disease.

The disease due to these worms is quite common. The worms enter the body as immature forms in the spring, when the animal is turned out on pasture. The first symptoms show in November or December, the disease being in a latent stage during the development of the worms. The first symptoms are diarrhea, loss of appetite, and emaciation. The animal becomes anemic. Secondary symptoms are edema and such complications as joint infection, colic due to embolism, and accidents from falls, hemorrhage from ruptured aneurisms, or perforation at the site of abscess. The animal may die, recover, or become a chronic sufferer, the internal injuries failing to make a satisfactory recovery even with the removal of the worms in chronic cases.

Treatment calls for the expulsion of the adult worms from the intestine, the development of the body resistance to repair the damage wrought by the developing worms, and the combating of complications. For the expulsion of the worms the use of carbon bisulphid in gelatin capsules, 2 to 5 grams, according to the size of the patient, for five days, followed by magnesium sulphate the sixth day, has been recommended. Owing to the difficulty and danger in the administration of carbon bisulphid in capsule, it is advisable to call in a veterinarian. Tonic treatment consists in the subcutaneous administration of artificial serum and caffein. The various complications of bacterial infection, colic, heart depression, etc., call for the attention of a veterinarian. Preventive measures consist in avoiding reinfection with worms so far as possible by using dry upland pasture in preference to low, wet land, and by rotating pastures or rotation of the stock on a given pasture. Horses may be alternated with cattle, sheep, or hogs to advantage, so far as parasites are concerned. Another feature, always of importance, is the provision of a pure, potable drinking water.

Bots (*Gastrophilus* spp.).—Bots (Pl. VI) are quite common in the stomach and upper part of the small intestine of the horse anywhere in the United States, one kind being occasionally found in the rectum. They attach to that portion of the mucous lining of the stomach nearest the esophagus or sometimes around the pyloric opening to the intestine or even in the upper intestine, and undoubtedly interfere with the proper functioning of the stomach and the health of the animal to a certain extent. The symptoms are rather vague as a rule, but the general result is a condition of unthriftiness.

A treatment which has been found effective consists in feeding lightly on the day preceding treatment, withholding food in the evening and giving an ounce of Barbados aloes or a pint of linseed oil. The next day give 3 drams of carbon bisulphid in a gelatin capsule at 6 o'clock, repeat the dose at 7 o'clock, and again at 8 o'clock, making a total of 9 drams altogether for an adult horse; half that amount will be sufficient for a yearling colt. As previously noted, there is some little difficulty and danger of accident in the administration of treatments of this character and it is advisable to call in a veterinarian.

Unless destroyed by treatment, the bots in the stomach of the horse pass out in the manure in the spring and burrow down into the soil an inch or two. Here they undergo a certain amount of development and finally emerge as adult flies. These bot flies mate and during the summer the eggs are deposited by the female on the forelegs and shoulders or around the chin, mouth and nostrils of the horse, the location and appearance of the eggs varying somewhat with different species of bot flies. These eggs or the young maggots escaping from them are ingested by the horse in licking the portions irritated by the movement of the escaping maggots, and when swallowed develop to form bots in the stomach. Careful currying, especially around the forequarters, is an aid in keeping down bot infestation, but this is not commonly feasible with horses on pasture, the ones most liable to become infested.

DISEASES OF THE RESPIRATORY ORGANS.

By W. H. Harbaugh, V. S.

[Revised by Leonard Pearson, B. S., V. M. D.]

The organs pertaining to the respiratory function may be enumerated in natural order as follows: The nasal openings, or nostrils; the nasal chambers, through which the air passes in the head; the sinuses in the head, communicating with the nasal chambers; the pharnyx, common to the functions of breathing and swallowing; the larynx, at the top of the windpipe; the trachea, or windpipe; the bronchi (into which the windpipe divides), two tubes leading from the windpipe to the right and left lungs, respectively; the bronchial tubes, which penetrate and convey air to all parts of the lungs; the lungs.

The pleura is a thin membrane that envelops the lung and lines the walls of the thoracic cavity. The diaphragm is a muscular structure, completely separating the contents of the thoracic cavity from those of the abdominal cavity. It is essentially a muscle of inspiration, and the principal one. Other muscles aid in the mechanism of respiration, but the diseases or injuries of them have nothing to do with the diseases under consideration.

Just within the nasal openings the skin becomes gradually but perceptibly finer, until it is succeeded by the mucous membrane. Near the junction of the skin and membrane is a small hole, presenting the appearance of having been made with a punch; this is the opening of the lachrymal duct, a canal that conveys the tears from the eyes. Within and above the nasal openings are the cavities, or fissures, called the false nostrils. The nasal chambers are completely separated, the right from the left, by a cartilaginous partition, the nasal septum. Each nasal chamber is divided into three continuous compartments by two thin, scroll-like turbinated bones.

The mucous membrane lining the nasal chambers, and, in fact, the entire respiratory tract, is much more delicate and more frequently diseased than the mucous membrane of any other part of the body. The sinuses of the head are compartments which communicate with the nasal chambers and are lined with a continuation of the same membrane that lines the nasal chambers; their presence increases the volume and modifies the form of the head without increasing its weight.

The horse, in a normal condition, breathes exclusively through the nostrils. The organs of respiration are quite liable to become dis-

95

eased, and, as many of the causes which lead to these attacks can be avoided, it is both important and profitable to know and study the causes.

CAUSES OF DISEASES OF RESPIRATORY ORGANS.

The causes of many of the diseases of these organs may be given under a common head, because even a simple cold, if neglected or badly treated, may run into the most complicated lung disease and terminate fatally. In the spring and fall, when the animals are changing their coats, there is a marked predisposition to contract disease, and consequently at those periods care should be taken to prevent other exciting causes.

Badly ventilated stables are a frequent source of disease. It is a mistake to think that country stables necessarily have purer air than city stables. Stables on some farms are so faultily constructed that it is almost impossible for the foul air to gain an exit. All stables should have a sufficient supply of pure air, and be so arranged that strong drafts can not blow directly on the animals. In ventilating a stable, it is best to arrange to remove air from near the floor and admit it through numerous small openings near the ceiling. The reason for this is that the coldest and most impure air in the stable is near the floor, while that which is warmest and purest, and therefore can least be spared, is near the top of the room. In summer, top exits and cross currents should be provided to remove excessive heat. Hot stables are almost always poorly ventilated, and the hot stable is a cause of disease on account of the extreme change of temperature that a horse is liable to when taken out, and extreme changes of temperature are to be avoided as certain causes of disease.

A cold, close stable is invariably damp, and is to be avoided as much as the hot, close, and foul one. Horses changed from a cold to a warm stable are more liable to contract cold than when changed from a warm to a cold one. Pure air is more essential than warmth, and this fact should be especially remembered when the stable is made close and foul to gain the warmth. It is more economical to keep the horse warm with blankets than to prevent the ingress of pure air in order to make the stable warm.

Stables should be well drained and kept clean. Some farmers allow large quantities of manure to accumulate in the stable. This is a pernicious practice, as the decomposing organic matter evolves gases that are predisposing or exciting causes of disease. When a horse is overheated, it is not safe to allow him to dry by evaporation; rubbing him dry and gradually cooling him out is the wisest treatment. When a horse is hot—covered with sweat—it is dangerous to allow him to stand in a draft; it is the best plan to walk him until his temperature moderates. In such cases a light blanket thrown over the animal may prevent a cold. Overwork or overexertion often causes the greater number of fatal cases of congestion of the lungs. Avoid prolonged or fast work when the horse is out of condition or unaccustomed to it. Animals that have been working in cold rains should be dried and cooled out and not left to dry by evaporation. When the temperature of the weather is at the extreme, either of heat or cold, diseases of the organs of respiration are most frequent.

It is not to be supposed that farmers can give their horses the particular attention given to valuable racing and pleasure horses, but they can most assuredly give them common-sense care, and this may often save the life of a valuable animal. If the owner properly considers his interests, he will study the welfare of his horses so that he may be able to instruct the servant in details of stable management.

WOUNDS ABOUT THE NOSTRILS.

Wounds in this neighborhood are common, and are generally caused by snagging on a nail or splinter or by the bite of another horse; or by getting " run into," or by running against something. Occasionally the nostril is so badly torn and lacerated that it is impossible to effect a cure without leaving the animal blemished for life, but in the majority of instances the blemish, or scar, is the result of want of conservative treatment. As soon as possible after the accident the parts should be brought together and held there by stitches. If too much time is allowed to elapse, the swelling of the parts will considerably interfere. Never cut away any skin that may be loose and hanging, or else a scar will certainly remain. Bring the parts in direct apposition and place the stitches from a quarter to a half-inch apart, as circumstances may demand. It is not necessary to have special surgeons' silk and needles for this operation; good linen thread or ordinary silk thread will answer. The wound afterwards only requires to be kept clean. For this purpose it should be cleansed and discharges washed away daily with a solution made of carbolic acid 1 part in 40 parts of water. If on account of the irritability the horse is inclined to rub the wound against some object, his head should be tied by means of two halter ropes attached to the opposite sides of the stall to prevent him from opening the wound. Except when at work or eating, the head should be so tied about 10 days.

TUMORS WITHIN THE NOSTRILS.

A small, globular tumor is sometimes found within the false nostril, under that part of the skin that is seen to puff or rise and fall when a horse is exerted and breathing hard. These tumors contain matter of a cheesy consistency.

54763°—23——7

Treatment.—If the tumor is well opened and the matter squeezed out, nature will perform a cure. If the opening is made from the outside through the skin, it should be at the most dependent part, but much the best way to open the tumor is from the inside. Quiet the animal, gently insert your finger up in the direction of the tumor, and you will soon discover that it is much larger inside than it appears to be on the outside. If necessary put a twitch on the ear of the horse to quiet him; run the index finger of your left hand against the tumor; now, with the right hand, carefully insert the knife by running the back of the blade along the index finger of the left hand until the tumor is reached; with the left index finger guide the point of the blade quickly and surely into the tumor; make the opening large. A little blood may flow for a while, but it is of no consequence. Squeeze out the matter and keep the part clean.

COLD IN THE HEAD, OR NASAL CATARRH.

Catarrh is an inflammation of a mucous membrane. It is accompanied with excessive secretion. In nasal catarrh the inflammation may extend from the membrane lining the nose to the throat, the inside of the sinuses, and to the eyes. The causes are the general causes of respiratory disease enumerated above. It is especially common in young horses and in horses not acclimated.

Symptoms.—The membrane at the beginning of the attack is dry, congested, and irritable; it is of a deeper hue than natural, pinkish red or red. Soon a watery discharge from the nostrils makes its appearance; the eyes may also be more or less affected and tears flow over the cheeks. The animal has some fever, which may be easily detected by means of a clinical thermometer inserted in the rectum or, roughly, by placing the finger in the mouth, as the feeling of heat conveyed to the finger will be greater than natural.

To become somewhat expert in ascertaining the changes of temperature in the horse it is only necessary to place the finger often in the mouths of horses known to be healthy. After you have become accustomed to the warmth of the mouth of the healthy animal you will have no difficulty in detecting a marked increase of the temperature. The animal may be dull; he sneezes or snorts, but does not cough unless the throat is affected; he expels the air forcibly through his nostrils, very often in a manner that may be aptly called "blowing his nose." A few days after the attack begins the discharge from the nostrils changes from a watery to that of a thick, mucilaginous state, of a yellowish-white color, and may be more or less profuse. Often the appetite is lost and the animal becomes debilitated.

Treatment.—This disease is not serious, but inasmuch as neglect or bad treatment may cause it to lead to something worse or become chronic it should receive proper attention. The animal should not be worked for a time. A few days of rest, with pure air and good feed, will be of greater benefit than most medication. The value of pure air can not be overestimated, but drafts must be avoided. The benefit derived from the inhalation of steam is considerable. This is effected by holding the horse's head over a bucketful of boiling water, so that the animal will be compelled to inhale steam with every inhalation of air. Stirring the hot water with a wisp of hay causes the steam to arise in greater abundance. One may cause the horse to put his nose in a bag containing cut hay upon which hot water has been poured, the bottom of the bag being stood in a bucket, but the bag must be of loose texture, as gunny sack, or, if of canvas, holes must be cut in the side to admit fresh air.

The horse may be made to inhale steam four or five times a day, about 15 or 20 minutes each time.

Particular attention should be paid to the diet. Give bran mashes, scalded oats, linseed gruel, and grass, if in season. If the horse evinces no desire for this soft diet, it is better to allow any kind of feed he will eat, such as hay, oats, corn, etc., than to keep him on short rations.

If the animal is constipated, relieve this symptom by injections (enemas) of warm water into the rectum three or four times a day, but do not administer purgative medicines, except of a mild character.

For simple cases the foregoing is all that is required, but if the appetite is lost and the animal appears debilitated and dull, give 3 ounces of the solution of acetate of ammonia and 2 drams of powdered chlorate of potassium diluted with a pint of water three times a day as a drench. Be careful when giving the drench; do not pound the horse on the gullet to make him swallow; be patient, and take time, and do it right.

If the weather is cold, blanket the animal and keep him in a comfortable stall. If the throat is sore, treat as advised for that ailment, to be described hereafter.

If, after 10 days or 2 weeks, the discharge from the nostrils continues, give one-half dram of reduced iron three times a day. This may be mixed with damp feed. Common cold should be thoroughly understood and intelligently treated in order to prevent more dangerous diseases.

CHRONIC CATARRH (OR NASAL GLEET, OR COLLECTION IN THE SINUSES).

This is a subacute or chronic inflammation of some part of the membrane affected in common cold, the disease just described. It is manifested by a persistent discharge of a thick white or yellowish-white matter from one or both nostrils. The commonest cause is a neglected or badly treated cold, and it usually follows those cases where the horse has suffered exposure, been overworked, or has not received proper feed, and, as a consequence, has become debilitated. It may occur as a sequel to influenza.

Other but less frequent causes for this affection are: Fractures of the bones that involve the membrane of the sinuses, and even blows on the head over the sinuses. Diseased teeth often involve a sinus and cause a fetid discharge from the nostril. Violent coughing is said to have forced particles of feed into the sinus, which acted as a cause of the disease. Tumors growing in the sinuses are known to have caused it. It is also attributed to disease of the turbinated bones. Absorption of the bones forming the walls of the sinuses has been caused by the pressure of pus collecting in them and by tumors filling up the cavity.

Symptoms.—Great caution must be exercised when examining these cases, for the horse may have glanders, while, on the other hand, horses have been condemned as glandered when really there was nothing ailing them but nasal gleet. This is not contagious, but may stubbornly resist treatment and last for a long time. In most cases the discharge is from one nostril only, which may signify that the sinuses on that side of the head are affected. The discharge may be intermittent; that is, quantities may be discharged at times and again little or none for a day or so. Such an intermittent discharge usually signifies disease of the sinuses. The glands under and between the bones of the lower jaw may be enlarged. The peculiar ragged-edged ulcer of glanders is not to be found on the membrane within the nostrils, but occasionally sores are to be seen there. If there is any doubt about it, the symptoms of glanders should be well studied in order that one may be competent to form a safe opinion.

The eye on the side of the discharging nostril may have a peculiar appearance and look smaller than its fellow. There may be an enlargement, having the appearance of a bulging out of the bone over the part affected, between or below the eyes. The breath may be offensive, which indicates decomposition of the matter or bones or disease of the teeth. A diseased tooth is further indicated by the horse holding his head to one side when eating, or by dropping the feed from the mouth after partly chewing it. When the bones between the eyes, below the eyes, and above the back teeth of the upper jaw are tapped on, a hollow, drumlike sound is emitted, but if the sinus is filled with pus or contains a large tumor the sound emitted will be the same as if a solid substance were struck; by this means the sinus affected may be located in some instances. The hair may be rough over the affected part, or even the bone may be soft to the touch and the part give somewhat to pressure or leave an impression where it is pressed upon with the finger.

Treatment.—The cause of the trouble must be ascertained before treatment is commenced. In the many cases in which the animal is in poor condition (in fact, in all cases) he should have the most nutritive feed and regular exercise. The feed, or box containing it, should be placed on the ground, as the dependent position of the head favors the discharge.

The cases that do not require a surgical operation must, as a rule, have persistent medical treatment. Mineral tonics and local medication are of the most value. For eight days give the following mixture: Reduced iron, 3 ounces; powdered nux vomica, 1 ounce. Mix and make into 16 powders; one powder should be mixed with the feed twice a day. Arsenious acid (white arsenic) in doses of from 3 to 6 grains three times daily is a good tonic for such cases. Sulphur burnt in the stable while the animal is there to inhale its fumes is also a valuable adjunct. Care should be taken that the fumes of the burning sulphur are sufficiently diluted with air so as not to suffocate the horse. Chlorid of lime sprinkled around the stall is good. Also keep a quantity of it under the hay in the manger so that the gases will be inhaled as the horse holds his head over the hay while eating. Keep the nostrils washed and the discharge cleaned away from the manger and stall. The horse may be caused to inhale the vapor of compound tincture of benzoin by pouring 2 ounces of this drug into hot water and fumigating in the usual way.

If the nasal gleet is the result of a diseased tooth, the latter must be removed. Trephining is the best possible way to remove it in such cases, as the operation immediately opens the cavity, which can be attended to direct. In all those cases of nasal gleet in which sinuses contain either tumors or collections of pus the only relief is by the trephine; and, no matter how thoroughly described, this is an operation that will be seldom attempted by the nonprofessional. It would therefore be a waste of time to give the modus operandi.

An abscess involving the turbinated bones is similar to the collection of pus in the sinuses and must be relieved by trephining.

THICKENING OF THE NASAL MEMBRANE.

This is sometimes denoted by a chronic discharge, a snuffling in the breathing, and a contraction of the nostril. It is a result of common cold and requires the same treatment as prescribed for nasal gleet, namely, the sulphate of iron, sulphate of copper, iodid of potassium, etc. The membranes of both sides may be affected, but one side only is the rule; the affected side may be easily detected by holding the hand tightly over one nostril at a time. When the healthy side is closed in this manner the breathing through the affected side will demonstrate a decreased caliber or an obstruction.

NASAL POLYPUS.

Tumors with narrow bases (somewhat pear-shaped) are occasionally found attached to the membrane of the nasal chambers, and are obstructions to breathing through the side in which they are located. They vary much in size; some are so small that their presence is not manifested, while others almost completely fill the chamber, thereby causing a serious obstruction to the passage of air. The stem, or base, of the tumor is generally attached high in the chamber, and usually the tumor can not be seen, but occasionally it increases in size until it can be observed within the nostril. Sometimes, instead of hanging down toward the nasal opening, it falls back into the pharynx. It causes a discharge from the nostril, a more or less noisy snuffling sound in breathing, according to its size, a discharge of blood (if it is injured), and sneezing. The side that it occupies can be detected in the same way as described for the detection of the affected side when the breathing is obstructed by a thickened membrane.

The only relief is removal of the polypus, which, like all other operations, should be done by an expert when it is possible to obtain one. The operation is performed by grasping the base of the tumor with suitable forceps and twisting it round and round until it is torn from its attachment, or by cutting it off with a noose of wire. The resulting hemorrhage is checked by the use of an astringent lotion, such as a solution of the tincture of iron, or by packing the nostrils with surgeon's gauze.

PHARYNGEAL POLYPUS.

This is exactly the same kind of tumor described as nasal polypus, the only difference being in the situation. Indeed, the stem of the tumor may be attached to the membrane of the nasal chamber, as before explained, or it may be attached in the fauces (opening of the back part of the mouth), and the body of the tumor then falls into the pharynx. In this situation it may seriously interfere with breathing. Sometimes it drops into the larynx, causing the most alarming symptoms. The animal coughs, or tries to cough, saliva flows from the mouth, the breathing is performed with the greatest difficulty and accompanied with a loud noise; the animal appears as if strangled and often falls exhausted. When the tumor is coughed out of the larynx the animal regains quickly and soon appears as if nothing were ailing. These sudden attacks and quick recoveries point to the nature of the trouble. The examination must be made by holding the animal's mouth open with a balling iron or speculum and running the hand back into the mouth. If the tumor is within reach, it must be removed in the same manner as though it were in the nose.

BLEEDING FROM THE NOSE.

This often occurs during the course of certain diseases, namely, influenza, bronchitis, purpura hemorrhagica, glanders, etc. But it also occurs independently of other affections and, as before mentioned, is a symptom of polypus, or tumor, in the nose.

Injuries to the head, exertion, violent sneezing—causing a rupture of a small blood vessel—also induce it. The bleeding is almost invariably from one nostril only, and is never very serious. The blood escapes in drops (seldom in a stream) and is not frothy, as when the hemorrhage is from the lungs. (See Bleeding from the lungs, p. 127.) In most cases bathing the head and washing out the nostril with cold water are all that is necessary. If the cause is known, you will be guided according to circumstances. If the bleeding continues, pour ice-cold water over the face, between the eyes and down over the nasal chambers. A bag containing ice in small pieces applied to the head is often efficient. If in spite of these measures the hemorrhage continues, plugging the nostrils with cotton, tow, or oakum, should be tried. A string should be tied around the plug before it is pushed up into the nostril, so that it can be safely withdrawn after 4 or 5 hours. If both nostrils are bleeding, only one nostril at a time should be plugged. If the hemorrhage is profuse and persistent, a drench composed of 1 dram of acetate of lead dissolved in 1 pint of water, or ergot, 1 ounce, should be given.

INFLAMMATION OF THE PHARYNX.

As already stated, the pharynx is common to the functions of both respiration and alimentation. From this organ the air passes into the larynx and thence onward to the lungs. In the posterior part of the pharynx is the superior extremity of the gullet, the canal through which the feed and water pass to the stomach. Inflammation of the pharynx is a complication of other diseases—namely, influenza, strangles, etc.—and is probably always more or less complicated with inflammation of the larynx. That it may exist as an independent affection there is no reason to doubt, and it is discussed as such with the diseases of the digestive tract.

SORE THROAT, OR LARYNGITIS.

The larynx is situated in the space between the lower jawbones just back of the root of the tongue. It may be considered as a box (somewhat depressed on each side), composed principally of cartilages and small muscles, and lined on the inside with a continuation of the respiratory mucous membrane. Posteriorly it opens into and is continuous with the windpipe. It is the organ of the voice, the vocal cords being situated within it; but in the horse this function is of little consequence. It dilates and contracts to a certain extent, thus regulating the volume of air passing through it. The mucous membrane lining it internally is so highly sensitive that if the smallest particle of feed happens to drop into it from the pharynx violent coughing ensues instantly and is continued until the source of irritation is ejected. This is a provision of nature to prevent foreign substances gaining access to the lungs. That projection called Adam's apple in the neck of man is the prominent part of one of the cartilages forming the larynx.

Inflammation of the larynx is a serious and sometimes fatal disease, and, as before stated, is usually complicated with inflammation of the pharynx, constituting what is popularly known as "sore throat." The chief causes are chilling and exposure.

Symptoms.—About the first symptom noticed is cough, followed by difficulty in swallowing, which may be due to soreness of the membrane of the pharynx, over which the feed or water must pass, or from the pain caused by the contraction of the muscles necessary to impel the feed or water onward to the gullet; or this same contraction of the muscles may cause a pressure on the larynx and produce pain. In many instances the difficulty in swallowing is so great that water, and in some cases feed, is returned through the nose. This, however, does not occur in laryngitis alone, but only when the pharynx is involved in the inflammation. The glands between the lower jawbones and below the ears may be swollen. Pressure on the larynx induces coughing. The head is more or less "poked out," and has the appearance of being stiffly carried. The membrane in the nose becomes red. A discharge from the nostrils soon appears. As the disease advances, the breathing may assume a more or less noisy character; sometimes a harsh, rasping snore is emitted with every respiration, the breathing becomes hurried, and occasionally the animal seems threatened with suffocation.

Treatment.—In all cases steam the nostrils, as has been advised for cold in the head. In bad cases cause the steam to be inhaled continuously for hours—until relief is afforded. Have a bucketful of fresh boiling water every fifteen or twenty minutes. In each bucketful of water put a tablespoonful of oil of turpentine, or compound tincture of benzoin, the vapor of which will be carried along with the steam to the affected parts and have a beneficial effect. In mild cases steaming the nostrils five, six, or seven times a day will suffice.

The animal should be placed in a comfortable, dry stall (a box stall preferred), and should have pure air to breathe. The body should be blanketed, and bandages applied to the legs. The diet should consist of soft feed—bran mashes, scalded oats, linseed gruel, and, best of all, fresh grass, if in season. The manger, or trough, should neither be too high nor too low, but a temporary one should be constructed at about the height he carries his head. Having to reach too high or too low may cause so much pain that the animal would rather forego satisfying what little appetite he may have than inflict pain by craning his head for feed or water. A supply of fresh water should be before him all the time; he will not drink too much, nor will the cold water hurt him. Constipation (if present) must be relieved by enemas of warm water, administered three or four times during the twenty-four hours.

A liniment composed of 2 ounces of olive oil and 1 each of solution of ammonia and tincture of cantharides, well shaken together, may be thoroughly rubbed in about the throat from ear to ear, and about 6 inches down over the windpipe, and in the space between the lower jaws. This liniment should be applied once a day for two or three days.

If the animal is breathing with great difficulty, persevere in steaming the nostrils, and dissolve 2 drams of chlorate of potassium in every gallon of water he will drink; even if he can not swallow much of it, and even if it is returned through the nostrils, it will be of some benefit to the pharynx as a gargle.

An electuary of acetate of potash, 2 drams, honey, and licorice powder may be spread on the teeth with a paddle every few hours. If the pain of coughing is great, 2 or 3 grains of morphin may be added to the electuary.

When the breathing begins to be loud, relief is afforded in some cases by giving a drench composed of 2 drams of fluid extract of jaborandi in half a pint of water. If benefit is derived, this drench may be repeated four or five hours after the first dose is given. It will cause a free flow of saliva from the mouth.

In urgent cases, when suffocation seems inevitable, the operation of tracheotomy must be performed. To describe this operation in words that would make it comprehensible to the general reader is a more difficult task than performing the operation, which, in the hands of the expert, is simple and attended with little danger.

The operator should be provided with a tracheotomy tube (to be purchased from any veterinary instrument maker) and a sharp knife, a sponge, and a bucket of clean cold water. The place to be selected for opening the windpipe is that part which is found, upon examination, to be least covered with muscles, about 5 or 6 inches below the throat. Right here, then, is the place to cut through. Have an assistant hold the animal's head still. Grasp your knife firmly in the right hand, select the spot and make the cut from above to below directly on the median line on the anterior surface of the windpipe. Make the cut about 2 inches long in the windpipe; this necessitates cutting three or four rings. One bold stroke is usually sufficient, but if it is necessary to make several other cuts to finish the operation, do not hesitate. Your purpose is to make a hole in the windpipe sufficiently large to admit the tracheotomy tube. It is quickly manifested when the windpipe is severed; the hot air rushes out, and when air is taken in it is sucked in with a noise. A slight hemorrhage may result (it never amounts to much), which is easily controlled by washing the wound with a sponge and cold water, but use care not to get any water in the windpipe. Do not neglect to instruct your assistant to hold the head down immediately after the operation, so that the neck will be in a horizontal line. This will prevent the blood from getting into the windpipe and will allow it to drop directly on the ground. If you have the self-adjustable tube, it retains its place in the wound without further trouble after it is inserted. The other kind requires to be secured in position by means of two tapes or strings tied around the neck. After the hemorrhage is somewhat abated, sponge the blood away and see that the tube is thoroughly clean, then insert it, directing the tube downward toward the lungs.

The immediate relief this operation affords is gratifying to behold. The animal, a few minutes before on the verge of death from suffocation, emitting a loud wheezing sound with every breath, with haggard countenance, body swaying, pawing, gasping, fighting for breath, now breathes tranquilly, and may be in search of something to eat.

The tube should be removed once a day and cleaned with carbolic-acid solution (1 to 20), and the discharge washed away from the wound with a solution of carbolic acid, 1 part to 40 parts water. Several times a day the hand should be held over the opening in the tube to test the animal's ability to breathe through the nostrils, and as soon as it is demonstrated that breathing can be performed in the natural way the tube should be removed, the wound thoroughly cleansed with carbolic-acid solution (1 to 40), and closed by inserting four or five stitches through the skin and muscle. Do not include the cartilages of the windpipe in the stitches. Apply the solution to the wound three or four times a day until healed. When the tube is removed to clean it the lips of the wound may be pressed together to ascertain whether or not the horse can breathe through the larynx. The use of the tube should be discontinued as soon as possible.

It is true that tracheotomy tubes are seldom to be found on farms, and especially when most urgently required. In such instances there is nothing left to be done but, with a strong needle, pass a waxed end or other strong string through each side of the wound, including the cartilage of the windpipe, and keep the wound open by tying the strings over the neck.

During the time the tube is used the other treatment advised must not be neglected. After a few days the discharge from the nostrils becomes thicker and more profuse. This is a good symptom and signifies that the acute stage has passed. At any time during the attack, if the horse becomes weak, give aromatic spirits of ammonia, 2 ounces in water. Do not be in a hurry to put the animal back to work, but give plenty of time for a complete recovery. Gentle and gradually increasing exercise may be given as soon as the horse is able to stand it. The feed should be carefully selected and of good quality. Tonics, as iron or arsenic, may be employed.

If abscesses form in connection with the disease they must be opened to allow the escape of pus, but do not rashly plunge a knife into swollen glands; wait until you are certain the swelling contains pus. The formation of pus may be encouraged by the constant application of poultices for hours at a time. The best poultice for the purpose is made of linseed meal, with sufficient hot water to make a thick paste. If the glands remain swollen for some time after the attack, rub well over them an application of the following: Biniodid of mercury, 1 dram; lard, 1 ounce; mix well. This may be applied once every day until the part is blistered.

Sore throat is also a symptom of other diseases, such as influenza, strangles, purpura hemorrhagica, etc., which diseases may be consulted under their proper headings.

After a severe attack of inflammation of the larynx the mucous membrane may be left in a thickened condition, or an ulceration of the part may ensue, either of which is liable to produce a chronic cough. For the ulceration it is useless to prescribe, because it can neither be diagnosed nor topically treated by the nonprofessional.

If a chronic cough remains after all the other symptoms have disappeared, it is advisable to give 1 dram of iodid of potassium dissolved in a bucketful of drinking water, one hour before feeding, three times a day for a month if necessary. Also rub in well the preparation of iodid of mercury (as advised for the swollen glands) about the throat, from ear to ear, and in the space between the lower jawbones. The application may be repeated every third day until the part is blistered.

SPASM OF THE LARYNX.

The symptoms are as follows: Sudden seizure by a violent fit of coughing; the horse may reel and fall, and after a few minutes recover and be as well as ever. The treatment recommended is this: Three drams of bromid of potassium three times a day, dissolved in the drinking water, or give as a drench in about a half pint of water for a week. Then give 1 dram of powdered nux vomica (either on the food or shaken with water as a drench) once a day for a few weeks.

CROUP AND DIPHTHERIA.

Neither of these diseases affects the horse, but these names are sometimes wrongly applied to severe laryngitis or pharyngitis, or to forage poisoning, in which the throat is paralyzed and becomes excessively inflamed and gangrenous.

THICK WIND AND ROARING.

Horses that are affected with chronic disease that causes a loud, unnatural noise in breathing are said to have thick wind, or to be roarers. This class does not include those affected with severe sore throat, as in these cases the breathing is noisy only during the attack of the acute disease.

Thick wind is caused by an obstruction to the free passage of the air in some part of the respiratory tract. Nasal polypi, thickening of the membrane, pharyngeal polypi, deformed bones, paralysis of the wing of the nostril, etc., are occasional causes. The noisy breathing of horses after having been idle and put to sudden exertion is not due to any disease and is only temporary. Very often a nervous, excitable horse will make a noise for a short time when started off, generally caused by the cramped position in which the head and neck are forced in order to hold him back.

Many other causes may occasion temporary, intermittent, or permanent noisy respiration, but chronic roaring is caused by paralysis of the muscles of the larynx; and almost invariably it is the muscles of the left side of the larynx that are affected.

In chronic roaring the noise is made when the air is drawn into the lungs; only when the disease is far advanced is a sound produced when the air is expelled, and even then it is not nearly so loud as during inspiration.

In a normal condition the muscles dilate the aperture of the larynx by moving the cartilage and vocal cord outward, allowing a sufficient volume of air to rush through. But when the muscles are paralyzed the cartilage and vocal cord that are normally controlled by the affected muscles lean into the tube of the larynx, so that when the air rushes in it meets this obstruction and the noise is produced. When the air is expelled from the lungs its very force pushes the cartilage and vocal cords out, and consequently noise is not produced in the expiratory act.

The paralysis of the muscles is due to derangement of the nerve that supplies them with energy. The muscles of both sides are not supplied by the same nerve; there is a right and a left nerve, each supplying its respective side. The reason why the muscles on the left side are the ones usually paralyzed is owing to the difference in the anatomical arrangement of the nerves. The left nerve is much longer and more exposed to interference than the right nerve.

In chronic roaring there is no evidence of any disease of the larynx other than the wasted condition of the muscles in question. The disease of the nerve is generally far from the larynx. Disease of parts contiguous to the nerve along any part of its course may interfere with its proper function. Enlargement of lymphatic glands within the chest through which the nerve passes on its way back to the larynx is the most frequent interruption of nervous supply, and consequently roaring. When roaring becomes confirmed, medical treatment is entirely useless, as it is impossible to restore the wasted muscle and at the same time remove the cause of the interruption of the nervous supply. Before roaring becomes permanent the condition may be benefited by a course of iodid of potassium, if caused by disease of the lymphatic glands. Electricity has been used with indifferent success. Blistering or firing over the larynx is, of course, not worthy of trial if the disease is due to interference of the nerve supply. The administration of strychnia (nux vomica) on the ground that it is a nerve tonic with the view of stimulating the affected muscles is treating only the result of the disease without considering the cause, and is therefore useless. The operation of extirpating the collapsed cartilage and vocal cord is believed to be the only relief, and, as this operation is critical and can be performed only by the skillful veterinarian, it will not be described here.

From the foregoing description of the disease it will be seen that the name "roaring," by which the disease is generally known, is only a symptom and not the disease. Chronic roaring is also in many cases accompanied with a cough. The best way to test whether a horse is a "roarer" is either to make him pull a load rapidly up a hill or over a sandy road or soft ground; or, if he is a saddle horse, gallop him up a hill or over soft ground. The object is to make him exert himself. Some horses require a great deal more exertion than others before the characteristic sound is emitted. The greater the distance he is forced, the more he will appear exhausted if he is a roarer; in bad cases the animal becomes utterly exhausted, the breathing is rapid and difficult, the nostrils dilate to the fullest extent, and the animal appears as if suffocation was imminent.

An animal that is a roarer should not be used for breeding purposes. The taint is transmissible in many instances.

Grunting.—A common test used by veterinarians when examining "the wind" of a horse is to see if he is a "grunter." This is a sound emitted during expiration when the animal is suddenly moved, or startled, or struck at. If he grunts he is further tested for roaring. Grunters are not always roarers, but, as it is a common thing for a roarer to grunt, such an animal must be looked upon with suspicion until he is thoroughly tried by pulling a load or galloped up a hill. The test should be a severe one. Horses suffering with pleurisy, pleurodynia, or rheumatism, and other affections accompanied with much pain, will grunt when moved, or when the pain is aggravated, but grunting under these circumstances does not justify the term of "grunter" being applied to the horse, as the grunting ceases when the animal recovers from the disease that causes the pain.

High blowing.—This term is applied to a noisy breathing made by some horses. It is distinctly a nasal sound, and must not be confounded with "roaring." The sound is produced by the action of the nostrils. It is a habit and not an unsoundness. Contrary to roaring, when the animal is put to severe exertion the sound ceases. An animal that emits this sound is called a "high blower." Some horses have naturally very narrow nasal openings, and they may emit sounds louder than usual in their breathing when exercised.

Whistling is only one of the variations of the sound emitted by a horse called a "roarer," and therefore needs no further notice, except to remind the reader that a whistling sound may be produced during an attack of severe sore throat or inflammation of the larynx, which passes away with the disease that causes it.

CHRONIC BRONCHITIS.

This may be due to the same causes as acute bronchitis or it may follow the latter disease. An attack of the chronic form is liable to be converted into acute bronchitis by a very slight cause. This chronic affection in most instances is associated with thickening of the walls of the tubes. Its course is slower, it is less severe, and is not accompanied with so much fever as the acute form. If the animal is exerted, the breathing becomes quickened and he soon shows signs of exhaustion. In many instances the animal keeps up strength and appearances moderately well, but in other cases the appetite is lost, flesh gradually disappears, and he becomes emaciated and debilitated. It is accompanied with a persistent cough, which in some cases is husky, smothered, or muffled, while in others it is hard and clear. A whitish matter, which may be curdled, is discharged from the nose. If the ear is placed against the chest behind the shoulder blade, the rattle of the air passing through the mucus can be heard within.

Treatment.—Rest is necessary, as even under the most favorable circumstances a cure is difficult to effect. The animal can not stand exertion and should not be compelled to undergo it. It should have much the same general care and medical treatment prescribed for the acute form. Arsenious acid in tonic doses (3 to 7 grains) three times daily may be given. As arsenic is irritant, it must be mixed with a considerable bulk of moist feed and never given alone. Arsenic may be given in the form of Fowler's solution, 1 ounce three times daily in the drinking water. An application of mustard applied to the breast is a beneficial adjunct. The diet should be the most nourishing. Bulky feed should not be given. Linseed mashes, scalded oats, and, if in season, grass and green-blade fodder are the best diet.

THE LUNGS.

The lungs (see Pl. VII) are the essential organs of respiration. They consist of two (right and left) spongy masses, commonly called the " lights," situated entirely within the thoracic cavity. On account of the space taken up by the heart, the left lung is the smaller. Externally, they are completely covered by the pleura. The structure of the lung consists of a light, soft, but very strong and remarkably elastic tissue, which can be torn only with difficulty. Each lung is divided into a certain number of lobes, which are subdivided into numberless lobules (little lobes). A little bronchial tube terminates in every one of these lobules. The little tube then divides into minute branches which open into the air cells (pulmonary vesicles) of the lungs. The air cells are little sacs having a diameter varying from one-seventieth to one two-hundredth of an inch; they have but one opening, the communication with the branches of the little bronchial tubes. Small blood vessels ramify in the walls of the air cells. The air cells are the consummation of the intricate structures forming the respiratory apparatus. They are of prime importance, all the rest being complementary. It is here that the exchange of gases takes place. As before stated, the walls of the cells are very thin; so, also, are the walls of the blood vessels. Through these walls escapes from the blood the carbonic acid gas that has been absorbed by the blood in its circulation through the different parts of the body; through these walls also the oxygen gas, which is the life-giving element of the atmosphere, is absorbed by the blood from the air in the air cells.

CONGESTION OF THE LUNGS.

Congestion is essentially an excess of blood in the vessels of the parts affected. Congestion of the lungs in the horse, when it exists as an independent affection, is generally caused by overexertion when the animal is not in a fit condition to undergo more than moderate exercise. Very often what is recognized as congestion of the lungs is but a symptom of exhaustion or dilatation of the heart.

The methods practiced by the trainers of running and trotting horses will give an idea of what is termed " putting a horse in condition " to stand severe exertion. The animal at first gets walking exercises, then after some time he is made to go faster and farther each day; the amount of work is daily increased until he is said to be " in condition." An animal so prepared runs no risk of being affected with congestion of the lungs, if he is otherwise healthy. On the other hand, if the horse is kept in the stable for the purpose of laying on fat or for want of something to do, the muscular system becomes soft, and the horse is not in condition to stand the severe exertion of going fast or far, no matter how healthy he may be in other respects. If such a horse be given a hard ride or drive, he may start off in high spirits, but soon becomes exhausted, and if he is pushed he will slacken his pace, show a desire to stop, and may stagger or even fall. Examination will show the nostrils dilated, the flanks heaving, the countenance haggard, and the appearance of suffocation. The heart and muscles were not accustomed to the sudden and severe strain put upon them; the heart became unable to perform its work; the blood accumulated in the vessels of the lungs, which eventually became engorged with the stagnated blood, constituting congestion of the lungs.

The animal, after having undergone severe exertion, may not exhibit alarming symptoms until returned to the stable; then he will be noticed standing with his head down, legs spread out, the eyes wildly staring or dull and sunken. The breathing is very rapid and almost gasping; in most cases the body is covered with perspiration, which, however, may soon evaporate, leaving the surface of the body and the legs and ears cold; the breathing is both abdominal and thoracic; the chest rises and falls and the flanks are powerfully brought into action. If the pulse can be felt at all it will be found beating very frequently, one hundred or so to a minute. The heart may be felt tumultuously thumping if the hand is placed against the chest behind the left elbow, or it may be scarcely perceptible. The animal may tremble all over. If the ear is placed against the side of the chest a loud murmur will be heard and perhaps a fine, crackling sound.

One can scarcely fail to recognize a case of congestion of the lungs when brought on by overexertion, as the history of the case indicates the nature of the ailment. In all cases of suffocation the lungs are congested. It is also seen in connection with other diseases.

Treatment.—If the animal is attacked by the disease while on the road, stop him immediately. Do not attempt to return to the stables. If he is in the stable, make arrangements at once to insure an unlimited supply of pure air. If the weather is warm, out in the open air is the best place, but if too cold let him stand with head to the door. Let him stand still; he has all he can do, if he obtains sufficient pure air to sustain life. If he is encumbered with harness or saddle, remove it at once and rub the body with cloths or wisps of hay or straw. This stimulates the circulation in the skin, and thus aids in relieving the lungs of the extra quantity of blood that is stagnated there. If you have three or four assistants, let them rub the body

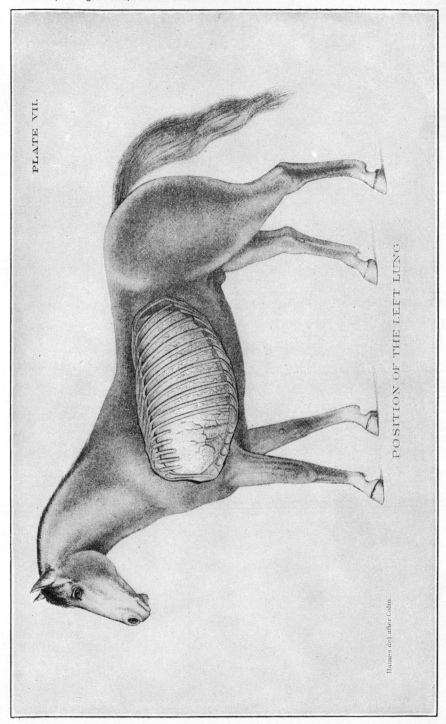

PLATE VII.

POSITION OF THE LEFT LUNG.

Hanos del. after Cohn.

and legs well until the skin feels natural; rub the legs until they are warm, if possible. When the circulation is reestablished, put bandages on the legs from the hoofs up as far as possible. Throw a blanket over the body and let the rubbing be done under the blanket. Diffusible stimulants are the medicines indicated—ether and aromatic spirits of ammonia. A drench of 2 ounces each of spirits of nitrous ether and alcohol, diluted with a pint of water, every hour until relief is afforded, is among the best remedies. Or give 1 ounce of tincture of arnica in a pint of water every hour until five or six doses have been given. If none of these remedies are at hand, 2 ounces of oil of turpentine, shaken with a half pint of milk, may be given once, but not repeated. The animal may be bled from the jugular vein. Do not take more than 5 or 6 quarts from the vein, and do not repeat the bleeding. The blood thus drawn will have a tarry appearance.

When the alarming symptoms have subsided active measures may be stopped, but care must be used in the general treatment of the animal for several days, for it must be remembered that congestion may be followed by pneumonia. The animal should have a comfortable stall, where he will not be subjected to drafts or sudden changes of temperature; he should be blanketed and the legs kept bandaged. The air should be pure, a plentiful supply of fresh, cold water always in the stall; and a diet composed principally of bran mashes, scalded oats, and, if in season, grass. When ready for use again the horse should at first receive only moderate exercise, which may be daily increased until he may safely be put to regular work.

PNEUMONIA, OR LUNG FEVER.

Pneumonia is inflammation of the lungs. The chief varieties of pneumonia are catarrhal—later discussed in connection with bronchitis, under the name of broncho-pneumonia—and the fibrinous or croupous variety. The latter form receives its names from the fact that the air spaces are choked with coagulated fibrin thrown out from the blood. This causes the diseased portions of the lungs to become as firm as liver, in which condition they are said to be hepatized. As air is excluded by the inflammatory product, the diseased lung will not float in water.

The inflammation usually begins in the lower part of the lung and extends upward. The first stage of the disease consists of congestion, or engorgement, of the blood vessels, followed by leakage of serum containing fibrin from the blood vessels into the air passages. The fluids thus escaping into the air cells and in the minute branches of the little bronchial tubes become coagulated.

54763°—23——8

The pleura covering the affected parts may be more or less inflamed. A continuance of the foregoing phenomena is marked by a further escape of the constituents of the blood, and a change in the membrane of the cells, which becomes swollen. The exudate that fills the air cells and minute bronchial branches undergoes disintegration and softening when healing commences.

The favorable termination of pneumonia is in resolution, that is, a restoration to health. This is gradually brought about by the exuded material contained in the air cells and lung tissues being broken down and softened and absorbed or expectorated through the nostrils. The blood vessels return to their natural state, and the blood circulates in them as before. In the cases that do not terminate so happily the lung may become gangrenous (or mortified), an abscess may form, or the disease may be merged into the chronic variety.

Pneumonia may be directly induced by any of the influences named as general causes for diseases of the organs of respiration, but in many instances it is from neglect. A common cold or sore throat may be followed by pneumonia if neglected or improperly treated. An animal may be debilitated by a cold, and when in this weakened state may be compelled to undergo exertion beyond his strength; or he may be kept in a badly ventilated stable, where the foul gases are shut in and the pure air is shut out; or the stable may be so open that parts of the body are exposed to drafts of cold air. An animal is predisposed to pneumonia when debilitated by any constitutional disease, and especially during convalescence if exposed to any of the exciting causes. Foreign bodies, such as feed accidentally getting into the lungs by way of the windpipe, as well as the inhalation of irritating gases and smoke, ofttimes produce fatal attacks of inflammation of the lung and bronchial tubes. Pneumonia is frequently seen in connection with other diseases, such as influenza, purpura hemorrhagica, strangles, glanders, etc. Pneumonia and pleurisy are most common during cold, damp weather, and especially during the prevalence of the cold north or northeasterly winds. Wounds puncturing the thoracic cavity may cause pneumonia.

Symptoms.—Pneumonia, when a primary disease, is ushered in by a chill, more or less prolonged, which in many cases is seen neither by the owner nor the attendant, but is overlooked. The breathing becomes accelerated, and the animal hangs its head and has a very dull appearance. The mouth is hot and has a sticky feeling to the touch; the heat conveyed to the finger in the mouth demonstrates a fever; if the thermometer is placed in the rectum the temperature will be found to have risen to 103° F. or higher. The pulse is frequent, beating from fifty or sixty to eighty or more a minute. There is usually a dry cough from the beginning, which, however, changes in character as the disease advances; for instance, it may become moist, or if pleurisy sets in, the cough will be peculiar to the latter affection; that is, cut short in the endeavor to suppress it. In some cases the discharge from the nostrils is tinged with blood, while in other cases it has the appearance of muco-pus. The appetite is lost to a greater or less extent, but the desire for water is increased, particularly during the onset of the fever. The membrane within the nostrils is red and at first dry, but sooner or later becomes moist. The legs are cold. The bowels are more or less constipated, and what dung is passed is uually covered with a slimy mucus. The urine is passed in smaller quantities than usual and is of a darker color.

The animal prefers to have the head where the freshest air can be obtained. When affected with pneumonia a horse does not lie down, but persists in standing from the beginning of the attack. If pneumonia is complicated with pleurisy, however, the horse may appear restless and lie down for a few moments to gain relief from the pleuritic pains, but he soon rises. In pneumonia the breathing is rapid and difficult, but when the pneumonia is complicated with pleurisy the ribs are kept as still as possible and the breathing is abdominal; that is, the abdominal muscles are now made to do as much of the work as they can perform. If pleurisy is not present there is little pain. To the ordinary observer the animal may not appear dangerously ill, as he does not show the seriousness of the ailment by violence, as in colic, but a careful observer will discover at a glance that the trouble is something more serious than a cold. By percussion it will be shown that some portions of the chest are less resonant than in health, indicating exclusion of air. If the air is wholly excluded the percussion is quite dull, like that elicited by percussion over the thigh.

By auscultation important information may be gained. When the ear is placed against the chest of a healthy horse, the respiratory murmur is heard more or less distinctly, according to the part of the chest that is beneath the ear. In the very first stage of pneumonia this murmur is louder and hoarser; also, there is a fine, crackling sound something similar to that produced when salt is thrown in a fire. After the affected part becomes solid there is an absence of sound over that particular part. After absorption begins one may again hear sounds that are of a more or less moist character and resemble bubbling or gurgling, which gradually change until the natural sound is heard announcing return to health.

When a fatal termination is approaching all the symptoms become intensified. The breathing becomes still more rapid and difficult; the flanks heave; the animal stares wildly about as if seeking aid to drive off the feeling of suffocation; the body is bathed with sweat; the horse staggers, but quickly recovers his balance; he may now, for the first time during the attack, lie down; he does so, however, in the hope of relief, which he fails to find, and with difficulty struggles to his feet; he pants; the nostrils flap; he staggers and sways from side to side and backward and forward, but still tries to retain the standing position, even by propping himself against the stall. It is no use, as after an exhausting fight for breath he goes down; the limbs stretch out and become rigid. In fatal cases death usually occurs in from 10 to 20 days after the beginning of the attack. On the other hand, when the disease is terminating favorably the signs are obvious. The fever abates and the animal gradually improves in appetite; he takes more notice of things around him; his spirits improve; he has a general appearance of returning health, and he lies down and rests. In the majority of cases pneumonia, if properly treated, terminates in recovery.

Treatment.—The comfort and surroundings of the patient must be attended to first. The quarters should be the best that can be provided. Pure air is essential. Avoid placing the animal in a stall where he may be exposed to drafts of cold air and sudden changes of temperature. It is much better for the animal if the air is cold and pure than if it is warm and foul. It is better to make the animal comfortable with warm clothing than to make the stable warm by shutting off the ventilation. From the start the animal should have an unlimited supply of fresh, cold drinking water. Blanket the body. Rub the legs until they are warm and then put bandages on them from the hoofs up to the knees and hocks. If warmth can not be reestablished in the legs by hand rubbing alone, apply dry, ground mustard and rub well in. The bandages should be removed once or twice every day, the legs well rubbed, and the bandages replaced. Much harm is often done by clipping off hair and rubbing in powerful blistering compounds. They do positive injury and retard recovery, and should not be allowed. Much benefit may be derived from hot application to the sides of the chest if the facilities are at hand to apply them. If the weather is not too cold, and if the animal is in a comfortable stable, the following method may be tried: Have a tub of hot water handy to the stable door; soak a woolen blanket in the water, then quickly wring as much water as possible out of it and wrap it around the chest. See that it fits closely to the skin; do not allow it to sag so that air may get between it and the skin. Now wrap a dry blanket over the wet hot one and hold in place with three girths. The hot blanket should be renewed every half hour, and while it is off being wetted and wrung the dry one should remain over the wet part of the chest to prevent reaction. The hot applications should be kept up for three or four hours, and when stopped the skin should be quickly rubbed as dry as possible, an application of alcohol rubbed over the wet part, and a dry blanklet snugly fitted over the animal. If the hot applications appear to benefit, they may be tried on three or four consecutive days. Unless every facility and circumstance favors the application of heat in the foregoing manner, it should not be attempted. If the weather is very cold or any of the details are omitted, more harm than good may result. Mustard may be applied by making a paste with a pound of freshly ground mustard mixed with warm water. This is to be spread evenly over the sides back of the shoulder blades and down to the median line below the chest. Care should be taken to avoid rubbing the mustard upon the thin skin immediately back of the elbow. The mustard-covered area should be covered with a paper and this with a blanket passed up from below and fastened over the back. The blanket and paper should be removed in from one to two hours. When pneumonia follows another disease, the system is always more of less debilitated and requires the careful use of stimulants from the beginning. To weaken the animal still further by bleeding him is one of the most effectual methods of retarding recovery, even if it does not hasten a fatal termination.

Another and oftentimes fatal mistake made by the nonprofessional is the indiscriminate and reckless use of aconite. This drug is one of the most active poisons, and should not be handled by anyone who does not thoroughly understand its action and uses. It is only less active than prussic acid in its poisonous effects. It is a common opinion, often expressed by nonprofessionals, that aconite is a stimulant. Nothing could be more erroneous; in fact, it is just the reverse. It is one of the most powerful sedatives used in the practice of medicine. In fatal doses it kills by paralyzing the very muscles used in breathing; it weakens the action of the heart, and should not be used. Do not give purgative medicines. If constipation exists, overcome it by an allowance of laxative diet, such as scalded oats, bran, and linseed mashes; also, grass, if in season. If the costiveness is not relieved by the laxative diet, give an enema of about a quart of warm water three or four times a day.

A diet consisting principally of bran mashes, scalded oats, and, when in season, grass or corn fodder is preferable if the animal retains an appetite; but if no desire is evinced for feed of this particular description, then the animal must be allowed to eat anything that will be taken spontaneously. Hay tea, made by pouring boiling water over good hay in a large bucket and allowing it to stand until cool, then straining off the liquid, will sometimes create a desire for feed. The animal may be allowed to drink as much of it as he desires. Corn on the cob is often eaten when everything else is refused. Bread may be tried; also apples or carrots. If the animal can be persuaded to drink milk, it may be supported by it for days. Three or four gallons of sweet milk may be given during the day, in which may be stirred three or four fresh eggs to each gallon. Some horses will drink milk, while others will refuse to touch it. It should be borne in mind that all feed must be taken by the horse as he desires it; none should be forced down him. If he will not eat, you will only have to wait until a desire is shown for feed. All kinds may be offered, first one thing and then another, but feed should not be allowed to remain long in trough or manger; the very fact of its constantly being before him will cause him to loathe it. When the animal has no appetite for anything the stomach is not in a proper state to digest food, and if it is poured or drenched into him it will only cause indigestion and aggravate the case. It is a good practice to do nothing when there is nothing to be done that will benefit. This refers to medicine as well as feed. Nothing is well done that is overdone.

There are many valuable medicines used for the different stages and different types of pneumonia, but in the opinion of the writer it is useless to refer to them here, as this work is intended for the use of those who are not sufficiently acquainted with the disease to recognize its various types and stages; therefore they would only confuse. If you can administer a ball or capsule, or have anyone at hand who is capable of doing it, a dram of sulphate of quinin in a capsule, or made into a ball, with sufficient linseed meal and molasses, given every three hours during the height of the fever, will do good in many cases. The ball of carbonate of ammonia, as advised in the treatment of bronchitis, may be tried if the animal is hard to drench. The heart should be kept strong by administering digitalis in doses of 2 drams of the tincture every three hours, or strychnia 1 grain, made into a pill with licorice powder, three times daily.

If the horse becomes very much debilitated, stimulants of a more pronounced character are required. The following drench is useful: Rectified spirits, 3 ounces; spirits of nitrous ether, 2 ounces; water, 1 pint. This may be repeated every four or five hours if it seems to benefit.

During the period of convalescence good nutritive feed should be allowed in a moderate quantity. Tonic medicines should be substituted for those used during the fever. The same medicines advised for the convalescing period of bronchitis are equally efficient in this case, especially the iodid of potash; likewise, the same general instructions apply here.

The chief causes of death in pneumonia are heart failure from exhaustion, suffocation, or blood poisoning from death (gangrene) of lung tissue. The greater the area of lung tissue diseased the greater the danger; hence double pneumonia is more fatal than pneumonia of one lung.

THE WINDPIPE.

The windpipe, or trachea as it is technically called, is the flexible tube that extends from the larynx, which it succeeds at the throat, to above the base of the heart in the chest, where it terminates by dividing into the right and left bronchi—the tubes going to the right and left lung, respectively. The windpipe is composed of about fifty incomplete rings of cartilage united by ligaments. A muscular layer is situated on the superior surface of the rings. Internally the tube is lined with a continuation of the mucous membrane that lines the entire respiratory tract, which here has very little sensibility in contrast to that lining the larynx, which is endowed with exquisite sensitiveness.

The windpipe is not subject to any special disease, but is more or less affected during laryngitis (sore throat), influenza, bronchitis, etc., and requires no special treatment. The membrane may be left in a thickened condition after these attacks. One or more of the rings may be accidentally fractured, or the tube may be distorted or malformed as the result of violent injury. After the operation of tracheotomy it is not uncommon to find a tumor or malformation as a result, or sequel, of the operation. In passing over this section attention is merely called to these defects, as they require no particular attention in the way of treatment. It may be stated, however, that any one of the before-mentioned conditions may constitute one of the causes of noisy respiration described as " thick wind."

GUTTURAL POUCHES.

These two sacs are situated above the throat, and communicate with the pharynx, as well as with the cavity of the tympanum of the ear. They are peculiar to solipeds. Normally, they contain air. Their function is unknown.

One or both guttural pouches may contain pus. The symptoms are as follows: Swelling on the side below the ear and an intermittent discharge of matter from one or both nostrils, especially when the head is depressed.

The swelling is soft, and, if pressed upon, matter will escape from the nose if the head is depressed. As before mentioned, these pouches communicate with the pharynx, and through this small opening matter may escape. A recovery is probable if the animal is turned out to graze, or if he is fed from the ground, as the dependent position of the head favors the escape of matter from the pouches. In addition to this, give the tonics recommended for nasal gleet. If this treatment fails, an operation must be performed, which should not be attempted by any one unacquainted with the anatomy of the part.

BRONCHITIS AND BRONCHO-PNEUMONIA.

Bronchitis is an inflammation of the bronchial tubes. When this inflammation extends to the air sacs at the termini of the smallest branches of the bronchial tubes, the disease is broncho-pneumonia. Bronchitis affecting the larger tubes is less serious than when the smaller are involved. The disease may be either acute or chronic. The causes are generally much the same as for other diseases of the respiratory organs, noticed in the beginning of this article. The special causes are these: The inhalation of irritating gases and smoke and fluids or solids gaining access to the parts. Bronchitis is occasionally associated with influenza and other specific fevers. It also supervenes on common cold or sore throat.

Symptoms.—The animal appears dull; the appetite is partially or wholly lost; the head hangs; the breathing is quickened; the cough, at first dry, and having somewhat the character of a "barking cough," is succeeded in a few days by a moist, rattling cough; the mouth is hot; the visible membranes in the nose are red; the pulse is frequent, and during the first stage is hard and quick, but as the disease advances becomes smaller and more frequent. There is a discharge from the nostrils that is at first whitish, but later becomes creamy or frothy, still later it is sometimes tinged with blood, and occasionally it may be of a brownish or rusty color. By auscultation, or placing the ear to the sides of the chest, unnatural sounds can now be heard. The air passing through the diseased tubes causes a wheezing sound when the small tubes are affected, and a hoarse, cooing, or snoring sound when the larger tubes are involved. After one or two days the dry stage of the disease is succeeded by a moist state of the membrane. The ear now detects a different sound, caused by the bursting of the bubbles as the air passes through the fluid, which is the exudate of inflammation and the augmented mucous secretions of the membrane. The mucus may be secreted in great abundance, which, by blocking up the tubes, may cause a collapse of a large extent of breathing surface. Usually the mucus is expectorated; that is, discharged through the nose. The matter is coughed up, and when it reaches the larynx much of it may be swallowed, and some is discharged from the nostrils. The horse, unlike the human being, can not spit, nor does the matter coughed up gain access to the mouth. If in serious cases all the symptoms become aggravated, the breathing is labored, short, and quick, it usually indicates that the inflammation has reached the breathing cells and that catarrhal pneumonia is established. In this case the ribs rise and fall much more than natural. This fact alone is enough to exclude the idea that the animal may be affected with pleurisy, because in that disease the ribs are kept in a fixed state as much as possible, and the breathing is accomplished to a great extent by aid of the abdominal muscles. The horse persists in standing throughout the attack. He prefers to stand with head to a door or window to gain all the fresh air possible, but if not tied may occasionally wander listlessly about the stall. The bowels most likely are constipated; the dung is covered with slimy mucus. The urine is decreased in quantity and darker in color than usual. The animal shows more or less thirst; in some cases the mouth is full of saliva. The discharge from the nose increases in quantity as the disease advances and inflammation subsides. This is rather a good symptom, as it shows that one stage has passed. The discharge then gradually decreases, the cough becomes less rasping, but of more frequent occurrence, until it gradually disappears with the return of health.

Bronchitis, affecting the smaller tubes, is one of the most fatal diseases, while that of the larger tubes is never very serious. It must be stated, however, that it is an exceedingly difficult matter for a nonexpert to discriminate between the two forms, and, further, it may as well be said here that he will have difficulty in discriminating between bronchitis and pneumonia.

Treatment.—The matter of first importance is to insure pure air to breathe, and next to make the patient's quarters as comfortable as possible. A well-ventilated box stall serves best for all purposes. Cover the body with a blanket, light or heavy, as the season of the year demands. Hand-rub the legs until they are warm, then wrap them in cotton and apply flannel or Derby bandages from the hoofs to the knees and hocks. If the legs can not be made warm with hand rubbing alone, apply dry mustard. Rub in thoroughly and then put the bandages on; also rub mustard paste well over the side of the chest, covering the space beginning immediately behind the shoulder blade and running back about eighteen inches, and from the median line beneath the breast to within ten inches of the ridge of the backbone. Repeat the application to the side of the chest about three days after the first one is applied.

Compel the animal to inhale steam from a bucketful of boiling water containing a tablespoonful of oil of turpentine and spirits of camphor, as advised for cold in the head. In serious cases the steam should be inhaled every hour, and in any case the oftener it is done the greater will be the beneficial results. Three times a day administer an electuary containing acetate of potash (2 drams), with licorice and molasses or honey. It is well to keep a bucketful of cold water before the animal all the time. If the horse is prostrated and has no appetite, give the following drench: Spirits of nitrous ether,

2 ounces; rectified spirits, 3 ounces; water, 1 pint. Repeat the dose every four or five hours if it appears to benefit. When the horse is hard to drench, give the following: Pulverized carbonate of ammonia, 3 drams; linseed meal and molasses sufficient to make the whole into a stiff mass; wrap it with a small piece of tissue paper and give as a ball. This ball may be repeated every four or five hours. When giving the ball care should be taken to prevent its breaking in the mouth, as in case of such accident it will make the mouth sore and prevent the animal from eating. If the bowels are constipated, give enemas of warm water. Do not give purgative medicines. Do not bleed the animal.

If the animal retains an appetite, a soft diet is preferable, such as scalded oats, bran mashes, and grass, if in season. If he refuses cooked feed, allow in small quantities anything he will eat. Hay, cob corn, oats, bread, apples, and carrots may be tried in turn. Some horses will drink sweet milk when they refuse all other kinds of feed, and especially is this the case if the drinking water is withheld for a while. One or 2 gallons at a time, four or five times a day, will support life. Bear in mind that when the disease is established recovery can not occur in less than two or three weeks, and more time may be necessary. Good nursing and patience are required.

When the symptoms have abated and nothing remains of the disease except the cough and a white discharge from the nostrils, all other medicines should be discontinued and a course of tonic treatment pursued. Give the following mixture: Reduced iron, 3 ounces; powdered gentian, 8 ounces; mix well together and divide into sixteen powders. Give a powder every night and morning mixed with bran and oats, if the animal will eat it, or shaken with about a pint of flaxseed tea and administered as a drench.

If the cough remains after the horse is apparently well, give 1 dram of iodid of potassium dissolved in a bucketful of drinking water one hour before each meal for two or three weeks if necessary. Do not put the animal to work too soon after recovery. Allow ample time to regain strength. This disease is prone to become chronic and may run into an incurable case of thick wind.

PLEURISY.

The thoracic cavity is divided into two lateral compartments, each containing one lung and a part of the heart. Each lung has its separate pleural membrane, or covering. The pleura is the thin, glistening membrane that covers the lung and also completely covers the internal walls of the chest. It is very thin, and to the ordinary observer appears to be part of the lung, which, in fact, it is for all practical purposes. The smooth, shiny surface of the lung, as well as the smooth, shiny surface so familiar on the rib, is the plura. In health this surface is always moist. A fluid is thrown off by the pleura, which causes the surface to be constantly moist. This is to prevent the effects of friction between the lungs and the walls of the chest and other contiguous parts which come in contact. It must be remembered that the lungs are dilating each time a breath is taken in, and contracting each time a breath of air is expelled. It may be readily seen that if it were not for the moistened state of the surface of the pleura the continual dilatation and contraction and the consequent rubbing of the parts against each other would cause serious friction.

Inflammation of this membrane is called pleurisy. Being so closely united with the lung, it can not always escape participation in the disease when the latter is inflamed. Pleurisy may be due to the same predisposing and exciting causes as mentioned in the beginning of this work as general causes for diseases of the organs of respiration, such as exposure to sudden changes of temperature, confinement in damp stables, etc. It may be caused also by wounds that penetrate the chest, for it must be remembered that such wounds must necessarily pierce the pleura. A fractured rib may involve the pleura. The inflammation following such wounds may be circumscribed; that is, confined to a small area surrounding the wound, or it may spread from the wound and involve a large portion of the pleura. The pleura may be involved secondarily when the heart or its membrane is the primary seat of the disease. It may occur in conjunction with bronchitis, influenza, and other diseases. Diseased growths that interfere with the pleura may induce pleurisy. The most frequent cause of pleurisy is an extension of inflammation from adjacent diseased lung. It is a common complication of pneumonia. Pleurisy will be described here as an independent affection, although it should be remembered that it is very often associated with the foregoing diseases.

The first lesion of pleurisy is overfilling of the blood vessels that ramify in this membrane and dryness of the surface. This is followed by the formation of a coating of coagulated fibrin on the diseased pleura and the transudation of serum which collects in the chest. This serum may contain flakes of fibrin and it may be straw colored or red from an admixture of blood. The quantity of this accumulation may amount to several gallons.

Symptoms.—When the disease exists as an independent affection it is ushered in by a chill, but this is usually overlooked. About the first thing noticed is the disinclination of the animal to move or turn around. When made to do so he grunts or groans with pain. He stands stiff; the ribs are fixed—that is, they move very little in the act of breathing—but the abdomen works more than natural; both the fore feet and elbows may be turned out; during the onset of the attack the animal may be restless and act as if he had a slight colic; he may even lie down, but does not remain long down, for when he finds no relief he soon gets up. After effusion begins these signs of restlessness disappear. Every movement of the chest causes pain; therefore the cough is peculiar; it is short and suppressed and comes as near being no cough as the animal can make it in his desire to suppress it. The breathing is hurried, the mouth is hot, the temperature being elevated from 102° or 103° to 105° F. Symptoms that usually accompany fever are present, such as costiveness, scanty, dark-colored urine, etc. The pulse is frequent, perhaps 70 or more a minute, and is hard and wiry. The legs and ears are cold.

Percussion is of valuable service in this affection. After effusion occurs the sound produced by percussing over the lower part of the chest is dull. By striking different parts one may come to a spot of greater or less extent where the blows cause much pain to be evinced. The animal may grunt or groan every time it is struck. Another method of detecting the affected part is to press the fingers between the ribs, each space in succession, beginning behind the elbow, until a place where the pressure causes more flinching than at any other part is reached. Auscultation is also useful. In the first stage, when the surfaces are dry and rough, one may hear, immediately under the ear, a distinct sound very much like that produced by rubbing two pieces of coarse paper together. No such friction sound occurs when the membrane is healthy, as the natural moisture, heretofore mentioned, prevents the friction. In many cases this friction is so pronounced that it may be felt by placing the hand over the affected part. When the dry stage is succeeded by the exudation of fluid this friction sound disappears. After the effusion into the cavity takes place sometimes there is heard a tinkling or metallic sound, due to dropping of the exudate from above into the collected fluid in the bottom of the cavity, as the collected fluid more or less separates the lung from the chest walls.

Within two or three days the urgent symptoms may abate owing to the exudation of the fluid and the subsidence of the pain. The fluid may now undergo absorption, and the case may terminate favorably within a week or 10 days.

If the quantity of the effusion is large its own volume retards the process of absorption to a great extent, and consequently convalescence is delayed. In severe cases the pulse becomes more frequent, the breathing more hurried and labored, the flanks work like bellows, the nostrils flap, the eyes stare wildly, the countenance expresses much anxiety, and general signs of dissolution are plain. After a time swellings appear under the chest and abdomen and down the legs. The accumulation in the chest is called hydrothorax, or dropsy of the chest. When this fluid contains pus the case usually proves fatal. The condition of pus within the cavity is called empyema.

Pleurisy may affect only a small area of one side or it may affect both sides. It is oftener confined to the right side.

Treatment.—The instructions in regard to the general management of bronchitis and pneumonia must be adhered to in the treatment of pleurisy. Comfortable quarters, pure air, warm clothing to the body and bandages to the legs, a plentiful supply of pure cold water, the laxative feed, etc., in this case are equally necessary and efficacious. The hot applications applied to the chest, as directed in the treatment of pneumonia, are very beneficial in pleurisy, and should be kept up while the symptoms show the animal to be in pain.

During the first few days, when pain is manifested by restlessness, apply hot packs to the sides diligently. After four or five days, when the symptoms show that the acute stage has somewhat subsided, mustard may be applied as recommended for pneumonia. From the beginning the following drench may be given every six hours, if the horse takes it kindly: Solution of the acetate of ammonia, 3 ounces; spirits of nitrous ether, 1 ounce; bicarbonate of potassium, 3 drams; water, 1 pint.

If the patient becomes debilitated, the stimulants as prescribed for pneumonia should be used according to the same directions. The same attention should be given to the diet. If the animal will partake of the bran mashes, scalded oats, and grass, it is the best; but if he refuses the laxative diet, then he should be tried with different kinds of feed and allowed whichever kind he desires.

In the beginning of the attack, if the pain is severe, causing the animal to lie down or paw, morphin may be given by the mouth in 5-grain doses, or the fluid extract of *Cannabis indica* may be used in doses of 2 to 4 drams.

If the case is not progressing favorably in ten or twelve days after the beginning of the attack, convalescence is delayed by the fluid in the chest failing to be absorbed. The animal becomes dull and weak and evinces little or no desire for feed. The breathing becomes still more rapid and difficult. An effort must now be made to excite the absorption of the effusion. An application of liniment or mild blister should be rubbed over the lower part of both sides and the bottom of the chest. The following drench may be given three times a day, for seven or eight days, if it is necessary and appears to benefit: Tincture of the perchlorid of iron, 1 ounce; tincture of gentian, 2 ounces; water, 1 pint. Also give 1 dram of iodid of potassium, dissolved in the drinking water, an hour before feeding every night and morning for a week or two.

Hydrothorax is sometimes difficult to overcome by means of the use of medicines alone, when the operation of tapping the chest is performed to allow an escape for the accumulated fluid. The operation is performed with a combined instrument called the trocar and cannula. The puncture is made in the lower part of the chest, in the space between the eighth and ninth ribs. Wounding of the intercostal artery is avoided by inserting the instrument as near as possible to the anterior edge of the rib. If the operation is of benefit, it is only so when performed before the strength is lowered beyond recovery. The operation merely receives a passing notice here, as it is not presumed that the nonprofessional will attempt it, although in the hands of the expert it is attended with little danger or difficulty.

We have described here bronchitis, pneumonia, and pleurisy mainly as they occur as independent diseases, but it should be remembered that they merge into each other and may occur together at one time. While it is true that much more might have been said in regard to the different stages and types of the affections, and also in regard to the treatment of each stage and each particular type, the plan adopted of advising plain, conservative treatment is considered the wisest on account of simplifying as much as possible a subject of which the reader is supposed to know very little.

PLEUROPNEUMONIA.

This is the state in which an animal is affected with pleurisy and pneumonia combined, which is not infrequently the case. At the beginning of the attack only one of the affections may be present, but the other soon follows. It has already been stated that the pleura is closely adherent to the lung. The pleura on this account is frequently more or less affected by the spreading of the inflammation from the lung tissue. There is a combination of the symptoms of both diseases, but to the ordinary observer the symptoms of pleurisy are the most obvious. The course of treatment to be pursued differs in no manner from that given for the affections when they occur independently. The symptoms will be the guide as to the advisability of giving oil and laudanum for the pain if the pleurisy is very severe. It should not be resorted to unless it is necessary to allay the pain.

BRONCHO-PLEUROPNEUMONIA.

This is the term or terms applied when bronchitis, pleurisy, and pneumonia all exist at once. It is impossible for one who is not an expert to diagnose the state with certainty. The apparent symptoms are the same as when the animal is affected with pleuropneumonia.

SUPPURATION AND ABSCESS IN THE LUNG.

There are instances, and especially when the surroundings of the patient have been bad or the disease is of an especially severe type, when pneumonia terminates in an abscess in the lung. Sometimes, when the inflammation has been extreme, suppuration in a large portion of the lung takes place. Impure air, the result of improper ventilation, is among the most frequent causes of this termination. The symptoms of suppuration in the lung are chronic pneumonia, a solidified area of lung tissue, continued low fever, and, in some cases, offensive smell of the breath, and the discharge of the matter from the nostrils.

MORTIFICATION.

Gangrene, or mortification, means the death of the part affected. Occasionally, owing to the intensity of the inflammation or bad treatment, pneumonia and pleuropneumonia terminate in mortification, which is soon followed by the death of the animal. Perhaps the most common cause of this complication is the presence of a foreign body in the lung, as food particles or medicine. Rough drenching or drenching through the nostrils may cause this serious condition.

HEMOPTYSIS, OR BLEEDING FROM THE LUNGS.

Bleeding from the lungs may occur during the course of congestion of the lungs, bronchitis, pneumonia, influenza, purpura hemorrhagica, or glanders. An accident or exertion may cause a rupture of a vessel. Plethora and hypertrophy of the heart predispose to it. Following the rupture of a vessel the blood may escape into the lung tissue and cause a serious attack of pneumonia, or it may fill up the bronchial tubes and prove fatal by suffocating the animal. When the hemorrhage is from the lung it is accompanied with coughing; the blood is frothy, of a bright red color, and comes from both nostrils; whereas when the bleeding is merely from a rupture of a vessel in some part of the head (hertofore described as bleeding from the nose) the blood is most likely to issue from one nostril only, and the discharge is not accompanied with coughing. The ear may be placed against the windpipe along its course, and if the blood is from the lungs a gurgling or rattling sound will be heard. When it occurs in connection with another disease it seldom requires special treatment. When caused by accident or overexertion the animal should be kept quiet. If the hemorrhage is profuse and continues for several hours, 1 dram of the acetate of lead dissolved in a pint of water may be given as a drench, or 1 ounce of the tincture of the perchlorid of iron, diluted with a pint of water, may be given instead of the lead. It is rare that the hemorrhage is so profuse as to require internal remedies. But hemorrhage into the lung may occur and cause death by suffocation without the least manifestation of it by the discharge of blood from the nose.

TUBERCULOSIS OF THE LUNGS.

Pulmonary consumption or tuberculosis has been recognized in the horse in a number of instances. The symptoms are as of chronic pneumonia or pleurisy. There is no treatment for the disease.

HEAVES, BROKEN WIND, OR ASTHMA.

Much confusion exists in the popular mind in regard to the nature of heaves. Many horsemen loosely apply the term to all ailments where the breathing is difficult or noisy. Scientific veterinarians are well acquainted with the phenomena and locality of the affection, but there is a great diversity of opinion as regards the exact cause. Asthma is generally thought to be caused by spasm of the small circular muscles that surround the bronchial tubes. The continued existence of this affection of the muscles leads to a paralysis of them, and the forced breathing to emphysema, which always accompanies heaves.

Heaves is usually associated with disorder of the function of digestion or to an error in the choice of feed. Feeding on clover hay or damaged hay or straw, too bulky and innutritious feed, and keeping the horse in a dusty atmosphere or a badly ventilated stable produce or predispose to heaves. Horses brought from a high to a low level are predisposed.

In itself broken wind is not a fatal disease, but death is generally caused by an affection closely connected with it. After death, if the organs are examined, the lesions found depend much upon the length of time broken wind has affected the animal. In recent cases very few changes are noticeable, but in animals that have been broken-winded for a long time the changes are well marked. The lungs are paler than natural, and of much less weight in proportion to the volume, as evidenced by floating them in water. The walls of the small bronchial tubes and the membrane of the larger tubes are thickened. The right side of the heart is enlarged and its cavities dilated. The stomach is enlarged and its walls stretched. The important change found in the lungs is a condition technically called pulmonary emphysema. This is of two varieties: First, what is termed " vesicular emphysema," which consists of an enlargement of the capacity of the air cells (air vesicles) by dilation of their walls. The second form is called interlobular, or interstitial, emphysema, and follows the first. In this variety the air finds its way into the lung tissue between the air cells or the tissue between the small lobules.

Symptoms.—Almost every experienced horseman is able to detect heaves. The peculiar movement of the flanks and abdomen point out the ailment at once. In recent cases, however, the affected animal does not always exhibit the characteristic breathing unless exerted to a certain extent. The cough which accompanies this disease is peculiar to it. It is difficult to describe, but the sound is short and something like a grunt. When air is inspired—that is, taken in—it appears to be done in the same manner as in health; it may possibly be done a little quicker than natural, but not enough to attract any notice. It is when the act of expiration (or expelling the air from the lungs) is performed that the great change in the breathing is perceptible. It must be remembered that the lungs have lost much of their elasticity, and in consequence of their power for contracting on account of the degeneration of the walls of the air cells, and also on account of the paralysis of muscular tissue before mentioned. The air passes into them freely, but the power to expel it is lost to a great extent by the lungs; therefore the abdominal muscles are brought into play. These muscles, especially in the region of the flank, are seen to contract, then pause for a moment, then complete the act of contracting, thus making a double bellowslike movement at each expiration, a sort of jerky motion with every breath. The double expiratory movement may also be detected by allowing the horse to exhale against the face or back of the hand. It will be observed that the expiratory current is not continuous, but is broken into two jets. When the animal is exerted a wheeezing noise accompanies the breathing. This noise may be heard to a less extent when the animal is at rest if the ear is applied to the chest.

As before remarked, indigestion is often present in these cases. The animal may have a depraved appetite, as shown by a desire to eat dirt and soiled bedding, which he often devours in preferencce to the clean feed in the trough or manger. The stomach is liable to be overloaded with indigestible feed. The abdomen may assume that form called "potbellied." The animal frequently passes wind of a very offensive odor. When first put to work dung is passed frequently; the bowels are often loose. The animal can not stand much work, as the muscular system is soft. Round-chested horses are said to be predisposed to the disease, and it is certain that in cases of long standing the chest usually becomes rounder than natural.

Certain individuals become very expert in managing a horse affected with heaves in suppressing the symptoms for a short time. They take advantage of the fact that the breathing is much easier when the stomach and intestines are empty. They also resort to the use of medicines that have a depressing effect. When the veterinarian is examining a horse for soundness, and he suspects that the animal has been "fixed," he usually gives the horse as much water as he will drink and then has him ridden or driven rapidly up a hill or on a heavy road. This will bring out the characteristic breathing of heaves if the horse is so afflicted, but will not cause the symptoms of heaves in a healthy horse. All broken-winded horses have the cough peculiar to the affection, but it is not regular. A considerable time may elapse before it is heard and then it may come on in paroxysms, especially when first brought out of the stable into the cold air, or when excited by work, or after a drink of cold water. The cough is usually the first symptom of the disease.

Treatment.—When the disease is established there is no cure for it. Proper attention paid to the diet will relieve the distressing symptoms to a certain extent, but they will undoubtedly reappear in their intensity the first time the animal overloads the stomach or is allowed food of bad quality. Clover hay or bulky feed which contains but little nutriment have much to do with the cause of the disease, and therefore should be entirely omitted when the animal is affected, as well as before. It has been asserted that the disease is unknown where clover hay is never used. The diet should be confined to feed of the best quality and in the smallest quantity. The bad effect of moldy or dusty hay, fodder, or feed of any kind can not be overestimated. A small quantity of the best hay once a day is sufficient. This should be cut and dampened. The animal should invariably be watered before feeding; never directly after a meal. The animal should not be worked immediately after a meal. Exertion, when the stomach is full, invariably aggravates the symptoms. Turning on pasture gives relief. Carrots, potatoes, or turnips chopped and mixed with oats or corn are a good diet. Half a pint to a pint of thick, dark molasses with each feed is useful.

Arsenic is efficacious in palliating the symptoms. It is best administered in the form of a solution of arsenic, as Fowler's solution or as the white powdered arsenious acid. Of the former the dose is 1 ounce to the drinking water three times daily; of the latter one may give 3 grains in each feed. These quantities may be cautiously increased as the animal becomes accustomed to the drug. If the bowels do not act regularly, a pint of raw linseed oil may be given once or twice a month, or a handful of Glauber's salt may be given in the feed twice daily, so long as necessary. It must, however, be borne in mind that all medicinal treatment is of secondary consideration; careful attention paid to the diet is of greatest importance. Broken-winded animals should not be used for breeding purposes. A predisposition to the disease may be inherited.

CHRONIC COUGH.

A chronic cough may succeed the acute disease of the respiratory organs, such as pneumonia, bronchitis, laryngitis, etc. It accompanies chronic roaring, chronic bronchitis, broken wind; it may succeed influenza. As previously stated, cough is but a symptom and not a disease in itself. Chronic cough is occasionally associated with diseases other than those of the organs of respiration. It may be a symptom of chronic indigestion or of worms. In such cases it is caused by a reflex nervous irritation. The proper treatment in all cases of chronic cough is to ascertain the nature of the disease of which it is a symptom, and then cure the disease if possible and the cough will cease.

The treatment of the affections will be found under their appropriate heads, to which the reader is referred.

PLEURODYNIA.

This is a form of rheumatism that affects the intercostal muscles; that is, the muscles between the ribs. The apparent symptoms are very similar to those of pleurisy. The animal is stiff and not inclined to turn round; the ribs are kept in a fixed state as much as possible. If the head is pulled round suddenly, or the affected side struck with the hand, or if the spaces between the ribs are pressed with the fingers, the animal will flinch and perhaps emit a grunt or groan expressive of much pain. It is distinguished from pleurisy by the absence of fever, cough, the friction sound, the effusion into the chest, and by the existence of rheumatism in other parts. The treatment for this affection is the same as for rheumatism affecting other parts.

WOUNDS PENETRATING THE WALLS OF THE CHEST.

A wound penetrating the wall of the chest admits air into the thoracic cavity outside the lung. This condition is known as pneumothorax and may result in collapse of the lung. The wound may be so made that when the walls of the chest are dilating a little air is sucked in, but during the contraction of the wall the contained air presses against the torn part in such manner as entirely to close the wound; thus a small quantity of air gains access with each inspiration, while none is allowed to escape until the lung is pressed into a very small compass and forced into the anterior part of the chest. The same thing may occur from a broken rib inflicting a wound in the lung. In this form the air gains access from the lung, and there may not be even an opening in the walls of the chest. In such cases the air may be absorbed, when a spontaneous cure is the result, but when the symptoms are urgent it is recommended that the air be removed by a trocar and cannula or by an aspirator.

It is evident that the treatment of wounds that penetrate the thoracic cavity should be prompt. It should be quickly ascertained whether or not a foreign body remains in the wound; then it should be thoroughly cleaned with a solution of carbolic acid, 1 part in 40 parts of water. The wound should then be closed immediately. If it is an incised wound, it should be closed with sutures or with adhesive plasters; if torn or lacerated, adhesive plaster may be used or a bandage around the chest over the dressing. At all events, air must be prevented from getting into the chest as soon and as effectually as possible. The after treatment of the wound should consist principally in keeping the parts clean with a solution of carbolic acid, and applying fresh dressing as often as required to keep the wound in a healthy condition. Care should be taken that the discharges from the wound have an outlet in the most dependent part. (See Wounds and their treatment, p. 484.) If pleurisy supervenes, it should be treated as advised under that head.

THUMPS, OR SPASM OF THE DIAPHRAGM.

"Thumps" is generally thought by the inexperienced to be a palpitation of the heart. While it is true that palpitation of the heart is sometimes called "thumps," it must not be confounded with the affection under consideration.

In the beginning of this article on the diseases of the organs of respiration, the diaphragm was briefly referred to as the principal and essential muscle of respiration. Spasmodic or irregular contractions of it in man are manifested by what is familiarly known as hiccoughs. Thumps in the horse is similar to hiccoughs in man, although in all cases the peculiar noise is not made in the throat of the horse.

There should be no difficulty in distinguishing this affection from palpitation of the heart. The jerky motion affects the whole body, and is not confined to the region of the heart. If one hand is placed on the body at about the middle of the last rib, while the other hand is placed over the heart behind the left elbow, it will be easily demonstrated that there is no connection between the thumping or jerking of the diaphragm and the beating of the heart. In fact, when the animal is affected with spasms of the diaphragm the beating of the heart is usually much weaker and less perceptible than natural. Thumps is produced by causes similar to those that produce congestion of the lungs and dilatation or palpitation of the heart, and may occur in connection with these conditions. If not relieved, death usually results from congestion or edema of the lungs, as the breathing is interfered with by the inordinate action of this important muscle of inspiration so much that proper aeration of the blood can not take place. The treatment should be as prescribed for congestion of the lungs, and, in addition, antispasmodics, such as 1 ounce of sulphuric ether in warm water or 3 drams of asafetida.

RUPTURE OF THE DIAPHRAGM.

Post-mortem examinations after colic or severe accident sometimes reveal rupture of the diaphragm. This may take place after death, from the generation of gases in the decomposing carcass, which distend the intestines so that the diaphragm is ruptured by the great pressure against it. The symptoms are intensely difficult respiration and great depression. There is no treatment.

DISEASES OF THE URINARY ORGANS.

By JAMES LAW, F. R. C. V. S.,
Formerly Professor of Veterinary Science, etc., in Cornell University.

USES OF THE URINARY ORGANS.

The urinary organs constitute the main channel through which are excreted the nitrogenous or albuminoid principles, whether derived directly from the feed or from the muscular and other nitrogenized tissues of the body. They constitute, besides, the channel through which are thrown out most of the poisons, whether taken in by the mouth or skin or developed in connection with faulty or natural digestion, blood-forming, nutrition, or tissue destruction; or, finally, poisons that are developed within the body, as the result of normal cell life or of the life of bacterial or other germs that have entered the body from without. Bacteria themselves largely escape from the body through the kidneys. To a large extent, therefore, these organs are the sanitary scavengers and purifiers of the system, and when their functions are impaired or arrested the retained poisons quickly show their presence in resulting disorders of the skin and connective tissue beneath it, of the nervous system, or other organs. Nor is this influence one-sided. Scarcely an important organ of the body can suffer derangement without entailing a corresponding disorder of the urinary system. Nothing can be more striking than the mutual balance maintained between the liquid secretions of the skin and kidneys during hot and cold weather. In summer, when so much liquid exhales through the skin as sweat, comparatively little urine is passed, whereas in winter, when the skin is inactive, the urine is correspondingly increased. This vicarious action of skin and kidneys is usually kept within the limits of health, but at times the draining off of the water by the skin leaves too little to keep the solids of the urine safely in solution, and these are liable to crystallize out and form stone and gravel. Similarly the passage, in the sweat, of some of the solids that normally leave the body, dissolved in the urine, serves to irritate the skin and produce troublesome eruptions.

PROMINENT CAUSES OF URINARY DISORDERS.

A disordered liver contributes to the production under different circumstances of an excess of biliary coloring matter which stains the urine; of an excess of hippuric acid and allied products which, being less soluble than urea (the normal product of tissue change),

134

favor the formation of stone, of taurocholic acid, and other bodies that tend when in excess to destroy the blood globules and to cause irritation of the kidneys by the resulting hemoglobin excreted in the urine, and of glycogen too abundant to be burned up in the system, which induces saccharine urine (diabetes). Any disorder leading to impaired functional activity of the lungs is causative of an excess of hippuric acid and allied bodies, of oxalic acid, of sugar, etc., in the urine, which irritate the kidneys, even if they do not produce solid deposits in the urinary passages. Diseases of the nervous system, and notably of the base of the brain and of the spinal cord, induce various urinary disorders, prominent among which are diabetes, chylous urine, and albuminuria. Certain affections, with imperfect nutrition or destructive waste of the bony tissues, tend to charge the urine with phosphates of lime and magnesia and endanger the formation of stone and gravel. In all extensive inflammations and acute fevers the liquids of the urine are diminished, while the solids (waste products), which should form the urinary secretion, are increased, and the surcharged urine proves irritant to the urinary organs or the retained waste products poison the system at large.

Diseases of the heart and lungs, by interfering with the free, onward flow of the blood from the right side of the heart, tend to throw that liquid back on the veins, and this backward pressure of venous blood strongly tends to disorders of the kidneys. Certain poisons taken with the feed and water, notably that found in magnesian limestone and those found in irritant, diuretic plants, are especially injurious to the kidneys, as are also various cryptogams, whether in musty hay or oats. The kidneys may be irritated by feeding green vegetables covered with hoar frost or by furnishing an excess of feed rich in phosphates (wheat bran, beans, peas, vetches, lentils, rape cake, cottonseed cake) or by a privation of water, which entails a concentrated condition and high density of the urine. Exposure in cold rain or snow storms, cold drafts of air, and damp beds are liable to further disorder an already overworked or irritable kidney. Finally, sprains of the back and loins may cause bleeding from the kidneys or inflammation.

The right kidney, weighing 23½ ounces, is shaped like a French bean, and extends from the loins forward to beneath the heads of the last two ribs. The left kidney (Pl. VIII) resembles a heart of cards, and extends from the loins forward beneath the head of the last rib only. Each consists of three distinct parts—(a) the external (cortical), or vascular part, in which the blood vessels form elaborate capillary networks within the dilated globular sacs which form the beginnings of the secreting (uriniferous) tubes and on the surface of the sinuous, secreting tubes leading from the sacs inward toward the second, or medullary, part of the organ; (b) the internal (medullary) part, made up in the main of blood vessels, lymphatics, and nerves extending between the notch on the inner border of the kidney to and from the outer vascular portion, in which the secretion of urine is almost exclusively carried on; and (d) a large, saccular reservoir in the center of the kidney, into which all uriniferous tubes pour their secretions and from which the urine is carried away through a tube g (ureter), which passes out of the notch at the inner border of the kidney and which opens by a valve-closed orifice into the roof of the bladder just in front of its neck. The bladder is a dilatable reservoir for the retention of the urine until the discomfort of its presence causes its voluntary discharge. It is kept closed by circular, muscular fibers surrounding its neck or orifice, and is emptied by looped, muscular fibers extending in all directions forward from the neck around the blind anterior end of the sac. From the bladder the urine escapes through a dilatable tube (urethra) which extends from the neck of the bladder backward on the floor of the pelvis, and in the male through the penis to its free end, where it opens through a pink, conical papilla. In the mare the uretha is not more than an inch in length, and is surrounded by the circular, muscular fibers closing the neck of the bladder. Its opening may be found directly in the median line of the floor of the vulva, about 4½ inches from its external opening.

GENERAL SYMPTOMS OF DISEASE.

These apply especially to acute inflammations and the irritation caused by stone. The animal moves stiffly on the hind limbs, strad-dles, and makes frequent attempts to pass urine, which may be in excess, deficient in amount, liable to sudden arrest in spite of the straining, passed in driblets, or entirely suppressed. Again, it may be modified in density or constituents. Difficulty in making a sharp turn, or in lying down and rising with or without groaning, drop-ping the back when mounted or when pinched on the loins is sugges-tive of kidney disease, and so to a less extent are swelled legs, dropsy, and diseases of the skin and nervous system. The oiled hand intro-duced through the rectum may feel the bladder beneath and detect any overdistention, swelling, tenderness, or stone. In ponies the kid-neys even may be reached.

EXAMINATION OF THE URINE.

In some cases the changes in the urine are the sole sign of disease. In health the horse's urine is of a deep amber color and has a strong odor. On a feed of grain and hay it may show a uniform transpar-ency, while on a green ration there in an abundant white deposit of carbonate of lime. Of its morbid changes the following are to be

PLATE VIII.

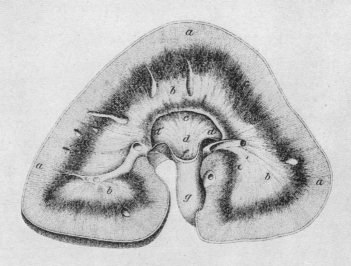

a, Cortical (or vascular) portion; b, Medullary (or tubular) portion; c, Peripheral portion of the latter; d, Interior of the pelvis; d, d, Arms of the pelvis; e, Border of the crest; f, Infundibulum; g, Ureter.

Geo. Marx. del. after D'Arboval. p. 669.

LONGITUDINAL SECTION THROUGH KIDNEY.

PLATE IX.

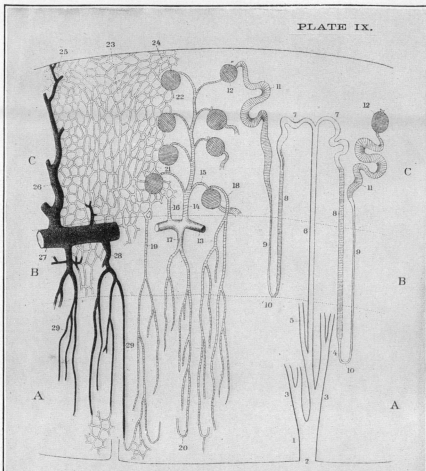

Structure of the Kidney. Diagrammatic.

a, Medullary layer; b, Boundary zone; c, Cortical layer; 1, Excretory tube; 2, Opening on the summit of renal papilla; 3, First branch of bifurcation; 4, Second branch of bifurcation; 5, Third branch of bifurcation; 6, Straight collecting tube; 7, Junctional tubule; 8, Ascending portion of Henle's loop; 9, Descending portion of Henle's loop; 10, Loop of Henle; 11, Convoluted tubule; 12, Malpighian corpuscle; 13, Renal artery; 14, Branch supplying the glomeruli; 15, Afferent vessel of the glomeruli; 16, Branch going directly to the capillaries; 17, Straight arterioles coming directly from the renal artery; 18, Straight arteriole coming from the afferent vessel of the glomerulus; 19, Straight arteriole coming from the capillary plexus; 20, Vascular loop of the pyramids; 21, Efferent vessel of the glomerulus going to the capillary plexus; 22, Capillary plexus of the glomerular part of the cortical substance; 23, Capillary plexus of the pyramids of Ferrein; 24, Cortical plexus of the kidney; 25, Venae stellatae; 26, Vein coming from the capillaries of the cortex; 27, Interlobular vein; 28, Vein receiving the venae rectae; 29, Venae rectae.

Note: The shaded part of the urinary ducts represent the part in which the epithelium is rodded and of a granular appearance.

Geo. Marx, after D'Arboval. p 372. 371.

MICROSCOPIC ANATOMY OF KIDNEY.

PLATE X.

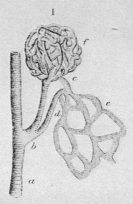

Renal Glomerulus.

a, Artery of the glomerulus; b, Branch supplying the afferent vessel of the glomerulus; c, Afferent vessel of the glomerule; d, Artery going directly to the capillary plexus of the cortical substance; e, Capillary plexus; f, Glomerulus.

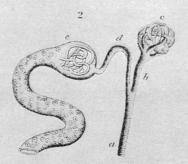

Renal Glomerulus with its afferent vessels and efferents.

a, Branch of renal artery; b, Afferent vessel of the glomerulus; c, Glomerulus; d, Afferent vessel going into corpuscle e, of Malpighi.

MICROSCOPIC ANATOMY OF KIDNEY.

looked for: (1) *Color:* White from deposited salts of lime; brown or red from blood clots or coloring matter; yellow or orange from bile or blood pigment; pale from excess of water; or variously colored from vegetable ingredients (santonin makes it red; rhubarb or senna, brown; tar or carbolic acid, green). (2) *Density:* The horse's urine may be 1.030 or 1.050, but it may greatly exceed this in diabetes and may sink to 1.007 in diuresis. (3) *Chemical reaction*, as ascertained by blue litmus or red test papers. The horse on vegetable diet has alkaline urine turning red test papers blue, while in the sucking colt and the horse fed on flesh or on his own tissue (in starvation or abstinence during disease) it is acid, turning blue litmus red. (4) *Organic constituents*, as when glairy from albumen coagulable by strong nitric acid and boiling, when charged with microscopic casts of the uriniferous tubes, with the eggs or bodies of worms, with sugar, blood, or bile. (5) *In its salts*, which may crystallize out spontaneously, or on boiling, or on the addition of chemical reagents.

Albuminous urine in the horse is usually glairy, so that it may be drawn out in threads, but its presence can always be tested as follows: If the liquid is opaque, it may be first passed through filter paper; if very dense and already precipitating its salts, it may be diluted with distilled water; add to the suspected liquid acetic acid drop by drop until it reddens the blue litmus paper; then boil gently in a test tube; if a precipitate is thrown down, set the tube aside to cool and then add strong nitric acid. If the precipitate is not dissolved, it is albumen; if dissolved it is probably urate or hippurate of ammonia. Albumen is normally present in advanced gestation; abnormally it is seen in diseases in which there occurs destruction of blood globules (anthrax, low fevers, watery states of the blood, dropsies), in diseases of the heart and liver which prevent the free escape of blood from the veins and throw back venous pressure on the kidneys, in inflammation of the lungs and pleuræ, and even tympany (bloating), doubtless from the same cause, and in all congestive or inflammatory diseases of the kidneys, acute or chronic.

Casts of the uriniferous tubes can be seen only by placing the suspected urine under the microscope. They are usually very elastic and mobile, waving about in the liquid when the cover glass is touched, and showing a uniform, clear transparency (waxy) or entangled circular epithelial cells or opaque granules or flattened, red-blood globules or clear, refrangent oil globules. They may be even densely opaque from crystals of earthy salts.

Pus cells may be found in the urine associated with albumen, and are recognized by clearing up, when treated with acetic acid, so that each cell shows two or three nuclei.

DIURESIS (POLYURIA, DIABETES INSIPIDUS, OR EXCESSIVE SECRETION OF URINE).

This consists in an excessive secretion of a clear, watery urine of a low specific gravity (1.007) with a correspondingly ardent thirst, a rapidly advancing emaciation, and great loss of strength and spirit.

Causes.—Its causes may be any agent—medicinal, alimentary, or poisonous—which unduly stimulates the kidneys; the reckless administration of diuretics, which form such a common constituent of quack horse powders; acrid diuretic plants in grass or hay; new oats still imperfectly cured; an excess of roots or other very watery feed; a full allowance of salt to animals that have become inordinately fond of it; but, above all, feeding on hay, grain, or bran which has not been properly dried and has become musty and permeated by fungi. Thus hay, straw, or oats obtained in wet seasons and heating in the rick or stack is especially injurious. Hence this malady, like coma somnolentum (sleepy staggers), is widespread in wet seasons, and especially in rainy districts.

Symptoms.—The horse drinks deep at every opportunity and passes urine on every occasion when stopped, the discharge being pale, watery, of a low density, and inodorous; in short, it contains a great excess of water and a deficiency of the solid excretions. So great is the quantity passed, however, that the small amount of solids in any given specimen amounts in 24 hours to far more than the normal—a fact in keeping with the rapid wasting of the tissues and extreme emaciation. The flanks become tucked up, the fat disappears, the bones and muscles stand out prominently, the skin becomes tense and hidebound, and the hair erect, scurfy, and deficient in luster. The eye becomes dull and sunken, the spirits are depressed, the animal is weak and sluggish, sweats on the slightest exertion, and can endure little. The subject may survive for months, or may die early of exhaustion. In the slighter cases, or when the cause ceases to operate, a somewhat tardy recovery may be made.

Treatment consists in stopping the ingestion of the faulty drugs, poisons, or feed, and supplying sound hay and grain free from all taint of heating or mustiness. A liberal supply of boiled flaxseed in the drinking water at once serves to eliminate the poison and to sheathe and protect the irritated kidneys. Tonics like sulphate or phosphate of iron (2 drams morning and evening) and powdered gentian or Peruvian bark (4 drams) help greatly by bracing the system and hastening repair. To these may be added agents calculated to destroy the fungus and eliminate its poisonous products. In that form which depends on musty food nothing acts better than large doses of iodid of potassium (2 drams), while in other cases creosote, carbolic acid (1 dram), or oil of turpentine (4 drams), properly diluted, may be resorted to.

SACCHARINE DIABETES (DIABETES MELLITUS, GLYCOSURIA, OR INOSURIA).

This is primarily a disease of the nervous system or liver rather than of the kidneys, yet, as the most prominent symptom is the sweet urine, it may be treated here.

Causes.—Its causes are varied, but resolve themselves largely into disorder of the liver or disorder of the brain. One of the most prominent functions of the liver is the formation of glycogen, a principle allied to grape sugar, and passing into it by further oxidation in the blood. This is a constant function of the liver, but in health the resulting sugar is burned up in the circulation and does not appear in the urine. On the contrary, when the supply of oxygen is defective, as in certain diseases of the lungs, the whole of the sugar does not undergo combustion and the excess is excreted by the kidneys. Also in certain forms of enlarged liver the quantity of sugar produced is more than can be disposed of in the natural way, and it appears in the urine. A temporary sweetness of the urine often occurs after a hearty meal on starchy feed, but this is due altogether to the superabundant supply of the sugar-forming feed, lasts for a few hours only, and has no pathological significance. In many cases of fatal glycosuria the liver is found to be enlarged, or at least congested, and it is found that the disorder can be produced experimentally by agencies which produce an increased circulation through the liver. Thus Bernard produced glycosuria by pricking the oblong medulla at the base of the brain close to the roots of the pneumogastric nerve, which happens to be also the nerve center (vasomotor) which presides over the contractions of the minute blood vessels. The pricking and irritation of this center leads to congestion of the liver and the excessive production of sugar. Irritation carried to this point through the pneumogastric nerve causes saccharine urine, and, in keeping with this, disease of the pancreas has been found in this malady. The complete removal of the pancreas, however, determines glycosuria, the organ having in health an inhibitive action on sugar production by the liver. The same result follows the reflection of irritation from other sources, as from different ganglia (corpora striata, optic thalami, pons, cerebellum, cerebrum) of the brain. Similarly it is induced by interruption of the nervous control along the vasomotor tracts, as in destruction of the upper or lower cervical sympathetic ganglion, by cutting the nervous branch connecting these two, in injury to the spinal marrow in the interval between the brain and the second or fourth dorsal vertebra, or in disease of the celiac plexus, which directly presides over the liver. Certain chemical poisons also cause saccharine urine, notably woorara, strychnia, morphia, phosphoric acid, alcohol, ether, quinia, chloroform, ammonia, arsenic, and phlorizin.

Symptoms.—The symptoms are ardent thirst and profuse secretion of a pale urine of a high density (1.060 and upward), rapid loss of condition, scurfy, unthrifty skin, costiveness or irregularity of the bowels, indigestion, and the presence, in the urine, of a sweet principle—grape sugar or inosite, or both. This may be most promptly detected by touching the tip of the tongue with a drop. Sugar may be detected simply by adding a teaspoonful of liquid yeast to 4 ounces of the urine and keeping it lightly stopped at a temperature of 70° to 80° F. for 12 hours, when the sugar will be found to have been changed into alcohol and carbon dioxid. The loss of density will give indication of the quantity of sugar transformed; thus a density of 1.035 in a urine which was formerly 1.060 would indicate about 15 grains of sugar to the fluid ounce.

Inosite, or muscle sugar, frequently present in the horse's urine, and even replacing the glucose, is not fermentable. Its presence may be indicated by its sweetness and the absence of fermentation or by Gallois's test. Evaporate the suspected urine at a gentle heat almost to dryness, then add a drop of a solution of mercuric nitrate and evaporate carefully to dryness, when a yellowish residue is left that is changed on further cautious heating to a deep rose color, which disappears on cooling and reappears on heating.

In advanced diabetes, dropsies in the limbs and under the chest and belly, puffy, swollen eyelids, cataracts, catarrhal inflammation of the lungs, weak, uncertain gait, and drowsiness may be noted.

Treatment is most satisfactory in cases dependent on some curable disease of liver, pancreas, lungs, or brain. Thus, in liver diseases, a run at pasture in warm weather, or in winter a warm, sunny, well-aired stable, with sufficient clothing and laxatives (sulphate of soda, 1 ounce daily) and alkalies (carbonate of potassium, one-fourth ounce) may benefit. To this may be added mild blistering, cupping, or even leeching over the last ribs. Diseases of the brain or pancreas may be treated according to their indications. The diet should be mainly albuminous, such as wheat bran or middlings, peas, beans, vetches, and milk. Indeed, an exclusive milk diet is one of the very best remedial agencies. It may be given as skimmed milk or buttermilk, and in the last case combines an antidiabetic remedy in the lactic acid. Under such an exclusive diet recent and mild cases are often entirely restored, though at the expense of an attack of rheumatism. Codeia, one of the alkaloids of opium, is strongly recommended by Tyson. The dose for the horse would be 10 to 15 grains thrice daily. In cases in which there is manifest irritation of the brain, bromid of potassium, 4 drams, or ergot one-half ounce, may be resorted to. Salicylic acid and salicylate of sodium have proved useful in certain cases; also phosphate of sodium. Bitter tonics (especially nux vomica one-half dram) are useful in improving the digestion and general health.

HEMATURIA (BLOODY URINE).

Cause.—As seen in the horse, bloody urine is usually the direct result of mechanical injuries, as sprains and fractures of the loins, lacerations of the sublumbar muscles (psoas), irritation caused by stone in the kidney, ureter, bladder, or urethra. It may, however, occur with acute congestion of the kidney, with tumors in its substance, or with papilloma or other diseased growth in the bladder. Acrid diuretic plants present in the feed may also lead to the escape of blood from the kidney. The predisposition to this affection is, however, incomparably less than in the case of the ox or the sheep, the difference being attributed to the greater plasticity of the horse's blood in connection with the larger quantity of fibrin.

The blood may be present in small clots or in more or less intimate admixture with the urine. Its condition may furnish some indication as to its source; thus, if from the kidneys it is more liable to be uniformly diffused through the urine, while as furnished by the bladder or passages clots are more liable to be present. Again, in bleeding from the kidney, minute, cylindrical clots inclosing blood globules and formed in the uriniferous tubes can be detected under the microscope. Precision also may be approximated by observing whether there is coexisting fracture, sprain of the loins, or stone or tumor in the bladder or urethra.

Treatment.—The disease being mainly due to direct injury, treatment will consist, first, in removing such cause whenever possible, and then in applying general and local styptics. Irritants in feed must be avoided, sprains appropriately treated, and stone in bladder or urethra removed. Then give mucilaginous drinks (slippery elm, linseed tea) freely, and styptics (tincture of chlorid of iron 3 drams, acetate of lead one-half dram, tannic acid one-half dram, or oil of turpentine 1 ounce). If the discharge is abundant, apply cold water to the loins and keep the animal perfectly still.

HEMOGLOBINURIA (AZOTURIA, AZOTEMIA, POISONING BY ALBUMINOIDS).

Like diabetes, this is rather a disease of the liver and blood-forming functions than of the kidney, but as prominent symptoms are loss of control over the hind limbs and the passage of ropy and dark-colored urine, the vulgar idea is that it is a disorder of the urinary organs. It is a complex affection directly connected with a plethora in the blood of nitrogenized constituents, with extreme nervous and muscular disorder and the excretion of a dense reddish or brownish urine. It is directly connected with high feeding, especially on highly nitrogenized feed (oats, beans, peas, vetches, cottonseed meal), and with a period of idleness in the stall under full rations. The disease is never seen at pasture, rarely under constant daily work, even though the feeding is high, and the attack is usually precipitated by taking the horse from the stable and subjecting it to exercise or work. The poisoning is not present when taken from the stable, as the horse is likely to be noticeably lively and spirited, but he will usually succumb under the first hundred yards or half mile of exercise. It seems as if the aspiratory power of the chest under the sudden exertion and accelerated breathing speedily drew from the gorged liver and abdominal veins (portal) the accumulated store of nitrogenous matter in an imperfectly oxidized or elaborated condition, and as if the blood, surcharged with these materials, were unable to maintain the healthy functions of the nerve centers and muscles. It has been noticed rather more frequently in mares than horses, attributable, perhaps, to the nervous excitement attendant on heat, and to the fact that the unmutilated mare is naturally more excitable than the docile gelding.

Lignières has found in hemoglobinuria a streptococcus which produced nephritis, bloody urine, and paraplegia in experimental animals, including horses.

Symptons.—In the milder forms this affection may appear as a lameness in one limb, from indefinite cause, succeeding to some sudden exertion and attended by a dusky-brown color of the membranes of the eye and nose and some wincing when the last ribs are struck. The severe forms come on after one or two days of rest on a full ration, when the animal has been taken out and driven one hundred paces or more. The fire and life with which he had left the stable suddenly give place to dullness and oppression, as shown in heaving flanks, dilated nostrils, pinched face, perspiring skin, and trembling body. The muscles of the loins or haunch become swelled and rigid, the subject moves stiffly or unsteadily, crouches behind, the limbs being carried semiflexed, and he soon drops, unable to support himself. When down, the body and limbs are moved convulsively, but there is no power of coordination of movement in the muscles. The pulse and breathing are accelerated, the eyes red with a tinge of brown, and the urine, if passed, is seen to be highly colored, dark brown, red, or black, but it contains neither blood clots nor globules. The color is mainly due to hemoglobin and other imperfectly elaborated constituents of the blood.

It may end fatally in a few hours or days, or a recovery may ensue, which is usually more speedy and perfect if it has set in at an early stage. In the late and tardy recoveries a partial paralysis of the hind limbs may last for months. A frequent sequel of these tardy cases is an extensive wasting of the muscles leading up from the front of the stifle (those supplied by the crural nerve) and a complete inability to stand.

Prevention.—The prevention of this serious affection lies in restricting the diet and giving daily exercise when the animal is not at work. A horse that has had one attack should never be left idle for a single day in the stall or barnyard. When a horse has been condemned to absolute repose on good feeding he may have a laxative (one-half to 1 pound Glauber's salt), and have graduated exercise, beginning with a short walk and increasing day by day.

Treatment.—The treatment of the mild cases may consist in a laxative, graduated daily exercise, and a daily dose of saltpeter (1 ounce). Sudden attacks will sometimes promptly subside if taken on the instant and the subject kept still and calmed by a dose of bromid of potassium (4 drams) and sweet spirits of niter (1 ounce). The latter has the advantage of increasing the secretion of the kidneys. Iodid of potassium in one-half ounce doses every four hours has succeeded well in some hands. In severe cases, as a rule, it is desirable to begin treatment by a dose of aloes (4 to 6 drams) with the above-named dose of bromid of potassium, and this latter may be continued at intervals of four or six hours, as may be requisite to calm the nervous excitement. Fomentations with warm water over the loins are always useful in calming the excitable conditions of the spinal cord, muscles, liver, and kidneys, and also in favoring secretion from the two latter. On the second day diuretics may be resorted to, such as saltpeter one-half ounce, and powdered colchicum one-half dram, to be repeated twice daily. A laxative may be repeated in three or four days should the bowels seem to demand it, and as the nervous excitement disappears any remaining muscular weakness or paralysis may be treated by one-half dram doses of nux vomica twice a day and a stimulating liniment (aqua ammonia and sweet oil in equal proportions) rubbed on the torpid muscles.

During the course of the disease friction to the limbs is useful, and in the advanced paralytic stage the application of electricity along the line of the affected muscles. When the patient can not stand he must have a thick, soft bed, and should be turned from side to side at least every twelve hours. As soon as he can be made to stand he may be helped up and even supported in a sling.

ACUTE INFLAMMATION OF THE KIDNEYS, OR ACUTE NEPHRITIS.

Inflammations of the kidneys have been differentiated widely, according as they were acute or chronic, parenchymatous or tubal, suppurative or not, with increased or shrunken kidney, etc. In a work like the present, however, utility will be consulted by classing all under acute or chronic inflammation.

Causes.—The causes of inflammation of the kidneys are extremely varied. Congestion occurs from the altered and irritant products passed through these organs during recovery from inflammations of other organs and during fevers. This may last only during the existence of its cause, or may persist and become aggravated. Heart disease, throwing the blood pressure back on the veins and kidneys, is another cause. Disease of the ureter or bladder, preventing the escape of urine from the kidney and causing increased fullness and tension in its pelvis and tubes, will determine inflammation. Decomposition of the detained urine in such cases and the production of ammonia and other irritants must also be named. In elimination of bacteria through the kidney, the latter is liable to infection with consequent inflammation. The advance of bacteria upward from the bladder to the kidneys is another cause. The consumption in hay or other fodder of acrid or irritant plants, including fungi, the absorption of cantharidine from a surface blistered by Spanish flies, the reckless administration of diuretics, the presence of stones in the kidney, exposure of the surface to cold and wet, and the infliction of blows or sprains on the loins, may contribute to its production. Liver disorders which throw on the kidneys the work of excreting irritant products, diseases of the lungs and heart from which clots are carried, to be arrested in the small blood vessels of the kidney, and injuries and paralysis of the spinal cord, are additional causes.

Symptoms.—The symptoms are more or less fever, manifest stiffness of the back and straddling gait with the hind limbs, difficulty in lying down and rising, or in walking in a circle, the animal sometimes groaning under the effort, arching of the loins and tucking up of the flank, looking back at the abdomen as if from colicky pain, and tenderness of the loins to pinching, especially just beneath the bony processes 6 inches to one side of the median line. Urine is passed frequently, a small quantity at a time, of a high color, and sometimes mixed with blood or even pus. Under the microscope it shows the microscopic casts referred to under general symptoms. If treated by acetic acid, boiling and subsequent addition of strong nitric acid, the resulting and persistent precipitate indicates the amount of albumen. The legs tend to swell from the foot up, also the dependent parts beneath the belly and chest, and effusions of liquid may occur within the chest or abdomen. In the male the alternate drawing up and relaxation of the testicles in the scrotum are suggestive, and in small horses the oiled hand introduced into the rectum may reach the kidney and ascertain its sensitiveness.

Treatment demands, first, the removal of any recognized cause. Then, if the suffering and fever are high, 2 to 4 quarts of blood may be abstracted from the jugular vein; in weak subjects or unless in high fever this should be omitted. Next relieve the kidneys so far as possible by throwing their work on the bowels and skin. A pint of castor oil is less likely than either aloes or salts to act on the kidneys. To affect the skin a warm stall and heavy clothing may be supplemented by dram doses of Dover's powder. Pain may be soothed by dram doses of bromid of potassium. Boiled flaxseed may be added to the drinking water, also thrown into the rectum as an injection, and blankets saturated with hot water should be persistently applied to the loins. This may be followed by a very thin pulp of the best ground mustard made with tepid water, rubbed in against the direction of the hair and covered with paper and a blanket. This may be kept on for an hour, or until the skin thickens and the hair stands erect. It may then be rubbed or sponged off and the blanket reapplied. When the action of the bowels has been started it may be kept up by a daily dose of 2 or 3 ounces of Glauber's salt.

During recovery a course of bitter tonics (nux vomica 1 scruple, ground gentian root 4 drams) should be given. The patient should also be guarded against cold, wet, and any active exertion for some time after all active symptoms have subsided.

CHRONIC INFLAMMATION OF THE KIDNEYS.

Causes.—Chronic inflammation of the kidneys is more commonly associated with albumen and casts in the urine than the acute form, and in some instances these conditions of the urine may be the only prominent symptoms of the disease. Though it may supervene on blow, injuries, and exposures, it is much more commonly connected with faulty conditions of the system—as indigestion, heart disease, lung or liver disease, imperfect blood formation, or assimilation; in short, it is rather the attendant on a constitutional infirmity than on a simple local injury.

It may be associated with various forms of diseased kidneys, as shrinkage (atrophy), increase (hypertrophy), softening, red congestion, white enlargement, etc., so that it forms a group of diseases rather than a disease by itself.

Symptoms.—The symptoms may include stiffness, weakness, and increased sensibility of the loins, and modified secretion of urine (increase or suppression), or the flow may be natural. Usually it contains albumen, the quantity furnishing a fair criterion of the gravity of the affection, and microscopic casts, also most abundant in bad cases. Dropsy, manifested in swelled legs, is a significant symptom, and if the effusion takes place along the lower line of the body or in chest or abdomen, the significance is increased. A scurfy, unthrifty skin, lack-luster hair, inability to sustain severe or continued exertion, poor or irregular appetite, loss of fat and flesh, softness of the muscles, and pallor of the eyes and nose are equally suggestive. So are skin eruptions of various kinds. Any one or more of these symptoms would warrant an examination of the urine for albumen and casts, the finding of which signifies renal inflammation.

54763°—23——10

Treatment of these cases is not always satisfactory, as the cause is liable to be maintained in the disorders of important organs elsewhere. If any such coincident disease of another organ or function can be detected, that should be treated first or simultaneously with this affection of the kidneys. In all cases the building up of the general health is important. Hence a course of tonics may be given (phosphate of iron 2 drams, nux vomica 20 grains, powdered gentian root 4 drams, daily) or 60 drops of sulphuric acid or nitrohydrochloric acid may be given daily in the drinking water. If there is any elevated temperature of the body and tenderness of the loins, fomentations may be applied, followed by a mustard pulp, as for acute inflammation, and even in the absence of these indications the mustard may be resorted to with advantage at intervals of a few days. In suppression of urine, fomentations with warm water or with infusion of digitalis leaves is a safer resort than diuretics, and cupping over the loins may also benefit. To apply a cup, shave the skin and oil it; then take a narrow-mouthed glass, rarify the air within it by introducing a taper in full flame for a second, withdraw the taper and instantly apply the mouth of the glass to the skin and hold it closely applied till the cooling tends to form a vacuum in the glass and to draw up the skin, like a sucker.

As in the acute inflammation, every attention must be given to secure warm clothing, a warm stall, and pure air.

TUMORS OF THE KIDNEYS.

Tumors, whether malignant or simple, would give rise to symptoms resembling some form of inflammation, and are not liable to be recognized during life.

PARASITES.

To parasites of the kidney belong the echinococcus, the larval, or bladder worm, stage of the small echinococcus tapeworm of the dog. *Dioctophyme renale*, the largest of roundworms, has been found in the kidney of the horse. Its presence can be certified only by the passage of its microscopic eggs or of the entire worm. Immature stages of roundworms, either *Strongylus equinus* or a related species. may be found in the renal artery or in the kidney itself.

SPASM OF THE NECK OF THE BLADDER.

This affection consists in spasmodic closure of the outlet from the bladder by tonic contraction of the circular muscular fibers. It may be accompanied with a painful contraction of the muscles on the body of the bladder; or, if the organ is already unduly distended, these will be affected with temporary paralysis. It is most frequent in the horse, but by no means unknown in the mare.

Causes.—The causes are usually hard and continuous driving without opportunity for passing urine, cold rainstorms, drafts of cold air when perspiring and fatigued, the administration of Spanish fly or the application of extensive blisters of the same, abuse of diuretics, the presence of acrid, diuretic plants in the fodder, and the presence of stone in the bladder. As most mares refuse to urinate while in harness, they should be unhitched at suitable times for urination. Spasms of the bowels are always attended by spasm of the bladder, hence the free passage of water is usually a symptom of relief.

Symptoms.—The symptoms are frequent stretching and straining to urinate, with no result or a slight dribbling only. These vain efforts are attended by pain and groaning. On resuming his natural position the animal is not freed from the pain, but moves uneasily, paws, shakes the tail, kicks at the abdomen with his hind feet, looks back to the flank, lies down and rises, arches the back, and attempts to urinate as before. If the oiled hand is introduced into the rectum the greatly distended bladder may be felt beneath, and the patient will often shrink when it is handled.

It is important to notice that irritation of the urinary organs is often present in impaction of the colon with solid matters, because the impacted intestine under the straining of the patient is forced backward into the pelvis and presses upon and irritates the bladder. In such cases the horse stands with his fore limbs advanced and the hind ones stretched back beyond the natural posture and makes frequent efforts to urinate, with varying success. Unpracticed observers naturally conclude that the secondary urinary trouble is the main and only one, and the intestinal impaction and obstruction is too often neglected until it is irremediable. In cases in which the irritation has caused spasm of the neck of the bladder and overdistention of that organ, the mistake is still more easily made; hence it is important in all cases to examine for the impacted bowel, forming a bend or loop at the entrance of the pelvis and usually toward the left side. The impacted intestine feels soft and doughy and is easily indented with the knuckles, forming a marked contrast with the tense, elastic, resilient, overdistended bladder.

It remains to be noted that similar symptoms may be determined by a stone or sebaceous mass, or stricture obstructing the urethra, or in the newborn by thickened mucus in that duct and by the pressure of hardened, impacted feces in the rectum. In obstruction, the hard, impacted body can usually be felt by tracing the urethra along the lower and posterior surface of the penis and forward to the median line of the floor of the pelvis to the neck of the bladder. That part of the urethra between the seat of obstruction and the bladder is usually distended with urine and feels enlarged, elastic, and fluctuating.

Treatment.—Treatment may be begun by taking the animal out of harness. This failing, spread clean litter beneath the belly or turn the patient out on the dung heap. Some seek to establish sympathetic action by pouring water from one vessel into another with dribbling noise. Others soothe and distract the attention by slow whistling. Friction of the abdomen with wisps of straw may succeed, or it may be rubbed with ammonia and oil. These failing, an injection of 2 ounces of laudanum or of an infusion of 1 ounce of tobacco in water may be tried. In the mare the neck of the bladder is easily dilated by inserting two oiled fingers and slightly parting them. In the horse the oiled hand introduced into the rectum may press from before backward on the anterior or blind end of the bladder. Finally, a well-oiled gum-elastic catheter may be entered into the urethra through the papilla at the end of the penis and pushed on carefully until it has entered the bladder. To effect this the penis must first be withdrawn from its sheath, and when the advancing end of the catheter has reached the bend of the urethra beneath the anus it must be guided forward by pressure with the hand, which guidance must be continued onward into the bladder, the oiled hand being introduced into the rectum for this purpose. The horse catheter, $3\frac{1}{2}$ feet long and one-third inch in diameter, may be bought of a surgical-instrument maker.

PARALYSIS OF THE BLADDER.

Paralysis of the body of the bladder with spasm of the neck has been described under the last heading, and may occur in the same way from overdistention in tetanus, acute rheumatism, paraplegia, and hemiplegia, in which the animal can not stretch himself to urinate, and in cystitis, affecting the body of the bladder but not the neck. In all these cases the urine is suppressed. It also occurs as a result of disease of the posterior end of the spinal marrow and with broken back, and is then associated with palsy of the tail, and, it may be, of the hind limbs.

Symptoms.—The symptoms are a constant dribbling of urine when the neck is involved, the liquid running down the inside of the thighs and irritating the skin. When the neck is unaffected the urine is retained until the bladder is greatly overdistended, when it may be expelled in a gush by the active contraction of the muscular walls of the abdomen; this never empties the bladder, however, and the oiled hand introduced through the rectum may feel the soft, flabby organ still half full of urine. This retained urine is liable to decompose and give off ammonia, which dissolves the epithelial cells, exposing the raw, mucous membrane and causing the worst type of cystitis.

Suppression and incontinence of urine are common also to obstruction of the urethra by stone or otherwise; hence this source of fallacy should be excluded by manual examination along the whole course of that duct.

Treatment.—Treatment is only applicable in cases in which the determining cause can be abated. In remedial sprains of the back or disease of the spinal cord these must have appropriate treatment, and the urine must be drawn off frequently with a catheter to prevent overdistention and injury to the bladder. If the paralysis persists after recovery of the spinal cord, or if it continues after relief of spasm of the neck of the bladder, apply a pulp of mustard and water over the back part of the belly in front of the udder, and cover with a rug until the hair stands erect. In the male the mustard may be applied between the thighs from near the anus downward. Daily doses of 2 drams extract of belladonna or of 2 grains powdered Spanish fly may serve to rouse the lost tone. These failing, a mild current of electricity daily may succeed.

INFLAMMATION OF THE BLADDER (CYSTITIS, OR UROCYSTITIS).

Cystitis may be slight or severe, acute or chronic, partial or general. It may be caused by abuse of diuretics, especially such as are irritating (cantharides, turpentine, copaiba, resin, etc.), by the presence of a stone or gravel in the bladder, the irritation of a catheter or other foreign body introduced from without, the septic ferment (bacterium) introduced on a filthy catheter, the overdistention of the bladder by retained urine, the extrication of ammonia from retained decomposing urine, resulting in destruction of the epithelial cells and irritation of the raw surface, and a too concentrated and irritating urine. The application of Spanish flies or turpentine over a too extensive surface, sudden exposure of a perspiring and tired horse to cold or wet, and the presence of acrid plants in the fodder may cause cystitis, as they may nephritis. Finally, inflammation may extend from a diseased vagina or urethra to the bladder.

Symptoms.—The symptoms are slight or severe colicky pains; the animal moves his hind feet uneasily or even kicks at the abdomen, looks around at his flank, and may even lie down and rise frequently. More characteristic are frequently repeated efforts to urinate, resulting in the discharge of a little clear, or red, or more commonly flocculent urine, always in jets, and accompanied with signs of pain, which persist after the discharge, as shown in continued straining, groaning, and perhaps in movements of the feet and tail. The penis hangs from the sheath, or in the mare the vulva is frequently opened and closed, as after urination. The animal winces when the abdomen is pressed in the region of the sheath or udder, and the bladder is found to be sensitive and tender when pressed with the oiled hand introduced through the rectum or vagina. In the mare the thickening of the walls of the bladder may be felt by introducing one finger through the urethra. The discharged urine, which may be turbid or even oily, contains an excess of mucus, with flat shreds of membrane, with scaly epithelial cells, and pus corpuscles, each showing two or more nuclei when treated with acetic acid, but there are no microscopic tubular casts, as in nephritis. If due to stone in the bladder. that will be found on examination through rectum or vagina.

Treatment implies, first, the removal of the cause, whether poisons in feed or as medicine, the removal of Spanish flies or other blistering agents from the skin, or the extraction of stone or gravel. If the urine has been retained and decomposed it must be completely evacuated through a clean catheter, and the bladder thoroughly washed out with a solution of 1 dram of borax in a quart of water. This must be repeated twice daily until the urine no longer decomposes, because so long as ammonia is developed in the bladder the protecting layer of epithelial cells will be dissolved and the surface kept raw and irritable. The diet must be light (bran mashes, roots, fresh grass), and the drink impregnated with linseed tea, or solution of slippery elm or marsh mallow. The same agents may be used to inject into the rectum, or they may even be used along with borax and opium to inject into bladder (gum arabic 1 dram, opium 1 dram. tepid water 1 pint). Fomentations over the loins are often of great advantage, and these may be followed or alternated with the application of mustard, as in paralysis; or the mustard may be applied on the back part of the abdomen below or between the thighs from the anus downward. Finally, when the acute symptoms have subsided, a daily dose of buchu 1 dram and nux vomica one-half dram will serve to restore lost tone.

IRRITABLE BLADDER.

Some horses, and especially mares, show an irritability of the bladder and nerve centers presiding over it by frequent urination in small quantities, though the urine is not manifestly changed in character and no more than the natural quantity is passed in the twenty-four hours. The disorder appears to have its source quite as frequently in the generative or nervous system as in the urinary. A troublesome and dangerous form is seen in mares, which dash off and refuse all control by the rein if driven with a full bladder, but usually prove docile if the bladder has been emptied before hitching. In other cases the excitement connected with getting the tail over the reins is a powerful determining cause. The condition is marked in many mares during the period of heat.

An oleaginous laxative (castor oil 1 pint) will serve to remove any cause of irritation in the digestive organs, and a careful dieting will avoid continued irritation by acrid vegetable agents. The bladder should be examined to see that there is no stone or other cause of irritation, and the sheath and penis should be washed with soapsuds, any sebaceous matter removed from the bilocular cavity at the end of the penis, and the whole lubricated with sweet oil. Irritable mares should be induced to urinate before they are harnessed, and those that clutch the lines under the tail may have the tail set high by cutting the cords on its lower surface, or it may be prevented from getting over the reins by having a strap carried from its free end to the breeching. Those proving troublesome when " in heat " may have 4-dram doses of bromid of potassium, or they may be served by the male or castrated. Sometimes irritability may be lessened by daily doses of belladonna extract (1 dram), or a better tone may be given to the parts by balsam copaiba (1 dram).

DISEASED GROWTHS IN THE BLADDER.

These may be of various kinds, malignant or simple. In the horse I have found villous growths from the mucous membrane especially troublesome. They may be attached to the mucous membrance by a narrow neck or by a broad base covering a great part of the organ.

Symptoms.—The symptoms are frequent straining, passing of urine and blood with occasionally gravel. An examination of the bladder with the hand in the rectum will detect the new growth, which may be distinguished from a hard, resistant stone. In mares, in which the finger can be inserted into the bladder, the recognition is still more satisfactory. The polypi attached by narrow necks may be removed by surgical operation, but for those with broad attachments treatment is eminently unsatisfactory.

DISCHARGE OF URINE BY THE NAVEL, OR PERSISTENT URACHUS.

This occurs only in the newborn, and consists in the nonclosure of the natural channel (urachus), through which the urine is discharged into the outer water bag (allantois) in fetal life. At that early stage of the animal existence the bladder resembles a long tube, which is prolonged through the navel string and opens into the outermost of the two water bags in which the fetus floats. In this way the urine is prevented from entering the inner water bag (amnion), where it would mingle with the liquids, bathing the skin of the fetus and cause irritation. At birth this channel closes up, and the urine takes the course normal to extrauterine life. Imperfect closure is more frequent in males than in females, because of the great length and small caliber of the male urethra and its consequent tendency to obstruction. In the female there may be a discharge of a few drops only at a time, while in the male the urine will be expelled in strong jets coincidently with the contractions of the bladder and walls of the abdomen.

The first care is to ascertain whether the urethra is pervious by passing a human catheter. This determined, the open urachus may be firmly closed by a stout, waxed thread, carried with a needle through the tissues back of the opening and tied in front of it so as to inclose as little skin as possible. If a portion of the naval string remains, the tying of that may be all sufficient. It is important to tie as early as possible so as to avoid inflammation of the navel from contact with the urine. In summer a little carbolic-acid water or tar water may be applied to keep the flies off.

EVERSION OF THE BLADDER.

This can occur only in the female. It consists in the turning of the organ outside in through the channel of the urethra, so that it appears as a red, pear-shaped mass hanging from the floor of the vulva and protruding externally between its lips. It may be a mass like the fist, or it may swell up to the size of an infant's head. On examining its upper surface the orifices of the urethra may be seen, one on each side, a short distance behind the neck, with the urine oozing from them drop by drop.

This displacement usually supervenes on a flaccid condition of the bladder, the result of paralysis, overdistention, or severe compression during a difficult parturition.

The protruding organ may be washed with a solution of 1 ounce of laudanum and a teaspoonful of carbolic acid in a quart of water, and returned by pressing a smooth, rounded object into the fundus and directing it into the urethra, while careful pressure is made on the surrounding parts with the other hand. If too large and resistant it may be wound tightly in a strip of bandage about 2 inches broad to express the great mass of blood and exudate and diminish the bulk of the protruded organ so that it can be easily pushed back. This method has the additional advantage of protecting the organ against bruises and lacerations in the effort made to return it. After the return, straining may be kept in check by giving laudanum (1 to 2 ounces) and by applying a truss to press upon the lips of the vulva. (See Eversion of the womb.) The patient should be kept in a stall a few inches lower in front than behind, so that the action of gravity will favor retention.

PLATE XI.

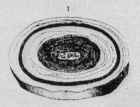

Phosphatic calculus, uric acid nucleus.

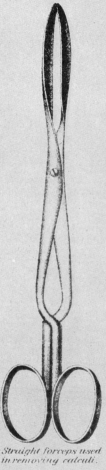

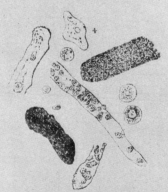

X 215

Calculus of oxalate of lime.

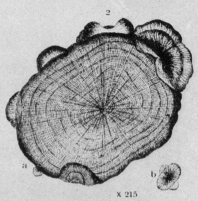

*Straight forceps used
in removing calculi.*

*Renal casts. Some deprived of
epithelium. Two are deeper-colored
from the presence of urate of soda.*

Haines.del.after Hurtrel D'Arboval.

CALCULI AND INSTRUMENT FOR REMOVAL.

INFLAMMATION OF THE URETHRA (URETHRITIS, OR GLEET).

This affection belongs quite as much to the generative organs, yet it can not be entirely overlooked in a treatise on urinary disorders. It may be induced by the same causes as cystitis (which see) ; by the passage and temporary arrest of small stones, or gravel; by the irritation caused by foreign bodies introduced from without; by blows on the penis by sticks, stones, or by the feet of a mare that kicks while being served; by an infecting inflammation contracted from a mare served in the first few days after parturition or one suffering from leucorrhea; by infecting matter introduced on a dirty catheter, or by the extension of inflammation from an irritated, bilocular cavity filled with hardened sebaceous matter, or from an uncleansed sheath.

Symptoms.—The symptoms are swelling, heat, and tenderness of the sheath and penis; difficulty, pain, and groaning in passing urine, which is liable to sudden temporary arrests in the course of micturition, and later a whitish, mucopurulent oozing from the papilla on the end of the penis. There is a tendency to erection of the penis, and in cases contracted from a mare the outer surface of that organ will show more or less extensive sores and ulcers. Stallions suffering in this way will refuse to mount or, having mounted, will fail to complete the act of coition. If an entrance is effected, infection of the mare is liable to follow.

Treatment in the early stages consists in a dose of physic (aloes 6 drams) and fomentations of warm water to the sheath and penis. If there is reason to suspect the presence of infection, inject the urethra twice daily with borax 1 dram, tepid water 1 quart. When the mucopurulent discharge indicates the supervention of the second stage a more astringent injection may be used (nitrate of silver 20 grains, water 1 quart), and the same may be applied to the surface of the penis and inside the sheath. Balsam of copaiba (1 dram daily) may also be given with advantage after the purulent discharge has appeared.

Every stallion suffering from urethritis should be withheld from service, as should mares with leucorrhea.

STRICTURE OF THE URETHRA.

This is a permanent narrowing of the urethra at a given point, the result of previous inflammation, caused by the passage or arrest of a stone, or gravel, by strong astringent injections in the early nonsecreting stage of urethritis, or by contraction of the lining membrane occurring during the healing of ulcers in neglected inflammations of that canal. The trouble is shown by the passage of urine in a fine stream, with straining, pain, and groaning, and by frequent painful

erections. It must be remedied by mechanical dilatation, with cathe-
ters just large enough to pass with gentle force, to be inserted once a
day, and to be used of larger size as the passage will admit them.
The catheter should be kept perfectly clean and washed in a borax
solution and well oiled before it is introduced.

URINARY CALCULI (STONE, OR GRAVEL).

These consist in some of the solids of the urine that have been
precipitated from the urine in the form of crystals, which remain
apart as a fine, powdery mass, or magma, or aggregate into calculi, or
stones, of varying size. (See Pl. XI.) Their composition is therefore determined in different animals by the salts or other constituents found dissolved in the healthy urine, and by the additional constituents which may be thrown off in solution in the urine in disease.
In this connection it is important to observe the following analysis
of the horse's urine in health:

Water	918. 5
Urea	13. 4
Uric acid and urates	.1
Hippuric acid	26. 4
Lactic acid and lactates	1. 2
Mucus and organic matter	22. 0
Sulphates (alkaline)	1. 2
Phosphates (lime and soda)	.2
Chlorids (sodium)	1. 0
Carbonates (potash, magnesia, lime)	16. 0
	1000. 0

The carbonate of lime, which is present in large quantity in the
urine of horses fed on green fodder, is practically insoluble, and
therefore forms in the passages after secretion, and its miscroscopic
rounded crystals give the urine of such horses a milky whiteness. It
is this material which constitutes the soft, white, pultaceous mass that
sometimes fills the bladder to repletion and requires to be washed
out. In hay-fed horses carbonates are still abundant, while in those
mainly grain-fed they are replaced by hippurates and phosphates—
the products of the wear of tissues—the carbonates being the result
of oxidation of the vegetable acids in the feed. Carbonate of lime,
therefore, is a very common constituent of urinary calculi in herbivora, and in many cases is the most abundant constituent.

Oxalate of lime, like carbonate of lime, is derived from the burning
up of the carbonaceous matter of the feed in the system, one important factor being the less perfect oxidation of the carbon. Indeed,
Füstenberg and Schmidt have demonstrated on man, horse, ox, and
rabbit that under the full play of the breathing (oxidizing) forces
oxalic acid, like other organic acids, is resolved into carbonic acid.

In keeping with this is the observation of Lehmann, that in all cases in which man suffered from interference with the breathing oxalate of lime appeared in the urine. An excess of oxalate of lime in the urine may, however, claim a different origin. Uric and hippuric acids are found in the urine of carnivora and herbivora, respectively, as the result of the healthy wear (disassimilation) of nitrogenous tissues. If these products are fully oxidized, however, they are thrown out in the form of the more soluble urea rather than as these acids. When uric acid out of the body is treated with peroxid of lead it is resolved into urea, allantoin, and oxalic acid, and Wœhler and Frerrichs found that the administration of uric acid not only increased the excretion of urea but also of oxalic acid. It may therefore be inferred that oxalic acid is not produced from the carbonaceous feed alone but also from the disintegration of the nitrogenous tissues of the body. An important element of its production is, however, the imperfect performance of the breathing functions, and hence it is liable to result from diseases of the chest (heaves, chronic bronchitis, etc.). This is, above all, liable to prove the case if the subject is fed to excess on highly carbonaceous feeds (grass and green feed generally, potatoes, etc.).

Carbonate of magnesia, another almost constant ingredient of the urinary calculi of the horse, is formed the same way as the carbonate of lime—from the excess of carbonaceous feed (organic acids) becoming oxidized into carbon dioxid, which unites with the magnesia derived from the feed.

The phosphates of lime and magnesia are not abundant in urinary calculi of the horse, the phosphates being present to excess in the urine in only two conditions—(a) when the ration is excessive and especially rich in phosphorus (wheat, bran, beans, peas, vetches, rape cake, oil cake, cottonseed cake) ; and (b) when, through the morbid, destructive changes in the living tissues, and especially of the bones, a great quantity of phosphorus is given off as a waste product. Under these conditions, however, the phosphates may contribute to the formation of calculi, and this, above all, is liable if the urine is retained in the bladder until it has undergone decomposition and given off ammonia. The ammonia at once unites with the phosphate of magnesia to form a double salt—phosphate of ammonia and magnesia—which, being insoluble, is at once precipitated. The precipitation of this salt is, however, rare in the urine of the horse, though much more frequent in that of man and sheep.

These are the chief mineral constituents of the urine which form ingredients in the horse's calculi, for though iron and manganese are usually present it is only in minute quantities.

The excess of mineral matter in a specimen of urine unquestionably contributes to the formation of calculi, just as a solution of such matters out of the body is increasingly disposed to throw them down in the form of crystals as it becomes more concentrated and approaches nearer to the condition of saturation. Hence, in considering the causes of calculi we can not ignore the factor of an excessive ration, rich in mineral matters and in carbonaceous matters (the source of carbonates and much of the oxalates), nor can we overlook the concentration of the urine that comes from dry feed and privation of water, or from the existence of fever which causes suspension of the secretion of water. In these cases, at least the usual quantity of solids is thrown off by the kidneys, and as the water is diminished there is danger of its approaching the point of supersaturation, when the dissolved solids must necessarily be thrown down. Hence, calculi are more common in stable horses fed on dry grain and hay, in those denied a sufficiency of water or that have water supplied irregularly, in those subjected to profuse perspiration (as in summer), and in those suffering from a watery diarrhea. On the whole, calculi are most commonly found in winter, because the horses are then on dry feeding, but such dry feeding is even more conducive to them in summer. when the condition is aggravated by the abundant loss of water by the skin.

In the same way the extreme hardness of the water in certain districts must be looked upon as contributing to the concentration of the urine and correspondingly to the production of stone. The carbonates, sulphates, etc., of lime and magnesia taken in the water must be again thrown out, and just in proportion as these add to the solids of the urine they dispose it to precipitate its least soluble constituents. Thus the horse is very subject to calculi on certain limestone soils, as over the calcareous formations of central and western New York, Pennsylvania, and Ohio, in America; of Norfolk, Suffolk, Derbyshire, Shropshire, and Gloucestershire, in England; of Poitou and Landes, in France; and Munich, in Bavaria.

The saturation of the urine from any or all of these conditions can only be looked on as an auxiliary cause, however, and not as in itself an efficient one, except on the rarest occasions. For a more direct and immediate cause we must look to the organic matter which forms a large proportion of all urinary calculi. This consists of mucus, albumen, pus, hyaline casts of the uriniferous tubes, epithelial cells, blood, etc., mainly agents that belong to the class of colloid or noncrystalline bodies. A horse may live for months and years with the urine habitually of a high density and having the mineral constituents in excess without the formation of stone or gravel; again, one with dilute urine of low specific gravity will have a calculus.

Rainey, Ord, and others furnish the explanation. They not only show that a colloid body, like mucus, albumen, pus, or blood, determined the precipitation or the crystalline salts in the solution, but they determined the precipitation in the form of globules, or spheres, capable of developing by further deposits into calculi. Heat intensifies this action of the colloids, and a colloid in a state of decomposition is specially active. The presence, therefore, of developing fungi and bacteria must be looked upon as active factors in causing calculi.

In looking, therefore, for the immediate causes of calculi we must consider especially all those conditions which determine the presence of albumen, blood, and excess of mucus, pus, etc., in the urine. Thus diseases of distant organs leading to albuminuria, diseases of the kidneys and urinary passages causing the escape of blood or the formation of mucus or pus, become direct causes of calculi. Foreign bodies of all kinds in the bladder or kidney have long been known as determining causes of calculi and as forming the central nucleus. This is now explained by the fact that these bodies are liable to carry bacteria into the passages and thus determine decomposition, and they are further liable to irritate the mucous membrane and become enveloped in a coating of mucus, pus, and perhaps blood.

The fact that horses, especially on the magnesian limestones, the same districts in which they suffer from goiter, appear to suffer from calculi may be similarly explained. The unknown poison which produces goiter presumably leads to such changes in the blood and urine as will furnish the colloid necessary for precipitation of the urinary salts in the form of calculi.

CLASSIFICATION OF URINARY CALCULI.

These have been named according to the place where they are found, renal (kidney), ureteric (ureter), vesical (bladder), urethral (urethra), and preputial (sheath, or prepuce). They have been otherwise named according to their most abundant chemical constituent, carbonate of lime, oxalate of lime, and phosphate of lime calculi. The stones formed of carbonates or phosphates are usually smooth on the surface, though they may be molded into the shape of the cavity in which they have been formed; thus those in the pelvis of the kidney may have two or three short branchlike prolongations, while those in the bladder are round, oval, or slightly flattened upon each other. Calculi containing oxalate of lime, on the other hand, have a rough, open, crystalline surface, which has gained for them the name of mulberry calculi, from a supposed resemblance to that fruit. These are usually covered with more or less mucus or blood, produced by the irritation of the mucous membrane by their rough surfaces. The color of calculi varies from white to yellow and deep brown, the shades depending mainly on the amount of the coloring matter of blood, bile, or urine which they may contain.

Renal calculi.—These may consist of minute, almost microscopic, deposits in the uriniferous tubes in the substance of the kidney, but more commonly they are large masses and lodged in the pelvis. The larger calculi, sometimes weighing 12 to 24 ounces, are molded in the pelvis of the kidney into a cylindroid mass, with irregular rounded swellings at intervals. Some have a deep brown, rough, crystalline surface of oxalate of lime, while others have a smooth, pearly white aspect from carbonate of lime. A smaller calculus, which has been called coralline, is also cylindroid, with a number of brown, rough, crystalline oxalate of lime branches and whitish depressions of carbonate. These vary in size from 15 grains to nearly 2 ounces. Less frequently are found masses of very hard, brownish white, rounded, pealike calculi. These are smoother, but on the surface crystals of oxalate of lime may be detected with a lens. Some renal calculi are formed of more distinct layers, more loosely adherent to one another, and contain an excess of mucus, but no oxalate of lime. Finally, a loose aggregation of small masses, forming a very friable calculus, is found of all sizes within the limits of the pelvis of the kidney. These, too, are in the main carbonate of lime (84 to 88 per cent) and without oxalate.

Symptoms of renal calculi are violent, colicky, pains, appearing suddenly, very often in connection with exhausting work or the drawing of specially heavy loads, and in certain cases disappearing with equal suddenness. The nature of the colic becomes more manifest if it is associated with stiffness of the back and hind limbs, frequent passage of urine, and, above all, the passage of gravel with the urine, especially at the time of the access of relief. The passage of blood and pus in the urine is equally significant. If the irritation of the kidney goes on to active inflammation, then the symptoms of nephritis are added.

Ureteric calculi.—These are so called because they are found in the passage leading from the kidney to the bladder. They are simply small, renal calculi which have escaped from the pelvis of the kidney and have become arrested in the ureter. They give rise to symptoms almost identical with those of renal calculi, with this difference, that the colicky pains, caused by the obstruction of the ureter by the impacted calculus, are more violent, and if the calculus passes on into the bladder the relief is instantaneous and complete. If the ureter is completely blocked for a length of time, the retained urine may give rise to destructive inflammation in the kidney, which may end in the entire absorption of that organ, leaving only a fibrous capsule containing an urinous fluid. If both the ureters are similarly blocked, the animal will die of uremic poisoning.

Treatment of renal and ureteric calculi.—Treatment is unsatisfactory, as it is only the small calculi that can pass through the ureters and escape into the bladder. This may be favored by agents which will relax the walls of the ureters by counteracting their spasm and even lessening their tone, and by a liberal use of water and watery fluids to increase the urine and the pressure upon the calculus from behind. One or two ounces of laudanum, or 2 drams of extract of belladonna, may be given and repeated as it may be necessary, the relief of the pain being a fair criterion of the abating of the spasm. To the same end use warm fomentations across the loins, and these should be kept up persistently until relief is obtained. These act not only by soothing and relieving the spasm and inflammation, but they also favor the freer secretion of a more watery urine, and thus tend to carry off the smaller calculi. To accomplish this object further give cool water freely, and let the feed be only such as contains a large proportion of liquid, gruels, mashes, turnips, beets, apples, pumpkins, ensilage, succulent grasses, etc. If the acute stage has passed and the presence of the calculus is manifested only by the frequent passage of urine with gritty particles, by stiffness of the loins and hind limbs, and by tenderness to pressure, the most promising resort is a long run at pasture where the grasses are fresh and succulent. The long-continued secretion of a watery urine will sometimes cause the breaking down of a calculus, as the imbibition of the less dense fluid by the organic, spongelike framework of the calculus causes it to swell and thus lessens its cohesion. The same end is sought by the long-continued use of alkalies (carbonate of potassium), and of acids (muriatic), each acting in a different way to alter the density and cohesion of the stone. It is only exceptionally, however, that any one of these methods is entirely satisfactory. If inflammation of the kidneys develops, treat as advised under that head.

Stone in the bladder (vesical calculus, or cystic calculus).—These may be of any size up to over a pound in weight. One variety is rough and crystalline and has a yellowish-white or deep-brown color. These contain about 87 per cent carbonate of lime, the remainder being carbonate of magnesia, oxalate of lime, and organic matter. The phosphatic calculi are smooth, white and formed of thin, concentric layers of great hardness extending from the nucleus outward. Besides the phosphate of lime they contain the carbonates of lime and magnesia and organic matter. In some cases the bladder contains and may be even distended by a soft, pultaceous mass made up of minute, round granules of carbonates of lime and magnesia. This, when removed and dried, makes a firm, white, and stony mass.

Sometimes this magma is condensed into a solid mass in the bladder by reason of the binding action of the mucus and other organic matter, and then forms a conglomerate stone of nearly uniform consistency and without stratification.

Symptoms of stone in the bladder.—The symptoms of stone in the bladder are more obvious than those of renal calculus. The rough, mulberry calculi especially lead to irritation of the mucous membrane and frequent passing of urine in small quantities and often mingled with mucus or blood or containing minute, gritty particles. At times the flow is suddenly arrested, though the animal continues to strain and the bladder is not quite emptied. In the smooth, phosphatic variety the irritation is much less marked and may even be altogether absent. With the pultaceous deposit in the bladder there is incontinence of urine, which dribbles away continually and keeps the hair on the inner side of the thighs matted with soft magma. In all cases alike the calculus may be felt by the examination of the bladder with the oiled hand in the rectum. The pear-shaped outline of the bladder can be felt beneath, and within it the solid, oval body. It is most easily recognized if the organ is half full of liquid, as then it is not grasped by the contracting walls of the bladder, but may be made to move from place to place in the liquid. If a pultaceous mass is present it has a soft, doughy feeling, and when pressed an indentation is left.

In the mare the hard stone may be touched by the finger introduced through the short urethra.

Treatment of stone in the bladder.—The treatment of stone in the bladder consists in the removal of the offending body; in the mare this is easily effected with the lithotomy forceps. These are slightly warmed and oiled, and carried forward along the floor of the passage of the vulva for 4 inches, when the orifice of the urethra will be felt exactly in the median line. Through this the forceps are gradually pushed with gentle, oscillating movement until they enter the bladder and strike against the hard surface of the stone. The stone is now grasped between the blades, care being taken to include no loose fold of the mucous membrane, and it is gradually withdrawn with the same careful, oscillating motions as before. Facility and safety in seizing the stone will be greatly favored by having the bladder half full of liquid, and if necessary one oiled hand may be introduced into the rectum or vagina to assist. The resulting irritation may be treated by an injection of laudanum, 1 ounce in a pint of tepid water.

The removal of the stone in the horse is a much more difficult proceeding. It consists in cutting into the urethra just beneath the anus and introducing the lithotomy forceps from this forward into the bladder, as in the mare. It is needful to distend the urethra with tepid water or to insert a sound or catheter to furnish a guide upon which the incision may be made, and in case of a large stone it may be needful to enlarge the passage by cutting in a direction upward and outward with a probe-pointed knife, the back of which is slid along in the groove of a director until it enters the bladder.

The horse may be operated upon in the standing position, being simply pressed against the wall by a pole passed from before backward along the other side of the body. The tepid water is injected into the end of the penis until it is felt to fluctuate under the pressure of the finger, in the median line over the bone just beneath the anus. The incision is then made into the center of the fluctuating canal, and from above downward. When a sound or catheter is used as a guide it is inserted through the penis until it can be felt through the skin at the point where the incision is to be made beneath the anus. The skin is then rendered tense by the thumb and fingers of the left hand pressing on the two sides of the sound, while the right hand, armed with a scalpel, cuts downward onto the catheter. This vertical incision into the canal should escape wounding any important blood vessel. It is in making the obliquely lateral incision in the subsequent dilatation of the urethra and neck of the bladder that such danger is to be apprehended.

If the stone is too large to be extracted through the urethra, it may be broken down with the lithotrite and extracted piecemeal with the forceps. The lithotrite is an instrument composed of a straight stem bent for an inch or more to one side at its free end so as to form an obtuse angle, and having on the same side a sliding bar moving in a groove in the stem and operated by a screw so that the stone may be seized between the two blades at its free extremity and crushed again and again into pieces small enough to extract. Extra care is required to avoid injury to the urethra in the extraction of the angular fragments, and the gravel or powder that can not be removed in this way must be washed out, as advised below.

When a pultaceous magma of carbonate of lime accumulates in the bladder it must be washed out by injecting water through a catheter by means of a force pump or a funnel, shaking it up with the hand introduced through the rectum and allowing the muddy liquid to flow out through the tube. This is to be repeated until the bladder is empty and the water comes away clear. A catheter with a double tube is sometimes used, the injection passing in through the one tube and escaping through the other. The advantage is more apparent than real, however, as the retention of the water until the magma has been shaken up and mixed with it hastens greatly its complete evacuation.

54763°—23——11

To prevent the formation of a new deposit any fault in feeding (dry grain and hay with privation of water, excess of beans, peas, wheat bran, etc.) and disorders of stomach, liver, and lungs must be corrected. Give abundance of soft drinking water, encouraging the animal to drink by a handful of salt daily. Let the feed be laxative, consisting largely of roots, apples, pumpkins, ensilage, and give daily in the drinking water a dram of either carbonate of potash or soda. Powdered gentian root (3 drams daily) will also serve to restore the tone of the stomach and system at large.

Urethral calculus (stone in the urethra).—This is less frequent in horses than in cattle and sheep, owing to the larger size of the urethra in the horse and the absence of the S-shaped curve and vermiform appendix. The calculi arrested in the urethra are never formed there, but consist of cystic calculi which have been small enough to pass through the neck of the bladder, but are too large to pass through the whole length of the urethra and escape. Such calculi therefore are primarily formed either in the bladder or kidney, and have the chemical composition of the other calculi found in those organs. They may be arrested at any point of the urethra, from the neck of the bladder back to the bend of the tube beneath the anus, and from that point down to the extremity of the penis. I have found them most frequently in the papilla on the extreme end of the penis, and immediately behind this.

Symptoms of urethral calculus.—The symptoms are violent straining to urinate, but without any discharge, or with the escape of water in drops only. Examination of the end of the penis will detect the swelling of the papilla or the urethra behind it, and the presence of a hard mass in the center. A probe inserted into the urethra will strike against the gritty calculus. If the stone has been arrested higher up, its position may be detected as a small, hard, sensitive knot on the line of the urethra, in the median line of the lower surface of the penis, or on the floor of pelvis in the median line from the neck of the bladder back to the bend of the urethra beneath the anus. In any case the urethra between the neck of the bladder and the point of obstruction is liable to be filled with fluid, and to feel like a distended tube, fluctuating on pressure.

Treatment of urethral calculus may be begun by an attempt to extract the calculi by manipulation of the papilla on the end of the penis. This failing, the calculus may be seized with a pair of fine-pointed forceps and withdrawn from the urethra; or, if necessary, a probe-pointed knife may be inserted and the urethra slightly dilated, or even laid open, and the stone removed. If the stone has been arrested higher up it must be extracted by a direct incision through the walls of the urethra and down upon the nodule. If in the free (protractile) portion of the penis, that organ is to be withdrawn from its sheath until the nodule is exposed and can be incised. If behind the scrotum, the incision must be made in the median line between the thighs and directly over the nodule, the skin having been rendered tense by the fingers and thumb of the left hand. If the stone has been arrested in the intrapelvic portion of the urethra, the incision must be made beneath the anus and the calculus extracted with forceps, as in stone in the bladder. The wound in the urethra may be stitched up, and usually heals slowly but satisfactorily. Healing will be favored by washing two or three times daily with a solution of a teaspoonful of carbolic acid in a pint of water.

Preputial calculus (*calculus in the sheath, or bilocular cavity*).— These are concretions in the sheath, though the term has been also applied to the nodule of sebaceous matter which accumulates in the blind pouches (bilocular cavity) by the sides of the papilla on the end of the penis. Within the sheath the concretion may be a soft, cheesy-like sebaceous matter, or a genuine calculus of carbonate, oxalate, phosphate and sulphate of lime, carbonate of magnesia, and organic matter. These are easily removed with the fingers, after which the sheath should be washed out with castile soap and warm water and smeared with sweet oil.

DISEASES OF THE GENERATIVE ORGANS.

By James Law, F. R. C. V. S.,

Formerly Professor of Veterinary Science, etc., in Cornell University.

CONGESTION AND INFLAMMATION OF THE TESTICLES, OR ORCHITIS.

In the prime of life, in vigorous health, and on stimulating feed, stallions are subject to congestion of the testicles, which become swollen, hot, and tender, but without any active inflammation. A reduction of the grain in the feed, the administration of 1 or 2 ounces of Glauber's salt daily in the feed, and the bathing of the affected organs daily with tepid water or alum water will usually restore them to a healthy condition.

When the factors producing congestion are extraordinarily potent, when there has been frequent copulation and heavy grain feeding, when the weather is warm and the animal has had little exercise, and when the proximity of other horses or mares excites the generative instinct without gratification, this congestion may grow to actual inflammation. Among the other causes of orchitis are blows and penetrating wounds implicating the testicles, abrasions of the scrotum by a chain or rope passing inside the thigh, contusions and frictions on the gland under rapid paces or heavy draft, compression of the blood vessels of the spermatic cord by the inguinal ring under the same circumstances, and, finally, sympathetic disturbance in cases of disease of the kidneys, bladder, or urethra. Stimulants of the generative functions, like rue, savin, tansy, cantharides, and damiana, may also be accessory causes of congestion and inflammation. Finally, certain specific diseases, like dourine, glanders, and tuberculosis, localized in the testicles, will cause inflammation.

Symptoms.—Apart from actual wounds of the parts, the symptoms of orchitis are swelling, heat, and tenderness of the testicles, straddling with the hind legs alike in standing and walking, stiffness and dragging of the hind limbs or of the limb on the affected side, arching of the loins, abdominal pain, manifested by glancing back at the flank, more or less fever, elevated body temperature, accelerated pulse and breathing, lack of appetite, and dullness. In bad

164

cases the scanty urine may be reddish and the swelling may extend to the skin and envelopes of the testicle, which may become thickened and doughy, pitting on pressure. The swelling may be so much greater in the convoluted excretory duct along the upper border of the testicle as to suggest the presence of a second stone. Even in the more violent attacks the intense suffering abates somewhat on the second or third day. If it lasts longer, it is liable to give rise to the formation of matter (abscess). In exceptional cases the testicle is struck with gangrene, or death. Improvement may go on slowly to complete recovery, or the malady may subside into a subacute and chronic form with induration. Matter (abscess) may be recognized by the presence of a soft spot, where pressure with two fingers will detect fluctuation from one to the other. When there is liquid exudation into the scrotum, or sac, fluctuation may also be felt, but the liquid can be made out to be around the testicle and can be pressed up into the abdomen through the inguinal canal. When abscess occurs in the cord the matter may escape into the scrotal sac and cavity of the abdomen and pyemia may follow.

Treatment consists in perfect rest and quietude, the administration of a purgative (1 to 1½ pounds Glauber's salt), and the local application of an astringent lotion (acetate of lead 2 drams, extract of belladonna 2 drams, and water 1 quart) upon soft rags or cotton wool, kept in contact with the part by a suspensory bandage. This bandage, of great value for support, may be made nearly triangular and tied to a girth around the loins and to the upper part of the same surcingle by two bands carried backward and upward between the thighs. In severe cases scarifications one-fourth inch deep serve to relieve vascular tension. When abscess is threatened its formation may be favored by warm fomentations or poultices, and on the occurrence of fluctuation the knife may be used to give free escape to the pus. The resulting cavity may be injected daily with a weak carbolic-acid lotion, or salol may be introduced. The same agents may be used on a gland threatened with gangrene, but its prompt removal by castration is to be preferred, antiseptics being applied freely to the resulting cavity.

SARCOCELE.

This is an enlarged and indurated condition of the gland, resulting from chronic inflammation, though it is often associated with a specific deposit, like glanders. In this condition the natural structure of the gland has given place to embryonal tissue (small, round cells, with a few fibrous bundles), and its restoration to health is very improbable. Apart from active inflammation, it may increase very slowly. The diseased testicle is enlarged, firm, nonelastic, and comparatively insensible. The skin of the scrotum is tense, and it may be edematous (pitting on pressure), as are the deeper envelopes and spermatic cord. If liquid is present in the sac, the symptoms are masked somewhat. As it increases it causes awkward, straddling, dragging movement of the hind limbs, or lameness on the affected side. The spermatic cord often increases at the same time with the testicle, and the inguinal ring being thereby stretched and enlarged, a portion of intestine may escape into the sac, complicating the disease with hernia.

The only rational and effective treatment is castration, and when the disease is specific (glanders, tuberculosis), even this may not succeed.

HYDROCELE, OR DROPSY OF THE SCROTUM.

This may be merely an accompaniment of dropsy of the abdomen, the cavity of which is continuous with that of the scrotum in horses. It may be the result, however, of local disease in the testicle, spermatic cord, or walls of the sac.

Symptoms.—The symptoms are enlargement of the scrotum, and fluctuation under the fingers, the testicle being recognized as floating in water. By pressure the liquid is forced, in a slow stream and with a perceptible thrill, into the abdomen. Sometimes the cord or the scrotum is thickened and pits on pressure.

Treatment may be the same as for ascites, yet when the effusion has resulted from inflammation of the testicle or cord, astringent applications (chalk and vinegar) may be applied to these. Then, if the liquid is not reabsorbed under diuretics and tonics, it may be drawn off through the nozzle of a hypodermic syringe which has been first passed through carbolic acid. In geldings it is best to dissect out the sacs.

VARICOCELE.

This is an enlargement of the venous network of the spermatic cord, and gives rise to general thickening of the cord from the testicle up to the ring. The same astringent dressings may be tried as in hydrocele, and, this failing, castration may be resorted to.

ABNORMAL NUMBER OF TESTICLES.

Sometimes one or both testicles are wanting; in most such cases, however, they are merely partially developed, and retained in the inguinal canal or abdomen (cryptorchid). In rare cases there may be a third testicle, the animal becoming to this extent a double monster. Teeth, hair, and other indications of a second fetus have likewise been found in the testicle or scrotum.

DEGENERATION OF THE TESTICLES.

The testicles may become the seat of fibrous, calcareous, fatty, cartilaginous, or cystic degeneration, for all which the appropriate treatment is castration. They also become the seat of cancer, glanders, or tuberculosis, and castration is requisite, though with less hope of arresting the disease. Finally, they may become infested with cystic tapeworms or the agamic stage of a strongyle (*Stronglyus edentatus*).

WARTS ON THE PENIS.

These are best removed by twisting them off, using the thumb and forefinger. They may also be cut off with scissors and the roots cauterized with nitrate of silver.

DEGENERATION OF PENIS (PAPILLOMA, OR EPITHELIOMA).

The penis of the horse is subject to great cauliflower-like growths on its free end, which extend back into the substance of the organ, obstruct the passage of urine, and cause very fetid discharges. The only resort is to cut them off, together with whatever portion of the penis has become diseased and indurated. The operation, which should be performed by a veterinary surgeon, consists in cutting through the organ from its upper to its lower aspect, twisting or tying the two dorsal arteries, and leaving the urethra longer by half an inch to 1 inch than the adjacent structures.

EXTRAVASATION OF BLOOD IN THE PENIS.

As the result of kicks, blows, or of forcible striking of the penis on the thighs of the mare which it has failed to enter, the penis may become the seat of effusion of blood from one or more ruptured blood vessels. This gives rise to a more or less extensive swelling on one or more sides, followed by some heat and inflammation, and on recovery a serious curving of the organ. The treatment in the early stages may be the application of lotions, of alum, or other astringents, to limit the effusion and favor absorption. The penis should be suspended in a sling.

PARALYSIS OF THE PENIS.

This results from blows and other injuries, and also in some cases from too frequent and exhausting service. The penis hangs from the sheath, flaccid, pendulous, and often cold. The passage of urine occurs with lessened force, and especially without the final jets. In cases of local injury the inflammation should first be subdued by astringent and emollient lotions, and in all cases the system should be invigorated by nourishing diet, while 30-grain doses of nux vomica are given twice a day. Finally, a weak current of electricity sent through the penis from just beneath the anus to the free portion of the penis, continued for 10 or 15 minutes and repeated daily, may prove successful.

SELF-ABUSE, OR MASTURBATION.

Some stallions acquire this vicious habit, stimulating the sexual instinct to the discharge of semen by rubbing the penis against the belly or between the fore limbs. The only remedy is a mechanical one, the fixing of a net under the penis in such fashion as to prevent the extension of the penis or so prick the organ as to compel the animal to desist through pain.

DOURINE.

This disease is discussed in the chapter on " Infectious Diseases."

CASTRATION.

CASTRATION OF STALLIONS.

This is usually done at 1 year old, but may be accomplished at a few weeks old at the expense of an imperfect development of the fore parts. The simplicity and safety of the operation are greatest in the young. The delay till 2, 3, or 4 years old will secure a better development and carriage of the fore parts. The essential part of castration is the safe removal or destruction of the testicle and the arrest or prevention of bleeding from the spermatic artery found in the anterior part of the cord. Into the many methods of accomplishing this limited space forbids us to enter here, so that but one, castration by clamps, will be noticed. The animal having been thrown on his left side, and the right hind foot drawn up on the shoulder, the exposed scrotum, penis, and sheath are washed with soap and water, any concretion of sebum being carefully removed from the bilocular cavity in the end of the penis. The left spermatic cord, just above the testicle, is now seized in the left hand, so as to render the skin tense over the stone, and the right hand, armed with the knife, makes an incision from before backward, about three-fourths of an inch from and parallel to the median line between the thighs, deep enough to expose the testicle and long enough to allow that organ to start out through the skin. At the moment of making this incision the left hand must grasp the cord very firmly, otherwise the sudden retraction of the testicle by the cremaster muscle may draw it out of the hand and upward through the canal and even into the abdomen. In a few seconds, when the struggle and retraction have ceased, the knife is inserted through the cord, between its anterior and posterior portions, and the latter, the one which the muscle retracts, is cut completely through. The testicle will now hang limp, and there is no longer any tendency to retraction. It should be pulled down until it will no longer hang loose below the wound and the clamps applied around the still attached portion of the cord, close up to the skin. The clamps, which may be made of any tough wood, are grooved along the center of the surfaces opposed to each other, thereby fulfilling two important indications—(a) enabling the clamps to hold more securely and (b) providing for the application of an antiseptic to the cord. For this purpose a dram of sulphate of copper may be mixed with an ounce of vaseline and pressed into the groove in the face of each clamp. In applying the clamp over the cord it should be drawn so close with pincers as to press out all blood from the compressed cord and destroy its vitality, and the cord applied upon the compressing clamps should be so hard-twined that it will not stretch later and slacken the hold. When the clamp has been fixed the testicle is cut off one-half to 1 inch below it, and the clamp may be left thus for 24 hours; then, by cutting the cord around one end of the clamp, the latter may be opened and the stump liberated without any danger of bleeding. Should the stump hang out of the wound it should be pushed inside with the finger and left there.

The young horse suffers less from castration than the old, and very rarely perishes. Good health in the subject is all important. Castration should never be attempted during the prevalence of strangles, influenza, catarrhal fever, contagious pleurisy, bronchitis, pneumonia, purpura hemorrhagica, or other specific disease, nor on subjects that have been kept in close, ill-ventilated, filthy buildings, where the system is liable to have been charged with putrid bacteria or other products. Warm weather is to be preferred to cold, but the fly time should be avoided or the flies kept at a distance by the application of a watery solution of tar, carbolic acid, or camphor to the wound.

CASTRATION OF CRYPTORCHIDS (RIDGLINGS).

This is the removal of a testicle or testicles that have failed to descend into the scrotum, but have been detained in the inguinal canal or inside the abdomen. The manipulation requires an accurate anatomical knowledge of the parts, and special skill, experience, and manual dexterity, and can not be made clear to the unprofessional mind in a short description. It consists, however, in the discovery and removal of the missing gland by exploring through the natural channel (the inguinal canal), or, in case it is absent, through the inguinal ring or through an artificial opening made in front and above that channel between the abdominal muscles and the strong fascia on the inner side of the thigh (Poupart's ligament). Whatever method is used, the skin, hands, and instruments should be rendered aseptic with a solution of mercuric chlorid 1 part, water 2,000 parts (a carbolic-acid lotion for the instruments), and the spermatic cord is best torn through by the écraseur. In many such cases, too, it is desirable to sew up the external wound and keep the animal still, to favor healing of the wound by adhesion.

CONDITIONS FOLLOWING CASTRATION.

Pain after castration.—Some horses are pained and very restless for several hours after castration, and this may extend to cramps of the bowels and violent colic. This is best kept in check by carefully rubbing the patient dry when he rises from the operation, and then leading him in hand for some time. If the pain still persists a dose of laudanum (1 ounce for an adult) may be given.

Bleeding after castration.—Bleeding from the wound in the scrotum and from the little artery in the posterior portion of the spermatic cord always occurs, and in warm weather may appear to be quite free. It scarcely ever lasts, however, more than 15 minutes, and is easily checked by dashing cold water against the part.

Bleeding from the spermatic artery in the anterior part of the cord may be dangerous when due precaution has not been taken to prevent it. In such case the stump of the cord should be sought for and the artery twisted with artery forceps or tied with a silk thread. If the stump can not be found, pledgets of tow wet with tincture of muriate of iron may be stuffed into the canal to favor the formation of clot and the closure of the artery.

Strangulated spermatic cord.—If in castration the cord is left too long, so as to hang out of the wound, the skin wound in contracting grasps and strangles it, preventing the free return of blood and causing a steadily advancing swelling. In addition the cord becomes adherent to the lips of the wound in the skin, whence it derives an increased supply of blood, and is thereby stimulated to more rapid swelling. The subject walks stiffly, with a straddling gait, loses appetite, and has a rapid pulse and high fever. Examination of the wound discloses the partial closure of the skin wound and the protrusion, from its lips, of the end of the cord, red, tense, and varying in size from a hazelnut upward. If there is no material swell- and little protrusion, the wound may be enlarged with the knife and the end of the cord broken loose from any connection with the skin and pushed up inside. If the swelling is larger, the mass constitutes a tumor and must be removed. (See below.)

Swelling of the sheath, penis, and abdomen.—This occurs in certain unhealthy states of the system, in unhealthful seasons, as the result of operating without cleansing the sheath and penis, or of keeping the subject in a filthy, impure building, as the result of infecting the wound by hands or instruments bearing septic bacteria, or as the result of premature closure of the wound, and imprisonment of matter.

Pure air and cleanliness of groin and wound are to be obtained. Antiseptics, like the mercuric-chlorid lotion (1 part to 2,000) are to be applied to the parts; the wound, if closed, is to be opened anew, any accumulated matter or blood washed out, and the antiseptic liquid freely applied. The most tense or dependent parts of the swelling in sheath or penis, or beneath the belly, should be pricked at intervals of 3 or 4 inches to a depth of half an inch, and antiseptics freely applied to the surface. Fomentations with warm water may also be used to favor oozing from the incisions and to encourage the formation of white matter in the original wounds, which must not be allowed to close again at once. A free, creamlike discharge implies a healthy action in the sore, and is the precursor of recovery.

Phymosis and paraphymosis.—In cases of swelling, as above, the penis may be imprisoned within the sheath (phymosis) or protruded and swollen so that it can not be retracted into it (paraphymosis). In these cases the treatment indicated above, and especially the scarifications, will prove a useful preliminary resort. The use of astringent lotions is always desirable, and in case of the protruded penis the application of an elastic or simple linen bandage, so as to press the blood and accumulated fluid out, will enable the operator to return it.

Tumors on the spermatic cord.—These are due to rough handling or dragging upon the cord in castration, to strangulation of unduly long cords in the external wound, to adhesion of the end of the cord to the skin, to inflammation of the cord succeeding exposure to cold or wet, or to the presence of infection (*Staphylococcus botriomyces*). These tumors give rise to a stiff, straddling gait, and may be felt as hard masses in the groin connected above with the cord. They may continue to grow slowly for many years until they reach a weight of 15 or 20 pounds, and contract adhesions to all surrounding parts. If disconnected from the skin and inguinal canal they may be removed in the same manner as the testicle, while if larger and firmly adherent to the skin and surrounding parts generally, they must be carefully dissected from the parts, the arteries being tied as they are reached and the cord finally torn through with an écraseur. When the cord has become swollen and indurated up into the abdomen such removal is impossible, though a partial destruction of the mass may still be attempted by passing white-hot, pointed irons upward toward the inguinal ring in the center of the thickened and indurated cord.

CASTRATION BY THE COVERED OPERATION.

This is only required in case of hernia or protrusion of bowels or omentum into the sac of the scrotum, and consists in the return of the hernia and the application of the caustic clamps over the cord and inner walls of the inguinal canal, so that the walls of the latter become adherent above the clamps, the canal is obliterated, and further protrusion is hindered. For the full description of this and of the operation for hernia for geldings, see remarks on hernia.

CASTRATION OF THE MARE.

Castration is a much more dangerous operation in the mare than in the females of other domesticated quadrupeds and should never be resorted to except in animals that become unmanageable on the recurrence of heat and that will not breed or that are utterly unsuited to breeding. Formerly the operation was extensively practiced in Europe, the incision being made through the flank, and a large proportion of the subjects perished. By operating through the vagina the risk can be largely obviated, as the danger of unhealthy inflammation in the wound is greatly lessened. The animal should be fixed in a trevis, with each foot fixed to a post and a sling placed under the body, or it may be thrown and put under chloroform. The manual operation demands special professional knowledge and skill, but it consists essentially in making an opening through the roof of the vagina just above the neck of the womb, then following with the hand each horn of the womb until the ovary on that side is reached and grasped between the lips of forceps and twisted off. It might be torn off by an écraseur especially constructed for the purpose. The straining that follows the operation may be checked by ounce doses of laudanum, and any risk of protrusion of the bowels may be obviated by applying the truss advised to prevent eversion of the womb. To further prevent the pressure of the abdominal contents against the vaginal wound the mare should be tied short and high for twenty-four or forty-eight hours, after which I have found it best to remove the truss and allow the privilege of lying down. Another important point is to give bran mashes and other laxative diet only, and in moderate quantity, for a fortnight, and to unload the rectum by copious injections of warm water in case impaction is imminent.

STERILITY.

Sterility may be in the male or in the female. If due to the stallion, then all the mares put to him remain barren; if the fault is in the mare, she alone fails to conceive, while other mares served by the same stallion get in foal.

In the stallion sterility may be due to the following causes: (a) Imperfect development of the testicles, as in cases in which they are retained within the abdomen; (b) inflammation of the testicles, resulting in induration; (c) fatty degeneration of the testicles, in stallions liberally fed on starchy feed and not sufficiently exercised; (d) fatty degeneration of the excretory ducts of the testicles (vasa deferentia); (e) inflammation or ulceration of these ducts; (f) inflammation or ulceration of the mucous membrane covering the penis; (g) injuries to the penis from blows (often causing paralysis); (h) warty growths on the end of the penis; (i) tumors of other kinds (largely pigmentary), affecting the testicles or penis; (j) nervous diseases which abolish the sexual appetite or that control the muscles which are essential to the act of coition; (k) azoturia with resulting weakness or paralysis of the muscles of the loins or the front of the thigh (above the stifle); (l) ossification (anchylosis) of the joints of the back or loins, which render the animal unable to rear or mount; (m) spavins, ringbones, or other painful affections of the hind limbs, the pain of which in mounting causes the animal to suddenly stop short in the act. In the first three of these only (a, b, and c) is there real sterility in the sense of the nondevelopment or imperfect development of the male vivifying element (spermatozoa). In the other examples the secretion may be imperfect in kind and amount, but as copulation is prevented it can not reach and impregnate the ovum.

In the mare barrenness is equally due to a variety of causes. In a number of breeding studs the proportion of sterile mares has varied from 20 to 40 per cent. It may be due to: (a) Imperfect development of the ovary and nonmaturation of ova; (b) cystic or other tumors of the ovary; (c) fatty degeneration of the ovary in very obese, pampered mares; (d) fatty degeneration of the excretory tubes of the ovaries (Fallopian tubes); (e) catarrh of the womb, with mucopurulent discharge; (f) irritable condition of the womb, with profuse secretion, straining, and ejection of the semen; (g) nervous irritability, leading to the same expulsion of the male element; (h) high condition (plethora), with profuse secretion and excitement; (i) low condition, with imperfect maturation of the ova and lack of sexual desire; (j) poor feeding, overwork, and chronic debilitating diseases, as leading to the condition just named; (k) closure of the neck of the womb, temporarily by spasm or permanently by inflammation and induration; (l) closure of the entrance to the vagina through imperforate hymen, a rare, though not unknown, condition in the mare; (m) acquired indisposition to breed, seen in old, hard-worked mares which are first put to the stallion when aged; (n) change of climate has repeatedly been followed by barrenness; (o) hybridity, which in male and female alike usually entails sterility.

Treatment.—The treatment of the majority of these conditions will be found dealt with in other parts of this work, so that it is only necessary here to name them as causes. Some, however, must be specially referred to in this place. Stallions with undescended testicles are beyond the reach of medicine, and should be castrated and devoted to other uses. Indurated testicles may sometimes be remedied in the early stages by smearing with a weak iodin ointment daily for a length of time, and at the same time invigorating the system by liberal feeding and judicious work. Fatty degeneration is best met by an albuminoid diet (wheat bran, cottonseed meal, rape cake) and constant, well-regulated work. Saccharine, starchy, and fatty food (potatoes, wheat, corn, etc.) are to be specially avoided. In the mare one diseased and irritable ovary should be removed, to do away with the resulting excitability of the remainder of the generative organs. An irritable womb, with frequent straining and the ejection of a profuse secretion, may sometimes be corrected by a restricted diet and full but well-regulated work. Even fatigue will act beneficially in some such cases, hence the practice of the Arab riding his mare to exhaustion just before service. The perspiration in such case, like the action of a purgative or the abstraction of blood just before service, benefits, by rendering the blood vessels less full, by lessening secretion in the womb and elsewhere, and thus counteracting the tendency to the ejection and loss of semen. If these means are ineffectual, a full dose of camphor (2 drams) or of salicin may at times assist. Low condition and anemia demand just the opposite kind of treatment—rich, nourishing, albuminoid feed, bitter tonics (gentian), sunshine, gentle exercise, liberal grooming, and supporting treatment generally are here in order.

Spasmodic closure of the neck of the womb is common and is easily remedied in the mare by dilatation with the fingers. The hand, smeared with belladonna ointment and with the fingers drawn into the form of a cone, is introduced through the vagina until the projecting, rounded neck of the womb is felt at its anterior end. This is opened by the careful insertion of one finger at a time, until the fingers have been passed through the constricted neck into the open cavity of the womb. The introduction is made with a gentle, rotary motion, and all precipitate violence is avoided, as abrasion, laceration, or other cause of irritation is likely to interfere with the retention of the semen and consequently with impregnation. If the neck of the womb is rigid and unyielding from the induration which follows inflammation—a rare condition in the mare, though common in the cow—more force will be requisite, and it may even be needful to incise the neck to the depth of one-sixth of an inch in four or more opposite directions prior to forcible dilatation. The incision may be made with a probe-pointed knife, and should be done by a professional man if possible. The subsequent dilatation may be best effected by the slow expansion of sponge or seaweed tents inserted into the narrow canal. In such cases it is best to let the wounds of the neck heal before putting to horse. An imperforate hymen may be freely incised in a crucial manner until the passage will admit the human hand. An ordinary knife may be used for this purpose, and after the operation the stallion may be admitted at once or only after the wounds have healed.

PREGNANCY.

INDICATIONS OF PREGNANCY.

As the mere fact of service by the stallion does not insure pregnancy, it is important that the result should be determined to save the mare from unnecessary and dangerous work or medication when actually in foal and to obviate wasteful and needless precautions when she is not.

The cessation and nonrecurrence of the symptoms of heat (horsing) are most significant, though not an infallible, sign of conception. If the sexual excitement speedily subsides and the mare persistently refuses the stallion for a month, she is probably pregnant. In very exceptional cases a mare, though pregnant, will accept a second or third service after weeks or months, and some mares will refuse the horse persistently, though conception has not taken place, and this in spite of warm weather, good condition of the mare, and liberal feeding. The recurrence of heat in the pregnant mare is most liable to take place in hot weather. If heat merely persists an undue length of time after service, or if it reappears shortly after, in warm weather and in a comparatively idle mare, on good feeding, it is less significant, while the persistent absence of heat under such conditions may be usually accepted as proof of conception.

An unwonted gentleness and docility on the part of a previously irritable or vicious mare, and supervening on service, is an excellent indication of pregnancy, the generative instinct which caused the excitement having been satisfied.

An increase of fat, with softness and flabbiness of muscle, a loss of energy, indisposition for active work, a manifestation of laziness, indeed, and of fatigue early and easily induced, when preceded by service, will usually imply conception.

Enlargement of the abdomen, especially in its lower third, with slight falling in beneath the loins and hollowness of the back are significant symptoms, though they may be entirely absent. Swelling and firmness of the udder, with the smoothing out of its wrinkles, is a suggestive sign, even though it appears only at intervals during gestation.

A steady increase in weight (1½ pounds daily) about the fourth or fifth month is a useful indication of pregnancy. So is a swollen and red or bluish-red appearance of the vaginal mucous membrane.

From the seventh or eighth month onward the foal may be felt by the hand (palm or knuckles) pressed into the abdomen in front of the left stifle. The sudden push displaces the foal toward the opposite side of the womb, and as it floats back its hard body is felt to strike against the hand. If the pressure is maintained the movements of the live foal are felt, and especially in the morning and after a drink of cold water or during feeding. A drink of cold water will often stimulate the fetus to movements that may be seen by the eye, but an excess of iced water may prove injurious, even to the causing of abortion. Cold water dashed on the belly has a similar effect on the fetus and is equally provocative of abortion.

Examination of the uterus with the oiled hand introduced into the rectum is still more satisfactory, and, if cautiously conducted, no more dangerous. The rectum must be first emptied and then the hand carried forward until it reaches the front edge of the pelvic bones below, and pressed downward to ascertain the size and outline of the womb. In the unimpregnated state the vagina and womb can be felt as a single rounded tube, dividing in front to two smaller tubes (the horns of the womb). In the pregnant mare not only the body of the womb is enlarged, but still more so one of the horns (right or left), and on compression the latter is found to contain a hard, nodular body, floating in a liquid, which in the latter half of gestation may be stimulated by gentle pressure to manifest spontaneous movements. By this method the presence of the fetus may be determined as early as the third month. If the complete, natural outline of the virgin womb can not be made out, careful examination should always be made on the right and left side for the enlarged horn and its living contents. Should there still be difficulty the mare should be placed on an inclined plane, with her hind parts lowest, and two assistants, standing on opposite sides of the body, should raise the lower part of the abdomen by a sheet passed beneath it. Finally the ear or stethoscope applied on the wall of the abdomen in front of the stifle may detect the beating of the fetal heart (one hundred and twenty-five a minute) and a blowing sound (the uterine sough), much less rapid and corresponding to the number of the pulse of the dam. It is heard most satisfactorily after the sixth or eighth month and in the absence of active rumbling of the bowels of the dam.

DURATION OF PREGNANCY.

Mares usually go about eleven months with young, though first pregnancies often last a year. Foals have lived when born at the three hundredth day, so with others carried till the four hundredth day. With the longer pregnancies there is a greater probability of male offspring.

HYGIENE OF THE PREGNANT MARE.

The pregnant mare should not be exposed to teasing by a young and ardent stallion, nor should she be overworked or fatigued, particularly under the saddle or on uneven ground. Yet exercise is beneficial to both mother and offspring, and in the absence of moderate work the breeding mare should be kept in a lot where she can take exercise at will.

The feed should be liberal, but not fattening—oats, bran, sound hay, and other feeds rich in the principles which form flesh and bone being especially indicated. All aliments that tend to indigestion are to be especially avoided. Thus rank, aqueous, rapidly growing grasses and other green feed, partially ripe rye grass, millet, Hungarian grass, vetches, peas, beans, or maize are objectionable, as is overripe, fibrous, innutritious hay, or that which has been injured and rendered musty by wet, or that which is infested with smut or ergot. Feed that tends to costiveness should be avoided. Water given often, and at a temperature considerable above freezing, will avoid the dangers of indigestion, which result from taking too much ice-cold water at one time. Very cold or frozen feed is objectionable in the same sense. Severe surgical operations and medicines that act violently on the womb, bowels, or kidneys are to be avoided as being liable to cause abortion. Constipation should be corrected, if possible, by bran mashes, carrots, or beets, seconded by exercise, and if a medicinal laxative is required it should be olive oil or other equally bland agent.

The stall of the pregnant mare should not be too narrow, so as to cramp her when lying down or to entail violent effort in getting up, and it should not slope too much from the front backward, as this throws the weight of the uterus back on the pelvis and endangers protrusions and even abortion. It is important to prevent prolonged, acute suffering by the pregnant mare, as certain troubles of the eyes, feet, and joints in the foals have been clearly traced to corresponding injured organs in herself. Sire and dam alike tend to

54763°—23——12

reproduce their individual defects which predispose to disease, but the dam is far more liable to perpetuate the evil in her progeny which was carried while she was individually enduring severe suffering caused by such defects. Hence, an active bone spavin or ringbone, causing lameness, is more objectionable than that in which the inflammation and lameness have both passed, and an active ophthalmia is more to be feared than even an old cataract. For this reason all active diseases in the breeding mare should be soothed and abated as early as possible.

EXTRA-UTERINE GESTATION.

It is rare in the domestic animals to find the fetus developed elsewhere than in the womb. The exceptional forms are those in which the sperm of the male, making its way through the womb and Fallopian tubes, impregnates the ovum prior to its escape, and in which the now vitalized and growing ovum, by reason of its gradually increasing size, becomes imprisoned and fails to escape into the womb. The arrest of the ovum may be in the substance of the ovary itself (ovarian pregnancy), in the Fallopian tube (tubal pregnancy), or when by its continuous enlargement it has ruptured its envelopes so that it escapes into the cavity of the abdomen, it may become attached to any part of the serous membrane and draw its nourishment directly from that (abdominal pregnancy). In all such cases there is an increase and enlargement of the capillary blood vessels at the point to which the embryo has attached itself so as to furnish the needful nutriment for the growing offspring.

All appreciable symptoms are absent, unless from the death of the fetus, or its interference with normal functions, general disorder and indications of parturition supervene. If these occur later than the natural time for parturition, they are the more significant. There may be general malaise, loss of appetite, elevated temperature, accelerated pulse, with or without distinct labor pains. Examination with the oiled hand in the rectum will reveal the womb of the natural, unimpregnated size and shape and with both horns of one size. Further exploration may detect an elastic mass apart from the womb, in the interior of which may be felt the characteristic solid body of the fetus. If the latter is still alive and can be stimulated to move, the evidence is even more perfect. The fetus may die and be carried for years, its soft structures becoming absorbed so as to leave only the bones, or by pressure it may form a fistulous opening through the abdominal walls, or less frequently through the vagina or rectum. In the latter cases the best course is to favor the expulsion of the foal and to wash out the resulting cavity with a solution of carbolic acid 1 part to water 50 parts. This may be repeated daily. When there is no spontaneous opening it is injudicious to interfere, as the danger from the retention of the fetus is less than that from septic fermentation in the enormous fetal sac when that has been opened to the air.

MOLES, OR ANIDIAN MONSTERS.

These are evidently products of conception, in which the impregnated ovum has failed to develop naturally, and presents only a chaotic mass of skin, hair, bones, muscles, etc., attached to the inner surface of the womb by an umbilical cord, which is itself often shriveled and wasted. They are usually accompanied with a well-developed fetus, so that the mole may be looked upon as a twin which has undergone arrest and vitiation of development. They are expelled by the ordinary process of parturition, and usually at the same time with the normally developed offspring.

CYSTIC DISEASE OF THE WALLS OF THE WOMB, OR VESICULAR MOLE.

This condition appears to be attributable to hypertrophy (enlargement) of the villi on the inner surface of the womb, which become greatly increased in number and hollowed out internally into a series of cysts, or pouches, containing liquid. Unlike the true mole, therefore, they appear to be disease of the maternal structure of the womb rather than of the product of conception. Rodet, in a case of this kind, which had produced active labor pains, quieted the disorder with anodynes and effected a recovery. When this can not be done, attempts may be made to remove the mass with the écraseur or otherwise, following it up with antiseptic injections, as advised under the last heading.

DROPSY OF THE WOMB.

This appears as a result of some disease of the walls of the womb, but has been frequently observed as the result of infection after sexual congress, and has, therefore, been confounded with pregnancy. The symptoms are those of pregnancy, but without any movements of the fetus and without the detection of any solid body in the womb when examined with the oiled hand in the rectum. At the end of four or eight months there are signs of parturition or of frequent straining to pass urine, and after a time the liquid is discharged clear and watery, or muddy, thick, and fetid. The hand introduced into the womb can detect neither fetus nor fetal membrane. If the neck of the womb closes, the liquid may accumulate a second time, or even a third, if no means are taken to disinfect it or to correct the tendency. The best resort is to remove any diseased product that may be found attached to the walls of the womb and to inject it daily with a warm solution of carbolic acid 2 drams, chlorid of zinc one-half dram, water 1 quart. A course of bitter tonics (gentian 2 drams, sulphate of iron 2 drams, daily) should be given, and a nutritious, easily digested, and slightly laxative diet allowed.

DROPSY OF THE AMNION.

This differs from simple dropsy of the womb in that the fluid collects in the inner of the two water bags (that in which the foal floats) and not in the otherwise void cavity of the womb. This affection can occur only in the pregnant animal, while dropsy of the womb occurs in the unimpregnated. The blood of the pregnant mare contains an excess of water and a smaller proportion of albumen and red globules, and when this condition is still further aggravated by poor feeding and other unhygienic conditions there is developed the tendency to liquid transudation from the vessels and dropsy. As the watery condition of the blood increases with advancing pregnancy, so dropsy of the amnion is a disease of the last four or five months of gestation. The abdomen is large and pendulous, and the swelling fluctuates under pressure, though the solid body of the fetus can still be felt to strike against the hand pressed into the swelling. If the hand is introduced into the vagina, the womb is found to be tense and round, with the projecting rounded neck effaced, while the hand in the rectum will detect the rounded, swollen mass of the womb so firm and tense that the body of the fetus can not be felt within it. The mare moves weakly and unsteadily on her limbs, having difficulty in supporting the great weight, and in bad cases there may be loss of appetite, stocking (dropsy) of the hind limbs, difficult breathing, and colicky pains. The tension may lead to abortion, or a slow, laborious parturition may occur at the usual time.

Treatment consists in relieving the tension and accumulation by puncturing the fetal membrane with a cannula and trocar introduced through the neck of the womb and the withdrawal of the trocar so as to leave the cannula in situ, or the membranes may be punctured with the finger and the excess of liquid allowed to escape. This may bring on abortion, or the womb may close and gestation continue to the full term. A course of tonics (gentian root 2 drams, sulphate of iron 2 drams, daily) will do much to fortify the system and counteract further excessive effusion.

DROPSY OF THE LIMBS, PERINEUM, AND ABDOMEN.

The disposition to dropsy often shows itself in the hind and even in the fore limbs, around and beneath the vulva (perineum), and beneath the abdomen and chest. The affected parts are swollen and pit on pressure, but are not especially tender, and subside more or less perfectly under exercise, hand rubbing, and bandages. In obstinate cases rubbing with the following liniment may be resorted to:

Compound tincture of iodin, 2 ounces; tannic acid, one-half dram; water, 10 ounces. It does not last more than a day or two after parturition.

CRAMPS OF THE HIND LIMBS.

The pressure of the distended womb on the nerves and blood vessels of the pelvis, besides conducing to dropsy, occasionally causes cramps of the hind limbs. The limb is raised without flexing the joints, the front of the hoof being directed toward the ground, or, the spasms occurring intermittently, the foot is kicked violently against the ground several times in rapid succession. The muscles are felt to be firm and rigid. The cramp may be promptly relieved by active rubbing or by walking the animal about, and it does not reappear after parturition.

CONSTIPATION.

This may result from compression by gravid womb, and is best corrected by a graduated allowance of boiled flaxseed.

PARALYSIS.

The pressure on the nerves of the pelvis is liable to cause paralysis of the hind limbs or of the nerve of sight. These are obstinate until after parturition, when they recover spontaneously, or under a course of nux vomica and (local) stimulating liniments.

PROLONGED RETENTION OF THE FETUS (FOAL).

Though far less frequently than in the case of the cow, parturition may not be completed at term, and the mare, to her serious and even fatal injury, may carry the foal in the womb for a number of months. Hamon records one case in which the mare died after carrying the fetus for 17 months, and Caillier a similar result after it had been carried 22 months. In these cases the fetus retained its natural form, but in one reported by Gohier the bones only were left in the womb amid a mass of apparently purulent matter.

Cause.—The cause may be any effective obstruction to the act of parturition, such as lack of contractile power in the womb, unduly strong (inflammatory) adhesions between the womb and the fetal membranes, wrong presentation of the fetus, contracted pelvis (from fracture or disease of the bones), or disease and induration of the neck of the womb.

The mere prolongation of gestation does not necessarily entail the death of the foal; hence the latter has been born alive at the four hundredth day. Even when the foal has perished putrefaction does not set in unless the membranes (water bags) have been ruptured and septic bacteria have been admitted to the interior of the womb. In the latter case a fetid decomposition advances rapidly, and the mare usually perishes from poisoning with the putrid matters absorbed.

At the natural period of parturition preparations are apparently made for that act. The vulva swells and discharges much mucus, the udder enlarges, the belly becomes more pendent, and the animal strains more or less. No progress is made, however; there is not even opening of the neck of the womb, and after a time the symptoms subside. The mare usually refuses the male, yet there are exceptions to this rule. If the neck of the womb has been opened and putrefying changes in its contents have set in, the mare loses appetite and condition, pines, discharges an offensive matter from the generative passages, and dies of inflammation of the womb and putrid infection. In other cases there is a slow wearing out of the strength, and she finally dies of exhaustion.

The treatment is such as will facilitate the expulsion of the fetus and its membranes and the subsequent washing out of the womb with disinfectants. So long as the mouth of the womb is closed time should be allowed for its natural dilatation, but if this does not come about after a day or two of straining, the opening may be smeared with extract of belladonna, and the oiled hand, with the fingers and thumb drawn into the form of a cone, may be inserted by slow oscillating movements into the interior of the womb. The water bags may now be ruptured, any malpresentation rectified (see "Difficult parturition"), and delivery effected. After removal of the membranes wash out the womb first with tepid water and then with a solution of 2 ounces of borax in half a gallon of water.

This injection may have to be repeated if a discharge sets in. The same course may be pursued even after prolonged retention. If the soft parts of the fetus have been absorbed and the bones only left, these must be carefully sought for and removed, and subsequent daily injections will be required for some time. In such cases, too, a course of iron tonics (sulphate of iron, 2 drams daily) will be highly beneficial in restoring health and vigor.

ABORTION.

Abortion is, strictly speaking, the expulsion of the impregnated ovum at any period from the date of impregnation until the foal can survive out of the womb. If the foal is advanced enough to live, it is premature parturition, and in the mare this may occur as early as the tenth month (three hundredth day).

The mare may abort by reason of almost any cause that very profoundly disturbs the system; hence, very violent inflammations of important internal organs (bowels, kidneys, bladder, lungs) may induce abortion. Profuse diarrhea, whether occurring from the reckless use of purgatives, the consumption of irritants in the feed, or a simple indigestion, is an effective cause. No less so is acute indigestion with evolution of gas in the intestines (bloating). The presence of stone in the kidneys, uterus, bladder, or urethra may induce so much sympathetic disorder in the womb as to induce abortion. In exceptional cases wherein mares come in heat during gestation, service by the stallion may cause abortion. Blows or pressure on the abdomen, rapid driving or riding of the pregnant mare, especially if she is soft and out of condition from idleness, the brutal use of the spur or whip, and the jolting and straining of travel by rail or boat are prolific causes. Bleeding the pregnant mare, a painful surgical operation, and the throwing and constraint resorted to for an operation are other causes. Traveling on heavy, muddy roads, slips and falls on ice, and jumping must be added. The stimulation of the abdominal organs by a full drink of iced water may precipitate a miscarriage, as may exposure to a cold rainstorm or a very cold night after a warm day. Irritant poisons that act on the urinary or generative organs, such as Spanish flies, rue, savin, tansy, cotton-root bark, ergot of rye or other grasses, the smut of maize and other grain, and various fungi in musty fodder are additional causes. Frosted or indigestible feed, and, above all, green succulent vegetables in a frozen state, have proved effective factors, and filthy, stagnant water is dangerous. Low condition in the dam and plethora have in opposite ways caused abortion, and hot, relaxing stables and lack of exercise strongly conduce to it. The exhaustion of the sire by too frequent service, entailing debility of the offspring and disease of the fetus or of its envelopes, must be recognized as a further cause.

The symptoms vary mainly according as the abortion is early or late in pregnancy. In the first month or two of pregnancy the mare may miscarry without observable symptoms, and the fact appears only by her coming in heat. If more closely observed a small clot of blood may be found behind her, in which a careful search reveals the rudiments of the foal. If the occurrence is somewhat later in gestation, there will be some general disturbance, loss of appetite, neighing, and straining, and the small body of the fetus is expelled, enveloped in its membranes. Abortions during the later stages of pregnancy are attended with greater constitutional disturbance, and the process resembles normal parturition, with the aggravation that more effort and straining is requisite to force the fetus through the comparatively undilatable mouth of the womb. There is the swelling of the vulva, with mucus or even bloody discharge; the abdomen droops, the flanks fall in, the udder fills, the mare looks at her flanks, paws with the fore feet and kicks with the hind, switches the tail, moves around uneasily, lies down and rises, strains, and, as in natural foaling, expels first mucus and blood, then the waters, and finally the fetus. This may occupy an hour or two, or it may be prolonged for a day or more, the symptoms subsiding for a time, only to reappear with renewed energy. If there is malpresentation of the fetus it will hinder progress until rectified, as in difficult parturition. Abortion may also be followed by the same accidents, as flooding, retention of the placenta, and leucorrhea.

The most important object in an impending abortion is to recognize it at as early a stage as possible, so that it may, if possible, be cut short and prevented. Any general, indefinable illness in a pregnant mare should lead to a close examination of the vulva as regards swelling, vascularity of its mucous membrane, and profuse mucus secretion, and, above all, any streak or staining of blood; also the condition of the udder, if that is congested and swollen. Any such indication, with colicky pains, straining, however little, and active movement of the fetus or entire absence of movement, are suggestive symptoms and should be duly counteracted.

The changes in the vulva and udder, with a soiled and bloody condition of the tail, may suggest an abortion already accomplished, and the examination with the hand in the vagina may detect the mouth of the womb soft and dilatable and the interior of the organ slightly filled with a bloody liquid.

Treatment should be preventive if possible, and would embrace the avoidance of all causes mentioned, and particularly of such as may seem to be particularly operative in the particular case. If abortions have already occurred in a stud, the especial cause in the matter of feed, water, exposure to injuries, overwork, lack of exercise, etc., may often be identified and removed. A most important point is to avoid all causes of constipation, diarrhea, indigestion, bloating, violent purgatives, diuretics or other potent medicines, painful operations, and slippery roads, unless well frosted.

When abortion is imminent, the mare should be placed alone in a roomy, dark, quiet stall, and have the straining checked by some sedative. Laudanum is usually at hand and may be given in doses of 1 or 2 ounces, according to size, and repeated after two or three hours, and even daily if necessary. Chloroform or chloral hydrate, 3 drams, may be substituted if more convenient. These should be given in a pint or quart of water, to avoid burning the mouth and throat. Or *Viburnum prunifolium* (black haw), 1 ounce, may be given and repeated if necessary to prevent straining.

When all measures fail and miscarriage proceeds, all that can be done is to assist in the removal of the fetus and its membranes, as in ordinary parturition. As in the case of retention of the fetus, it may be necessary after delivery to employ antiseptic injections into the womb to counteract putrid fermentation. This, however, is less necessary in the mare than in the cow, in which the prevalent contagious abortion must be counteracted by the persistent local use of antiseptics. After abortion a careful hygiene is demanded, especially in the matter of pure air and easily digestible feed. The mare should not be served again for a month or longer, and in no case until after all discharge from the vulva has ceased.

INFECTIOUS ABORTION IN MARES.

This disease is discussed in the chapter on " Infectious Diseases."

PARTURITION.

SYMPTOMS OF PARTURITION.

As the period of parturition approaches, the swelling of the udder bespeaks the coming event, the engorgement in exceptional cases extending forward on the lower surface of the abdomen and even into the hind limbs. For about a week a serous fluid oozes from the teat and concretes as a yellow, waxlike mass around its orifice. About 24 hours before the birth this gives place to a whitish, milky liquid, which falls upon and mats the hairs on the inner sides of the legs. Another symptom is enlargement of the vulva, with redness of its lining membrane, and the escape of glairy mucus. The belly droops, the flanks fall in, and the loins may even become depressed. Finally the mare becomes uneasy, stops feeding, looks anxious, whisks her tail, and may lie down and rise again. In many mares this is not repeated, but they remain down; violent contractions of the abdominal muscles ensue; after two or three pains the water bags appear and burst, followed by the fore feet of the foal, with the nose between the knees, and by a few more throes the fetus is expelled. In other cases the act is accomplished standing. The whole act may not occupy more than 5 or 10 minutes. This, together with the disposition of the mare to avoid observation, renders the act one that is rarely seen by the attendants.

The navel string, which connects the foal to the membranes, is ruptured when the fetus falls to the ground, or when the mare rises, if she has been down, and the membranes are expelled a few minutes later.

NATURAL PRESENTATION.

When there is a single foal, the common and desirable presentation is with the fore feet first, the nose between the knees, and with the front of the hoofs and knees and the forehead directed upward toward the anus, tail, and croup. (Plate XII, fig. 1.) In this way the natural curvature of the body of the fetus corresponds to the curve of the womb and genital passages, and particularly of the bony pelvis, and the foal passes with much greater ease than if placed with its back downward toward the udder. When there is a twin birth the second foal usually comes with its hind feet first, and the backs of the legs, the points of the hocks, and the tail and croup are turned upward toward the anus and tail of the mare. (Plate XII, fig. 2.) In this way, even with a posterior presentation, the curvature of the body of the foal still corresponds to that of the passages, and its expulsion may be quite as easy as in anterior presentation. Any presentation aside from these two may be said to be abnormal and will be considered under "Difficult parturition."

PREMATURE LABOR PAINS.

These may be brought on by any violent exertion, use under the saddle, or in heavy draft, or in rapid paces, or in travel by rail or sea, blows, kicks, crushing by other animals in a doorway or gate. Excessive action of purgative or diuretic agents, or of agents that irritate the bowels or kidneys, like arsenic, paris green, all caustic salts and acids, and acrid and narcotico-acrid vegetables, is equally injurious. Finally, the ingestion of agents that stimulate the action of the gravid womb (ergot of rye or of other grasses, smut, various fungi of fodders, rüe, savin, cotton root, etc.) may bring on labor pains prematurely.

Besides the knowledge that parturition is not yet due, there will be less enlargement, redness, and swelling of the vulva, less mucous discharge, less filling of the udder, and fewer appearances of wax and probably none of milk from the ends of the teats. The oiled hand introduced into the vulva will not enter with the ease usual at full term, and the neck of the womb will be felt not only closed, but with its projecting papillæ, through which it is perforated, not yet flattened down and effaced, as at full term. The symptoms are, indeed, those of threatened abortion, but at such an advanced stage of gestation as is compatible with the survival of the offspring.

Treatment.—The treatment consists in the separation of the mare, in a quiet, dark, secluded place, from all other animals, and the free use of antispasmodics and anodynes. Opium in dram doses every two hours, or laudanum in ounce doses at similar intervals, will often suffice. When the more urgent symptoms have subsided these doses may be repeated thrice a day till all excitement passes off or until the passages have become relaxed and prepared for parturition. *Viburnum prunifolium* (black haw), in ounce doses, may be added if necessary. Should parturition become inevitable, it may be favored and any necessary assistance furnished.

DIFFICULT PARTURITION.

With natural presentation this is a rare occurrence. The great length of the fore limbs and face entail, in the anterior presentation, the formation of a long cone, which dilates and glides through the passages with comparative ease. Even with the hind feet first a similar conical form is presented, and the process is rendered easy and quick. Difficulty and danger arise mainly from the act being brought on prematurely before the passages are sufficiently dilated, from narrowing of the pelvic bones or other mechanical obstruction in the passages, from monstrous distortions or duplications in the fetus, or from the turning back of one of the members so that the elongated conical or wedge-shaped outline is done away with. Prompt as is the normal parturition in the mare, however, difficult and delayed parturitions are surrounded by special dangers and require unusual precautions and skill. From the proclivity of the mare to unhealthy inflammations of the peritoneum and other abdominal organs, penetrating wounds of the womb or vagina are liable to prove fatal. The contractions of the womb and abdominal walls are so powerful as to exhaust and benumb the arm of the assistant and to endanger penetrating wounds of the genital organs. By reason of the looser connection of the fetal membranes with the womb, as compared with those of ruminants, the violent throes early detach these membranes throughout their whole extent, and the foal, being thus separated from the mother and thrown on its own resources, dies at an early stage of any protracted parturition. The foal rarely survives four hours after the onset of parturient throes. From the great length of the limbs and neck of the foal it is extremely difficult to secure and bring up limb or head which has been turned back when it should have been presented. When assistance must be rendered, the operator should don a thick woolen undershirt with the sleeves cut out at the shoulders. This protects the body and leaves the whole arm free for manipulation. Before inserting the arm it should be smeared with lard. This protects the skin against septic infection and favors the introduction of the hand and arm. The hand should be inserted with the thumb and fingers drawn together like a cone. Whether standing or lying, the mare should be turned with head downhill and hind parts raised as much as possible. The contents of the abdomen gravitating forward leave much more room for manipulation. Whatever part of the foal is presented (head, foot) should be secured with a cord and running noose before it is pushed back to search for the other missing parts. Even if a missing part is reached, no attempt should be made to bring it up during a labor pain. Pinching the back will sometimes check the pains and allow the operator to secure and bring up the missing member. In intractable cases a large dose of chloral hydrate (1 ounce in a quart of water) or the inhalation of chloroform and air (equal proportions) to insensibility may secure a respite, during which the missing members may be replaced. If the waters have been discharged and the mucus dried up, the genital passages and body of the fetus should be lubricated with lard or oil before any attempt at extraction is made. When the missing member has been brought up into position and presentation has been rendered natural, traction on the fetus must be made only during a labor pain. If a mare is inclined to kick, it may be necessary to apply hobbles to protect the operator.

DIFFICULT PARTURITION FROM NARROW PELVIS.—A disproportion between the fetus got by a large stallion and the pelvis of a small dam is a serious obstacle to parturition, sometimes seen in the mare. This is not the rule, however, as the foal up to birth usually accommodates itself to the size of the dam, as illustrated in the successful crossing of Percheron stallions on mustang mares. If the disproportion is too great the only resort is embryotomy.

FRACTURED HIP BONES.—More commonly the obstruction comes from distortion and narrowing of the pelvis as the result of fractures. (Plate XIII, fig. 2.) Fractures at any point of the lateral wall or floor of the pelvis are repaired with the formation of an extensive bony deposit bulging into the passage of the pelvis. The displacement of the ends of the broken bone is another cause of constriction, and between the two conditions the passage of the fetus may be rendered impossible without embryotomy. Fracture of the sacrum (the continuation of the backbone forming the croup) leads to the depression of the posterior part of that bone in the roof of the pelvis and the narrowing of the passage from above downward by a bony ridge presenting its sharp edge forward.

In all cases in which there has been injury to the bones of the pelvis the obvious precaution is to withhold the mare from breeding and to use her for work only.

If a mare with a pelvis thus narrowed has got in foal inadvertently, abortion may be induced in the early months of gestation by slowly introducing the oiled finger through the neck of the womb and following this by the other fingers until the whole hand has been introduced. Then the water bags may be broken, and with the escape of the liquid the womb will contract on the solid fetus and labor pains will ensue. The fetus being small will pass easily.

TUMORS IN THE VAGINA AND PELVIS.—Tumors of various kinds may form in the vagina or elsewhere within the pelvis, and when large enough will obstruct or prevent the passage of the fetus. Gray mares, which are so subject to black pigment tumors (melanosis) on the tail, anus, and vulva, are the most liable to suffer from this. Still more rarely the wall of the vagina becomes relaxed, and being pressed by a mass of intestines will protrude through the lips of the vulva as a hernial sac, containing a part of the bowels. If a tumor is small it may only retard and not absolutely prevent parturition. A hernial protrusion of the wall of the vagina may be pressed back and emptied, so that the body of the fetus engaging in the passage may find no further obstacle. When a tumor is too large to allow delivery the only resort is to remove it, but before proceeding it must be clearly made out that the obstruction is a mass of diseased tissue, and not a sac containing intestines. If the tumor hangs by a neck it can usually be most safely removed by the écraseur, the chain being passed around the pedicel and gradually tightened until that is torn through.

HERNIA OF THE WOMB.—The rupture of the musculo-fibrous floor of the belly and the escape of the gravid womb into a sac formed by the peritoneum and skin hanging toward the ground is described by all veterinary obstetricians, yet it is very rarely seen in the mare. The form of the fetus can be felt through the walls of the sac, so that it is easy to recognize the condition. Its cause is usually external violence, though it may start from an umbilical hernia. When the period of parturition arrives, the first effort should be to return the fetus within the proper abdominal cavity, and this can sometimes be accomplished with the aid of a stout blanket gradually tightened around the belly. This failing, the mare may be placed on her side or back and gravitation brought to the aid of manipulation in effecting the return. Even after the hernia has been reduced the relaxed state of the womb and abdominal walls may serve to hinder parturition, in which case the oiled hand must be introduced through the vagina, the fetus brought into position, and traction coincident with the labor pains employed to produce delivery.

TWISTING OF THE NECK OF THE WOMB.—This condition is very uncommon in the mare, though occasionally seen in the cow, owing to the greater laxity of the broad ligaments of the womb in that animal. It consists in a revolution of the womb on its own axis, so that its right or left side will be turned upward (quarter revolution), or the lower surface may be turned upward and the upper surface downward (half revolution). The effect is to throw the narrow neck of the womb into a series of spiral folds, turning in the direction in which the womb has revolved, closing the neck and rendering distention and dilatation impossible.

The period and pains of parturition arrive, but in spite of continued efforts no progress is made, neither water bags nor liquids appearing. The oiled hand introduced into the closed neck of the womb will readily detect the spiral direction of the folds on its inner surface.

The method of relief which I have successfully adopted in the cow may be equally effective in the mare. The dam is placed (with her head uphill) on her right side if the upper folds of the spiral turn toward the right, and on her left side if they turn toward the left, and the oiled hand is introduced through the neck of the womb and a limb or other part of the body of the fetus is seized and pressed against the wall of the womb, while two or three assistants turn the animal over on her back toward the other side. The object is to keep the womb stationary while the animal is rolling. If success attends the effort, the constriction around the arm is suddenly relaxed, the spiral folds are effaced, and the water bags and fetus press forward into the passage. If the first attempt does not succeed, it may be repeated again and again until success crowns the effort. Among my occasional causes of failure have been the prior death and decomposition of the fetus, with the extrication of gas and over-distention of the womb, and the supervention of inflammation and inflammatory exudation around the neck of the womb, which hinders untwisting. The first of these conditions occurs early in the horse from the detachment of the fetal membranes from the wall of the womb; and as the mare is more subject to fatal peritonitis than the cow, it may be concluded that both these sources of failure are more probable in the former subject.

When the case is intractable, though the hand may be easily introduced, the instrument shown in Plate XIV, figure 7, may be used. Each hole at the small end of the instrument has passed through it a stout cord with a running noose, to be passed around two feet or other portion of the fetus which it may be possible to reach. The cords are then drawn tight and fixed around the handle of the instrument; then, by using the cross handle as a lever, the fetus and womb may be rotated in a direction opposite to that causing the obstruction. During this process the hand must be introduced to feel when the twist has been undone. This method may be supplemented, if necessary, by rolling the mare as described above.

EFFUSION OF BLOOD IN THE VAGINAL WALLS.—This is common as a result of difficult parturition, but it may occur from local injury before that act, and may seriously interfere with it. This condition is easily recognized by the soft, doughy swelling so characteristic of blood clots, and by the dark-red color of the mucous membrane. I have laid open such swellings with the knife as late as 10 days before parturition, evacuated the clots, and dressed the wound daily with an astringent lotion (sulphate of zinc 1 dram, carbolic acid 1 dram, water 1 quart). A similar resort might be had, if necessary, during parturition.

CALCULUS (STONE) AND TUMOR IN THE BLADDER.—The pressure upon the bladder containing a stone or a tumor may prove so painful that the mare will voluntarily suppress the labor pains. Examination of the bladder with the finger introduced through the urethra will detect the offending agent. A stone should be extracted with forceps. (See "Lithotomy.") The large papillary tumors which I have met with in the mare's bladder have been invariably delicate in texture and could be removed piecemeal by forceps. Fortunately, mares affected in this way rarely breed.

FECAL IMPACTION OF THE RECTUM.—In some animals, with more or less paralysis or weakness of the tail and rectum, the rectum may become so impacted with solid feces that the mare is unable to discharge them, and the accumulation both by reason of the mechanical obstruction and the pain caused by pressure upon it will impel the animal to cut short all labor pains. The rounded swelling surrounding the anus will at once suggest the condition, when the obstruction may be removed by the well-oiled or well-soaped hand.

SPASM OF THE NECK OF THE WOMB.—This occurs in the mare of specially excitable temperament, or under particular causes of irritation, local or general. Labor pains, though continuing for some time, produce no dilatation of the neck of the womb, which will be found firmly closed so as to admit but one or two fingers; this, although the projection at the mouth of the womb may have been entirely effaced, so that a simple round opening is left, with rigid margins.

The simplest treatment consists in smearing this part with solid extract of belladonna, and after an interval inserting the hand with fingers and thumb drawn into the form of a cone, rupturing the membranes and bringing the fetus into position for extraction, as advised under "Prolonged retention of the fetus." Another mode is to insert through the neck of the womb an ovoid rubber bag, empty, and furnished with an elastic tube 12 feet long. Carry the free end of this tube upward to a height of 8, 10, or 12 feet, insert a filler into it, and proceed to distend the bag with tepid or warm water.

FIBROUS BANDS CONSTRICTING OR CROSSING THE NECK OF THE WOMB.— These, occurring as the result of disease, have been several times observed in the mare. They may exist in the cavity of the abdomen and compress and obstruct the neck of the womb, or they may extend from side to side of the vagina across and just behind the neck of the womb. In the latter position they may be felt and quickly remedied by cutting them across. In the abdomen they can be reached only by incision, and two alternatives are presented: (1) To perform embryotomy and extract the fetus piecemeal, and (2) to make an incision into the abdomen and extract by the Cæsarean operation, or simply to cut the constricting band and attempt delivery by the usual channel.

FIBROUS CONSTRICTION OF VAGINA OR VULVA.—This is probably always the result of direct mechanical injury and the formation of rigid cicatrices which fail to dilate with the remainder of the passages at the approach of parturition. The presentation of the fetus in the natural way and the occurrence of successive and active labor pains without any favorable result will direct attention to the rigid and unyielding cicatrices which may be incised at one, two, or more points to a depth of half an inch or more, after which the natural expulsive efforts will usually prove effective. The resulting wounds may be washed frequently with a solution of 1 part of carbolic acid to 50 parts of water, or of 1 part of mercuric chlorid to 1,000 parts of water.

FETUS ADHERENT TO THE WALLS OF THE WOMB.—In inflammation of the mucous membrane lining the cavity of the womb and implicating the fetal membranes the resulting embryonic tissue sometimes establishes a medium of direct continuity between the womb and fetal membranes; the blood vessels of the one communicate freely with those of the other and the fibers of the one are prolonged into the other. This causes retention of the membranes after birth, and a special risk of bleeding from the womb, and of septic poisoning. In exceptional cases the adhesion is more extensive and binds a portion of the body of the foal firmly to the womb. In such cases it has repeatedly been found impossible to extract the foal until such adhesions were broken down. If they can be reached with the hand and recognized, they may be torn through with the fingers or with a blunt hook, after which delivery may be attempted with hope of success.

EXCESSIVE SIZE OF FETUS.—It would seem that a small mare may usually be safely bred to a large stallion, yet this is not always the case, and when the small size is an individual rather than a racial characteristic or the result of being very young, the rule can not be expected to hold. There is always great danger in breeding the young, small, and undeveloped female, and the dwarfed representative of a larger breed, as the offspring tend to partake of the large race characteristics and to show them even prior to birth. When impregnation has occurred in the very young or in the dwarfed female there are two alternatives—to induce abortion or to wait until there are attempts at parturition and to extract by embryotomy if impracticable otherwise.

CONSTRICTION OF A MEMBER BY THE NAVEL STRING.—In man and animals alike the winding of the umbilical cord around a member of the fetus sometimes leads to the amputation of the latter. It is also known to get wound around the neck or a limb at birth, but in the mare this does not seriously impede parturition, as the loosely attached membranes are easily separated from the womb and no strangulation or retarding occurs. The foal may, however, die from the cessation of the placental circulation unless it is speedily delivered.

WATER IN THE HEAD (HYDROCEPHALUS) OF THE FOAL.—This consists in the excessive accumulation of liquid in the ventricles of the brain so that the cranial cavity is enlarged and constitutes a great, projecting, rounded mass occupying the space from the eyes upward. (See

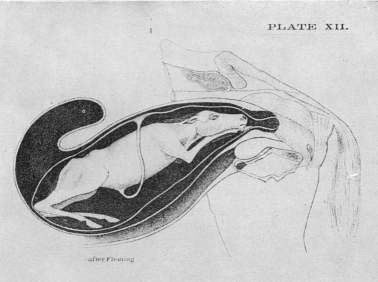

PLATE XII.

1

after Fleming

Vertebro Sacral presentation

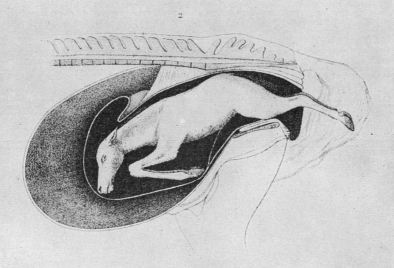

2

Lumbo Sacral presentation

Haines del.

NORMAL PRESENTATIONS.

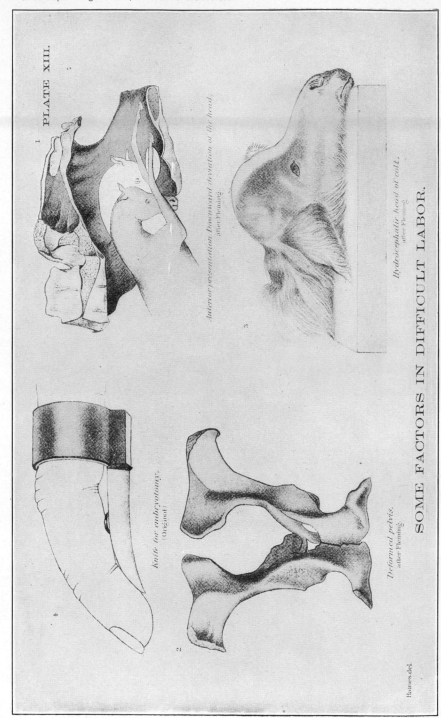

PLATE XIII.

Anteror presentation downward deviation of the head, after Fleming.

Hydrocephalic head of colt, after Fleming

Knife for embryotomy, (Original)

Deformed pelvis, after Fleming

SOME FACTORS IN DIFFICULT LABOR.

Haines, del.

PLATE XIV.

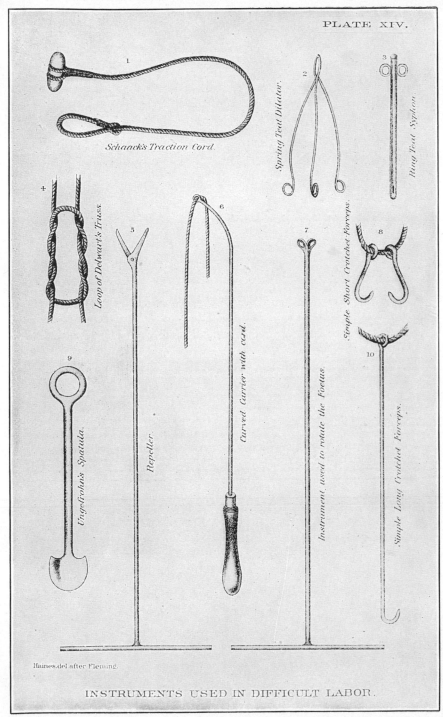

1. Schaack's Traction Cord.
2. Spring Teat Dilator.
3. Ring Teat Syphon.
4. Loop of Detwart's Truss.
5. Repeller.
6. Curved Carrier with cord.
7. Instrument used to rotate the Foetus.
8. Simple Short Crotchet Forceps.
9. Ungefrohn's Spatula.
10. Simple Long Crotchet Forceps.

Haines.del after Fleming.

INSTRUMENTS USED IN DIFFICULT LABOR.

Plate XIII, fig. 3.) With an anterior presentation (fore feet and nose) this presents an insuperable obstacle to progress, as the diseased cranium is too large to enter the pelvis at the same time with the fore arms. With a posterior presentation (hind feet) all goes well until the body and shoulders have passed out, when progress is suddenly arrested by the great bulk of the head. In the first case, the oiled hand introduced along the face detects the enormous size of the head, which may be diminished by puncturing it with a knife or trocar and cannula in the median line, evacuating the water and pressing in the thin, bony walls. With a posterior presentation, the same course must be followed; the hand passed along the neck will detect the cranial swelling, which may be punctured with a knife or trocar. Oftentimes with an anterior presentation the great size of the head leads to its displacement backward, and thus the fore limbs alone engage in the passages. Here the first object is to seek and bring up the missing head, and then puncture it as above suggested.

ASCITES, OR DROPSY OF THE ABDOMEN IN THE FOAL.—The accumulation of liquid in the abdominal cavity of the fetus is less frequent, but when present it may arrest parturition as completely as will hydrocephalus. With an anterior presentation the foal may pass as far as the shoulders, but behind this all efforts fail to effect a further advance. With a posterior presentation the hind legs as far as the thighs may be expelled, but at this point all progress ceases. In either case the oiled hand, passed inward by the side of the foal, will detect the enormous distension of the abdomen and its soft, fluctuating contents. The only course is to puncture the cavity and evacuate the liquid. With the anterior presentation this may be done with a long trocar and cannula, introduced through the chest and diaphragm, or with a knife an incision may be made between the first two ribs and the lungs and heart cut or torn out, when the diaphragm will be felt projecting strongly forward, and may be easily punctured. Should there not be room to introduce the hand through the chest, the oiled hand may be passed along beneath the breast bone and the adbomen punctured. With a posterior presentation the abdomen must be punctured in the same way, the hand, armed with a knife protected in its palm, being passed along the side of the flank or between the hind limbs. It should be added that moderate dropsy of the abdomen is not incompatible with natural delivery, the liquid being at first crowded back into the portion of the belly still engaged in the womb, and passing slowly from that into the advanced portion as soon as that has cleared the narrow passage of the pelvis and passed out where it can expand.

GENERAL DROPSY OF THE FETUS.—In this case the tissues generally are distended with liquid, and the skin is found at all points tense and rounded, and pitting on pressure with the fingers. In some such cases delivery may be effected after the skin has been punctured at narrow intervals to allow the escape of the fluid and then liberally smeared with fresh lard. More commonly, however, it can not be reached at all points to be so punctured nor sufficiently reduced to be extracted whole, and resort must be had to embryotomy.

EMPHYSEMA, OR SWILLING OF THE FETUS WITH GAS.—This has been described as occuring in a living fetus, but I have met with it only in the dead and decomposing foal after futile efforts had been made for several days to effect delivery. These cases are very difficult, as the foal is inflated to such extent that it is impossible to advance it into the passages, and the skin of the fetus and the walls of the womb and vagina have become so dry that it is impracticable to cause the one to glide on the other. The hair comes off any part that may be seized, and the case is rendered the more offensive and dangerous by the very fetid liquids and gases. The only resort is embryotomy, by which I have succeeded in saving a valuable mare that had carried a colt in this condition for four days.

CONTRACTIONS OF MUSCLES.—The foal is not always developed symmetrically, but certain groups of muscles are liable to remain short, or to shorten because of persistent spasmodic contraction, so that even the bones become distorted and twisted. This is most common in the neck. The bones of this part and even of the face are drawn to one side and shortened, the head being held firmly to the flank and the jaws being twisted to the right or left. In other cases the flexor muscles of the fore limbs are contracted so that the latter are strongly bent at the knee. In neither of these cases can the distorted part be extended and straightened, so that body or limbs must necessarily present double, and natural delivery is rendered impossible. The bent neck may sometimes be straightened after the muscles have been cut on the side to which it is turned, and the bent limbs after the tendons on the back of the shank bone have been cut across. Failing to accomplish this, the next resort is embryotomy.

INCLOSED OVUM, OR TUMORS OF THE FETUS.—Tumors or diseased growths may form on any part of the foal, internal or external, and by their size impede or hinder parturition. In some cases what appears as a tumor is an imprisoned and undeveloped ovum which has grafted itself on the fetus. These are usually sacculated, and may contain skin, hair, muscle, bone, and other natural tissues. The only course to be pursued in such cases is to excise the tumor, or, if this is not feasible, to perform embryotomy.

MONSTROSITIES.—Monstrosity in the foal is an occasional cause of difficult parturition, especially such monsters as show excessive development of some part of the body, a displacement or distortion of parts, or a redundancy of parts, as in double monsters. Monsters may be divided into—

(1) Monsters with absence of parts—absence of head, limb, or other organ.

(2) Monsters with some part abnormally small—dwarfed head, limb, trunk, etc.

(3) Monsters through unnatural division of parts—cleft head, trunk, limbs, etc.

(4) Monsters through absence of natural divisions—absence of mouth, nose, eyes, anus, confluent digits, etc.

(5) Monsters through fusion of parts—one central eye, one nasal opening, etc.

(6) Monsters through abnormal position or form of parts—curved spine, face, limb, etc.

(7) Monsters through excess of formation—enormous head, supernumerary digits, etc.

(8) Monsters through imperfect differentiation of sexual organs—hermaphrodites.

(9) Double monsters—double-headed, double-bodied, extra limbs, etc.

Causes.—The causes of monstrosities appear to be very varied. Some monstrosities, like extra digits, absence of horns or tail, etc., run in families and are produced almost as certainly as color or form. Others are associated with too close breeding, the powers of symmetrical development being interfered with, just as in other cases a sexual incompatibility is developed, near relatives failing to breed with each other. Mere arrest of development of a part may arise from accidental disease of the embryo; hence vital organs are left out, or portions of organs, like the dividing walls of the heart, are omitted. Sometimes an older fetus is inclosed in the body of another, each having started independently from a separate ovum, but the one having become embedded in the semifluid mass of the other and having developed there simultaneously with it, but not so largely nor perfectly. In many cases of redundance of parts the extra part or member has manifestly developed from the same ovum and nutrient center with the normal member to which it remains adherent, just as a new tail will grow out in a newt when the former has been cut off. In the early embryo, with its great powers of development, this factor can operate to far greater purpose than in the adult animal. Its influence is seen in the fact pointed out by St. Hilaire that such redundant parts are nearly always connected with the corresponding portions in the normal fetus. Thus superfluous legs or digits are attached to the normal ones, double heads or tails are connected to a common neck or rump, and double bodies are attached to each other by corresponding points, navel to navel, breast to breast, back to back. All this suggests the development of extra parts from the same primary layer of the impregnated and developing ovum. The effect of disturbing conditions in giving such wrong directions to the developmental forces is well shown in the experiments of St. Hilaire and Valentine in varnishing, shaking, and otherwise breaking up the natural connections in eggs, and thereby determining the formation of monstrosities at will. So, in the mammal, blows and other injuries that detach the fetal membranes from the walls of the womb or that modify their circulation by inducing inflammation are at times followed by the development of a monster. The excitement, mental and physical, attendant on fright occasionally acts in a similar way, acting probably through the same channels.

The monstrous forms liable to interfere with parturition are such as, from contracted or twisted limbs or spine, must be presented double; where supernumerary limbs, head, or body must approach the passages with the natural ones; where a head or other member has attained to an unnatural size; where the body of one fetus has become inclosed in or attached to another, etc.

Extraction is sometimes possible by straightening the members and obtaining such a presentation as will reduce the presenting mass to its smallest and most wedgelike dimensions. To effect this it may be needful to cut the flexor tendons of bent limbs or the muscles on the side of a twisted neck or body; one or more of the manipulations necessary to secure and bring up a missing member may be required. In most cases of monstrosity by excess, however, it is needful to remove the superfluous parts, in which case the general principles employed for embryotomy must be followed. The Cæsarean section, by which the fetus is extracted through an incision in the walls of the abdomen and womb, is inadmissible, as it practically entails the sacrifice of the mare, which should never be done for the sake of a monster. (See "Embryotomy," p. 202.)

ENTRANCE OF TWINS INTO THE PASSAGE AT ONCE.—Twins are rare in the mare, and still more rare is the impaction of both at once into the pelvis. The condition would be easily recognized by the fact that two fore limbs and two hind would occupy the passage at once, the front of the hoofs of the fore feet being turned upward and those of the hind feet downward. If both belonged to one foal, they would be turned in the same direction. Once recognized, the condition is easily remedied by passing a rope with a running noose round each foot of the foal that is furthest advanced or that promises to be most easily extracted, and to push the members of the other fetus back into the depth of the womb. As soon as the one fetus is fully engaged into the passage it will hold its place and its delivery will proceed in the natural way.

ABNORMAL PRESENTATIONS.

(Pls. XV–XVIII.)

Abnormal presentations may be tabulated as follows:

Anterior presentations.	Fore limbs	Incompletely extended. Flexor tendons shortened.
		Crossed over the neck.
		Bent back at the knee.
		Bent back from the shoulder.
	Head	Bent downward on the neck.
		Head and neck turned back beneath the breast.
		Turned to one side.
		Turned upward and backward on the back.
	Hind limbs	Hind feet engaged in the pelvis.
	Transverse	Back of foal to side of pelvis.
	Inverted	Back of foal to floor of pelvis.
Posterior presentations.	Hind limbs	Bent on itself at the hock.
		Bent at the hip.
	Transverse	Back of foal to side of pelvis.
	Inverted	Back of foal to floor of pelvis.
Transverse presentation of body		With back and loins presented.
		With breast and belly presented.

FORE LIMBS INCOMPLETELY EXTENDED.—In cases of this kind, not only are the back tendons behind the knee and shank bone unduly short, but the sinew extending from the front of the shoulder blade over the front of the elbow and down to the head of the shank bone is also shortened. The result is that the fore limb is bent at the knee and the elbow is also rigidly bent. The condition obstructs parturition by the feet becoming pressed against the floor of the pelvis or by the elbow pressing on its anterior brim. Relief is to be obtained by forcible extension. A rope with a running noose is passed around each fetlock and a repeller (see Plate XIV) planted in the breast is pressed in a direction upward and backward while active traction is made on the ropes. If the feet are not thereby raised from the floor of the pelvis the palm of the hand may be placed beneath them to protect the mucous membrane until they have advanced sufficiently to obviate this danger. In the absence of a repeller, a smooth rounded fork handle may be employed. If the shortening is too great to allow of the extension of the limbs in this way, the tense tendons may be cut across behind the shank bone and in front of the elbow, and the limb will be easily straightened out. This is most easily done with an embryotomy knife furnished with a ring for the middle finger, so that the blade may be protected in the palm of the hand. (See Plate XIII, fig. 4.)

FORE LIMB CROSSED OVER BACK OF NECK.—With the long fore limbs of the foal this readily occurs, and the resulting increase in thickness, both at the head and shoulder, offers a serious obstacle to progress. (See Plate XV, fig. 2.) The hand introduced into the passage detects the head and one fore foot, and farther back on the same side of the head the second foot, from which the limb may be traced obliquely across the back of the neck.

If parturition continues to make progress the displaced foot may bruise and lacerate the vagina. By seizing the limb above the fetlock it may be easily pushed over the head to the proper side, when parturition will proceed normally.

FORE LIMB BENT AT KNEE.—The nose and one fore foot present, and on examination the knee of the missing fore limb is found farther back. (Plate XV, fig. 1.) First place a noose each on the presenting pastern and lower jaw, and push back the body of the fetus with a repeller, while the operator seizing the shank of the bent limb extends it so as to press back the knee and bring forward the fetlock and foot. As progress is made little by little the hand is slid down from the region of the knee to the fetlock, and finally that is secured and brought up into the passage, when parturition will proceed without hindrance. If both fore limbs are bent back the head must be noosed and the limbs brought up as above, one after the other. It is usually best to employ the left hand for the right fore limb, and the right hand for the left fore limb.

FORE LIMB TURNED BACK FROM SHOULDERS.—In this case, on exploration by the side of the head and presenting limb, the shoulder only can be reached at first. (Plate XV, fig 4.) By noosing the head and presenting fore limb, they may be drawn forward into the pelvis, and the oiled hand being carried along the shoulder in the direction of the missing limb is enabled to reach and seize the forearm just below the elbow. The body is now pushed back by the assistants pressing on the head and presenting limb or on a repeller planted in the breast until the knee can be brought up into the pelvis, after which the procedure is the same as described in the last paragraph.

HEAD BENT DOWN BETWEEN FORE LIMBS.—This may be so that the poll or nape of the neck, with the ears, can be felt far back between the fore limbs, or so that only the upper border of the neck can be reached, head and neck being bent back beneath the body. With the head only bent on the neck, noose the two presenting limbs, then introduce the hand between them until the nose can be seized in the palm of the hand. Next have the assistants push back the presenting limbs, while the nose is strongly lifted upward over the brim of the pelvis. This accomplished, it assumes the natural position and parturition is easy.

When both head and neck are bent downward it may be impossible to reach the nose. If, however, the labor has only commenced, the limbs may be drawn upon until the operator can reach the ear, by dragging on which the head may be so far advanced that the fingers may reach the orbit; traction upon this while the limbs are being pushed back may bring the head up so that it bends on the neck only, and the further procedure will be as described in the last paragraph.

If the labor has been long in progress and the fetus is jammed into the pelvis, the womb emptied of the waters, and firmly contracted on its solid contents, the case is incomparably more difficult. The mare may be chloroformed and turned on her back with hind parts elevated, and the womb may be injected with sweet oil. Then, if the ear can be reached, the correction of the malpresentation may be attempted as above described. Should this fail, one or more sharp hooks may be inserted in the neck as near the head as can be reached, and ropes attached to these may be dragged on, while the body of the foal is pushed back by the fore limbs or by a repeller. Such repulsion should be made in a direction obliquely upward toward the loins of the mother, so as to rotate the fetus in such a way as to bring the head up. As this is accomplished a hold should be secured nearer and nearer to the nose, with hand or hook, until the head can be straightened out on the neck.

All means failing, it becomes necessary to remove the fore limbs (embryotomy) so as to make more space for bringing up the head. If, even then, this can not be accomplished, it may be possible to push the body backward and upward with the repeller until the hind limbs are brought to the passage, when they may be noosed and delivery effected with the posterior presentation.

HEAD TURNED ON SHOULDERS.—In this case the fore feet present, and the oiled hand passed along the fore arms in search of the missing head finds the side of the neck turned to one side, the head being perhaps entirely out of reach. (Plate XVIII, fig. 1.) To bring the head forward it may be desirable to lay the mare on the side opposite to that to which the head is turned, and even to give chloroform or ether. Then the feet being noosed, the body of the fetus is pushed by the hand or repeller forward and to the side opposite to that occupied by the head until the head comes within reach, near the entrance of the pelvis. If such displacement of the fetus is difficult, it may be facilitated by a free use of oil or lard. When the nose can be seized it can be brought into the passage, as when the head is turned down. If it can not be reached, the orbit may be availed of to draw the head forward until the nose can be seized or the lower jaw noosed. In very difficult cases a rope may be passed around the neck by the hand or with the aid of a curved carrier (Plate XIV), and traction may be made upon this while the body is being rotated to the other side. In the same way in bad cases a hook may be fixed in the orbit or even between the bones of the lower jaw to assist in bringing the head up into position. Should all fail, the amputation of the fore limbs may be resorted to, as advised under the last heading.

HEAD TURNED UPWARD ON BACK.—This differs from the last malpresentation only in the direction of the head, which has to be sought above rather than at one side, and is to be secured and brought forward in a similar manner. (Plate XVIII, fig. 2.) If a rope can be passed around the neck it will prove most effectual, as it naturally slides nearer to the head as the neck is straightened and ends by bringing the head within easy reach.

HIND FEET ENGAGED IN PELVIS.—In this case fore limbs and head present naturally, but the hind limbs bent forward from the hip and the loins arched allow the hind feet also to enter the passages, and the further labor advances the more firmly does the body of the foal become wedged into the pelvis (Plate XVII, fig. 2.) The condition is to be recognized by introducing the oiled hand along the belly of the fetus, when the hind feet will be felt advancing. An attempt should at once be made to push them back, one after the other, over the brim of the pelvis. Failing in this, the mare may be turned on her back, head downhill, and the attempt renewed. If it is possible to introduce a straight rope carrier, a noose passed through this may be put on the fetlock and the repulsion thereby made more effective. In case of continued failure the anterior presenting part of the body may be skinned and cut off as far back toward the pelvis as possible (see "Embryotomy"); then nooses are placed on the hind fetlocks and traction is made upon these while the quarters are pushed back into the womb. Then the remaining portion is brought away by the posterior presentation.

ANTERIOR PRESENTATION WITH BACK TURNED TO ONE SIDE.—The diameter of the axis of the foal, like that of the pelvic passages, is from above downward, and when the fetus enters the pelvis with this greatest diameter engaged transversely or in the narrow diameter of the pelvis, parturition is rendered difficult or impossible. In such a case the pasterns and head may be noosed, and the passages and engaged portion of the foal freely lubricated with lard, the limbs may be crossed over each other and the head, and a movement of rotation effected in the fetus until its face and back are turned up toward the croup of the mother; then parturition becomes natural.

BACK OF FOAL TURNED TO FLOOR OF PELVIS.—In a roomy mare this is not an insuperable obstacle to parturition, yet it may seriously impede it, by reason of the curvature of the body of the foal being opposite to that of the passages, and the head and withers being liable to arrest against the border of the pelvis. Lubrication of the passage with lard and traction of the limbs and head will usually suffice with or without the turning of the mare on her back.

In obstinate cases two other resorts are open: First, to turn the foal, pushing back the fore parts and bringing up the hind so as to make a posterior presentation, and, second, the amputation of the fore limbs, after which extraction will usually be easy.

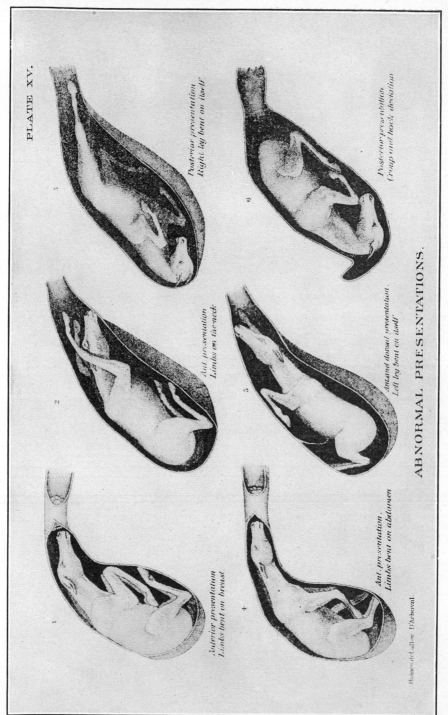

PLATE XV.

Posterior presentation
Right leg bent on itself.

Posterior presentation
Croup and back deviation

Ant. presentation
Limbs on tierneck

Ant and dorsal presentation
Left leg bent on itself

Anterior presentation
Limbs bent on breast.

Ant. presentation.
Limbs bent on abdomen

Raines del after l'Arboval.

ABNORMAL PRESENTATIONS.

PLATE XVI.

1

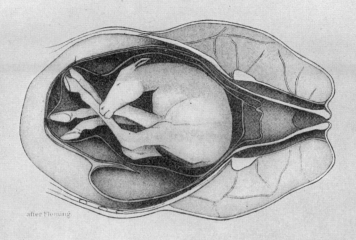

Transverse presentation – Upper view.

2

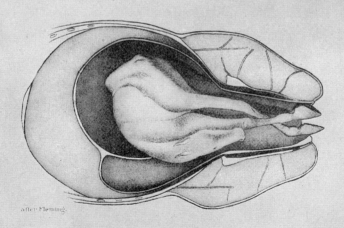

Sterno-abdominal presentation – Head and Feet engaged.

ABNORMAL PRESENTATIONS.

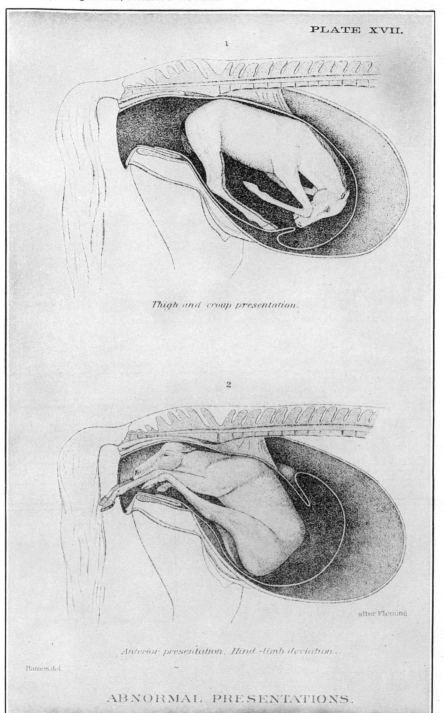

PLATE XVII.

1

Thigh and croup presentation.

2

after Fleming

Anterior presentation. Hind-limb deviation.

Haines.del.

ABNORMAL PRESENTATIONS.

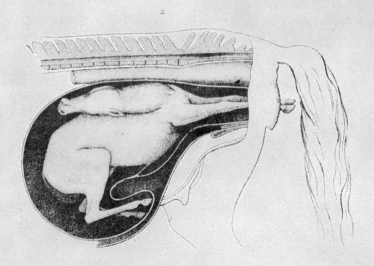

PLATE XVIII.

1

Anterior presentation. Head turned on side.

2

Anterior presentation. Head turned on back.

Haines.del.

ABNORMAL PRESENTATIONS.

HIND PRESENTATION WITH LEG BENT AT HOCK.—In this form the quarters of the foal with the hind legs bent up beneath them present, but can not advance through the pelvis by reason of their bulk. (PlateXV, fig. 3.) The oiled hand introduced can recognize the outline of the buttocks, with the tail and anus in the center and the sharp points of the hocks beneath. First pass a rope around each limb at the hock, then with hand or repeller push the buttocks backward and upward, until the feet can be brought up into the passages. To this the great length of the shank and pastern in the foal is a serious obstacle, and in all cases the foot should be protected in the palm of the hand while being brought up over the brim of the pelvis; otherwise the womb may be torn. When the pains are too violent and constant to allow effective manipulation, some respite may be obtained by the use of chloroform or morphin and by turning the mare on her back, but too often the operator fails and the foal must be sacrificed. Two courses are still open: First, to cut through the cords behind and above the hock and extend the upper part of the limb, leaving the hock bent, and extract in this way, and, second, to amputate the hind limbs at the hip joint and remove them separately, after which the body may be extracted.

HIND PRESENTATION WITH LEGS BENT FORWARD FROM HIP.—This is merely an aggravated form of the presentation last described. (Plate XVII, fig. 1.) If the mare is roomy, a rope may be passed around each thigh and the body pushed upward and forward, so as to bring the hocks and heels upward. If this can be accomplished, nooses are placed on the limb further and further down until the fetlock is reached and brought into position. If failure is met with, then amputation at the hips is the last resort.

HIND PRESENTATIONS WITH BACK TURNED SIDEWAYS OR DOWNWARD.— These are the counterparts of similar anterior presentations and are to be managed in the same way.

PRESENTATION OF THE BACK.—This is rare, yet not unknown, the foal being bent upon itself with the back, recognizable by its sharp row of spines, presented at the entrance of the pelvis and the head and all four feet turned back into the womb. (Plate XVI, fig. 1.) The body of the fetus may be extended across the opening transversely, so that the head corresponds to one side (right or left), or it may be vertical, with the head above or below.

In any such position the object should be to push the body of the fetus forward and upward or to one side, as may best promise to bring up the fore or hind extremities, and bring the latter into the passage so as to constitute a normal anterior or posterior presentation. This turning of the fetus may be favored by a given position of the mother, by the free use of oil or lard on the surface of the fetus, and by the use of a propeller.

PRESENTATION OF BREAST AND ABDOMEN.—This is the reverse of the back presentation, the foal being extended across in front of the pelvic opening, but with the belly turned toward the passages and with all four feet engaged in the passage. (Plate XVI, fig. 2.) The most promising course is to secure the hind feet with nooses and then push the fore feet forward into the womb. As soon as the fore feet are pushed forward clear of the brim of the pelvis, traction is made on the hind feet so as to bring the thighs into the passage and prevent the reentrance of the fore limbs. If it proves difficult to push the fore limbs back, a noose may be passed around the fetlock of each and the cord drawn through the eye of a rope carrier, by means of which the members may be easily pushed back.

EMBRYOTOMY.

Embryotomy consists in the dissection of the fetus, so as to reduce its bulk and allow of its exit through the pelvis. The indications for its adoption have been furnished in the foregoing pages. The operation will vary in different cases according to the necessity for the removal of one or more parts in order to secure the requisite reduction in size. Thus it may be needful to remove head and neck, one fore limb or both, one hind limb or both, to remove different parts of the trunk, or to remove superfluous (monstrous) parts. Some of the simplest operations in embryotomy (incision of the head in hydrocephalus, incision of the belly in dropsy) have already been described. It remains to notice the more difficult procedures which can be best undertaken by the skilled anatomist.

Amputation of the head.—This is easy when both fore limbs are turned back and the head alone has made its exit in part. It is more difficult when the head is still retained in the passages or womb, as in double-headed monsters. The head is secured by a hook in the lower jaw, or in the orbit, or by a halter, and the skin is divided circularly around the lower part of the face or at the front of the ears, according to the amount of head protruding. Then an incision is made backward along the line of the throat, and the skin dissected from the neck as far back as possible. Then the muscles and other soft parts of the neck are cut across, and the bodies of two vertebræ (neck bones) are severed by cutting completely across the cartilage of the joint. The bulging of the ends of the bones will serve to indicate the seat of the joint. The head and detached portion of the neck may now be removed by steady pulling. If there is still an obstacle, the knife may be again used to sever any obstinate connections. In the case of a double-headed monster, the whole of the second neck must be removed with the head. When the head has been detached, a rope should be passed through the eyeholes, or through an artificial opening in the skin, and tied firmly around the skin, to be employed as a means of traction when the missing limbs or the second head have been brought up into position.

Amputation of the hind limb.—This may be required when there are extra hind limbs or when the hind limbs are bent forward at hock or hip joint. In the former condition the procedure resembles that for removal of a fore limb, but requires more anatomical knowledge. Having noosed the pastern, a circular incision is made through the skin around the fetlock, and a longitudinal one from that up to the groin, and the skin is dissected from the limb as high up as can be reached, over the croup, if possible. Then cut through the muscles around the hip joint, and, if possible, the two interarticular ligaments of the joint (pubofemoral and round), and extract the limb by strong dragging.

Amputation of the fore limbs.—This may usually be begun on the fetlock of the limb projecting from the vulva. An embryotomy knife is desirable. This knife consists of a blade with a sharp, slightly hooked point, and one or two rings in the back of the blade large enough to fit on the middle finger, while the blade is protected in the palm of the hand. (See Plate XIII, fig. 4.) Another form has the blade inserted in a mortise in the handle, from which it is pushed out by a movable button when wanted. First place a noose around the fetlock of the limb to be amputated, cut the skin circularly entirely around the fetlock, then make an incision on the inner side of the limb from the fetlock up to the breastbone. Next dissect the skin from the limb, from the fetlock up to the breastbone on the inner side, and as far up on the shoulder blade as possible on the outer side. Finally, cut through the muscles attaching the limb to the breastbone, and employ strong traction on the limb, so as to drag out the whole limb, shoulder blade included. The muscles around the upper part of the shoulder blade are easily torn through and need not be cut, even if that were possible. In no case should the fore limb be removed unless the shoulder blade is taken with it, as that furnishes the greatest obstruction to delivery, above all when it is no longer advanced by the extension of the fore limb, but is pressed back so as to increase the already thickest posterior portion of the chest. The preservation of the skin from the whole limb is advantageous in various ways; it is easier to cut it circularly at the fetlock than at the shoulder; it covers the hand and knife in making the needful incisions, thus acting as a protection to the womb; and it affords a means of traction on the body after the limb has been removed. In dissecting the skin from the limb the knife is not needful at all points; much of it may be stripped off with the fingers or knuckles, or by a blunt, iron spud pushed up inside the hide, which is meanwhile held tense to render the spud effective.

In case the limb is bent forward at the hock, a rope is passed round that and pulled so as to bring the point of the hock between the lips of the vulva. The hamstring and the lateral ligaments of the hock are now cut through, and the limbs extended by a rope tied round the lower end of the long bone above (tibia). In case it is still needful to remove the upper part of the limb, the further procedure is the same as described in the last paragraph.

In case the limb is turned forward from the hip, and the fetus so wedged into the passage that turning is impossible, the case is very difficult. I have repeatedly succeeded by cutting in on the hip joint and disarticulating it, then dissecting the muscles back from the upper end of the thigh bone. A noose was placed around the neck of the bone and pulled on forcibly, while any unduly resisting structures were cut with the knife.

Cartwright recommends to make free incisions round the hip joints and tear through the muscles when they can not be cut; then with cords round the pelvic bones, and hooks inserted in the openings in the floor of the pelvis to drag out the pelvic bones; then put cords around the heads of the thigh bones and extract them; then remove the intestines; finally, by means of the loose, detached skin, draw out the body with the remainder of the hind limbs bent forward beneath it.

Reuff cuts his way into the pelvis of the foal, and with a knife separates the pelvic bones from the loins, then skinning the quarter draws out these pelvic bones by means of ropes and hooks, and along with them the hind limbs.

The hind limbs having been removed by one or the other of these procedures, the loose skin detached from the pelvis is used as a means of traction and delivery is effected. In case of a monstrosity with extra hind limbs, it may be possible to bring these up into the passage and utilize them for traction.

Removal of the abdominal viscera.—In case the belly is unduly large, from decomposition, tumors, or otherwise, it may be needful to lay it open with the knife and cut or tear out the contents.

Removal of the thoracic viscera.—To diminish the bulk of the chest it has been found advisable to cut out the breastbone, remove the heart and lungs, and allow the ribs to collapse with the lower free ends overlapping each other.

Dissection of the trunk.—In case it becomes necessary to remove other portions of the trunk, we should follow the general rule of preserving the skin so that all manipulations can be made inside this as a protector, that it may remain available as a means of exercising traction on the remaining part of the body, and as a covering to protect the vaginal walls against injuries from bones while such part is passing.

FLOODING, OR BLEEDING FROM THE WOMB.

This is rare in the mare, but not unknown, in connection with a failure of the womb to contract on itself after parturition, or with eversion of the womb (casting the withers), and congestion or laceration. If the blood accumulates in the flaccid womb, the condition may be suspected only by reason of the rapidly advancing weakness, swaying, unsteady gait, hanging head, paleness of the eyes and other mucous membranes, and weak, small, failing pulse. The hand introduced into the womb detects the presence of the blood partly clotted. If the blood escapes by the vulva, the condition is evident.

Treatment consists in evacuating the womb of its blood clots, giving a large dose of powdered ergot of rye, and in the application of cold water or ice to the loins and external generative organs. Besides this, a sponge impregnated with a strong solution of alum, or, still better, with tincture of muriate of iron, may be introduced into the womb and squeezed so as to bring the liquid in contact with the walls generally.

EVERSION OF THE WOMB.

If the womb fails to contract after difficult parturition, the afterpains will sometimes lead to the fundus passing into the body of the organ and passing through that and the vagina until the whole inverted organ appears externally and hangs down on the thighs. The result is rapid engorgement and swelling of the organ, impaction of the rectum with feces, and distention of the bladder with urine, all of which conditions seriously interfere with the return of the mass. In returning the womb the standing is preferable to the recumbent position, as the abdomen is more pendent and there is less obstruction to the return. It may, however, be necessary to put hobbles on the hind limbs to prevent the mare from kicking. A clean sheet should be held beneath the womb, and all filth, straw, and foreign bodies washed from its surface. Then with a broad, elastic (indiarubber) band, or in default of that a long strip of calico 4 or 5 inches wide, wind the womb as tightly as possible, beginning at its most dependent part (the extremity of the horn). This serves two good ends. It squeezes out into the general circulation the enormous mass of blood which engorged and enlarged the organ, and it furnishes a strong protective covering for the now delicate, friable organ, through which it may be safely manipulated without danger of laceration. The next step may be the pressure on the general mass while those portions next the vulva are gradually pushed in with the hands; or the extreme lowest point (the end of the horn) may be turned within itself and pushed forward into the vagina by the closed fist, the return being assisted by manipulations by the other hand, and even by those of assistants. By either mode the manipulations may be made with almost perfect safety so long as the organ is closely wrapped in the bandage. Once a portion has been introduced into the vagina the rest will usually follow with increasing ease, and the operation should be completed with the hand and arm extended the full length within the womb and moved from point to point so as to straighten out all parts of the organ and insure that no portion still remain inverted within another portion. Should any such partial inversion be left it will give rise to straining, under the force of which it will gradually increase until the whole mass will be protruded as before. The next step is to apply a truss as an effectual mechanical barrier to further escape of the womb through the vulva. The simplest is made with two 1-inch ropes, each about 18 feet long, each doubled and interwoven at the bend, as seen in Plate XIV, figure 4. The ring formed by the interlacing of the two ropes is adjusted around the vulva, the two ends of the one rope are carried up on the right and left of the tail and along the spine, being wound around each other in their course, and are finally tied to the upper part of the collar encircling the neck. The remaining two ends, belonging to the other rope, are carried downward and forward between the thighs and thence forward and upward on the sides of the belly and chest to be attached to the right and left sides of the collar. These ropes are drawn tightly enough to keep closely applied to the opening without chafing, and will fit still more securely when the mare raises her back to strain. It is desirable to tie the mare short so that she may be unable to lie down for a day or two, and she should be kept in a stall with the hind parts higher than the fore. Violent straining may be checked by full doses of opium (one-half dram), and any costiveness or diarrhea should be obviated by a suitable laxative or binding diet.

In some mares the contractions are too violent to allow of the return of the womb, and full doses of opium one-half dram, laudanum 2 ounces, or chloral hydrate 1 ounce, may be demanded, or the mare must be rendered insensible by ether or chloroform.

RUPTURE, OR LACERATION, OF THE WOMB.

This may occur from the feet of the foal during parturition, or from ill-directed efforts to assist, but it is especially liable to take place in the everted, congested, and friable organ. The resultant dangers are bleeding from the wound, escape of the bowels through the opening and their fatal injury by the mare's feet or otherwise, and peritonitis from the extension of inflammation from the wound and from the poisonous action of the septic liquids of the womb escaping into the abdominal cavity. The first object is to close the wound, but unless in eversion of the womb this is practically impossible. In the last-named condition the wound must be carefully and accurately sewed up before the womb is returned. After its return, the womb must be injected daily with an antiseptic solution (borax, one-half ounce, or carbolic acid, 3 drams to a quart of tepid water). If inflammation threatens, the abdomen may be bathed continuously with hot water by means of a heavy woolen rag, and large doses of opium (one-half dram) may be given twice or thrice daily.

RUPTURES OF THE VAGINA.

These are attended with dangers similar to those belonging to rupture of the womb, and in addition by the risk of protrusion of the bladder, which appears through the lips of the vulva as a red, pyriform mass. Sometimes such lacerations extend downward into the bladder, and in others upward into the terminal gut (rectum). In still other cases the anus is torn so that it forms one common orifice with the vulva.

Too often such cases prove fatal, or at least a recovery is not attained, and urine or feces or both escape freely into the vagina. The simple laceration of the anus is easily sewed up, but the ends of the muscular fibers do not reunite and the control over the lower bowel is never fully reacquired. The successful stitching up of the wound communicating with the bladder or the rectum requires unusual skill and care, and though I have succeeded in a case of the latter kind, I can not advise the attempt by unprofessional persons.

BLOOD CLOTS IN THE WALLS OF THE VAGINA.

(See " Effusion of blood in the vaginal walls," p. 190.)

LAMINITIS, OR FOUNDER, FOLLOWING PARTURITION.

This sometimes follows on inflammation of the womb, as it frequently does on disorder of the stomach. Its symptoms agree with those of the common form of founder, and treatment need not differ.

INFLAMMATION OF THE WOMB AND PERITONEUM.

These may result from injuries sustained by the womb during or after parturition, from exposure to cold or wet, or from the irritant infective action of putrid products within the womb. Under the inflammation the womb remains dilated and flaccid, and decomposition of its secretions almost always occurs, so that the inflammation tends to assume a putrid character and general septic infection is likely to occur.

Symptoms.—The symptoms are ushered in by shivering, staring coat, small, rapid pulse, elevated temperature, accelerated breathing, loss of appetite, with arched back, stiff movement of the body, looking back at the flanks, and uneasy motions of the hind limbs, discharge from the vulva of a liquid at first watery, reddish, or yellowish, and later it may be whitish or glairy, and fetid or not in different cases. Tenderness of the abdomen shown on pressure is especially characteristic of cases affecting the peritoneum or lining of the belly, and is more marked lower down. If the animal survives, the inflammation tends to become chronic and attended by a whitish mucopurulent discharge. If, on the contrary, it proves fatal, death is preceded by extreme prostration and weakness from the general septic poisoning.

Treatment.—In treatment the first thing to be sought is the removal of all offensive and irritant matters from the womb through a caoutchouc tube introduced into the womb, and into which a funnel is fitted. Warm water should be passed until it comes away clear. To insure that all the womb has been washed out, the oiled hand may be introduced to carry the end of the tube into the two horns successively. When the offensive contents have been thus removed, the womb should be injected with a quart of water holding in solution 1 dram permanganate of potash, or, in the absence of the latter, 2 teaspoonfuls of carbolic acid, twice daily. Fomentation of the abdomen, or the application of a warm flaxseed poultice, may greatly relieve. Acetanilid, in doses of half an ounce, twice or thrice a day, or sulphate of quinia in doses of one-third ounce, may be employed to reduce the fever. If the great prostration indicates septic poisoning, large doses (one-half ounce) bisulphite of soda, or salicylate of soda, or sulphate of quinin may be resorted to.

LEUCORRHEA.

This is a white, glutinous, chronic discharge, the result of a continued, subacute inflammation of the mucous membrane of the womb. Like the discharge of acute inflammation, it contains many forms of bacteria, by some of which it is manifestly inoculable on the penis of the stallion, producing ulcers and a specific, gonorrheal discharge.

Treatment may consist in the internal use of tonics (sulphate of iron, 3 drams, daily) and the washing out of the womb, as described under the last heading, followed by an astringent antiseptic injection (carbolic acid, 2 teaspoonfuls; tannic acid, ½ dram; water, 1 quart). This may be given two or three times a day.

DISEASES OF THE UDDER AND TEATS.
CONGESTION AND INFLAMMATION OF THE UDDER.

This is comparatively rare in the mare, though in some cases the udder becomes painfully engorged before parturition, and a doughy swelling, pitting on pressure, extends forward on the lower surface of the abdomen. When this goes on to active inflammation, one or both of the glands becomes enlarged, hot, tense, and painful; the milk is dried up or replaced by a watery or reddish, serous fluid, which at times becomes fetid; the animal walks lame, loses appetite, and shows general disorder and fever. The condition may end in recovery, in abscess, induration, or gangrene, and, in some cases, may lay the foundation for a tumor of the gland.

Treatment.—The treatment is simple so long as there is only congestion. Active rubbing with lard or oil, or, better, camphorated oil, and the frequent drawing off of the milk, by the foal or with the hand, will usually bring about a rapid improvement. When active inflammation is present, fomentation with warm water may be kept up for an hour and followed by the application of the camphorated oil, to which has been added some carbonate of soda and extract of belladonna. A dose of laxative medicine (4 drams Barbados aloes) will be of service in reducing fever, and one-half ounce saltpeter daily will serve a similar end. In case the milk coagulates in the udder and can not be withdrawn, or when the liquid becomes fetid, a solution of 20 grains carbonate of soda and 10 drops carbolic acid dissolved in an ounce of water should be injected into the teat. In doing this it must be noted that the mare has three separate ducts opening on the summit of each teat and each must be carefully injected. To draw off the fetid product it may be needful to use a small milking tube, or spring teat dilator designed by the writer. (Plate XIV, figs. 2 and 3.) When pus forms and points externally and can not find a free escape by the teat, the spot where it fluctuates must be opened freely with the knife and the cavity injected daily with the carbolic-acid lotion. When the gland becomes hard and indolent, it may be rubbed daily with iodin ointment 1 part, vaseline 6 parts.

TUMORS OF THE UDDER.

As the result of inflammation of the udder it may become the seat of an indurated diseased growth, which may go on growing and seriously interfere with the movement of the hind limbs. If such swellings do not give way in their early stages to treatment by iodin, the only resort is to cut them out with a knife. As the gland is often implicated and has to be removed, such mares can not in the future suckle their colts and therefore should not be bred.

SORE TEATS, SCABS, CRACKS, WARTS.

By the act of sucking, especially in cold weather, the teats are subject to abrasions, cracks, and scabs, and as the result of such irritation, or independently, warts sometimes grow and prove troublesome. The warts should be clipped off with sharp scissors and their roots burned with a solid pencil of lunar caustic. This is best done before parturition to secure healing before suckling begins. For sore teats use an ointment of vaseline 1 ounce, balsam of tolu 5 grains, and sulphate of zinc 5 grains.

DISEASES OF THE NERVOUS SYSTEM.

By M. R. TRUMBOWER, V. S.

[Revised by John R. Mohler, A. M., V. M. D.]

ANATOMY AND PHYSIOLOGY OF THE BRAIN AND NERVOUS SYSTEM.

(Pl. XIX.)

The nervous system may be regarded as consisting of two sets of organs, peripheral and central, the function of one being to establish a communication between the centers and the different parts of the body, and that of the other to generate nervous force. The whole may be arranged under two divisions: First, the cerebrospinal system; second, the sympathetic or ganglionic system. Each is possessed of its own central and peripheral organs.

In the first, the center is made up of two portions—one large and expanded (the brain) placed in the cranial cavity; the other elongated (spinal cord), continuous with the brain, and lodged in the canal of the vertebral column. The peripheral portion of this system consists of the cerebrospinal nerves, which leave the axis in symmetrical pairs and are distributed to the skin, the voluntary muscles, and the organs.

In the second, the central organ consists of a chain of ganglia, connected by nerve cords, which extends on each side of the spine from the head to the rump. The nerves of this system are distributed to the involuntary muscles, mucous membrane, viscera, and blood vessels.

The two systems have free intercommunication, ganglia being at the junctions.

Two substances, distinguishable by their color, namely, the white or medullary and the gray or cortical substance, enter into the formation of nervous matter. Both are soft, fragile, and easily injured, in consequence of which the principal nervous centers are well protected by bony coverings. The nervous substances present two distinct forms—nerve fibers and nerve cells. An aggregation of nerve cells constitutes a nerve ganglion.

The nerve fibers represent a conducting apparatus and serve to place the central nervous organs in connection with peripheral end organs. The nerve cells, however, besides transmitting impulses, act as physiological centers for automatic, or reflex, movements, and also for the sensory, perceptive, trophic, and secretory functions. A nerve consists of a bundle of tubular fibers, held together by

210

areolar tissue, each fiber of which is inclosed in a sheath—the neurilemma. Nerve fibers possess no elasticity, but are very strong. Divided nerves do not retract.

Nerves are thrown into a state of excitement when stimulated, and are, therefore, said to possess excitable or irritable properties. The stimuli may be applied to, or may act upon, any part of the nerve. Nerves may be paralyzed by continuous pressure being applied. When the nerves divide into branches, there is never any splitting up of their ultimate fibers, nor yet is there ever any coalescing of them; they retain their individuality from their source to their termination.

Nerves which convey impressions to the centers are termed sensory, or centripetal, and those which transmit stimulus from the centers to organs of motion are termed motor, or centrifugal. The function of the nervous system may, therefore, be defined in the simplest terms, as follows: It is intended to associate the different parts of the body in such a manner that stimulus applied to one organ may excite or depress the activity of another.

The brain is that portion of the cerebro-spinal axis within the cranium, which may be divided into four parts—the medulla oblongata, the cerebellum, the pons Varolii, and the cerebrum—and it is covered by three membranes, called the meninges. The outer of these membranes, the dura mater, is a thick, white, fibrous membrane which lines the cavity of the cranium, forming the internal periosteum of the bones; it is continuous with the spinal cord to the extremity of the canal. The second, the arachnoid, is a delicate serous membrane, and loosely envelops the brain and spinal cord; it forms two layers, having between them the arachnoid space which contains the cerebro-spinal fluid, the use of which is to protect the spinal cord and brain from pressure. The third, or inner, the pia mater, is closely adherent to the entire surface of the brain, but is much thinner and more vascular than when it reaches the spinal cord, which it also envelops, and is continued to form the sheaths of the spinal nerves.

The medulla oblongata is the prolongation of the spinal cord, extending to the pons Varolii. This portion of the brain is very large in the horse: it is pyramidal in shape, the narrowest part joining the cord.

The pons Varolii is the transverse projection on the base of the brain, between the medulla oblongata and the peduncles of the cerebrum.

The cerebellum is lodged in the posterior part of the cranial cavity, immediately above the medulla oblongata; it is globular or elliptical in shape, the transverse diameter being greatest. The body of the cerebellum is composed of gray matter externally and of white matter in the center. The cerebellum has the function of coordinating movements; that is, of so associating them as to cause them to accomplish a definite purpose. Injuries to the cerebellum cause disturbances of the equilibrium but do not interfere with the will power or intelligence.

The cerebrum, or brain proper, occupies the anterior portion of the cranial cavity. It is ovoid in shape, with an irregular, flattened base, and consists of lateral halves or hemispheres. The greater part of the cerebrum is composed of white matter. The hemispheres of the cerebrum are usually said to be the seat of all psychical activities. Only when they are intact are the process of feeling, thinking, and willing possible. After they are destroyed the organism comes to be like a complicated machine, and its activity is only the expression of the internal and external stimuli which act upon it.

The spinal cord, or spinal marrow, is that part of the cerebro-spinal system which is contained in the spinal canal of the backbone, and extends from the medulla oblongata to a short distance behind the loins. It is an irregularly cylindrical structure, composed of two lateral, symmetrical halves. The spinal cord terminates posteriorly in a pointed extremity, which is continued by a mass of nerve trunks—cauda equinæ. A transverse section of the cord reveals that it is composed of white matter externally and of gray matter internally. The spinal cord does not fill the whole spinal canal. The latter contains, besides, a large venous sinus, fatty matter, the membranes of the cord, and the cerebrospinal fluid.

The spinal nerves, forty-two or forty-three in number, arise each by two roots, a superior or sensory, and an inferior or motor. The nerves originating from the brain are twenty-four in number, and arranged in pairs, which are named first, second, third, etc., counting from before backward. They also receive special names, according to their functions or the parts to which they are distributed, viz:

1. Olfactory.	7. Facial.
2. Optic.	8. Auditory.
3. Oculo-motor.	9. Glossopharyngeal.
4. Pathetic.	10. Pneumogastric.
5. Trifacial.	11. Spinal accessory.
6. Abducens.	12. Hypoglossal.

INFLAMMATION OF THE BRAIN AND ITS MEMBRANES (ENCEPHA-LITIS, MENINGITIS, CEREBRITIS).

Inflammation may attack these membranes singly, or any one of the anatomical divisions of the nerve matter, or it may invade the whole at once. Practical experience, however, teaches us that primary inflammation of the dura mater is of rare occurrence, except in direct mechanical injuries to the head or diseases of the bones of the cranium. Neither is the arachnoid often affected with acute inflammation, except as a secondary result. The pia mater is most commonly the seat of inflammation, acute and subacute, but from its intimate relation with the surface of the brain the latter very soon becomes involved in the morbid changes. Practically, we can not separate inflammation of the pia mater from that of the brain proper. Inflammation may, however, exist in the center of the great nerve masses—the cerebrum, cerebellum, pons Varolii, or medulla at the base of the brain—without involving the surface. When, therefore, inflammation invades the brain and its enveloping membranes it is properly called encephalitis; when the membranes alone are affected it is called meningitis, or the brain substance alone cerebritis. Since all the conditions merge into one another and can scarcely be recognized separately during the life of the animal, they may here be considered together.

Causes.—Exposure to extreme heat or cold, sudden and extreme changes of temperature, excessive continued cerebral excitement, too much nitrogenous feed, direct injuries to the brain, such as concussion, or from fracture of the cranium, overexertion, sometimes as sequelæ to influenza, pyemia, poisons having a direct influence upon the encephalic mass, extension of inflammation from neighboring structures, food poisoning, tumors, parasites, metastatic abscesses, etc.

Symptoms.—The diseases here grouped together are accompanied with a variety of symptoms, almost none of which, however, are associated so definitely with a special pathological process as to point unmistakably to a given lesion. Usually the first symptoms indicate mental excitement, and are followed by symptoms indicating depression. Acute encephalitis may be ushered in by an increased sensibility to noises, with more or less nervous excitability, contraction of the pupils of the eyes, and a quick, hard pulse. In very acute attacks these symptoms, however, are not always noted. This condition will soon be followed by muscular twitchings, convulsive or spasmodic movements, eyes wide open with shortness of sight. The animal becomes afraid to have his head handled. Convulsions and delirium will develop, with inability of muscular control, or stupor and coma may supervene. When the membranes are greatly implicated, convulsions and delirium with violence may be expected, but if the brain substances are principally affected stupor and coma will be the prominent symptoms. In the former condition the pulse will be quick and hard; in the latter, soft and depressed, with often a dilatation of the pupils, and deep, slow, stertorous breathing. The symptoms may follow one another in rapid succession, and the disease approach a fatal termination within 12 hours. In subacute attacks the symptoms are better defined, and the animal seldom dies before the third day. Within three or four days gradual improvement may become manifest, or cerebral softening with partial paral-

ysis may occur. In all cases of encephalitis there is a marked rise in
temperature from the very onset of the disease, with a tendency to
increase until the most alarming symptoms develop, succeeded by a
decrease when coma becomes manifest. The violence and character of
the symptoms greatly depend upon the extent and location of the
structures involved. Thus, in some cases there may be marked paralysis of certain muscles, while in others there may be spasmodic rigidity of muscles in a certain region. Very rarely the animal becomes
extremely violent early in the attack, and by rearing up, striking
with the fore feet, or falling over, may do himself great injury.
Usually, however, the animal maintains the standing position, propping himself against the manger or wall, until he falls from inability
of muscular control, or from unconsciousness. Occasionally, in his
delirium, he may go through a series of automatic movements, such
as trotting or walking, and, if loose in a stall, will move around persistently in a circle. Early and persistent constipation of the bowels
is a marked symptom in nearly all acute affections of the brain; retention of the urine, also, is frequently observed.

Following these symptoms there are depression, loss of power and
consciousness, lack of ability or desire to move, and usually fall of
temperature. At this stage the horse stands with legs propped, the
head hanging or resting on the manger, the eyes partly closed, and
does not respond when spoken to or when struck with a whip.

Chronic encephalitis or meningitis may succeed the acute stage,
or may be due to stable miasma, blood poison, narcotism, lead poisoning, etc. This form may not be characterized in its initial stages by
excitability, quick and hard pulse, and high fever. The animal
usually appears at first stupid; eats slowly; the pupil of the eye does
not respond to light quickly; the animal often throws his head up
or shakes it as if suffering sudden twinges of pain. He is slow and
sluggish in his movements, or there may be partial paralysis of one
limb, one side of the face, neck, or body. These symptoms, with
some variations, may be present for several days and then subside,
or the disease may pass into the acute stage and terminate fatally.
Chronic encephalitis may effect an animal for ten days or two weeks
without much variation in the symptoms before the crisis is reached.
If improvement commences, the symptoms usually disappear in the
reverse order to that in which they developed, with the exception of
the paralytic effects, which remain intractable or permanent. Paralysis of certain sets of muscles is a very common result of chronic,
subacute, and acute encephalitis, and is due to softening of the brain
or to exudation into the cavities of the brain or arachnoid space.

Softening and abscess of the brain are terminations of cerebritis.
It may also be due to an insufficient supply of blood as a result

of diseased cerebral arteries and of apoplexy. The symptoms are drowsiness, vertigo, or attacks of giddiness, increased timidity, or fear of familiar objects, paralysis of one limb, hemiplegia, imperfect control of the limbs, and usually a weak, intermittent pulse. In some cases the symptoms are analogous to those of apoplexy. The character of the symptoms depends upon the seat of the softening or abscess within the brain.

Cerebral sclerosis sometimes follows inflammation in the structure of the brain affecting the connective tissues, which eventually become hypertrophied and press upon nerve cells and fibers, causing their ultimate disappearance, leaving the parts hard and indurated. This condition gives rise to a progressive paralysis and may extend along a certain bundle of fibers into the spinal cord. Complete paralysis almost invariably supervenes and causes death.

Lesions.—On making post-mortem examinations of horses which have died in the first stages of either of these diseases we find an excessive engorgement of the capillaries and small blood vessels, with correspondingly increased redness and changes in both the contents and the walls of the vessels. If death has occurred at a later period of the disease, it will be found that, in addition to the redness and engorgement, an exudation of the contents of the blood vessels into the tissues and upon the surfaces of the inflamed parts has supervened. If the case has been one of encephalitis, there will usually be found more or less watery fluid in the ventricles (natural cavities in the brain), in the subarachnoid space, and a serous exudation between the convolutions and interstitial spaces of the gray matter under the membranes of the brain. The quantity of fluid varies in different cases. Exudations of a membranous character may be present, and are found attached to the surfaces of the pia mater.

In meningitis, especially in chronic cases, in addition to the serous effusion, there are changes which may be regarded as characteristic in the formation of a delicate and highly vascular layer or layers of membrane or organized structure on the surface of the dura mater, and also indications of hemorrhages in connection with the membranous formations. Hematoma, or blood tumors, may be found embedded in this membrane. In some cases the hemorrhages are copious, causing paralysis or apoplexy, followed by speedy death. The meningitis may be suppurative. In this case a puslike exudate is found between the membranes covering the brain.

In cerebritis, or inflammation of the interior of the brain, there is a tendency to softening and suppuration and the formation of abscesses. In some cases the abscesses are small and numerous, surrounded with a softened condition of the brain matter, and sometimes we may find one large abscess. In cases of recent development the walls of the abscesses are fringed and ragged and have no lining membrane. In older or chronic cases the walls of the abscesses are generally lined with a strong membrane, often having the appearance of a sac or cyst, and the contents have a very offensive odor.

Treatment.—In all acute attacks of inflammation involving the membranes or cerebral masses, it is the pressure from the distended and engorged blood vessels and the rapid accumulation of inflammatory products that endangers the life of the animal in even the very early stage of the disease. The earlier the treatment is commenced to lessen the danger of fatal pressure from the engorged blood vessels, the less effusion and smaller number of inflammatory products we have to contend with later. The leading object, then, to be accomplished in the treatment of the first stage of encephalitis, meningitis, or cerebritis, and before a dangerous degree of effusion or exudation has taken place, is to relieve the engorgement of the blood vessels and thereby lessen the irritation or excitability of the affected structures. If the attempt to relieve the engorgement in the first stage has been only partially successful, and the second stage, with its inflammatory products and exudations, whether serous or plastic, has set in, then the main objects in further treatment are to keep up the strength of the animal and hasten the absorption of the exudative products as much as possible. To obtain these results, when the animal is found in the initial stage of the disease, if there is unnatural excitability or stupor with increase of temperature and quickened pulse, we should apply cold to the head in the form of cold water or ice. For this purpose cloths or bags may be used, and they should be renewed as often as necessary. If the disease is still in its early stages and the animal is strong, bleeding from the jugular vein may be beneficial. Good results are to be expected only during the stage of excitement, while there is a strong, full pulse and the mucous membranes of the head are red from a plentiful supply of blood. The finger should be kept on the pulse and the blood allowed to flow until there is distinct softening of the pulse. As soon as the animal recovers somewhat from the shock of the bleeding the following medicine should be made into a ball or dissolved in a pint of warm water and be given at one dose: Barbados aloes, 7 drams; calomel, 2 drams; powdered ginger, 1 dram; tincture of aconite, 20 drops.

The animal should be placed in a cool, dark place, as free from noise as possible. When the animal becomes thirsty half an ounce of bromid of potash may be dissolved in the drinking water every six hours. Injections of warm water into the rectum may facilitate the action of the purgative. Norwood's tincture of veratrum viride, in 20-drop doses, should be given every hour and 1 dram of solid extract of belladonna every four hours until the symptoms become modified and the pulse regular and full.

PLATE XIX.

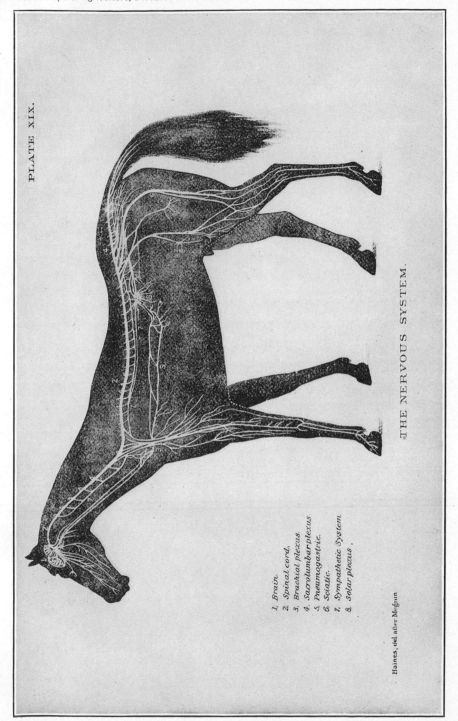

1. Brain.
2. Spinal cord.
3. Brachial plexus.
4. Sacrolumbar plexus.
5. Pneumogastric.
6. Sciatic.
7. Sympathetic System.
8. Solar plexus.

Haines, del. after McGunn.

THE NERVOUS SYSTEM.

If this treatment fails to give relief, the disease will pass into the advanced stages, or, if the animal has been neglected in the early stages, the treatment must be supplanted with the hypodermic injection of ergotin, in 5-grain doses, dissolved in 1 dram of water, every six hours. The limbs may be poulticed above the fetlocks with mustard. Warm blanketing, to promote perspiration, is to be observed always when there is no excessive perspiration.

If the disease becomes chronic (encephalitis or meningitis), we must place our reliance upon alteratives and tonics, with such incidental treatment as special symptoms may demand. Iodid of potassium in 2-dram doses should be given three times a day and 1 dram of calomel once a day to induce absorption of effusions or thickened membranes. Tonics, in the form of iodid of iron in 1-dram doses, to which is added 2 drams of powdered hydrastis, may also be given every six or eight hours, as soon as the active fever has abated. After the disappearance of the acute symptoms, blisters (cantharides ointment) may be applied behind the poll. When paralytic effects remain after the disappearance of all other symptoms, sulphate of strychnia in 2-grain doses, in combination with the other tonics, may be given twice a day and be continued until it produces muscular twitching. In some cases of paralysis, as of the lips or throat, benefit may be derived from the moderate use of the electric battery. Many of the recoveries will, however, under the most active and early treatment, be but partial, and in all cases the animals become predisposed to subsequent attacks. A long time should be allowed to pass before the animal is exposed to severe work or great heat. When the disease depends upon mechanical injuries, they have to be treated and all causes of irritation to the brain removed. If it is due to stable miasma, uremic poisoning, pyemia, influenza, rheumatism, toxic agents, etc., they should receive prompt attention for their removal or mitigation.

Cerebral softening, abscess, and sclerosis are practically inaccessible to treatment, otherwise than such relief as may be afforded by the administration of opiates and general tonics, and, in fact, the diagnosis is largely presumptive.

CONGESTION OF THE BRAIN, OR MEGRIMS.

Congestion of the brain consists in an accumulation of blood in the vessels, also called hyperemia, or engorgement. It may be active or passive—active when there is an undue accumulation of blood or diminished arterial resistance, and passive when it accumulates in the vessels of the brain, owing to some obstacle to its return by the veins.

Causes.—Active cerebral congestion may be from hypertrophy of the left ventricle of the heart, excessive exertion, the influence of extreme heat, sudden and great excitement, artificial stimulants, etc. Passive congestion may be produced by any mechanical obstruction which prevents the proper return of blood through the veins to the heart, such as a small or ill-fitting collar, which often impedes the blood current, tumors or abscesses pressing on the vein in its course, and organic lesions of the heart with regurgitation.

Extremely fat animals with short, thick necks are peculiarly subject to attacks of cerebral congestion. Simple congestion, however, is merely a functional affection, and in a slight or moderate degree involves no immediate danger. Extreme engorgement, on the contrary, may be followed by rupture of previously weakened arteries and capillaries and cause immediate death, designated then as a stroke of apoplexy.

Symptoms.—Congestion of the brain is usually sudden in its manifestation and of short duration. The animal may stop very suddenly and shake its head or stand quietly braced, then stagger, make a plunge, and fall. The eyes are staring, breathing hurried and stertorous, and the nostrils widely dilated. This may be followed by coma, violent convulsive movements, and death. Generally, however, the animal gains relief in a short time, but may remain weak and giddy for several days. If it is due to organic change of the heart or the disease of the blood vessels in the brain, then the symptoms may be of slow development, manifested by drowsiness, dimness or imperfect vision, difficulty in voluntary movements, diminished sensibility of the skin, loss of consciousness, delirium, and death. In milder cases effusion may take place in the arachnoid spaces and ventricles of the brain, followed by paralysis and other complications.

Pathology.—In congestion of the brain the cerebral vessels are loaded with blood, the venous sinuses distended to an extreme degree, and the pressure exerted upon the brain constitutes actual compression, giving rise to the symptoms just mentioned. On postmortem examinations this engorgement is found universal throughout the brain and its membranes, which serves to distinguish it from inflammations of these structures, in which the engorgements are confined more or less to circumscribed portions. A prolonged congestion may, however, lead to active inflammation, and in that case we find serous and plastic exudations in the cavities of the brain. In addition to the intensely engorged condition of the vessels we find the gray matter of the brain redder than natural. In cases in which several attacks have occurred the blood vessels are often found permanently dilated.

Treatment.—The animal should be taken out of harness at once, with prompt removal of all mechanical obstructions to the circulation. If it is caused by venous obstruction by too tight a collar, the loosening of the collar will give immediate relief. The horse should be bled freely from the jugular vein. If due to tumors or abscesses, a surgical operation becomes necessary to afford relief. To revive the animal if it becomes partially or totally unconscious, cold water should be dashed on the head. Give a purge of Glauber's salt. If the limbs are cold, tincture of capsicum or strong mustard water should be applied to them. If symptoms of paralysis remain after two or three days, an active cathartic and iodid of potassium will be indicated, to be given as prescribed for inflammation of the brain. In confirmed cases, treatment is not advisable, as there is considerable danger to the owner should an attack occur in a crowded street.

Prevention.—Well-adjusted collar, with strap running from the collar to the girth, to hold down the collar when pulling upgrade; regular feed and exercise, without allowing the animal to become excessively plethoric; moderate checking, allowing a free-and-easy movement of the head; well-ventilated stabling, proper cleanliness, pure water, etc.

SUNSTROKE, HEAT STROKE, OR HEAT EXHAUSTION.

The term sunstroke is applied to affections occasioned not exclusively by exposure to the sun's rays, as the word signifies, but by the action of great heat combined generally with humid atmosphere. Exhaustion produced by long-continued heat is often the essential factor, and is called heat exhaustion. Horses on the race track undergoing protracted and severe work in hot weather often succumb to heat exhaustion. Draft horses which do not receive proper care in watering, feeding, and rest in shady places and are exposed for many hours to the direct rays of the sun suffer very frequently from sunstroke.

Symptoms.—Sunstroke is manifested suddenly. The animal stops, drops his head, begins to stagger, and soon falls to the ground unconscious. The breathing is marked with great stertor, the pulse is very slow and irregular, cold sweats break out in patches on the surface of the body, and the animal often dies without having recovered consciousness.

The temperature becomes very high, reaching 105° to 109° F.

In heat exhaustion the animal usually requires urging for some time prior to the appearance of any other symptoms, generally perspiration is checked, and then the horse becomes weak in its gait, the breathing hurried or panting, eyes watery or bloodshot, nostrils dilated and highly reddened, assuming a dark, purple color; the pulse is rapid and weak, the heart bounding, followed by unconsciousness and death. If recovery takes place, convalescence extends over a long period of time, during which incoordination of movement may persist.

Pathology.—Sunstroke, virtually active congestion of the brain, often accompanied with effusion and blood extravasation, characterizes this condition, with often rapid and fatal lowering of all the vital functions. In many instances the death may be due to the complete stagnation in the circulation of the brain, inducing anemia, or want of nourishment of that organ. In other cases it may be directly due to the excessive compression of the nerve matter controlling the heart's action, and cause paralysis of that organ. There are also changes in the composition of the blood.

Treatment.—The animal should be placed in shaded surroundings. Under no circumstances is bloodletting permissible in sunstroke. Ice or very cold water should be applied to the head and along the spine, and half an ounce of carbonate of ammonia or 6 ounces of whisky should be given in 1 pint of water. Cold water may be used as an enema and should also be showered upon the body of the horse from the hose or otherwise. This should be continued until the temperature is down to 103° F. Brisk friction of the limbs and the application of spirits of camphor often yields good results. The administration of the stimulants should be repeated in one hour if the pulse has not become stronger and slower. In either case, when reaction has occurred, preparations of iron and general tonics may be given during convalescence: Sulphate of iron, 1 dram; gentian, 3 drams; red cinchona bark, 2 drams; mix and give in feed morning and evening.

Prevention.—In very hot weather horses should have wet sponges or light sunshades on the head when at work, or the head may be sponged with cold water as many times a day as possible. Proper attention should be given to feeding and watering, never in excess. During the warm months all stables should be cool and well ventilated, and if an animal is debilitated from exhaustive work or disease it should receive such treatment as will tend to build up the system. Horses should be permitted to drink as much water as they want while they are at work during hot weather.

An animal which has been affected with sunstroke is very liable to have subsequent attacks when exposed to the necessary exciting causes.

APOPLEXY OR CEREBRAL HEMORRHAGE.

Apoplexy is often confounded with cerebral congestion, but true apoplexy always consists in rupture of cerebral blood vessels, with blood extravasation and formation of blood clot.

Causes.—Two causes are involved in the production of apoplexy, the predisposing and the exciting. The predisposing cause is degeneration, or disease which weakens the blood vessel; the exciting cause is any one which tends to induce cerebral congestion.

Symptoms.—Apoplexy is characterized by a sudden loss of sensation and motion, profound coma, and stertorous, difficult breathing. The action of the heart is little disturbed at first, but soon becomes slower, then quicker and feebler, and after a little time ceases. If the rupture is one of a small artery and the extravasation limited, sudden paralysis of some part of the body is the result. The extent and location of the paralysis depend upon the location within the brain which is functionally deranged by the pressure of the extravasated blood; hence these conditions are very variable.

In the absence of any premonitory symptoms or an increase of temperature in the early stage of the attack, we may be reasonably certain in making the distinction between this disease and congestion of the brain, or sunstroke.

Pathology.—In apoplexy there is generally found an atheromatous condition of the cerebral vessels, with weakening and degeneration of their walls. When a large artery has been ruptured it is usually followed by immediate death, and large rents may be found in the cerebrum, with great destruction of brain tissue, induced by the forcible pressure of the liberated blood. In small extravasations producing local paralysis without marked general disturbance the animal may recover after a time; in such cases gradual absorption of the clot takes place. In large clots atrophy of the brain substances may follow, or softening and abscess from want of nutrition may result, and render the animal worthless, ultimately resulting in death.

Treatment.—Place the animal in a quiet, cool place and avoid all stimulating feed. Administer, in the drinking water or feed, 2 drams of the iodid of potassium twice a day for several weeks if necessary. Medical interference with sedatives or stimulants is more liable to be harmful than of benefit, and bloodletting in an apoplectic fit is extremely hazardous. From the fact that cerebral apoplexy is due to diseased or weakened blood vessels, the animal remains subject to subsequent attacks. For this reason treatment is very unsatisfactory.

COMPRESSION OF THE BRAIN.

Causes.—In injuries from direct violence a piece of broken bone may press upon the brain, and, according to its size, the brain is robbed of its normal space within the cranium. It may also be due to an extravasation of blood or to exudation in the subdural or arachnoid spaces. Death from active cerebral congestion results through compression. The occurrence may sometimes be traced to the direct cause, which will give assurance for the correct diagnosis.

Symptoms.—Impairment of all the special senses and localized paralysis. All the symptoms of lessened functional activity of the brain are manifested to some degree. The paralysis remains to be our guide for the location of the cause, for it will be found that the paralysis occurs on the opposite side of the body from the location of the injury, and the parts suffering paralysis will denote, to an expert veterinarian or physician, the part of the brain which is suffering compression.

Treatment.—Trephining, by a skillful operator, for the removal of the cause when due to depressed bone or the presence of foreign bodies. When the symptoms of compression follow other acute diseases of the brain, apoplectic fits, etc., the treatment must be such as the exigencies of the case demands.

CONCUSSION OF THE BRAIN.

This is generally caused by falling over backward and striking the poll, or perhaps falling forward on the nose, by a blow on the head, etc. Train accidents during shipping often cause concussion of the brain.

Symptoms.—Concussion of the brain is characterized by giddiness, stupor, insensibility, or loss of muscular power, succeeding immediately upon a blow or severe injury involving the cranium. The animal may rally quickly or not for hours; death may occur on the spot or after a few days. When there is only slight concussion or stunning, the animal soon recovers from the shock. When more severe, insensibility may be complete and continue for a considerable time; the animal lies as if in a deep sleep; the pupils are insensible to light; the pulse fluttering or feeble; the surface of the body cold, muscles relaxed, and the breathing scarcely perceptible. After a variable interval partial recovery may take place, which is marked by paralysis of some parts of the body, often of a limb, the lips, ear, etc. Convalescence is usually tedious, and frequently permanent impairment of some organs remains.

Pathology.—Concussion produces laceration of the brain, or at least a jarring of the nervous elements, which, if not sufficiently severe to produce sudden death, may lead to softening or inflammation, with their respective symptoms of functional derangement.

Treatment.—The first object in treatment will be to establish reaction or to arouse the feeble and weakening heart. This can often be accomplished by dashing cold water on the head and body of the animal; frequent injections of weak ammonia water, ginger tea, or oil and turpentine should be given per rectum. In the majority of cases this will soon bring the horse to a state of consciousness. In more severe cases mustard poultices should be applied along the spine and above the fetlocks. As soon as the animal gains partial consciousness stimulants, in the form of whisky or capsicum tea, should be given. Owing to severity of the structural injury to the brain or the possible rupture of blood vessels and blood extravasation, the reaction may often be followed by encephalitis or cerebritis, and will then have to be treated accordingly. For this reason the stimulants should not be administered too freely, and they must be abandoned as soon as reaction is established. There is no need for further treatment unless complications develop as a secondary result. Bleeding, which is so often practiced, proves almost invariably fatal in this form of brain affection. We should also remember that it is never safe to drench a horse with large quantities of medicine when he is unconscious, for he is very liable to draw the medicine into the lungs in inspiration.

Prevention.—Young horses, when harnessed or bitted for the first few times, should not have their heads checked high, for it frequently causes them to rear up, and, being unable to control their balance, they are liable to fall over sideways or backwards, thus causing brain concussion when they strike the ground.

ANEMIA OF THE BRAIN.

This is a physiological condition in sleep. It is considered a disease or may give rise to disease when the circulation and blood supply of the brain are interfered with. In some diseases of the heart the brain becomes anemic, and fainting fits occur, with temporary loss of consciousness. Tumors growing within the cranium may press upon one or more arteries and stop the supply of blood to certain parts of the brain, thus inducing anemia, ultimately atrophy, softening, or suppuration. Probably the most frequent cause is found in plugging, or occlusion, of the arteries by a blood clot.

Symptoms.—Imperfect vision, constantly dilated pupils, frequently a feeble and staggering gait, and occasionally cramps, convulsions, or epileptic fits occur.

Pathology.—The exact opposite of cerebral hyperemia. The blood vessels are found empty, the membranes blanched, and the brain substance softened.

Treatment.—Removal of the remote cause when possible. General tonics, nutritious feed, rest, and removal from all causes of nervous excitement.

HYDROCEPHALUS, OR DROPSY OF THE BRAIN.

This condition consists in an unnatural collection of fluid about or in the brain. Depending upon the location of the fluid, we speak of external and internal hydrocephalus.

External hydrocephalus is seen chiefly in young animals. It comsists in a collection of fluid under the meninges, but outside the brain proper. This defect is usually congenital. It is accompanied with an enlargement of the skull, especially in the region of the forehead. The pressure of the fluid may cause the bones to soften. The disease is incurable and usually fatal.

Internal hydrocephalus is a disease of mature horses, and consists in the accumulation of an excessive quantity of fluid in the cavities or ventricles of the cerebrum. The cause of this accumulation may be a previous inflammation, a defect in the circulation of blood through the brain, heat stroke, overwork, excessive nutrition, or long-continued indigestion. Common, heavy-headed draft horses are predisposed to this condition.

Symptoms.—The symptoms are an expression of dullness and stupidity, and from their nature this disease is sometimes known as "dumminess" or "immobility." A horse so afflicted is called a "dummy." Among the symptoms are loss of intelligence, stupid expression, poor memory, etc. The appetite is irregular; the horse may stop chewing with a wisp of hay protruding from his lips; he seems to forget that it is there. Unnatural positions are sometimes assumed, the legs being placed in clumsy and unusual attitudes. Such horses are difficult to drive, as they do not respond readily to the word, to pressure of the bit, or to the whip. Gradually the pulse becomes weaker, respiration becomes faster, and the subject loses weight. Occasionally there are periods of great excitement due to temporary congestion of the brain. At such times the horse becomes quite uncontrollable. A horse so afflicted is said to have "staggers." The outlook for recovery is not good.

Treatment is merely palliative. Regular work or exercise and nutritious feed easy of digestion, with plenty of fresh water, are strongly indicated. Intensive feeding should not be practiced. The bowels should be kept open by the use of appropriate diet or by the use of small regular doses of Glauber's salt.

TUMORS WITHIN THE CRANIUM.

Tumors within the cranial cavity and the brain occur not infrequently, and give rise to a variety of symptoms, imperfect control of voluntary movement, local paralysis, epilepsy, etc. Among the more common tumors are the following:

Osseous tumors, growing from the walls of the cranium, are not very uncommon.

Dentigerous cysts, containing a formation identical to that of a tooth, growing from the temporal bone, sometimes are found lying loose within the cranium.

Tumors of the choroid plexus, known as brain sand, are frequently met with on post-mortem examinations, but seldom give rise to any appreciable symptoms during life. They are found in horses at all ages, and are slow of development. They are found in one or both of the lateral ventricles, enveloped in the folds of the choroid plexus.

Melanotic tumors have been found in the brain and meninges in the form of small, black nodules in gray horses, and in one instance are believed to have induced the condition known as stringhalt.

Fibrous tumors may develop within or from the meningeal structures of the brain.

Gliomatous tumor is a variety of sarcoma very rarely found in the structure of the cerebellum.

Treatment for tumors of the brain is impossible.

SPASMS, OR CRAMPS.

Spasm is a marked symptom in many diseases of the brain and of the spinal cord. Spasms may result from irritation of the motor nerves as conductors, or may result from irritation of any part of the sympathetic nervous system, and they usually indicate an excessive action of the reflex motor centers. Spasms may be induced by various medicinal agents given in poisonous doses, or by effete materials in the circulation, such as nux vomica or its alkaloid strychnia, lead preparations, or an excess of the urea products in the circulation, etc. Spasms may be divided into two classes: Tonic spasm, when the cramp is continuous or results in persistent rigidity, as in tetanus; clonic spasm, when the cramping is of short duration, or is alternated with relaxations. Spasms may affect involuntary as well as the voluntary muscles, the muscles of the glottis, intestines, and even the heart. They are always sudden in their development.

Spasm of the glottis.—This is manifested by a strangling respiration; a wheezing noise is produced in the act of inspiration; extreme anxiety and suffering for want of air. The head is extended, the body profusely perspiring; pulse very rapid; soon great exhaustion becomes manifest; the mucous membranes become turgid and very dark colored, and the animal thus may suffocate in a short time.

Spasm of the intestines.—(See "Cramp colic," p. 74.)

Spasm of the neck of the bladder.—This may be due to spinal irritation or a reflex from intestinal irritation, and is manifested by frequent but ineffectual attempts to urinate.

Spasm of the diaphragm, or thumps.—Spasmodic contraction of the diaphragm, the principal muscle used in respiration, is generally occasioned by extreme and prolonged speeding on the race track or road. The severe strain thus put upon this muscle finally induces irritation of the nerves controlling it, and the contractions become very forcible and violent, giving the jerking character known among horsemen as "thumps." This condition may be distinguished from violent beating of the heart by feeling the pulse beat at the angle of the jaw, and at the same time watching the jerking movement of the body, when it will be discovered that the two bear no relation to each other. (See "Palpitation of the heart," p. 259.)

Spasm of the thigh, or cramp of a hind limb.—This is frequently witnessed in horses that stand on sloping plank floors—generally in cold weather—or it may come on soon after severe exercise. It is probably due to an irritation of the nerves of the thigh. In cramps of the hind leg the limb becomes perfectly rigid, and attempts to flex are unsuccessful; the animal stands on the affected limb, but is unable to move it; it is unnaturally cold; it does not, however, appear to cause much suffering unless attempts are made to change position. This cramp may be of short duration—a few minutes—or it may persist for several days. This condition is often taken for a dislocation of the stifle joint. In the latter the foot is extended backward, and the horse is unable to advance it, but drags the limb. An examination of the joint also reveals a change in form. Spasms may affect the eyelids, by closure or by retraction. Spasm of the sterno-maxillaris muscle has been witnessesd, and the animal was unable to close the jaws until the muscle became relaxed.

Treatment of spasms.—An anodyne liniment, composed of chloroform 1 part and soap liniment 4 parts, applied to cramped muscles will usually cause relaxation. This may be used when single external muscles are affected. In spasms of the glottis, inhalation of sulphuric ether will give quick relief. In spasm of the diaphragm, rest and the administration of half an ounce of chloroform in 3 ounces of whisky, with a pint of water added, will generally suffice to bring relief, or if this fails give 5 grains of sulphate of morphia by hypodermic injection. If spasms result from organic disease of the nervous system, the latter should receive such treatment as its character demands. In cramp of the leg, compulsory movement usually causes relaxation very quickly; therefore the animal should be led out of the stable and be forced to run or trot. Sudden, nervous excitement caused by a crack of the whip or smart blow will often bring about immediate relief. Should this fail, the anodyne liniment may be used along the inside of the thigh, and chloroform, ether, or laudanum given internally. An ounce of the chloral hydrate will certainly relieve the spasm when given internally, but the cramp may return soon after the effect has passed off, which in many cases it does very quickly.

Convulsions.—Although there is no disease of the nervous system which can be properly termed convulsive, or justify the use of the word convulsion to indicate any particular disease, yet it is often such a prominent symptom that a few words may not be out of place.

General, irregular muscular contractions of various parts of the body, with unconsciousness, characterize what we regard as convulsions, and like ordinary spasms are dependent upon some disease or irritation of the nervous structures, chiefly of the brain. No treatment is required; in fact, a general convulsion must necessarily be self-limited in its duration. Suspending, as it does, respiratory movements, checking the oxygenation and decarbonization of the blood, the rapid accumulation of carbonic-acid gas in the blood and the exclusion of oxygen quickly puts the blood in a condition to produce the most reliable and speedy sedative effect upon the nerve excitability that could be found, and consequently furnishes its own remedy so far as the continuance of the convulsive paroxysm is concerned. Whatever treatment is instituted must be directed toward a removal of the cause of the convulsive paroxysm.

CHOREA, OR ST. VITUS'S DANCE.

Chorea is characterized by involuntary contractions of voluntary muscles. This disease is an obscure disorder, which may be from pressure upon a nerve, cerebral or spinal sclerosis, small aneurisms in the brain, etc. Choreic symptoms have been produced by injecting granules of starch into the arteries entering the brain. Epilepsy and other forms of convulsions simulate chorea in appearance.

Stringhalt is by some termed "chorea." This is manifested by a sudden jerking up of one or both hind legs when the animal is walking. This symptom may be very slight in some horses, but has a tendency to increase with age. In some the catching up of the affected leg is very violent, and when it is lowered to the ground the motion is equally sudden and forcible, striking the foot to the ground like a pile driver. Very rarely chorea may be found to affect one of the fore legs, or the muscles of one side of the neck or the upper part of the neck. Involuntary jerking of the muscles of the hip or thigh is seen occasionally, and is termed "shivering" by horsemen.

Chorea is often associated with a nervous disposition, and is not so frequent in animals with a sluggish temperament. The involuntary muscular contractions cause no pain, and do not appear to produce much exhaustion of the affected muscles, although the jerking may be regular and persistent whenever the animal is in motion.

Treatment.—In a few cases, early in the appearance of this affection, general nerve tonics may be of benefit, viz: iodid of iron, 1 dram; pulverized nux vomica, 1 dram; pulverized scutellaria (skullcap), 1 ounce. Mix and give in the feed once a day for two weeks. Arsenic in the form of Fowler's solution is often beneficial. If the cause is connected with organic brain lesions, treatment is usually unsuccessful.

EPILEPSY, OR FALLING FITS.

The cause of epilepsy is seldom traceable to any special brain lesions. In a few cases it accompanies disease of the pituitary body, which is located in the under surface of the brain. Softening of the brain may give rise to this affection. Attacks may occur only once or twice a year or they may be of frequent recurrence.

Symptoms.—No premonitory symptoms precede an epileptic fit. The animal suddenly staggers; the muscles become cramped; the jaws may be spasmodically opened and closed, and the tongue become lacerated between the teeth; the animal foams at the mouth and falls in a spasm. The urine flows involuntarily, and the breathing may be temporarily arrested. The paroxysm soon passes off, and the animal gets on its feet in a few minutes after the return of consciousness.

Treatment.—Dashing cold water on the head during the paroxysm. After the recovery 1 dram of oxid of zinc may be given in the feed twice a day for several weeks, or benefit may be derived from the tonic prescribed for chorea.

PARALYSIS, OR PALSY.

Paralysis is a weakness or cessation of the muscular contraction by diminution of loss of the conducting power or stimulation of the motor nerves. Paralytic affections are of two kinds, the complete and the incomplete. The former includes those in which both motion and sensibility are affected; the latter those in which only one or the other is lost or diminished. Paralysis may be general or partial. The latter is divided into hemiplegia and paraplegia. When only a small portion of the body is affected, as the face, a limb, the tail, it is designated by the term local paralysis. When the irritation extends from the periphery of the center it is termed reflex paralysis.

Causes are much varied. Most of the acute affections of the brain and spinal cord may lead to paralysis. Injuries, tumors, disease of the blood vessels of the brain, etc., all have a tendency to produce suspension of the conducting motive power to the muscular structures. Pressure upon, or the severing of, a nerve causes a paralysis of the parts to which such a nerve is distributed. Apoplexy may be termed a general paralysis, and in nonfatal attacks is a frequent cause of the various forms of palsy.

GENERAL PARALYSIS.—This can not take place without producing immediate death. The term is, however, usually applied to paralysis of the four extremities, whether any other portions of the body are involved or not. This form of palsy is due to compression of the brain by congestion of its vessels, large clot formation in apoplexy, concussion, or shock, or any disease in which the whole brain structure is involved in functional disturbance.

HEMIPLEGIA (PARALYSIS OF ONE SIDE OR HALF OF THE BODY).—Hemiplegia is frequently the result of a tumor in the lateral ventricles of the brain, softening of one hemisphere of the cerebrum, pressure from extravasated blood, fracture of the cranium, or it may be due to poisons in the blood or to reflex origin. When hemiplegia is due to or the result of a prior disease of the brain, especially of an inflammatory character, it is seldom complete; it may affect only one limb and one side of the head, neck, or muscles along the back, and may pass off in a few days after the disappearance of all the other evidences of the primary affection. In most cases, however, hemiplegia arises from emboli obstructing one or more blood vessels of the brain, or the rupture of some vessel the wall of which had become weakened by degeneration and the extravasation of blood. Sensibility in most cases is not impaired, but in some there is a loss of sensibility as well as of motion. In some cases the bladder and rectum are involved in the paralysis.

Symptoms.—In hemiplegia the attack may be very sudden, and the animal fall, powerless to move one side of the body; one side of the lips will be relaxed; the tongue may hang out on one side of the mouth; the tail curved around sideways; an inability to swallow feed or water may be present, and often the urine dribbles away as fast as it collects in the bladder. Sensibility of the affected side may be entirely lost or only partial; the limbs may be cold and sometimes unnaturally warm. In cases wherein the attack is not so severe the animal may be able to maintain the standing position, but will have great difficulty in moving the affected side. In such cases the animal may recover from the disability. In the more severe, in which there is complete loss of power of movement, recoveries are rare.

PARAPLEGIA (TRANSVERSE PARALYSIS OF THE HIND EXTREMITIES).— Paralysis of the hind extremities is usually due to some injury or inflammation affecting the spinal cord. (See " Spinal meningitis," p. 232, and "Myelitis," p. 233.) It may also be due to a reflex irritation from disease of peripheral nerves, to spinal irritation or congestion caused by blood poisons, etc.

Symptoms.—When due to mechanical injury of the spinal cord, from a broken back or spinal hemorrhage, it is generally progressive in its character, although it may be sudden. When it is caused by agents in the bood, it may be intermittent or recurrent.

Paraplegia is not difficult to recognize, for it is characterized by a weakness and imperfect control of the hind legs and powerless tail. The urine usually dribbles away as it is formed and the manure is pushed out, ball by ball, without any voluntary effort, or the passages may cease entirely. When paraplegia is complete, large and ill-conditioned sores soon form on the hips and thighs from chafing and bruising, which have a tendency quickly to weaken the animal and necessitate his destruction.

LOCOMOTOR ATAXIA, OR INCOORDINATION OF MOVEMENT.—This is characterized by an inability to control properly the movement of the limbs. The animal appears usually perfectly healthy, but when he is led out of his stall his legs have a wobbly movement and he will stumble or stagger, especially in turning. When this is confined to the hind parts it may be termed a modified form of paraplegia, but often it may be seen to affect nearly all the voluntary muscles when they are called into play, and must be attributed to some pressure exerted on the base of the brain.

LOCAL PARALYSIS.—This is frequently met with in horses. It may affect many parts of the body, even vital organs, and it is verv frequently overlooked in diagnosis.

FACIAL PARALYSIS.—This is a frequent type of local paralysis, and is due to impairment of function of the motor nerve of the facial muscles, the portio dura. The cause may exist at the base of the brain, compression along its course after it leaves the medulla oblongata, or to a bruise after it spreads out on the great masseter muscle.

Symptoms.—A flaccid condition of the cheek muscles, pendulous lips, inability to grasp the feed, often a slow and weak movement in chewing, and difficulty and slowness in drinking.

LARYNGISMUS PARALYTICUS, OR ROARING.—This condition is characterized by roaring, and is usually caused by an inflamed or hypertrophied bronchial gland pressing against the left recurrent laryngeal nerve, which interferes with its conducting power. A similar condition is occasionally induced in acute pleurisy, when the recurrent nerve becomes involved in the diseased process or compressed by plastic exudation.

PARALYSIS OF THE RECTUM AND TAIL.—This is generally the result of a blow or fall on the rump, which causes a fracture of the sacrum bone and injury to the nerves supplying the tail and part of the rectum and muscles belonging thereto. This fracture would not be suspected were it not for the loss of motion of the tail.

INTESTINAL PARALYSIS.—Characterized by persistent constipation; frequently the strongest purgatives have no effect whatever on the movement of the bowels. In the absence of symptoms of indigestion, or special diseases implicating the intestinal canal, torpor of the bowels must be attributed to deficient innervation. This condition may depend upon brain affections or be due to reflex paralysis. Sudden checks of perspiration may induce excessive action of the bowels or paralysis.

PARALYSIS OF THE BLADDER.—This usually affects the neck of the bladder, and is characterized by incontinence of urine; the urine dribbles away as fast as it is secreted. The cause may be of reflex origin, disease of the rectum, tumors growing within the pelvic cavity, injury to the spinal cord, etc.

PARALYSIS OF THE OPTIC NERVE (AMAUROSIS).—A paralysis of eyesight may occur very suddenly from rupture of a blood vessel in the brain, acute local congestion of the brain, the administration of excessive doses of belladonna or its alkaloid atropia, etc. In amaurosis the pupil is dilated to its full extent; the eye looks clear, but does not respond to light.

Paralysis of hearing, of the external ear, of the eyelid, partial paralysis of the heart and organs of respiration, of the blood vessels from injury to the vasomotor nerves of the esophagus, or loss of deglutition, palsy of the stomach, all may be manifested when the supply of nervous influence is impaired or suspended.

TREATMENT FOR PARALYSIS.—In all paralytic affections there may be anesthesia, or impairment of sensibility, in addition to the loss of motion, or there may be hyperesthesia, or increased sensibility, in connection with the loss of motion. These conditions may call for special treatment in addition to that for loss of motion. If hyperesthesia is well marked local anodynes may be needed to relieve suffering. Chloroform liniment or hypodermic injections of from 3 to 5 grains of sulphate of morphia will allay local pain. If there is marked anesthesia, or loss of sensibility, it may become necessary to secure the animal in such way that he can not suffer serious injury from accidents which he can not avoid or feel. In the treatment of any form of paralysis we must always refer to the cause, and attempt its removal if it can be discovered. In cases in which the cause can not be determined we have to rely solely upon a general external and internal treatment. Externally, fly blisters or strong, irritant liniments may be applied to the paralyzed parts. In hemiplegia they should be applied along the bony part of the side of the neck; in paraplegia, across the loins. In some cases hot-water cloths will be beneficial. Internally, it is well to administer 1 dram of powdered nux vomica or 2 grains of sulphate of strychnia twice a day until twitching of some of the voluntary muscles occurs; then discontinue it for several days, and then commence again with a smaller dose, gradually increasing it until twitching recurs. Iodid of potassium in 1 to 2 dram doses two or three times daily may be used with the hope that it will favor the absorption of the clot or obstruction to the nervous current. In some cases Fowler's solution of arsenic in teaspoonful doses twice a day in the drinking water proves beneficial. Occasionally benefit may be derived from the application of the electric current, especially in cases of roaring, facial paralysis, paralysis of the eyelid, etc. Nutritious but not two bulky feed, good ventilation, clean stabling, moderate exercise if the animal is capable of taking it, good grooming, etc., should be observed in all cases.

SPINAL MENINGITIS, OR INFLAMMATION OF THE MEMBRANES ENVELOPING THE SPINAL CORD.

This may be induced by the irritant properties of blood poisons, exhaustion and exposure, spinal concussion, all forms of injury to the spine, tumors, caries of the vertebræ, rheumatism, etc.

Symptoms.—A chill may be the precursor, a rise in temperature, or a general weakness and shifting of the legs. Soon a painful, convulsive twitching of the muscles sets in, followed by muscular rigidity along the spine, in which condition the animal will move very stiffly and evince great pain in turning. Evidences of paralysis or paraplegia develop, retention or incontinence of urine, and oftentimes sexual excitement is present. The presence of marked fever at the beginning of the attack, associated with spinal symptoms, should lead us to suspect spinal meningitis or myelitis. These two conditions usually appear together, or myelitis follows inflammation of the meninges so closely that it is almost impossible to separate the two; practically it does not matter much, for the treatment will be about the same in both cases. Spinal meningitis generally becomes chronic, and is then marked principally by paralysis of that portion, or parts of it, posterior to the seat of the disease.

Pathology.—In spinal meningitis we find essentially the same condition as in cerebral meningitis; there is an effusion of serum between the membranes, and often a plastic exudation firmly adherent to the pia mater serves to maintain a state of paralysis for a long time after the acute symptoms have disappeared by compressing the cord. Finally, atrophy, softening, and even abscess may develop within the cord. Unlike in man, it is usually found localized in horses.

Treatment.—Bags filled with ice should be applied along the spine, to be followed later by strong blisters. The fever should be controlled as early as possible by giving 20 drops of Norwood's tincture of veratrum viride every hour until the desired result is obtained. One dram of the fluid extract of belladonna, to control pain and vascular excitement of the spinal cord, may be given every five or six hours until the pupils of the eyes become pretty well dilated. If the pain is very intense 5 grains of sulphate of morphia should be injected hypodermically. The animal must be kept as free from excitement as possible. If the urine is retained in the bladder it must be drawn off every four or six hours. In very acute attacks the disease generally proves fatal in a few days. If, however, the animal grows better, some form of paralysis is liable to remain for a long time, and the treatment will have to be directed then toward a removal of the exudative products and a strengthening of the system and stimulation of the nervous functions. To induce absorption, iodid of potassium in 2-dram doses, dissolved in the drinking water, may be given twice a day. To strengthen the system, iodid of iron 1 dram twice a day and 1 dram of nux vomica once a day may be given in the feed. Electricity to the paralyzed and weakened muscles is advisable; the current should be weak, but be continued for half an hour two or three times daily. If the disease is due to a broken back, caries of the vertebræ, or some other irremediable cause, the animal should be destroyed at once.

MYELITIS, OR INFLAMMATION OF THE SUBSTANCE OF THE SPINAL CORD.

This is a rare disease, except as a secondary result of spinal meningitis or injuries to the spine. Poisoning by lead, arsenic, mercury, phosphorus, carbonic-acid gas, etc., has been known to produce it. Myelitis may be confined to a small spot in the cord or may involve the whole for a variable distance. It may lead to softening abscess or degeneration.

Symptoms.—The attack may begin with a chill or convulsion; the muscles twitch or become cramped very early in the disease, and the bladder usually is affected at the outset, in which there may be either retention or incontinence of urine. These conditions are followed by complete or partial paralysis of the muscles posterior to the locality of the inflamed cord, and the muscles begin to waste away rapidly. The paralyzed limb becomes cold and dry, due to the suspension of proper circulation; the joints may swell and become edematous; vesicular eruptions appear on the skin; and frequently gangrenous sloughs form on the paralyzed parts. It is exceedingly seldom that recovery takes place. In a few instances it may assume a chronic type, when all the symptoms become mitigated, and thus continue for some time, until septicemia, pyemia, or exhaustion causes death.

Pathology.—The inflammation may involve nearly the whole length of the cord, but generally it is more intense in some places than others; when due to mechanical injury, the inflammation may remain confined to a small section. The cord is swollen and congested, reddened, often softened and infiltrated with pus cells, and the nerve elements are degenerated.

Treatment.—Similar to that of spinal meningitis.

SPINAL CONGESTION.

This condition consists in an excess of blood. As the blood vessels of the pia mater are the principal source of supply to the spinal cord, hyperemia of the cord and of the meninges usually go together. The symptoms are, therefore, closely allied to those of spinal meningitis and congestion. When the pia mater is diseased, the spinal cord is almost invariably affected also.

Cause.—Sudden checking of the perspiration, violent exercise, blows, and falls.

Symptoms.—The symptoms may vary somewhat with each case, and closely resemble the first symptoms of spinal meningitis, spinal tumors, and myelitis. First, some disturbance in movement, lowering the temperature, and partial loss of sensibility posterior to the seat of the congestion. If in the cervical region, it may cause interference in breathing and the action of the heart. When in the region of the loins, there may be loss of control of the bladder. When the congestion is sufficient to produce compression of the cord, paraplegia may be complete. Usually fever, spasms, muscular twitching, or muscular rigidity are absent, which will serve to distinguish spinal congestion from spinal meningitis.

Treatment.—Hot-water applications to the spine, 1-dram doses fluid extract of belladonna repeated every four hours, and tincture of aconite root 20 drops every hour until the symptoms become ameliorated. If no inflammatory products occur, the animal is likely to recover.

SPINAL ANEMIA.

This may be caused by extreme cold, exhausting diseases, spinal embolism or plugging of a spinal blood vessel, an interference with the circulation through the abdominal aorta, from compression, thrombosis, or aneurism of that vessel; the spinal vessels may be caused to contract through vasomotor influence, a result of peripheral irritation of some nerve.

Spinal anemia causes paralysis of the muscles used in extending the limbs. When the bladder is affected, it precedes the weakness of motion, while in spinal congestion it follows, and increased sensibility, in place of diminished sensibility, as in spinal congestion, is observed. Pressure along the spine causes excessive pain.

If the exciting cause can be removed, the animal recovers; if this fails, the spinal cord may undergo softening.

SPINAL COMPRESSION.

When caused by tumors or otherwise, when pressure is slight, it produces a paralysis of the muscles used in extending a limb and contraction of those which flex it. When compression is great it causes complete loss of sensibilty and motion posterior to the compressed part of the cord.

Compression of a lateral half of the cord produces motor paralysis, disturbance of the circulation, and difficulty of movement, an increased sensibility on the side corresponding to the compressed section, and a diminished sensibility and some paralysis on the opposite side.

Treatment.—When it occurs as a sequence of a preceding inflammatory disease, iodid of potassium and general tonics are indicated. When due to tumors growing within the spinal canal, or to pressure from displaced bone, no form of treatment will result in any benefit.

SPINAL HEMORRHAGE.

This may occur from changes in the wall of the blood vessels, in connection with tumors, acute myelitis, traumatic injuries, etc. The blood may escape through the pia mater into the subarachnoid cavity, and large clots be formed.

Symptoms.—The symptoms are largely dependent upon the seat and extent of the hemorrhage, as they are principally owing to the compression of the cord. A large clot may produce sudden paraplegia, accompanied with severe pain along the spine; usually, however, the paralysis of both motion and sensation is not very marked at first; on the second or third day fever is liable to appear, and increased or diminished sensibility along the spine posterior to the seat of the clot. When the bladder and rectum are involved in the symptoms it indicates that the spinal cord is compressed.

Treatment.—In the occurrence of injuries to the back of a horse, whenever there is any evidence of paralysis, it is always advisable to apply bags of ice along the spine to check or prevent hemorrhage or congestion, and 2 drams of the fluid extract of ergot and 20 drops of tincture of digitalis may be given every hour until three doses have been taken. Subsequently tincture of belladonna in half-ounce doses may be given three times a day. If there is much pain, 5 grains of sulphate of morphia, injected under the skin, will afford relief and lessen the excitability of the animal. In all cases the animal should be kept perfectly quiet.

SPINAL CONCUSSION.

This is rarely observed in the horse, and unless it is sufficiently severe to produce well-marked symptoms it would not be suspected. It may occur in saddle horses from jumping, or it may be produced by falling over an embankment, or a violent fall upon the haunches may produce it. Concussion may be followed by partial paralysis or spinal hemorrhage; generally, however, it is confined to a jarring and some disturbance of the nerve elements of the cord, and the paralytic effect which ensues soon passes off. Treatment consists in rest until the animal has completely recovered from the shock. If secondary effects follow from hemorrhage or compression, they have to be treated as heretofore directed.

SPINAL TUMORS.

Within the substance of the cord glioma or the mixed gliosarcomata are found to be the most frequent, tumors may form from the meninges and the vertebræ, being of a fibrous or bony nature, and affect the spinal cord indirectly by compression. In the meninges we may find glioma, cancers, and psammoma, fibromata; aneurisms of the spinal arteries have been discovered in the spinal canal.

Symptoms.—Tumors of the spinal canal cause symptoms of spinal irritation or compression of the cord. The gradual and slow development of symptoms of paralysis of one or both hind limbs or certain muscles may lead to a suspicion of spinal tumors. The paralysis induced is progressive, but not usually marked with atrophy of the muscles or increased sensibility along the spine. When the tumor is within the spinal cord itself all the symptoms of myelitis may be present.

Treatment.—General tonics and 1-dram doses of nux vomica may be given; iodid of iron or iodid of potassium in 1-dram doses, three times a day in feed, may, in a very few cases, give some temporary benefit. Usually the disease progresses steadily until it proves fatal.

NEURITIS, OR INFLAMMATION OF A NERVE.

This is caused by a bruise or wound of a nerve or by strangulation in a ligature when the nerve is included in the ligation of an artery. The changes in an inflamed nerve are an enlargement, reddening of the nerve sheath, spots of extravasated blood, and sometimes an infiltration of serum mixed with pus.

Symptoms.—Acute pain of the parts supplied by the nerve and absence of swelling or increased heat of the part.

Treatment.—Hypodermic injections of from 3 to 5 grains of morphia to relieve pain, hot fomentations, and rest. If it is due to an inclusion of a ligature, the nerve should be divided above and below the ligature.

NEUROMA, OR TUMOR OF A NERVE.

Neuroma may be from enlargement of the end of a divided nerve or due to fibrous degeneration of a nerve which has been bruised or wounded. Its most frequent occurrence is found after the operation of neurotomy for foot lameness, and it may appear after the lapse of months or even years. Neuroma usually develops within the sheath of the nerve with or without implicating the nerve fibers. It is oval, running lengthwise with the direction of the nerve.

Symptoms.—Pain of the affected limb or part is manifested, more especially after resting a while, and when pressure is made upon the tumor it causes extreme suffering.

Treatment.—Excision of the tumor, including part of the nerve above and below, and then treat it like any other simple wound.

INJURIES TO NERVES.

These may consist in wounding, bruising, laceration, stretching, compression, etc. The symptoms which are produced will depend upon the extent, seat, and character of the injury. Recovery may quickly take place, or it may lead to neuritis, neuroma, or spinal or cerebral irritation, which may result in tetanus, paralysis, and other serious derangements. In all diseases, whether produced by some form of external violence or intrinsic causes, the nerves are necessarily involved, and sometimes it is to a primary injury of them that the principal fault in movement or change of nutrition of a part is due. It is often difficult or impossible to discover that an injury to a nerve has been inflicted, but whenever this is possible it may enable us to remedy that which otherwise would result in permanent evil. Treatment should consist in relieving compression, in hot fomentations, the application of anodyne liniments, excision of the injured part, and rest.

FORAGE POISONING, OR SO-CALLED CEREBROSPINAL MENINGITIS.

This disease prevails among horses in nearly all parts of the United States. Its appearance in America is by no means of recent occurrence, for the malady was reported by Large in 1847, by Michener in 1850, and by Liautard in 1869 as appearing in both sporadic and enzootic form in several of the Eastern States. Since then the disease has occurred periodically in many States in all sections of the country, and has been the subject of numerous investigations and publications by a number of the leading men of the veterinary profession. It is prevalent with more or less severity every year in certain parts of the United States, and during the year 1912 the Bureau of Animal Industry received urgent requests for help from Colorado, Georgia, Iowa, Kansas, Kentucky, Louisiana, Maryland, Missouri, Nebraska, New Jersey, North Carolina, Oregon, South Carolina, South Dakota, Virginia, and West Virginia. While in 1912 the brunt of the disease seemed to fall on Kansas and Nebraska, other States were also seriously afflicted. In previous years, for instance in 1882, as well as in 1897, the horses of southeastern Texas were reported to have died by the thousand, and in the following year the horses of Iowa were said to have "died like rats." However, Kansas seems to have had more than her share of this trouble, as a severe outbreak that extended over almost the entire State occurred in 1891, while in 1902, in 1906, and again in 1912 the disease recurred with equal severity in various portions of the State.

This condition consists in a poisoning and depression of the nervous system from eating or drinking feed or water containing poison generated by mold or bacteria. It has been shown to be owing to eating damaged ensilage, corn, brewers' grains, oats, etc., or to drinking stagnant pond water or water from a well contaminated by surface drainage. Horses at pasture may contract the disease when the growth of grass is so profuse that it mats together and the lower part dies and ferments or becomes moldy.

In England a similar disease has been called "grass staggers," due to eating rye grass when it is ripening or when it is cut and eaten while it is heating and undergoing fermentation. In eastern Pennsylvania it was formerly known by the name of "putrid sore throat" and "choking distemper." A disease similar in many respects which is very prevalent in Virgina, especially along the eastern border, is commonly known by the name of "blind staggers," and in many of the Southern States this has been attributed to the consumption of worm-eaten corn. Horses of all ages and mules are subject to this disease.

Symptoms and lesions.—The symptoms which typify sporadic or epidemic cerebrospinal meningitis in man are not witnessed among horses, namely, excessive pain, high fever, and early muscular rigidity. In the recognition of the severity of the attack we may divide the symptoms into three grades. In the most rapidly fatal attacks the animal may first indicate it by weak, staggering gait, partial or total inability to swallow solids or liquids, impairment of eyesight; twitching of the muscles and slight cramps may be observed. As a rule, the temperature is not elevated—indeed, it is sometimes below normal. This is soon followed by a paralysis of the whole body, inability to stand, delirium in which the animal sometimes goes through a series of automatic movements as if trotting or running; the delirium may become very violent and the unconscious animal may bruise his head very seriously in his struggles; but usually a deep coma renders him quiet until he expires. Death in these cases usually takes place in from 4 to 24 hours from the time the first symptoms become manifest. The pulse is variable during the progress of the disease; it may be almost imperceptible at times, and then again very rapid and irregular; the respirations generally are quick and catching. In the next form in which this disease may develop it first becomes manifest by a difficulty in swallowing and slowness in mastication, and a weakness which may be first noticed in the strength of the tail; the animal will be unable to switch it or to offer resistance when we bend it up over the croup. The pulse is often a little slower than normal. There is no evidence of pain; the respirations are unchanged, and the temperature little less than normal; the bowels may be somewhat constipated. These symptoms may remain unchanged for two or three days and then gradual improvement may take place, or the power to swallow may become entirely lost and the weakness and uncertainty in gait more and more perceptible; then sleepiness or coma may appear; the pulse becomes depressed, slow, and weak, the breathing stertorous, and paroxysms of delirium develop, with inability to stand, and some rigidity of the spinal muscles or partial cramp of the neck and jaws. In such cases death may occur in from 6 to 10 days from the commencement of the attack. In many cases there is no evidence of pain, spasm, or fever at any time during the progress of the disease, and finally profound coma develops and death follows, painless and without a struggle.

In the last or mildest form the inability of voluntary control of the limbs becomes but slightly marked, the power of swallowing never entirely lost, and the animal has no fever, pain, or unconscious movements. Generally the animal will begin to improve about the fourth day and recovers.

In a few cases the spinal symptoms, manifested by paraplegia, may be the most prominent symptoms; in others they may be altogether absent and the main symptoms may be difficulty in mastication and swallowing; rarely it may affect one limb only. In all cases in which coma remains absent for six or seven days the animal is likely to recover. When changes toward recovery take place, the symptoms usually leave in the reverse order to that in which they developed, but local paralysis may remain for some time, rarely persistent.

On post-mortem the number of lesions observable to the naked eye is in marked contrast to the severity of the symptoms noted. The pharynx and larynx are inflamed in many cases, and sometimes coated with a yellowish-white glutinous deposit, extending at times over the tongue and occasionally a little way down the trachea. The lungs are normal, except from complications following drenching or recumbence for a long period. The heart is usually normal in appearance, except an occasional cluster of hemorrhagic points on the outer surface, while the blood is dark and firmly coagulated. The lining of the stomach indicates a subacute gastritis, while occasionally an erosion is noted. An edema is observed in the submucosa of such cases. The first few inches of the small intestines likewise may show slight inflammation in certain cases, while in others it is quite severe; otherwise the digestive tract appears normal, excluding the presence of varying numbers of bots, *Strongylus vulgatus*, and a few other nematodes. The liver is congested and swollen in some cases, while it appears normal in others. The spleen is, as a rule, normal, and at times the kidneys are slightly congested. The bladder is often distended with dark-colored urine, and occasionally a marked cystitis has been observed. The adipose tissue throughout the carcass may show a pronounced icteric appearance in certain cases. On removing the bones of the skull the brain appears to be normal macroscopically in a few instances, but in most cases the veins and capillaries of the meninges of the cerebrum, cerebellum, and occasionally the medulla is distinctly dilated and engorged, and in a few cases there are pronounced lesions of a leptomeningitis. An excessive quantity of cerebrospinal fluid is present in most of the cases. On the floor of the lateral ventricles of several brains there was noted a slight softening caused by hemorrhages into the brain substance. There is always an abundance of fluid in the subarachnoid spaces, ventricles, and at the base of the brain, usually of the color of diabetic urine, and containing a limited number of flocculi, but in a few cases it was slightly blood tinged. The spinal cord was not found involved in the few cases examined.

Treatment.—One attack of the disease does not confer immunity. Horses have been observed which have recovered from two attacks, and still others that recovered from the first but died as a result of the second attack.

Inasmuch as a natural immunity does not appear after an attack of cerebrospinal meningitis, it might be anticipated that serum of recovered cases would possess neither curative nor prophylactic qualities. Nevertheless, experiments have been made along these lines with serum from recovered cases, but without any positive results. Similar investigations have been conducted by others in Europe with precisely the same results. With the tendency of the disease to produce pathological lesions in the central nervous system, it seems scarcely imaginable that a medicinal remedy will be found to heal these foci, and even when recovery takes place considerable disturbance in the functions, as blindness, partial paralysis, dumbness, etc., is liable to remain. Indeed, when the disease once becomes established in an animal, drugs seem to lose their physiological action. Therefore, with all the previously mentioned facts before us, it is evident that the first principle in the treatment of this disease is prevention, which consists in the exercise of proper care in feeding only clean, well-cured forage and grain and pure water. These measures when faithfully carried out check the development of additional cases of the disease upon the affected premises.

While medicinal treatment has proved unsatisfactory in most cases, nevertheless the first indication is to clean out the digestive tract thoroughly, and to accomplish this prompt measures must be used early in the disease. Active and concentrated remedies should be given, preferably subcutaneously or intravenously, owing to the great difficulty in swallowing, even in the early stage. Arecolin in one-half grain doses, subcutaneously, has given as much satisfaction as any other drug. After purging the animal the treatment is mostly symptomatic. Intestinal disinfectants, particularly calomel, salol, and salicylic acid, have been recommended, and mild, antiseptic mouth washes are advisable. Antipyretics are of doubtful value, as better results are obtained, if the temperature is high, by copious cold-water injections. An ice pack applied to the head is beneficial in case of marked psychic disturbance. One-ounce doses of chloral hydrate per rectum should be given if the patient is violent or if muscular spasms are severe. If the temperature becomes subnormal, the animal should be warmly blanketed, and if much weakness is shown this should be combated with stimulants, such as strychnin, camphor, alcohol, atropin, or aromatic spirits of ammonia. Early in the disease urotropin (hexamethylenamin) in doses of 25 grains, dissolved in water and given by the mouth every two hours, appeared to have been responsible for the recovery of some cases of the malady. During convalescence tonic treatment is indicated.

Hygienic measures needful.—Whenever this disease appears in a stable all the animals should be removed as soon as possible. They should be provided with clean, well-ventilated, and well-drained stables, and each animal should receive a laxative and be fed feed and given water from a new, clean source. The abandoned stable should be thoroughly cleansed from all waste matters, receive a coat of whitewash containing 4 ounces of carbolic acid to the gallon of water and should have time to dry thoroughly before the horses are replaced. A complete change of feed is of the very greatest importance on account of the belief that the cause resides in diseased grain, hay, and grass.

TETANUS, OR LOCKJAW.

This disease is characterized by spasms affecting the muscles of the face, neck, body, and limbs and of all muscles supplied by the cerebrospinal nerves. The spasms or muscular contractions are rigid and persistent, yet mixed with occasional more intense contractions of convulsive violence.

Causes.—This disease is caused by a bacillus that is often found in the soil, in manure, and in dust. This germ forms spores at the end of the organism and grows only in the absence of oxygen. It produces a powerful nerve poison, which causes the symptoms of tetanus. The germ itself multiplies at the point where it is introduced, but its poison is absorbed and is carried by the blood to all parts of the body, and thus the nervous system is poisoned. Deep wounds infected by this germ are more dangerous than superficial wounds, because in them the germ is more remote from the oxygen of the air. Hence, nail pricks, etc., are especially dangerous. In the majority of instances the cause of tetanus can be traced to wounds, especially pricks and wounds of the feet or of tendinous structures. It sometimes follows castration, docking, the introduction of setons, inclusion of a nerve in a ligature, etc. It may come on a long time after the wound is healed—three or four months. Horses with a nervous, excitable disposition are more predisposed than those of a more sluggish nature. Stallions are more subject to develop tetanus as the result of wounds than geldings, and geldings more than mares.

Symptoms.—The attacks may be acute or subacute. In an acute attack the animal usually dies within four days. The first symptoms which attract the attention of the owner is difficulty in chewing and swallowing, an extension of the head and protrusion over the inner part of the eye of the membrana nictitans, or haw. An examination of the mouth will reveal an inability to open the jaws to their full extent, and the endeavor to do so will produce great nervous excitability and increased spasm of the muscles of the jaw and neck. The muscles of the neck and along the spine become rigid and the legs are moved in a stiff manner. The slightest noise or disturbance throws the animal into increased spasm of all the affected muscles. The tail is usually elevated and held immovable; the bowels become constipated early in the attack. The temperature and pulse are not much changed. These symptoms in the acute type become rapidly aggravated until all the muscles are rigid—in a state of tonic spasm—with a continuous tremor running through them; a cold perspiration breaks out on the body; the breathing becomes painful from the spasm of the muscles used in respiration; the jaws are completely set, eyeballs retracted, lips drawn tightly over the teeth, nostrils dilated, and the animal presents a picture of the most extreme agony until death relieves him. The pulse, which at first was not much affected, will become quick and hard, or small and thready when the spasm affects the muscles of the heart. In the subacute cases the jaws may never become entirely locked; the nervous excitability and rigidity of the muscles are not so great. There is, however, always some stiffness of the neck or spine manifest in turning; the haw is turned over the eyeball when the nose is elevated. It is not uncommon for owners to continue such animals at their work for several days after the first symptoms have been observed. All the symptoms may gradually increase in severity for a period of ten days, and then gradually diminish under judicious treatment, or they may reach the stage wherein all the characteristics of acute tetanus become developed. In some cases, however, we find the muscular cramps almost solely confined to the head or face, perhaps involving those of the neck. In such cases we have complete trismus (lockjaw), and all the head symptoms are acutely developed. On the contrary, we may find the head almost exempt in some cases, and have the body and limbs perfectly rigid and incapable of movement without falling.

Tetanus may possibly be confounded with spinal meningitis, but the character of the spasm-locked jaw, retraction of the eyeballs, the difficulty in swallowing due to spasms of the muscles of the pharynx, and above all, the absence of paralysis, should serve to make the distinction.

Prevention.—When a valuable horse has sustained a wound that it is feared may be followed by tetanus, it is well to administer a dose of tetanus antitoxin. This is injected beneath the skin with a hypodermic syringe. A very high degree of protection may in this way be afforded. This antitoxin should be administered only by a competent veterinarian.

Treatment.—The animal should be placed in a box stall without bedding, as far as possible from other horses. If in a country district, the animal should be put into an outbuilding or shed, where the noise of other animals will not reach it; if the place is moderately dark, it is all the better; in fly time it should be covered with a light sheet. The attendant must be very careful and quiet to prevent all unnecessary excitement and increase of spasm. Tetanus antitoxin appears to be useful as a remedy in some cases, if given in very large quantities early in the disease; otherwise it is useless. Subcutaneous injections of carbolic acid in glycerin and water (carbolic acid 30 grains, glycerin and water each 1 ounce) appear to be useful in some cases. Injections should be given twice daily.

A cathartic, composed of Barbados aloes 6 to 8 drams, with which may be mixed 2 drams of the solid extract of belladonna, should be given at once. This is best given in a ball form; if, however, the animal is greatly excited by the attempt or can not swallow, the ball may be dissolved in 2 ounces of olive oil and thrown on the back of the tongue with a syringe. If the jaws are set, or nearly so, an attempt to administer medicine by the mouth should not be made. In such cases one-quarter of a grain of atropia, with 5 grains of sulphate of morphia, should be dissolved in 1 dram of pure water and injected under the skin. This should be repeated sufficiently often to keep the animal continually under its effect. This will usually mitigate the severity of the spasmodic contraction of the affected muscles and lessen sensibility to pain. Good results may be obtained sometimes by the rectal injection of the fluid extract of belladonna and of cannabis indica, of each 1 dram, every four or six hours. This may be diluted with a quart of milk. When the animal is unable to swallow liquids, oatmeal gruel and milk should be given by injection per rectum to sustain the strength of the animal. A pailful of cool water should be constantly before him, placed high enough for him to reach it without special effort; even if drinking is impossible, the laving of the mouth is refreshing. Excellent success frequently may be obtained by clothing the upper part of the head, the neck, and greater part of the body in woolen blankets kept saturated with very warm water. This treatment should be continued for six or eight hours at a time. It often relaxes the cramped muscles and gives them rest and the animal almost entire freedom from pain; but it should be used every day until the acute spasms have permanently subsided in order to be of any lasting benefit.

Recently subcutaneous injections of brain emulsion have been recommended. It is thought that the tetanus toxin will attach itself to the brain cells so injected and thus free the system of this poison. When it is due to a wound, the wound should be thoroughly cleaned and disinfected with carbolic acid. If from a wound which has healed, an excision of the cicatrix may be beneficial. In all cases it is not uncommon to have a partial recovery followed by relapse when the animal becomes excited from any cause.

RABIES, HYDROPHOBIA, OR MADNESS.

This disease does not arise spontaneously among horses, but is the result of a bite from a rabid animal—generally a dog or cat. The development of the disease follows the bite in from three weeks to three months—very rarely in two weeks. (See also p. 559.)

Symptoms.—The first manifestation of the development of this disease may be an increased excitability and viciousness; very slight noises or the approach of a person incites the animal to kick, strike, or bite at any near object. Very often the horse will bite his own limbs or sides, lacerating the flesh and tearing the skin. The eyes appear staring, bloodshot; the ears are on the alert to catch all sounds; the head is held erect. In some cases the animal will continually rub and bite the locality of the wound inflicted by the rabid animal. This symptom may precede all others. Generally the bowels become constipated and the animal makes frequent attempts at urination, which is painful, and the urine very dark colored. The furious symptoms appear in paroxysms; at other times the animal may eat and drink, although swallowing appears to become painful toward the latter stage of the disease, and may cause renewed paroxysms. The muscles of the limbs or back may be subject to intermittent spasms, or spasmodic tremors; finally, the hind limbs become paralyzed, breathing very difficult, and convulsions supervene, followed by death. The pulse and respirations are increased in frequency from the outset of the attack. Rabies may possibly be mistaken for tetanus. In the latter disease we find tonic spasms of the muscles of the jaws, or stiffness of the neck or back very early in the attack, and evidence of viciousness is absent.

Treatment.—As soon as the true nature of the disease is ascertained the animal should be killed.

Prevention.—When a horse is known to have been bitten by a rabid animal, immediate cauterization of the wound with a red-hot iron may possibly destroy the virus before absorption of it takes place.

PLUMBISM, OR LEAD POISONING.

This disease is not of frequent occurrence. It may be due to the habitual drinking of water which has been standing in leaden conductors or in old paint barrels, etc. It has been met with in enzootic form near smelting works, where, by the fumes arising from the works, lead in the form of oxid, carbonate, or sulphate was deposited on the grass and herbage which the horses ate.

Symptoms.—Lead poisoning produces derangement of the functions of digestion and locomotion, or it may affect the lungs principally. In whatever system of organs the lead is mostly deposited there we have the symptoms of nervous debility most manifest. If in the lungs, the breathing becomes difficult and the animal gets out of breath very quickly when compelled to run. Roaring, also, is very frequently a symptom of lead poisoning. When it affects the stomach, the animal gradually falls away in flesh, the hair becomes rough, the skin tight, and colicky symptoms develop. When the deposit is principally in the muscles, partial or complete paralysis gradually develops. When large quantities of lead have been taken in and absorbed, symptoms resembling epilepsy may result, or coma and delirium develop and prove fatal. In lead poisoning there is seldom any increase in temperature. A blue line forms along the gums of the front teeth, and the breath assumes a peculiarly offensive odor. Lead can always be detected in the urine by chemical tests.

Treatment.—The administration of 2-dram doses of iodid of potassium three times a day is indicated. This will form iodid of lead in the system, which is rapidly excreted by the kidneys. If much muscular weakness or paralysis is present, sulphate of iron in 1-dram doses and strychnia in 2-grain doses may be given twice a day. In all cases of suspected lead poisoning all utensils which have entered into the supply of feed or water should be examined for the presence of soluble lead. If it occurs near lead works, great care must be given to the supply of uncontaminated fodder, etc.

UREMIA.

Uremic poisoning may affect the brain in nephritis, acute albuminuria, or when, from any cause, the functions of the kidneys become impaired or suppressed and urea (a natural product) is no longer eliminated from these organs, causing it to accumulate in the system and give rise to uremic poisoning.

Uremic poisoning is usually preceded by dropsy of the limbs or abdomen; a peculiar, fetid breath is often noticed; then drowsiness, attacks of diarrhea, and general debility ensue. Suddenly extreme stupor or coma develops; the surface of the body becomes cold; the pupils are insensible to light; the pulse slow and intermitting; the breathing labored, and death supervenes. The temperature throughout the disease is seldom increased, unless the disease becomes complicated with acute, inflammatory disease of the brain or respiratory organs, which often occur as a result of the urea in the circulation. Albumen and tube casts may frequently be found in the urine. The disease almost invariably proves fatal.

Treatment must be directed to a removal of the cause.

ELECTRIC SHOCK.

Electric shock, from coming in contact with electric wires, is becoming a matter of rather frequent occurrence, and has a similar effect upon the animal system as a shock from lightning. Two degrees of electric or lightning shock may be observed, one producing temporary contraction of muscles and insensibility, from which recovery is possible, the other killing directly, by producing a condition of nervous and general insensibility. In shocks which are not immediately fatal the animal is usually insensible, the respiration slow, labored, or gasping, the pulse slow, feeble, and irregular, and the pupils dilated and not sensitive, or they may be contracted and sensitive. The temperature is lowered. There may be a tendency to convulsions or spasms. The predominating symptoms are extreme cardiac and respiratory depression.

Treatment.—Sulphate of atropia should be given hypodermically in one-quarter grain doses every hour or two hours until the heart beats are invigorated, the number and fullness of the respirations increased, and consciousness returns. Stimulating injections per rectum may also be useful in arousing the circulation; for this purpose whisky or ammonia water may be used.

DISEASES OF THE HEART, BLOOD VESSELS, AND LYMPHATICS.

By M. R. TRUMBOWER, V. S.

[Revised by Leonard Pearson, B. S., V. M. D.]

ANATOMY AND PHYSIOLOGY OF THE HEART AND BLOOD VESSELS.

(Pls. XX and XXI.)

The heart is a hollow, muscular organ, situated a little to the left of the center of the chest. Its impulse is felt on the left side on account of its location and from the rotary movement of the organ in action. It is cone-shaped, with the base upward; the apex points downward, backward, and to the left side. It extends from about the third to the sixth ribs, inclusive. The average weight is about 7 to 8 pounds. In horses used for speed the heart is relatively larger, according to the weight of the animal, than in horses used for slow work. It is suspended from the spine by the large blood vessels and held in position below by the attachment of the pericardium to the sternum. It is inclosed in a sac, the pericardium, which is composed of a dense fibrous membrane lined by a delicate serous membrane, which is reflected over the heart; the inner layer is firmly adherent to the heart, the outer to the fibrous sac, and there is an intervening space, known as the pericardial space, in which a small amount of serum—a thin translucent liquid—is present constantly.

The heart is divided by a shallow fissure into a right and left side; each of these is again subdivided by a transverse partition into two compartments which communicate. Thus there are four cardiac cavities—the superior, or upper, ones called the auricles; the inferior, or lower, ones the ventricles. These divisions are marked on the outside by grooves, which contain the cardiac blood vessels, and are generally filled with fat.

The right side of the heart may be called the venous side, the left the arterial side, named from the kind of blood which passes through them. The auricles are thin-walled cavities placed at the base, and are connected with the great veins—the venæ cavæ and pulmonary veins—through which they receive blood from all parts of the body. The auricles communicate with the ventricles each by a large aper-

247

ture, the auriculo-ventricular orifice, which is furnished with a remarkable mechanism of valves, allowing the transmission of blood from the auricles into the ventricles, but preventing a reverse course. The ventricles are thick-walled cavities, forming the more massive portion of the heart toward the apex. They are separated by a partition, and are connected with the great arteries—the pulmonary artery and the aorta—by which they send blood to all parts of the body. At the mouth of the aorta and at the mouth of the pulmonary artery is an arrangement of valves in each case which prevents the reflux of blood into the ventricles. The auriculo-ventricular valve in the left side is composed of two flaps, hence it is called the bicuspid valve; in the right side this valve has three flaps and is called the tricuspid valve. The flaps which form these valves are connected with a tendinous ring between the auricles and ventricles; and each flap of the auriculo-ventricular valves is supplied with tendinous cords, which are attached to the free margin and under-surface, so as to keep the valves tense when closed—a condition which is produced by the shortening of muscular pillars with which the cords are connected. The arterial openings, both on the right and on the left side, are provided with three-flapped semilunar-shaped valves, to prevent the regurgitation of blood when the ventricles contract. The veins emptying into the auricles are not capable of closure, but the posterior vena cava has an imperfect valve at its aperture.

The inner surface of the heart is lined by a serous membrane, the endocardium, which is smooth and firmly adherent to the muscular structure of the heart. This membrane is continuous with the lining membrane of the blood vessels, and it enters into the formation of the valves.

The circulation through the heart is as follows: The venous blood is carried into the right auricle by the anterior and posterior venæ cavæ. It then passes through the right auriculo-ventricular opening into the right ventricle, thence through the pulmonary artery to the lungs. It returns by the pulmonary veins to the left auricle, then is forced through the auriculo-ventricular opening into the left ventricle, which propels it through the aorta and its branches into the system, the veins returning it again to the heart. The circulation, therefore, is double, the pulmonary, or lesser, being performed by the right side, and the systemic, or greater, by the left side.

As the blood is forced through the heart by forcible contractions of its muscular walls, it has the action of a force pump, and gives the impulse at each beat, which we call the pulse—the dilatation of the arteries throughout the system. The contraction of the auricles is quickly followed by that of the ventricles, and then a slight pause occurs; this takes place in regular rhythmical order during health.

PLATE XX.

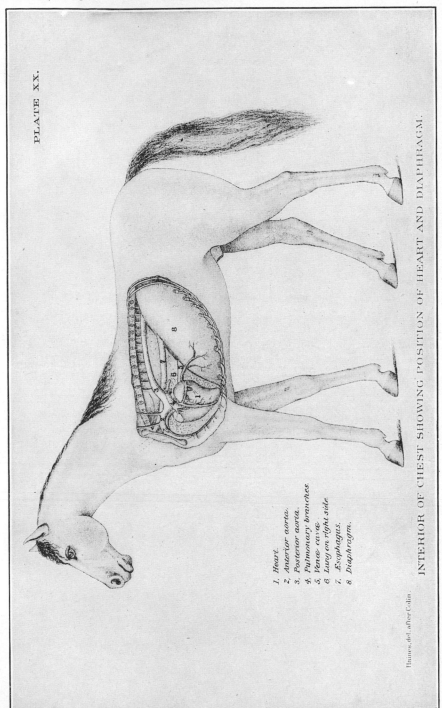

1. Heart.
2. Anterior aorta.
3. Posterior aorta.
4. Pulmonary branches.
5. Vena cava.
6. Lung on right side.
7. Esophagus.
8. Diaphragm.

Haines, del. after Colin.

INTERIOR OF CHEST SHOWING POSITION OF HEART AND DIAPHRAGM.

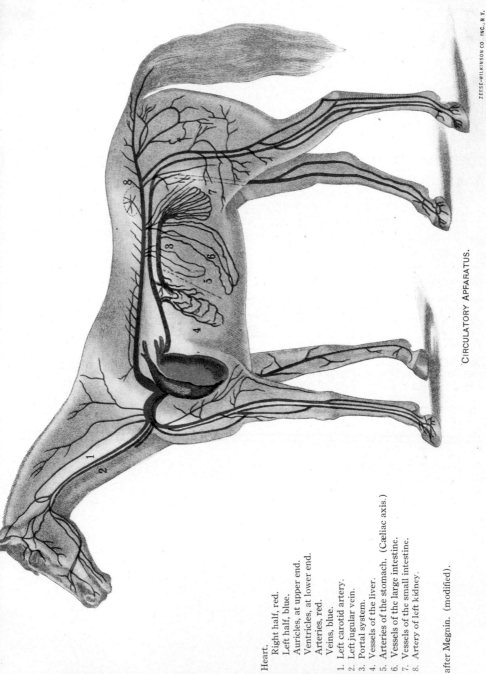

ZEESE-WILKINSON CO · INC., N Y.

CIRCULATORY APPARATUS.

Heart.
   Right half, red.
   Left half, blue.
   Auricles, at upper end.
   Ventricles, at lower end.
   Arteries, red.
   Veins, blue.
1. Left carotid artery.
2. Left jugular vein.
3. Portal system.
4. Vessels of the liver.
5. Arteries of the stomach. (Cæliac axis.)
6. Vessels of the large intestine.
7. Vessels of the small intestine.
8. Artery of left kidney.

Haines after Megnin. (modified).

The action of the heart is governed and maintained by the pneumo-gastric nerve (tenth pair of cranial nerves); it is the inhibitory nerve of the heart, and regulates, slows, and governs its action. When the nerve is cut, the heartbeats increase rapidly, and, in fact, the organ works without control. When the nerve is unduly irritated the holdback, or inhibitory force, is increased, and the heart slows up in the same measure. The left cavities of the heart, the pulmonary veins, and the aorta, or systemic artery, contain red or florid blood, fit to circulate through the body. The right cavities of the heart, with the venæ cavæ, or systemic veins, the pulmonary artery, contain dark blood, which must be transmitted through the lungs for reno-vation.

The arteries, commencing in two great trunks, the aorta and the pulmonary artery, undergo division, as in the branching of a tree. Their branches mostly come off at acute angles, and are commonly of uniform diameter in each case, but successively diminish after and in consequence of division, and in this manner gradually merge into the capillary system of blood vessels. As a general rule, the combined area of the branches is greater than that of the vessels from which they emanate, and hence the collective capacity of the arterial system is greatest at the capillary vessels. The same rule applies to the veins. The effect of the division of the arteries is to make the blood move more slowly along their branches to the capillary vessels, and the effect of the union of the branches of the veins is to accelerate the speed of the blood as it returns from the capillary vessels to the venous trunks.

In the smaller vessels a frequent running together, or anastomosis, occurs. This admits of a free communication between the currents of blood, and must tend to promote equability of distribution and of pressure, and to obviate the effects of local interruption. The arteries are highly elastic, being extensile and retractile both in length and breadth. During life they are also contractile, being provided with muscular tissue. When cut across they present, although empty, an open orifice; the veins, on the other hand, collapse.

In most parts of the body the arteries are inclosed in a sheath formed of connective tissue, but are connected so loosely that, when the vessel is cut across, its ends readily retract some distance within the sheath. Independently of this sheath, arteries are usually de-scribed as being formed of three coats, named, from the relative positions, external, middle, and internal. This applies to their struc-ture so far as it is discernible by the naked eye. The internal, serous, or tunica intima, is the thinnest, and is continuous with the lining membrane of the heart. It is made up of two layers—an inner, con-sisting of a layer of epithelial scales, and an outer, transparent, whitish, highly elastic, and perforated. The middle coat, tunica

media, is elastic, dense, and of a yellow color, consisting of nonstri-
ated muscular and elastic fibers, thickest in the largest arteries and
becoming thinner in the smaller. In the smallest vessels it is
almost entirely muscular. The external coat, tunica adventitia, is
composed mainly of fine and closely woven bundles of white connective tissue, which chiefly run diagonally or obliquely around the
vessel. In this coat the nutrient vessels, the vasa vasorum, form a
capillary network, from which a few penerate as far as the muscular
coat.

The veins differ from arteries in possessing thinner walls, less
elastic and muscular tissue, and for the most part a stronger tunica
adventitia. They collapse when cut across or when they are empty.
The majority of veins are provided with valves; these are folds of
the lining membrane, strengthened by fibrous tissue. They favor the
course of the blood and prevent its reflux. The nerves which supply
both the arteries and the veins come from the sympathetic system.
The smaller arteries terminate in the system of minute vessels known
as the capillaries, which are interposed between the termination of
the arteries and the commencement of the veins. Their average
diameter is about one three-thousandth of an inch.

DISEASES OF THE HEART AND BLOOD VESSELS.

In considering diseases of the heart we meet with many difficulties,
depending much upon the position which this organ occupies in the
animal. The shoulders cover so much of the anterior portion of the
chest, and often in very heavy-muscled horses the chest walls are so
thick that a satisfactory examination of the heart is attended with
difficulty. Diseases of the heart are not uncommon among horses;
the heart and its membranes are frequently involved in diseases of
the respiratory organs, diseases of the kidneys, rheumatism, influenza, etc. Some of the diseases of this organ are never suspected by
the ordinary observer during life, and are so difficult to diagnose
with any degree of certainty that we will have to confine ourselves
to a general outline, giving attention to such symptoms as may serve
to lead to a knowledge of their existence, with directions for treatment, care, etc.

Nervous affections often produce prominent heart symptoms by
causing functional disturbance of that organ, which, if removed, will
leave the heart restored to perfect vigor and normal action. Organic
changes involving the heart or valves, however, usually grow worse
and eventually prove fatal. Therefore it is necessary that we arrive
at an appreciation of the true nature and causes so that we may be
able to form a true estimate of the possibilities for recovery or en-
couragement for medical treatment.

Disease of the heart may occur at any age, but it is witnessed most frequently in young horses, which, when being trained for fast work, are often subjected to excessive hardship and fatigue. Nervous or timid animals also suffer from such diseases more frequently than those of a sluggish disposition. Any cause which induces a violent or sudden change in the circulation may result in injury to the heart. Symptoms which may frequently denote disease of the heart are difficult breathing or short-windedness, dropsies of the limbs, habitual coldness of the extremities, giddiness or fainting attacks, inability to stand work, although the general appearance would indicate strength and ability, etc.

MYOCARDITIS, OR INFLAMMATION OF THE MUSCULAR STRUCTURE OF THE HEART.

The heart muscle sometimes becomes inflamed as a complication or result of the existence of general or febrile and of infectious diseases. Severe influenza or infectious pneumonia is not infrequently followed by myocarditis. By extension of inflammation of the endocardium or pericardium the muscle of the heart may become involved. Over-exertion or especially hard work continued for a long time may cause this muscle to become inflamed.

Symptoms.—Inflammation of the heart muscle is shown by inability to contract forcibly. This results in a rapid but weak, soft pulse and irregular heart sounds. The pulse may be quite irregular as a result of the irregular, tumultuous action of the heart. There is great general weakness, shortness of breath, and rapid respiratory movements. In some cases, where the muscle is very much softened and weakened, or, perhaps when an abscess forms in the wall of the heart, the course of the disease is very rapid and terminates suddenly from paralysis or rupture of the heart.

Alterations.—The heart muscle has a brownish or yellowish, boiled appearance, and is so brittle that it tears easily. There may be a spotted appearance of the muscle from the intense changes in structure in small areas. These small areas may be due to suppuration, in which case they have the characteristics of small abscesses. This last condition is seen in pyemia (blood poisoning). If the disease is of long duration, the fibrous tissue in the wall of the heart may increase to such an extent as to produce an unnatural hardness of the wall.

Treatment.—In this disease the nutrition and strength of the heart should be kept up as much as possible with good food, good care, and heart tonics and stimulants. The horse should be tempted to eat such foods as he will take; he should be kept in an airy box stall; his legs should be well rubbed as often as necessary to keep them warm and bandaged loosely with flannel bandages. Internally the horse may have strychnia in 2-grain doses twice daily, whisky in 4-ounce doses every two to four hours, digitalis in the form of the tincture in doses of 1 dram every three to six hours. Artificial Carlsbad salts in heaping tablespoonful doses in the feed may be given three times daily for a couple of weeks. Rest is of the greatest importance and should be allowed for a few weeks after recovery seems to be complete.

ENDOCARDITIS, OR INFLAMMATION OF THE LINING MEMBRANE OF THE HEART.

Endocarditis frequently occurs as a complication of rheumatism, some of the specific or zymotic fevers, specific poisoning, etc. This is a more frequent disease among horses than is generally known, and often gives rise to symptoms which at first are obscure and unnoticed.

In influenza we may find the heart becoming involved in the disease, in consequence of the morbid material conveyed through the heart in the blood stream. In view of the fact that many affections in even remote portions of the body may be traced directly to a primary endocardial disease, we shall feel justified in inviting special attention to this disease.

Endocarditis may be acute, subacute, or chronic. In acute inflammation we find a thickening and a roughened appearance of the endocardium throughout the cavities of the heart. This condition may be followed by a coagulation of fibrin upon the inflamed surface, which adheres to it, and by attrition soon becomes worked up into shreddy-like granular elevations. This may lead to a formation of fibrinous clots in the heart and sudden death early in the disease the second or third day.

Subacute endocarditis, which is the most common form, may not become appreciable for several days after its commencement. It is characterized by being confined to one or more anatomical divisions of the heart, and all the successive morbid changes follow each other in a comparatively slow process. Often we would not be led to suspect heart affection were it not for the distress in breathing, which it generally occasions when the animal is exercised, especially if the valves are much involved. When coagula or vegetations form upon the inflamed membrane, either in minute shreds or patches, or when formation of fibrinous clots occurs in the cavity affected, some of these materials may be carried from the cavity of the heart by the blood current into remote organs, constituting emboli that are liable to suddenly plug vessels and thereby interrupt important functions. In the great majority of either acute or subacute grades of endocarditis, whatever the exciting cause, the most alarming symptoms disappear in a week or 10 days, often leaving, however, such changes in the interior lining or valvular structures as to cause impairment in the circulation for a much longer period of time. These changes usually consist of thickening or induration of the inflamed structures. But while the effects of the inflammation in the membrane lining the walls of the ventricles may subside to such a degree as to cause little or no inconvenience, or even wholly disappear, yet after the valvular structures have been involved, causing them to be thicker, less flexible than normal, they usually remain, obstructing the free passage of the blood through the openings of the heart, thereby inducing secondary changes, which take place slowly at first, but ultimately seriously impair the animal's usefulness. What was but a slight obstruction to the circulation during the first few weeks after the subsidence of the cardiac inflammatory attack becomes in process of time so much increased as to induce increased growth in the muscular structure of the heart, constituting hypertrophy of the walls of the ventricles, more particularly of the left, with corresponding fullness of the left auricle and pulmonary veins, thereby producing fullness of the capillaries in the lungs, pressure upon the air cells, difficult or asthmatic breathing—greatly increased in attempts to work—until in a few months many of these cases become entirely disabled for work. Sometimes, too, dropsical effusions in the limbs or into the cavities of the body result from the irregular and deficient circulation. Derangement of the urinary secretion, with passive congestion of the kidneys, may also appear.

Endocardial inflammation is seldom fatal in its early stages, but in many cases the recovery is incomplete, for a large proportion is left with some permanent thickening of the valves, which constitutes the beginning of valvular disease.

Symptoms.—Endocarditis may be ushered in by a chill, with sudden and marked rise in temperature. The pulse rapidly decreases in strength or may become irregular, while the heart beats more or less tumultuously. In the early stages soft-blowing sounds may be heard by placing the ear over the heart on the left side, which correspond in number and rhythm to the heart's action. Excessive pain, though not so great as in acute pleuritis, is manifested when the animal is compelled to trot; very often difficulty in breathing, or shortness of breath, on the slightest exertion develops early in the attack. When the valves are involved in the inflammatory process the visible mucous membranes become either very pale or very dark colored, and fainting may occur when the head is suddenly elevated. When the valves of the right side are affected we may find a regurgitant pulsation in the jugular vein. Occasionally it happens that the heart contracts more frequently than the pulse beats—that is, there may be twice as many contractions of the heart in a minute as there are pulse waves in the arteries. The pulse is always very fast. In some cases we find marked lameness of the left shoulder, and when the animal is turned short to the left side he may groan with pain, and the heart's action become violently excited, although pressure against the chest wall will not produce pain unless roughly applied. The animal is not disposed to eat or drink much; the surface of the body and legs are cold—rarely excessively hot—and frequently the body of the animal is in a subdued tremor. In nearly all cases there is partial suppression of the urinary secretion. The symptoms may continue with very little modification for three or four days, sometimes seven days, without any marked changes. If large fibrinous clots form in the heart the change will be sudden and quickly prove fatal unless they become loosened and are carried away in the circulation; then apoplexy may result from the plugging of arteries too small to give further transmission. If the animal manifests symptoms of improvement, the changes usually are slow and steady until he feels apparently as well as ever, eats well, and moves freely in his stall or yard. When he is taken out, however, the seeming strength often proves deceptive, as he may quickly weaken if urged into a fast gait, the breathing becomes quickened with a double flank movement as in heaves, and all the former symptoms reappear in a modified degree. An examination at this stage may reveal valvular insufficiency, cardiac hypertrophy, or pulmonary engorgement.

In fatal cases of endocarditis death often occurs about the fourth day, from the formation of heart clot or too great embarrassment of the circulation. Endocarditis may be suspected in all cases where plain symptoms of cardiac affection are manifested in animals affected with influenza, rheumatism, or any disease in which the blood may convey septic matter.

Acute endocardial inflammation may be distinguished from pleuritis by the absence of any friction murmur, absence of pain when the chest wall is percussed, and the absence of effusion in the cavity of the chest. It may be distinguished from pericarditis by the absence of the friction sounds and want of an enlarged area of dullness on percussion.

Treatment.—The objects to be attained by treatment will be to remove or mitigate as much as possible the cause inducing the disease; to find a medicine which will lessen the irritability of the heart without weakening it; and, last, to maintain a free urinary secretion and prevent exudation and hypertrophy. So long as there is an increase of temperature, with some degree of scantiness of the urine, it may be safe to believe that there is some degree of inflammatory action existing in the cardiac structures, and as long as any evidence of inflammatory action remains, however moderate in degree, there is a tendency to increase or hypertrophy of the connective tissue of the heart or valves, thereby rendering it almost certain that the structural changes will become permanent unless counteracted by persistent treatment and complete rest.

The tincture of digitalis, in 20-drop doses, repeated every hour, is perhaps the most reliable agent we know to control the irritability of the heart, and this also has a decided influence upon the urinary secretion. After the desired impression upon the heart is obtained the dose may be repeated every two or three hours, or as the case may demand. Tincture of strophanthus, in 2-dram doses, will quiet the tumultuous action of the heart in some cases where the digitalis fails. Bleeding, blistering, and stimulating applications to the chest should be avoided. They serve to irritate the animal and can do no possible good. Chlorate of potassium in 2-dram doses may be given in the drinking water every four hours for the first five or six days, and then be superseded by the nitrate of potassium in half-ounce doses for the following week or until the urinary secretion becomes abnormally profuse. Where the disease is associated with rheumatism, 2-dram doses of salicylate of soda may be substituted for the chlorate of potassium. To guard against chronic induration of the valves, the iodid of potassium, in 1 to 2 dram doses, should be given early in the disease and may be repeated two or three times a day for several weeks. When chronic effects remain after the acute stage has passed this drug becomes indispensable.

When dropsy of the limbs develops, it is due to weakened circulation or functional impairment of the kidneys. When there is much weakness in the action of the heart, or general debility is marked, the iodid of iron, in 1-dram doses, combined with hydrastis, 3 drams, may be given three times a day. Arsenic, in 5-grain doses twice a day, will give excellent results in some cases of weak heart associated with difficult breathing. In all cases absolute rest and warm stabling, with comfortable clothing, become necessary, and freedom from work should be allowed for a long time after all symptoms have disappeared.

PERICARDITIS, OR INFLAMMATION OF THE SAC INCLOSING THE HEART.

Causes.—Pericarditis may be induced by cold and damp stabling, exposure and fatigue, from wounds caused by broken ribs, etc. Generally, however, it is associated with an attack of influenza, rheumatism, pleuritis, etc.

Symptoms.—Usually the disease manifests itself abruptly by a brief stage of chills coincident with pain in moving, a short painful cough, rapid and short breathing, and high temperature, with a rapid and hard pulse. In the early stages of the disease the pulse is regular in beat; later, when there is much exudation present in the pericardial sac, the heartbeat becomes muffled, and may be of a double or rebounding character. By placing the ear against the left side of the chest behind the elbow a rasping sound may be heard, corresponding to the frequency of the heartbeat. This is known as a friction sound. Between the second and fourth days this sound may disappear, due to a distension of the pericardium by an exudate or serous effusion. As soon as this effusion partly fills the pericardium, percussion will reveal an abnormally increased area of dullness over the region of the heart, the heartbeats become less perceptible than in health, and in some cases a splashing or flapping sound may become audible.

If the effusion becomes absorbed, the friction sound usually recurs for a short time; this friction may often be felt by applying the hand to the side of the chest. In a few cases clonic spasms of the muscles of the neck may be present. In acute pericarditis, when the effusion is rapid and excessive, the animal may die in a few days or recovery may begin equally as early. In subacute or in chronic cases the effusion may slowly become augmented until the pressure upon the lungs and interference with the circulation become so great that death will result. Whether the attack is acute, subacute, or chronic, the characteristic symptoms which will guide us to a correct diagnosis are the friction sound, which is always synchronous with the heart's action, the high temperature with hard, irritable pulse, and, in cases of pericardial effusion, the increased area of dullness over the cardiac region. When the disease is associated with influenza or rheumatism, some of the symptoms may be obscure, but a careful examination will reveal sufficient evidence upon which to base a diagnosis. When pericarditis develops as a result of or in connection with pleuritis, the distinction may not be very clearly definable, neither will many recover. When it results from a wound or broken rib, it almost invariably proves fatal.

Pathology.—Pericarditis may at all times be regarded as a very serious affection. At first we will find an intense injection or accumulation of blood in the vessels of the pericardium, giving it a red and swollen appearance, during which we have the friction sound. In 24 to 48 hours this engorgement is followed by an exudation of sero-fibrinous fluid, the fibrinous portion of which may soon form a coating over the internal surface of the pericardial sac, and may ultimately form a union of the opposing surfaces. Generally this adhesion will only be found to occupy a portion of the surfaces. As the serous or watery portion of this effusion is absorbed, the distinctness of the friction sound recurs, and may remain perceptible in a varied degree for a long time. When the serous effusion is very great, the pressure exerted upon the heart weakens its action, and may produce death soon; when it is not so great, it may cause dropsies of other portions of the body. When the adhesions of the pericardial sac to the body of the heart are extensive, they generally lead to increased growth, or hypertrophy, of the heart, with or without dilatation of its cavities; when they are but slight, they may not cause any inconvenience.

Treatment.—In acute or subacute pericarditis the tincture of digitalis may be given in 20 to 30 drop doses every hour until the pulse and temperature become reduced. Carbonate of ammonia may be given regularly as a stimulant. Bandages should be applied to the legs; if the legs are very cold, tincture of capsicum should be first applied; the body should be warmly clothed in blankets, to promote perspiration. When the suffering from pain is very severe, 10 grains of morphin may be given by the mouth once or twice a day; nitrate of potassium, half an ounce, in drinking water, every six hours; after the third day, iodid of potassium, in 2-dram doses, may be substituted. Cold packs to the chest in the early stages of the disease may give marked relief, or, late in the disease, smart blisters may be applied to the sides of the chest with benefit. If the disease becomes chronic, iodid of iron and gentian to support the strength will be indicated, but the iodid of potassium, in 1 or 2 dram doses, two or three times a day, must not be abandoned so long as there is an evidence of effusion or plastic exudate accumulating in the pericardial sac. Where the effusion is great and threatens the life of the patient, tapping by an expert veterinarian may save the animal.

VALVULAR DISEASE OF THE HEART.

Acute valvular disease can not be distinguished from endocarditis, and chronic valvular affections are generally the result of endocardial inflammation. The valves of the left side are the most subject— the bicuspid or mitral and the aortic or semilunar. The derangement may consist of mere inflammation and swelling, or the edges of the valves may become covered by the organization of the exudation, thus narrowing the passage. Valvular obstruction and adhesions may occur or the tendinous cords may be lengthened or shortened, thus obstructing the orifices and permitting the regurgitation of blood. In protected cases the fibrous tissue of the valves may be transformed into fibro-cartilage or bone, or there may be deposits of salts of lime beneath the serous membrane, which may terminate in ulceration, rupture, or fissures. Sometimes the valves become covered by fibrinous, fleshy, or hard vegetations, or excrescences. In cases of considerable dilatation of the heart there may be atrophy and shrinking of the valves.

Symptoms.—Valvular disease may be indicated by a venous pulse, jerking pulse, intermittent pulse, irregular pulse; palpitation; constant abnormal fullness of the jugular veins; difficulty of breathing when the animal becomes excited or is urged out of a walk or into a fast trot; attacks of vertigo; congestion of the brain; dropsical swelling of the limbs. A blowing, cooing, or bubbling murmur may sometimes be heard by placing the ear over the heart on the left side of the chest.

Hypertrophy, or dilatation, or both, usually follow valvular disease.

Treatment.—When the pulse is irregular or irritable, tonics, such as preparations of iron, gentian, and ginger, may be given. When the action of the heart is jerking or violent, 20 to 30 drop doses of tincture of digitalis or of veratrum viride may be given until these symptoms abate. As the disease nearly always is the result of endocarditis, the iodid of potassium and general tonics, sometimes stimulants, when general debility supervenes, may be of temporary benefit. Very few animals recover or remain useful for any length of time after once marked organic changes have taken place in the valvular structure of the heart.

ADVENTITIOUS GROWTHS IN THE HEART.

Fibrous, cartilaginous, and bony formations have been observed in some rare instances in the muscular tissue. Isolated calcareous masses have sometimes been embedded in the cardiac walls. Fibrinous coagula and polypous concretions may be found in the cavities of the heart. The former consist of coagulated fibrin, separated from the mass of blood, of a whitish or yellowish white color, translucent, of a jellylike consistence, and having a nucleus in the center. They may slightly adhere to the surface of the cavity, from which they can easily be separated without altering the structure of the endocardium. They probably result from an excess of coagulability of fibrin, which is produced by an organization of the lymph during exudation. They are usually found in the right auricle and ventricle.

Polypous concretions are firmer than in the preceding, more opaque, of a fibrous texture, and may be composed of successive layers. In some instances they are exceedingly minute, while in others they almost fill one or more of the cavities. Their color is usually white, but occasionally red from the presence of blood. They firmly adhere to the endocardium, and when detached from it give it a torn appearance. Occasionally, a vascular communication seems to exist between them and the substance of the heart. They may be the result of fibrinous exudation from inflammation of the inner surface of the heart or the coagulation of a portion of the blood which afterwards contracts adhesion with the heart. These concretions prove a source of great inconvenience and often danger, no matter how formed. They cause a diminution in the cavity in which they are found, thus narrowing the orifice through which the blood passes, or preventing a proper coaptation of the valves, which may produce most serious valvular disease.

Symptoms.—These are frequently uncertain; they may, however, be suspected when the action of the heart suddenly becomes embarrassed with irregular and confused pulsations, great difficulty of breathing, and the usual signs dependent upon the imperfect arterialization of the blood.

Treatment.—Stimulants, whisky, or carbonate of ammonia may be of service.

PALPITATION OF THE HEART.

This is a tumultuous and usually irregular beating of the heart. It may be due to a variety of causes, both functional and organic. It may occur as a result of indigestion, fright, increased nervousness, sudden excitement, excessive speeding, etc. (See "Thumps," p. 225.)

Symptoms.—The heart may act with such violence that each beat may jar the whole body of the animal; very commonly it may be heard at a short distance away from the animal. It can usually be traced very readily to the exciting cause, which we may be able to avoid or overcome in the future and thereby obviate subsequent attacks. Rest, a mild stimulant, or a dose or two of tincture of digitalis or opium will generally give prompt relief. When it is due to organic impairment of the heart it must be regarded as a symptom, not as a matter of primary specific treatment.

SYNCOPE, OR FAINTING.

Actual fainting rarely occurs among horses. It may, however, be induced by a rapid and great loss of blood, pain of great intensity, a mechanical interference with the circulation of the brain, etc.

Symptoms.—Syncope is characterized by a decrease or temporary suspension of the action of the heart and respiration, with partial or total loss of consciousness. It generally occurs suddenly, though there may be premonitory symptoms, as giddiness, or vertigo, dilated pupil, staggering, blanching of the visible mucous membranes, a rapidly sinking pulse, and dropping to the ground. The pulse is feeble or ceases to beat; the surface of the body turns cold; breathing is scarcely to be perceived, and the animal may be entirely unconscious. This state is uncertain in duration—generally it lasts only a few minutes; the circulation becomes restored, breathing becomes more distinct, and consciousness and muscular strength return. In cases attended with much hemorrhage or organic disease of the heart, the fainting fit may be fatal; otherwise it will prove but a transient occurrence. In paralysis of the heart the symptoms may be exactly similar to syncope. Syncope may be distinguished from apoplexy by the absence of stertorous breathing and lividity of the visible mucous membranes.

Treatment.—Dash cold water on the head; administer a stimulant—half an ounce of carbonate of ammonia. Prevent the animal from getting up too soon, or the attack may immediately recur. Afterwards, if the attack was due to weakness from loss of blood, impoverished blood, or associated with debility, general tonics, rest, and nourishing food are indicated.

HYPERTROPHY OF THE HEART, OR CARDIAC ENLARGEMENT.

Hypertrophy of the heart implies augmentation of bulk in its muscular substance, with or without dilatation or contraction of its cavities. It may exist with or without other cardiac affections. In valvular disease or valvular insufficiency hypertrophy frequently results as a consequence of increased demand for propelling power. The difficulties with which it is most frequently connected are dilatation and ossification of the valves. It may also occur in connection with atrophied kidneys, weak heart, etc. It may be caused by an increased determination of blood to the organ or from a latent form of myocarditis, and it may arise from a long-continued increase of action dependent upon nervous disease. All the cavities of the heart may have their walls hypertrophied or the thickening may involve one or more. While the wall of a ventricle is thickened, its cavity may retain its normal size (simple hypertrophy) or be dilated (eccentric hypertrophy), or it may be contracted (concentric hypertrophy). Hypertrophy of both ventricles increases the length and breadth of the heart. Hypertrophy of the left ventricle alone increases its length; of the right ventricle alone increases its breadth toward the right side. Hypertrophy with dilatation may affect the chambers of the heart conjointly or separately. This form is by far the most frequent variety of cardiac enlargement. When the entire heart is affected, it assumes a globular appearance, the apex being almost obliterated and situated transversely in the chest. The bulk may become three or four times greater than the average heart.

Symptoms.—In hypertrophy of the heart, in addition to the usual symptoms manifested in organic diseases of the heart, there is a powerful and heaving impulse at each beat, which may be felt on the left side, often also on the right. These pulsations are regular, and when full and strong at the jaw there is a tendency to active congestion of the capillary vessels, which frequently give rise to local inflammation, active hemorrhage, etc. If the pulse is small and feeble at the jaw, we may conclude that there is some obstacle to the escape of the blood from the left ventricle into the aorta, which has given rise to the hypertrophy. In case of hypertrophy with dilatation, the impulse is not only powerful and heaving, but it is diffused over the whole region of the heart, and the normal sounds of the heart are greatly increased in intensity. Percussion reveals an enlarged area of dullness, while the impulse is usually much stronger than normal. Dropsy of the pericardium will give the same wide space of dullness, but the impulse and sound are lessened. An animal with a moderate degree of enlargement may possibly live a number of years and be capable of ordinary work; it depends largely upon concomitant disease. As a rule, an animal affected with hypertrophy of the heart will soon be incapacitated for work, and becomes useless and incurable.

Treatment.—If the cause can be discovered and is removable, it should be done. The iodid of potassium, in cases of valvular thickening, may be of some benefit if continued for a sufficient length of time; it may be given in 2-dram doses, twice a day, for a month or more. The tincture of digitalis may be given, in cases where the pulse is weak, in doses of 2 teaspoonfuls three times daily. This remedy should not be continued if the pulse becomes irregular. General tonics, freedom from excitement or fatigue, avoidance of bulky food, good ventilation, etc., are indicated.

DILATATION OF THE HEART.

This is an enlargement, or stretching, of the cavities of the heart, and may be confined to one or extend to all. Two forms of dilatation may be mentioned—simple dilatation, where there is normal thickness of the walls, and passive, or attenuated, dilatation, where the walls are simply distended or stretched out without any addition of substance.

Causes.—Any cause producing constant and excessive exertion of the heart may lead to dilatation. Valvular disease is the most frequent cause. General anemia predisposes to it by producing relaxation of muscular fiber. Changes in the muscular tissue of the heart walls, serous infiltration from pericarditis, myocarditis, fatty degeneration and infiltration, and atrophy of the muscular fibers may all lead to dilatation.

Symptoms.—The movements of the heart are feeble and prolonged, a disposition to staggering or vertigo, dropsy of the limbs, very pale or very dark-colored membranes, and difficult breathing on the slightest excitement.

Treatment.—General tonics, rich feed, and rest.

FATTY DEGENERATION OF THE HEART.

Fatty degeneration may involve the whole organ, or may be limited to its walls, or even to circumscribed patches. The latter is situated at the exterior, and gives it a mottled appearance. When generally involved it is flabby or flaccid, and in extreme cases collapses when emptied or cut. Upon dissection the interior of the ventricles is observed to be covered with buff-colored spots of a singular zigzag form. This appearance may be noticed beneath the pericardium, and pervading the whole thickness of the ventricular walls, and in extreme cases those of the fleshy columns in the interior of the heart. These spots are found to be degenerated muscular fibers and colonies of oil globules. Fatty degeneration is often associated with other morbid conditions of the heart, such as obesity, dilatation, rupture, aneurism, etc. It may be connected with fatty diseases of other organs, such as the liver, kidneys, etc. When it exists alone its presence is seldom suspected previous to death. It may be secondary to hypertrophy of the heart, to myocarditis, or to pericarditis. It may be due to deteriorated conditions of the blood in wasting diseases, excessive hemorrhages, etc., or to poisoning with arsenic and phosphorus.

Symptoms.—The most prominent symptoms of fatty degeneration are a feeble action of the heart, a remarkably slow pulse, general debility, and attacks of vertigo. It may exist for a long time, but is apt to terminate suddenly in death upon the occurrence of other diseases, surgical operations, etc. It may involve a liability to sudden death from rupture of the ventricular walls.

Treatment.—Confinement in feed to oats, wheat or rye bran, and timothy hay. Twenty drops of sulphuric acid may be given in drinking water three times a day, and hypophosphite of iron in 2-dram doses, mixed with the feed, twice a day. Other tonics and stimulants as they may be indicated.

RUPTURE OF THE HEART.

This may occur as the result of some previous disease, such as fatty degeneration, dilatation with weakness of the muscular walls, etc. It may be caused by external violence, a crushing fall, pressure of some great weight, etc. Usually death follows a rupture very quickly, though an animal may live for some time when the rent is not very large.

WEAKNESS OF THE HEART.

This may arise from general debility, the result of exhausting disease, overwork, or heart strain, or loss of blood. It is indicated by a small, feeble, but generally regular pulse, coldness of the body, etc.

Treatment should be directed to support and increase the strength of the animal by tonics, rest, and nutritious feed. Carbonate of ammonia may be given to stimulate the heart's action and to prevent the formation of heart clot.

CONGESTION OF THE HEART.

Congestion, or an accumulation of the blood in the cavities of the heart, may occur in consequence of fibrinous deposits interfering with the free movements of the valves, usually the product of endocarditis or as a result of excessive muscular exertion.

Symptoms are great difficulty of breathing, paleness of the visible mucous membranes, great anxiety, frequently accompanied by a general tremor and cold perspiration, followed by death. It usually results in death very quickly.

CYANOSIS OF NEWBORN FOALS.

This is a condition sometimes found in foals immediately after birth, and is due to nonclosure of the foramen ovale, which allows a mixture of the venous with the arterial blood in the left cavities of the heart. It is characterized by a dark purple or bluish color of the visible mucous membranes, shortness of breath, and a general feebleness. Foals thus affected generally live only a few hours after birth.

DISEASES OF ARTERIES, OR ARTERITIS AND ENDARTERITIS.

Inflammation of arteries is rarely observed in the horse as a primary affection. Direct injuries, such as blows, may produce a contusion and subsequent inflammation of the wall of an artery; severe muscular strain may involve an arterial trunk; hypertrophy of the heart, by increasing arterial tension, may result in the production of a general endarteritis. Septic infection may affect the inner coat and ultimately involve all three, or it may be the result of an inflammation in the vicinity of the vessels, etc. Inflammation of arteries, whatever the cause may be, often leads to very serious results in the development of secondary changes in their walls. Arteritis may be acute, subacute, or chronic; when the inner coat alone is affected it is known as endarteritis.

Symptoms.—Arteritis is characterized by a painful swelling along the inflamed vessel, throbbing pulse, coldness of the parts supplied by the inflamed vessel, sometimes the formation of gangrenous sloughs, suppuration, abscess, etc. In an inflammation of the iliac arteries we find coldness and excessive lameness or paralysis of one or both hind limbs.

Pathology.—In acute arteritis we find swelling along the vessel, loss of elasticity, friability, and thickening of the walls; a roughness and loss of gloss of the inner coat, with the formation of coagula or pus in the vessel. Subacute or chronic arteritis may affect only the outer coat (periarteritis), both the outer and middle coat, or the inner coat alone (endarteritis); and by weakening the respective coats leads to rupture, aneurism, or to degenerations, such as bony, calcareous, fatty, atheromatous, etc. It may also lead to sclerosis or increase of fibrous tissue, especially in the kidneys, when it may result in the condition known as arterio-capillary fibrosis. Chronic endarteritis is fruitful in the production of thrombus and atheroma. Arteritis may be limited to single trunks or it may affect, more or less, all the arteries of the body. Arteries which are at the seat of chronic endarteritis are liable to suffer degenerative changes, consisting chiefly of fatty degeneration, calcification, or the breaking down of the degenerated tissue, and the formation of erosions or ulcerlike openings in the inner coat. These erosions are frequently called atheromatous ulcers, and fragments of tissue from these ulcers may be carried into the circulation, forming emboli. Fibrinous thrombi are apt to form upon the roughened surface of the inner coat or upon the surface of the erosions.

Fatty degeneration and calcification of the middle and outer coats may occur, and large, hard, calcareous plates project inward, upon which thrombi may form or may exist in connection with atheroma of the inner coat. When there is much thickening and increase of new tissue in the wall of the affected artery it may encroach upon the capacity of the vessel, and even lead to obliteration. This is often associated with interstitial inflammation of glandular organs.

Treatment.—Carbonate of potassium in 1-dram doses, to be given in 4 ounces liquor acetate of ammonia every six hours; scalded bran sufficient to produce loosening of the bowels, and complete rest; externally, applications of hot water or hot hop infusion.

ATHEROMA.

Atheroma is a direct result of an existing chronic endarteritis, the lining membrane of the vessels being invariably involved to a greater or less degree. It is most frequently found in the arteries, although the veins may develop an atheromatous condition when exposed to any source of prolonged irritation. Atheroma may affect arteries in any part of the body; in some instances almost every vessel is diseased, in others only a few, or even parts of one vessel. It is a very common result of endocarditis extending into the aorta, which we find perhaps the most frequent seat of atheroma. As a result of this condition the affected vessel becomes impaired in its contractile power, loses its natural strength, and, in consequence of its inability to sustain its accustomed internal pressure, undergoes in many cases dilatation at the seat of disease, constituting aneurism. In an atheromatous vessel, calcareous deposits soon occur, which render it rigid, brittle, and subject to ulceration or rupture. In such vessels the contractility is destroyed, the middle coat atrophied and beyond repair. Atheroma in the vessels of the brain is a frequent cause of cerebral apoplexy. No symptoms are manifested by which we can recognize this condition during life.

CONSTRICTION OF AN ARTERY.

This is usually the result of arteritis, and may partly or wholly be impervious to the flow of blood. When this occurs in a large vessel it may be followed by gangrene of the parts; usually, however, collateral circulation will be established to nourish the parts previously supplied by the obliterated vessel. In a few instances constriction of the aorta has produced death.

ANEURISM.

Aneurism is usually described as true or false. True aneurism is a dilatation of the coats of an artery over a larger or smaller part of its course. Such dilatations are usually due to chronic endarteritis and atheroma. False aneurism is formed after a puncture of an artery by a dilatation of the adhesive lymph by which the puncture was united.

Symptoms.—If the aneurism is seated along the neck or a limb it appears as a tumor in the course of an artery and pulsating with it. The tumor is round, soft, and compressible, and yields a peculiar fluctuation upon pressure. By applying the ear over it a peculiar purring or hissing sound may sometimes be heard. Pulsation, synchronous with the action of the heart, is the diagnostic symptom. It is of a slow, expansive, and heavy character, as if the whole tumor were enlarging under the hand. Aneurisms seated internally may occupy the cavity of the cranium, chest, or abdomen. As regards the first, little is known during life, for all the symptoms which they produce may arise from other causes. Aneurism of the anterior aorta may be situated very closely to the heart or in the arch, and it is very seldom that we can distinguish it from disease of the heart. The tumor may encroach upon the windpipe and produce difficulty in breathing, or it may produce pressure upon the vena cava or the thoracic duct, obstructing the flow of blood and lymph. In fact, whatever parts the aneurism may reach or subject to its pressure, may have their functions suspended or disturbed. When the tumor in the chest is large, we generally find much irregularity in the action of the heart; the superficial veins of the neck are distended, and there is usually dropsical swelling under the breast and of the limbs. There may be a very troublesome cough without any evidence of lung affection. Sometimes pulsation of the tumor may be felt at the lower part of the neck where it joins the chest. When the aneurism occurs in the posterior aorta no diagnostic symptoms are appreciable; when it occurs in the internal iliac arteries an examination per rectum will reveal it.

There is one form of aneurism which is not infrequently overlooked, affecting the anterior mesenteric artery, primarily induced by a worm—*Strongylus vulgaris*. This worm produces an arteritis, with atheroma, degeneration, and dilatation of the mesenteric arteries, associated with thrombus and aneurism. The aneurism gives rise to colic, which appears periodically in a very violent and often persistent type. Ordinary colic remedies have no effect, and after a time the animal succumbs to the disease. In all cases of animals which are habitually subject to colicky attacks, parasitic aneurism of the anterior mesenteric artery may be suspected. (See p. 92.)

Pathology.—Aneurisms may be diffuse or sacculated. The diffuse consists in a uniform dilatation of all the coats of an artery, so that it assumes the shape of a cylindrical swelling. The wall of the aneurism is atheromatous, or calcified; the middle coat may be atrophied. The sacculated, or circumscribed, aneurism consists either in a dilatation of the entire circumference of an artery over a short portion of its length, or in a dilatation of only a small portion of one side of the wall. Aneurism may become very large; as it increases in size it presses upon and causes the destruction of neighboring tissues. The cavity of the aneurismal sac is filled with fluid or clotted blood or with layers of fibrin which adhere closely to its wall. Death is produced usually by the pressure and interference of the aneurism with adjoining organs or by rupture. In worm aneurism we usually find large thrombi within the aneurismal dilatation of the artery, which sometimes plug the whole vessel or extend into the aorta. Portions of this thrombus, or clot, may be washed away and produce embolism of a smaller artery. The effect in either case is to produce anemia of the intestinal canal, serous or bloody exudation in its walls, which leads to paralysis of the intestine and resultant colicky symptoms.

Treatment.—The only treatment advisable is to extirpate or ligate the tumor above and below.

RUPTURE OF AN ARTERY.

Endarteritis, with its subsequent changes in the walls of arteries, is the primary cause of rupture in the majority of instances. The rupture may be partial, involving only one or two coats, and will then form an aneurism. If complete, it may produce death when it involves a large vessel, especially if it is situated in one of the large cavities permitting an excessive escape of blood. Rupture may be produced by mechanical violence or accident.

Symptoms.—In fatal rupture, associated with profuse bleeding, the animal becomes weak, the visible mucous membranes become blanched, the breathing hurried or gasping, pupils dilated, staggering in gait, syncope, death. When the hemorrhage is limited the symptoms may not become noticeable; if it is near the surface of the body a round or diffuse swelling or tumor may form, constituting a hygroma. If the rupture is associated with an external wound, the bleeding artery should be ligated, or where a bandage is applicable, pressure may be applied by tight bandaging. As a secondary result of rupture of an artery we may have formation of abscess, gangrene of a part, etc.

Treatment.—When rupture of a deep-seated artery is suspected, large doses of fluid extract of ergot may be given to produce contraction of the blood vessels. Tannin and iron are also useful. The animal should be allowed to have as much water as he desires. Afterwards stimulants and nourishing feed are indicated.

THROMBUS AND EMBOLISM.

By thrombosis is generally understood the partial or complete closure of a vessel by a morbid product developed at the site of the obstruction. The coagulum, which is usually fibrinous, is known as a thrombus. The term " embolism " designates an obstruction caused by any body detached and transported from the interior of the heart or of some vessel. Thrombi occur as the result of an injury to the wall of the vessel or may follow its compression or dilatation; they may result from some alteration of the wall of the vessel by disease or by the retardation of the circulation. These formations may occur during life, in the heart, arteries, veins, or in the portal system. When a portion of fibrin coagulates in one of the arteries and is carried along by the circulation, it will be arrested, of course, in the capillaries, if not before; when in the veins, it may not be stopped until it reaches the lungs; and when in the portal system the capillaries of the liver will prevent its further progress. The formation of thrombi may act primarily by causing partial or complete obstruction, and, secondarily, either by larger or smaller fragments becoming detached from their end and by being carried along by the circulation of the blood to remote vessels, embolism; or by the coagulum becoming softened and converted into pus, constituting suppurative phlebitis. These substances occur most frequently in those affections characterized by great exhaustion or debility, such as pneumonia, purpura hemorrhagica, endocarditis, phlebitis, puerperal fever, hemorrhages, etc. These concretions may form suddenly and produce instantaneous death by retarding the blood current, or they may arise gradually, in which case the thrombi may be organized and attached to the walls of the heart, or they may soften, and fragments of them (emboli) may be carried away. The small, wartlike excrescences occurring sometimes in endocarditis may occasionally form a foundation on which a thrombi may develop.

Symptoms.—When heart clot, or thrombus, exists in the right side, the return of blood from the body and the aeration in the lungs is impeded, and if death occurs, it is owing to syncope rather than to strangulation in pulmonary respiration. There will be hurried and gasping breathing, paleness and coldness of the surface of the body, a feeble and intermittent or fluttering pulse, and fainting. When a fibrinous coagulum is carried into the pulmonary artery from the right side of the heart, the indications are a swelling and infiltration of the lungs and pulmonary apoplexy. When the clot is situated in the left cavities of the heart or in the aorta, death, if it occurs, takes place either suddenly or at the end of a few hours from coma.

Pathology.—When a coagulum is observed in the heart it may become a question whether it was formed during life or after death. The loose, dark coagula so often found after death are polypi. If the deposition has taken place during the last moments of life, the fibrin will be isolated and soft, but not adherent to the walls; if it be isolated, dense, and adherent or closely intertwined with the muscles of the papillæ and tendinous cords, the deposition has occurred more or less remote from the act of dying. Occasionally the fibrin may be seen lining one of the cavities of the heart, like a false endocardium, or else forming an additional coat to the aorta or other large vessels without producing much obstruction. Thrombi, in some instances, soften in their centers, and are then observed to contain a puslike substance. If this softening has extended considerably, an outer shell, or cyst, only may remain. The sources of danger exist not only in the interruption of the circulation of the blood, but also in a morbid state of the system, produced by the disturbed nutrition of a limb or organ, as well as the mingling of purulent and gangrenous elements with the blood.

Treatment.—The urgent symptoms should be relieved by rest, stimulants, and the use of agents which will act as solvents to the fibrinous clots. Alkalis are specially useful for this purpose. Carbonate of ammonia may be administered in all cases of thrombus, and should be continued for a long time in small doses several times a day. In cases of great debility associated with a low grade of fever, stimulants and tonics, and nitro-muriatic acid as an antiseptic, may be beneficial.

DISEASES OF VEINS, OR PHLEBITIS.

Inflammation of veins may be simple or diffuse. In simple phlebitis the disease of the vein is confined to a circumscribed or limited portion of a vein; in diffuse it involves the vein for a long distance; it may even extend from a limb or foot to the heart.

Causes.—Phlebitis may be induced by contusions or direct injuries, an extension of inflammation from surrounding tissue, such as in abscess, formation of tumor, or malignant growth. It is often due to embolism of infective material, gangrenous matter, etc. Bloodletting from the jugular vein is occasionally followed by dangerous phlebitis.

Symptoms.—The symptoms vary according to the extent and severity of the inflammation. In most cases the vein is swollen, thickened, and indurated to such a degree as to resemble an artery. A diffused swelling, with great tenderness, may extend along the affected vessel and the animal manifest all the symptoms connected with acute fever and general functional disturbance.

Pathology.—The disease is only serious when large veins are affected. The coats undergo the same changes as in arteritis; clots of blood and lymph plug the inflamed vessel, and, if the inflammatory process continues, these are converted into pus, which ruptures the vessel and produces a deep abscess; or it may be carried away in the circulation and produce metastatic abscess in the lungs or other remote organs. In mild cases the clots may become absorbed and the vessel restored to health. Phlebitis in the course of the veins of the limbs frequently leads to numerous abscesses, which may be mistaken for farcy ulcerations. A very common result of phlebitis is an obliteration of the affected portion of the vein, but as collateral circulation is readily established this is seldom of any material inconvenience.

Treatment.—Phlebitis should be treated by the application of a smart blister along the course of the inflamed vessel; early opening of any abscesses which may form; the animal should have complete rest, and the bowels be kept loose with bran mashes. When the fever runs high, half-ounce doses of nitrate of potassium may be given in the drinking water, which may be changed in two or three days for 1-dram doses of the iodid of potassium. If the animal becomes debilitated, carbonate of ammonia, 1 dram, and powdered gentian, 3 drams, may be given every six hours.

VARICOSE VEINS, VARIX, OR DILATATION OF VEINS.

This may be a result of weakening of the coats from inflammatory disease and degeneration. It may also be due to mechanical obstruction from internal or external sources. It is sometimes found in the vein which lies superficial over the inside of the hock joint, and may be due to the pressure of a spavin. Occasionally it may be observed in stallions, which are more or less subject to varicocele, or dilatation of the veins of the testicular cord. Hemorrhoidal veins, or piles, are occasionally met with, generally in horses which run at pasture. Varicose veins may ulcerate and form an abscess in the surrounding tissues, or they may rupture from internal blood pressure and the blood form large tumors where the tissues are soft.

Treatment.—Stallions which manifest a tendency to varicocele should wear suspensory bags when they are exercised. Piles may often be reduced by astringent washes—tea made from white-oak bark or a saturated solution of alum. The bowels should be kept loose with bran mashes and the animal kept quiet in the stable.

When varicose veins exist superficially and threaten to produce inconvenience, they may be ligated above and below and thus obliterated. Sometimes absorption may be induced by constant bandages.

AIR IN VEINS, OR AIR EMBOLISM.

It was formerly supposed that the entrance of air into a vein at the time of the infliction of a wound or in blood-letting was extremely dangerous and very often produced sudden death by interfering with the circulation of the blood through the heart and lungs. Danger from air embolism is exceedingly doubtful, unless great quantities were forced into a large vein by artificial means.

PURPURA HEMORRHAGICA.

Purpura hemorrhagica usually occurs as a sequel to debilitating diseases, such as strangles, influenza, etc. It may, however, arise in the absence of any previous disease in badly ventilated stables, among poorly fed horses, and in animals subject to exhausting work and extreme temperatures. The disease is probably due to some as yet undiscovered infectious principle. Its gravity does not depend so much upon the amount of blood extravasated as it does upon the disturbance or diminished action of the vaso-motor centers.

Symptoms.—This disease becomes manifested by the occurrence of sudden swellings on various parts of the body, on the head or lips, limbs, abdomen, etc. These swellings may be diffused or very markedly circumscribed, though in the advanced stages they cover large areas. They pit on pressure and are but slightly painful to the touch. The limbs may swell to a very large size, the nostrils may become almost closed, and the head and throat may swell to the point of suffocation. The swellings not infrequently disappear from one portion of the body and develop on another, or may recede from the surface and invade the intestinal mucous membrane. The mucous lining of the nostrils and mouth show more or less dark-red or purple spots. There may be a discharge of blood-colored serum from the nostrils; the tongue may be swollen so as to prevent eating or closing of the jaws. In the most intense cases, within from twenty-four to forty-eight hours bloody serum may exude through the skin over the swollen parts, and finally large gangrenous sloughs may form. The temperature is never very high, the pulse is frequent and compressible, and becomes feebler as the animal loses strength. A cough is usually present. The urine is scanty and high colored, and when the intestines are much affected a bloody diarrhea may set in, with colicky pains. Some of the internal organs become implicated in the disease, the lungs may become edematous, extravasation may occur in the intestinal canal, or effusion of serum into the cavity of the chest or abdomen; occasionally the brain becomes affected. A few cases run a mild course and recovery may commence in three or four days; generally, however, the outlook is unfavorable. In severe cases septic poisoning is liable to occur, which soon brings the case to a fatal issue.

Pathology.—On section we find the capillaries dilated, the connective tissue filled with a coagulable or coagulated lymph, and frequently we may discover gangrenous spots beneath the skin or involving the skin. The lymphatic glands are swollen and inflamed. Extensive extravasations of blood may be found embedded between the coats of the intestines, or excessive effusion into the substance of the lungs.

Treatment.—Diffusible stimulants and tonics should be given from the start. Carbonate of ammonia, 1 dram, fluid extract of red cinchona bark, 2 drams, and tincture of ginger half an ounce, with half a pint of water; thin gruel or milk should be given every four or six hours. But especial care should be exercised to avoid injury by drenching. If the horse has difficulty in getting the head up and swallowing, smaller doses must be given with a small hard-rubber syringe. Sulphate of iron in 1-dram doses may be dissolved in water and given every six hours. Chlorate of potassium, in 2-ounce doses, may be given every eight or twelve hours. Colloidal silver may be administered intravenously in doses of from 5 to 12 grains. Washings with lead and alum water are useful and may be repeated several times each day. If the swellings are very great, they may be incised freely and the resulting wounds should be washed at least twice daily with a warm 3 per cent solution of carbolic acid or other good antiseptic. Tracheotomy may be necessary. Complications, when they arise, must be treated with proper circumspection.

DISEASES OF THE LYMPHATIC SYSTEM.

The lymphatic, or absorbent, system is connected with the bloodvascular system, and consists of a series of tubes which absorb and convey to the blood certain fluids. These tubes lead to lymphatic glands, through which the fluids pass to reach the right lymphatic vein and thoracic duct, both of which enter the venous system near the heart. Through the excessively thin walls of the capillaries the fluid part of the blood transudes to nourish the tissues outside the capillaries; at the same time fluid passes from the tissues into the blood. The fluid, after it passes into the tissues, constitutes the lymph, and acts like a stream irrigating the tissue elements. Much of the surplus of this lymph passes into the lymph vessels, which in their commencement can hardly be treated as independent structures, since their walls are so closely joined with the tissues through which they pass, being nothing more than spaces in the connective tissue until they reach the larger lymph vessels, which finally empty into lymph glands. These lymph glands are structures so placed that the lymph flowing toward the larger trunks passes through them, undergoing a sort of filtration. From the fact of this arrangement lymph glands are subject to inflammatory diseases in the vicinity of diseased structures, because infective material being conveyed in the lymph stream lodges in the glands and produces irritation.

LOCAL INFLAMMATION AND ABSCESS OF LYMPHATIC GLANDS.

Acute inflammation of the lymph glands usually occurs in connection with some inflammatory process in the region from which its lymph is gathered. Several or all of the glands in a cluster may become affected, as in strangles, nasal catarrh, or nasal gleet, diseased or ulcerated teeth, the lymph glands between the branches of the lower jaw almost invariably become affected, which may lead to suppuration or induration. Similar results obtain in other portions of the body; in pneumonia the bronchial glands become affected; in pharyngitis the postpharyngeal glands lying above the trachea become affected, etc.

Symptoms.—The glands swell and become painful to the touch, the connective tissue surrounding them becomes involved, suppuration usually takes place, and one or more abscesses form. If the inflammation is of a milder type, resolution may take place and the swelling recede, the exudative material being absorbed, and the gland restored without the occurrence of suppuration. In the limbs a whole chain of the glands along the lymphatic vessels may become affected, as in farcy, phlebitis, or septic poisoning.

Treatment.—Fomentation with hot water and the application of camphorated soap liniment or camphorated oil may produce a revulsive action and prevent suppuration. If there is any indication of abscess forming, poultices of linseed meal and bran made into a paste with hot water should be applied, or a mild blistering ointment rubbed in over the swollen gland. As soon as fluctuation can be felt a free opening must be made for the escape of the contained pus. The wound may subsequently be washed out with a solution of chlorid of zinc, 5 grains to the ounce of water, three times a day.

LYMPHANGITIS.

Specific inflammation of the lymphatic structures usually affects the hind legs; very seldom a fore leg. This disease is very sudden in its attack, exceedingly painful, accompanied by a high temperature and great general disturbance.

Causes.—Horses of lymphatic or sluggish temperament are predisposed to this affection. It usually attacks well-fed animals, and in such cases may be due to an excess of nutritive elements in the blood. Sudden changes in work or in the habits of the animal may induce an attack.

Symptoms.—It is usually ushered in by a chill, rise in temperature, and some uneasiness; in a very short time this is followed by lameness in one leg and swelling on the inside of the thigh. The swelling gradually surrounds the whole limb and continues on downward until it reaches the foot. The limb is excessively tender to the touch, the animal perspires, the breathing is accelerated, pulse hard and quick, and the temperature may reach 106° F The bowels early become very constipated and urine scanty. The symptoms usually are on the increase for about two days, then they remain stationary for the same length of time; the fever then abates; the swelling recedes and becomes less painful. It is very seldom, though, that all the swelling leaves the leg; generally it leaves some permanent enlargement, and the animal becomes subject to recurrent attacks. Occasionally the inguinal lymphatic glands (in the groin) undergo suppuration, and pyemia may supervene and prove fatal. In severe cases the limb becomes denuded of hair in patches, and the skin remains indurated with a fibrous growth, which is known by the name of elephantiasis.

Treatment.—The parts should be bathed freely and frequently with water as hot as the hand can bear and then fomented with vinegar and water, equal parts, to which add 2 ounces of nitrate of potassium for each gallon. This should be applied frequently, after the hot water, for the first day. Afterwards the leg may be dried with a woolen cloth and bathed with camphorated soap liniment. Internally administer artificial Carlsbad salts in 2 to 4 ounce doses three times daily. Feed lightly and give complete rest. This treatment, if instituted early in the attack, very frequently brings about a remarkable change within 24 hours.

DISEASES OF THE EYE.

By James Law, F. R. C. V. S.,

Formerly Professor of Veterinary Science, etc., Cornell University.

We can scarcely overestimate the value of sound eyes in the horse, and hence all diseases and injuries which seriously interfere with vision are matters of extreme gravity and apprehension, for should they prove permanent they invariably depreciate the selling price to a considerable extent. A blind horse is always dangerous in the saddle or in single harness, and he is scarcely less so when, with partially impaired vision, he sees things imperfectly, in a distorted form or in a wrong place, and when he shies or avoids objects which are commonplace or familiar. When we add to this that certain diseases of the eyes, like recurring inflammation (moon blindness), are habitually transmitted from parent to offspring, we can realize still more fully the importance of these maladies. Again, as a mere matter of beauty, a sound, full, clear, intelligent eye is something which must always add a high value to our equine friends and servants.

STRUCTURE OF THE EYE.

(Pl. XXII.)

THE EYEBALL.

A full description of the structure of the eye is incompatible with our prescribed limits, and yet a short description is absolutely essential to the clear understanding of what is to follow.

The horse's eye is a spheroidal body, flattened behind, and with its posterior four-fifths inclosed by an opaque, white, strong fibrous membrane (the sclera), on the inner side of which is laid a more delicate, friable membrane, consisting mainly of blood vessels and pigment cells (the choroid), which in its turn is lined by the extremely delicate and sensitive expansion of the nerve of sight (the retina). The anterior fifth of the globe of the eye bulges forward from what would have been the direct line of the sclera, and thus forms a segment of a much smaller sphere than is inclosed by the sclera. Its walls, too, have in health a perfect translucency, from which it has derived the name of transparent cornea. This transparent coat is composed, in the main, of fibers with lymph interspaces,

274

and it is to the condition of these and their condensation and compression that the translucency is largely due. This may be shown by compressing with the fingers the eye of an ox which has just been killed, when the clear transparent cornea will suddenly become clouded over with a whitish-blue opacity, and this will remain until the compression is interrupted. The interior of the eye contains three transparent media for the refraction of the rays of light on their way from the cornea to the visual nerve. Of these media the anterior one (aqueous humor) is liquid, the posterior (vitreous humor) is semisolid, and the intermediate one (crystalline lens) is solid. The space occupied by the aqueous humor corresponds nearly to the portion of the eye covered by the transparent cornea. It is, however, divided into two chambers, anterior and posterior, by the iris, a contractile curtain with a hole in the center (the pupil), and which may be looked on as in some sense a projection inward of the vascular and pigmentary coat from its anterior margin at the point where the sclera or opaque outer coat becomes continuous with the cornea or transparent one. This iris, or curtain, besides its abundance of blood vessels and pigment, possesses two sets of muscular fibers, one set radiating from the margin of the pupil to the outer border of the curtain at its attachment to the sclera and choroid, and the other encircling the pupil in the manner of a ring. The action of the two sets is necessarily antagonistic, the radiating fibers dilating the pupil and exposing the interior of the eye to view, while the circular fibers contract this opening and shut out the rays of light. The form of the pupil in the horse is ovoid, with its longest diameter from side to side, and its upper border is fringed by several minute, black bodies (corpora nigra) projecting forward and serving to some extent the purpose of eyebrows in arresting and absorbing the excess of rays of light which fall upon the eye from above. These pigmentary projections in front of the upper border of the pupil are often mistaken for the products of disease or injury in place of the normal and beneficent protectors of the nerve of sight which they are. Like all other parts, they may become the seat of disease, but so long as they and the iris retain their clear, dark aspect, without any tints of brown or yellow, they may be held to be healthy.

The vitreous or semisolid refracting medium occupies the posterior part of the eye—the part corresponding to the sclera, choroid, and retina—and has a consistency corresponding to that of the white of an egg, and a power of refraction of the light rays correspondingly greater than the aqueous humor.

The third or solid refracting medium is a biconvex lens, with its convexity greatest on its posterior surface, which is lodged in a depression in the vitreous humor, while its anterior surface corresponds to the opening of the pupil. It is inclosed in a membranous covering (capsule) and is maintained in position by a membrane (suspensory ligament) which extends from the margin of the lens outward to the sclera at the point of junction of the choroid and iris. This ligament is, in its turn, furnished with radiating, muscular fibers, which change the form or position of the lens so as to adapt it to see with equal clearness objects at a distance or close by.

Another point which strikes the observer of the horse's eye is that in the darkness a bright, bluish tinge is reflected from the widely dilated pupil. This is owing to a comparative absence of pigment in the choroid coat inside the upper part of the eyeball, and enables the animal to see and advance with security in darkness where the human eye would be of little use. The lower part of the cavity of the horse's eye, into which the dazzling rays fall from the sky, is furnished with an intensely black lining, by which the rays penetrating the inner nervous layer are instantly absorbed.

MUSCLES OF THE EYE.

These consist of four straight muscles, two oblique, and one retractor. The straight muscles pass from the depth of the orbit forward on the inner, outer, upper, and lower sides of the eyeball, and are fixed to the anterior portion of the fibrous (sclerotic) coat, so that in contracting singly they respectively turn the eye inward, outward, upward, and downward. When all act together they draw the eyeball deeply into its socket. The retractor muscle also consists of four muscular slips, repeating the straight muscles on a smaller scale, but as they are only attached on the back part of the eyeball they are less adapted to roll the eye than to draw it down into its socket. The two oblique muscles rotate the eye on its own axis, the upper one turning its outer surface upward and inward, and the lower one turning it downward and inward.

THE HAW (THE WINKING CARTILAGE, OR CARTILAGO NICTITANS).

This is a structure which, like the retractor muscle, is not found in the eye of man, but it serves in the lower animals to assist in removing foreign bodies from the front of the eyeball. It consists, in the horse, of a cartilage of irregular form, thickened inferiorly and posteriorly where it is intimately connected with the muscles of the eyeball and the fatty material around them, and expanded and flattened anteriorly where its upper surface is concave, and, as it were, molded on the lower and inner surface of the eyeball. Externally it is covered by the mucous membrane which lines the eyelids and extends over the front of the eye. In the ordinary restful state of the eye the edge of this cartilage should just appear as a thin fold of membrane at the inner angle of the eye, but when the eyeball is drawn deeply into the orbit the cartilage is pushed forward, outward, and upward

PLATE XXII.

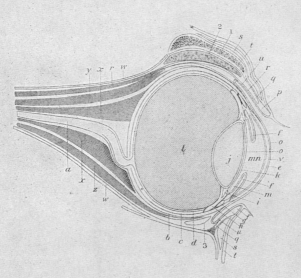

Theoretical Section of the Horse's Eye.

a, Optic nerve; b, Sclerotic; c, Choroid; d, Retina; e, Cornea; f, Iris;
g,h, Ciliary circle, (or ligament,) and processes given off by the choroid,
though represented as isolated from it, in order to indicate their limits
more clearly; i, Insertion of the ciliary processes on the crystalline lens;
j, Crystalline lens; k, Crystalline capsule; l, Vitreous body; m,n, Anterior
and posterior chambers; o, Theoretical indication of the membrane of
the aqueous humour; p,p, Tarsi; q,q, Fibrous membrane of the eyelids;
r, Elevator muscle of the upper eyelid; s,s, Orbicularis muscle of the
eyelids; t,t, Skin of the eyelids; u, Conjunctiva; v, Epidermic layer of
this membrane covering the Cornea; x, Posterior rectus muscle;
y, Superior rectus muscle; z, Inferior rectus muscle; w, Fibrous
sheath of the orbit (or orbital membrane).

Geo. Marx. del. alter D'Arboval. p. 371.

DIAGRAMMATIC VERTICAL SECTION THROUGH HORSE'S EYE.

over it until the entire globe may be hidden from sight. This protrusion of the cartilage so as to cover the eye may be induced in the healthy eye by pressing the finger and thumb on the upper and lower lids, so as to cause retraction of the eyeball into the socket. When foreign bodies, such as sand, dust, and chaff, or other irritants, have fallen on the eyeball or eyelids it is similarly projected to push them off, their expulsion being further favored by a profuse flow of tears.

This is seen, to a lesser extent, in all painful inflammations of the eye, and to a very marked degree in lockjaw, when the spasm of the muscles of the eyeball draws the latter deeply into the orbit and projects forward the masses of fat and the cartilage. The brutal practice of cutting off this apparatus whenever it is projected necessitates this explanation, which it is hoped may save to many a faithful servant a most valuable appendage. That the cartilage and membrane may become the seat of disease is undeniable, but so long as its edge is thin and even and its surface smooth and regular the mere fact of its projection over a portion of the eyeball is no evidence of disease in its substance, nor any warrant for its removal. It is usually but the evidence of the presence of some pain in another part of the eye, which the suffering animal endeavors to assuage by the use of this beneficent provision. For the diseases of the cartilage itself, see "Encephaloid cancer."

LACRIMAL APPARATUS.

This consists, first, of a gland for the secretion of the tears, and, second, of a series of canals for the conveyance of the superfluous tears into the cavity of the nose.

The gland is situated above the outer part of the eyeball, and the tears which have flowed over the eye and reached the inner angle are there directed by a small, conical papilla (lacrimal caruncle) into two minute orifices, and thence by two ducts (lacrimal) to a small pouch (lacrimal sac) from which a canal leads through the bones of the face into the nose. This opens in the lower part of the nose on the floor of the passage and a little outside the line of union of the skin which lines the false nostril with the mucous membrane of the nose. In the ass and mule this opening is situated on the roof instead of the floor of the nose, but still close to the external opening.

EXAMINATION OF THE EYE.

To avoid unnecessary repetition the following general directions are given for the examination of the eye: The eye, and to a certain extent the mucous membrane lining the eyelids, may be exposed to view by gently parting the eyelids with the thumb and forefinger pressed on the middle of the respective lids. The pressure, it is true, causes the protrusion of the haw over a portion of the lower and inner part of the eye, but by gentleness and careful graduation of the pressure this may be kept within bounds, and oftentimes even the interior of the eye can be seen. As a rule it is best to use the right hand for the left eye, and the left hand for the right, the finger in each case being pressed on the upper lid while the thumb depresses the lower one. In cases in which it is desirable to examine the inner side of the eyelid further than is possible by the above means, the upper lid may be drawn down by the eyelashes with the one hand and then everted over the tip of the forefinger of the other hand, or over a probe laid flat against the middle of the lid. When the interior of the eye must be examined it is useless to make the attempt in the open sunshine or under a clear sky. The worst cases, it is true, can be seen under such circumstances, but for the slighter forms the horse should be taken indoors, where all light from above will be shut off, and should be placed so that the light may fall on the eye from the front and side. Then the observer, placing himself in front of the animal, will receive the reflected rays from the cornea, the front of the lens and the back, and can much more easily detect any cloudiness, opacity, or lack of transparency. The examination can be made much more satisfactory by placing the horse in a dark chamber and illuminating the eye by a lamp placed forward and outward from the eye which is to be examined. Any cloudiness is thus easily detected, and any doubt may be resolved by moving the lamp so that the image of the flame may be passed in succession over the whole surface of the transparent cornea and of the crystalline lens. Three images of the flame will be seen, the larger one upright, reflected from the anterior surface of the eye; a smaller one upright, reflected from the anterior surface of the lens; and a second small one inverted from the back surface of the lens.

So long as these images are reflected from healthy surfaces they will be clear and perfect in outline, but as soon as one strikes on an area of opacity it will become diffused, cloudy, and indefinite. Thus, if the large, upright image becomes hazy and imperfect over a particular spot of the cornea, that will be found to be the seat of disease and opacity. Should the large image remain clear, but the small upright one become diffuse and indefinite over a given point, it indicates opacity on the front of the capsule of the lens. If both upright images remain clear while the inverted one becomes indistinct at a given point, then the opacity is in the substance of the lens itself or in the posterior part of its capsule.

If in a given case the pupil remains so closely contracted that the deeper parts of the eye can not be seen, the eyelids may be rubbed with extract of belladonna, and in a short time the pupil will be found widely dilated.

DISEASES OF THE EYELIDS.

CONGENITAL DISORDERS.

Some faulty conditions of the eyelids are congenital, as division of an eyelid in two, after the manner of harelip, abnormally small opening between the lids, often connected with imperfect development of the eye, and closure of the lids by adhesion. The first is to be remedied by paring the edges of the division and then bringing them together, as in torn lids. The last two, if remediable at all, require separation by the knife, and subsequent treatment with a cooling astringent eyewash.

NERVOUS DISORDERS.

SPASM OF EYELIDS may be owing to constitutional susceptibility, or to the presence of local irritants (insects, chemical irritants, sand, etc.) in the eye, to wounds or inflammation of the mucous membrane, or to disease of the brain. When due to local irritation it may be temporarily overcome by instilling a few drops of a 4 per cent solution of cocaine into the eye, when the true cause may be ascertained and removed. The nervous or constitutional disease must be treated according to its nature.

DROOPING EYELIDS, OR PTOSIS.—This is usually present in the upper lid, or is at least little noticed in the lower. It is sometimes but a symptom of paralysis of one-half of the face, in which case the ear, lips, and nostrils on the same side will be found soft, drooping, and inactive, and even the half of the tongue may partake of the palsy. If the same condition exists on both sides, there is difficult, snuffling breathing, from the air drawing in the flaps of the nostrils in inspiration, and all feed is taken in by the teeth, as the lips are useless. In both there is a free discharge of saliva from the mouth during mastication. This paralysis is a frequent result of injury, by a poke, to the seventh nerve, as it passes over the back of the lower jaw. In some cases the paralysis is confined to the lid, the injury having been sustained by the muscles which raise it, or by the supraorbital nerve, which emerges from the bone just above the eye. Such injury to the nerve may have resulted from fracture of the orbital process of the frontal bone above the eyeball.

The condition may, however, be due to spasm of the sphincter muscle, which closes the lids, or to inflammation of the upper lid, usually a result of blows on the orbit. In the latter case it may run a slow course with chronic thickening of the lid.

The paralysis due to the poke may be often remedied, first, by the removal of any remaining inflammation by a wet sponge worn beneath the ear and kept in place by a bandage; secondly, when all inflammation has passed, by a blister on the same region, or by rubbing it daily with a mixture of olive oil and strong aqua ammonia in equal proportions. Improvement is usually slow, and it may be months before complete recovery ensues.

In paralysis from blows above the eyes the same treatment may be applied to that part.

Thickening of the lid may be treated by painting with tincture of iodin, and that failing, by cutting out an elliptical strip of the skin from the middle of the upper lid and stitching the edges together.

INFLAMMATION OF THE EYELIDS.

The eyelids suffer more or less in all severe inflammations of the eye, whether external or internal, but inasmuch as the disease sometimes starts in the lids and at other times is exclusively confined to them, it deserves independent mention.

Among the causes may be named: Exposure to drafts of cold air, or to cold rain or snow storms; the bites or stings of mosquitoes, flies, or other insects; snake bites, pricks with thorns, blows of whip or club; accidental bruises against the stall or ground, especially during the violent struggles of colic, enteritis, phrenitis (staggers), and when thrown for operations. It is also a result of infecting inoculations, as of erysipelas, anthrax, boil, etc., and is noted by Leblanc as especially prevalent among horses kept on low, marshy pastures. Finally, the introduction of sand, dust, chaff, beards of barley and seeds of the finest grasses, and the contact with irritant, chemical powders, liquids, and gases (ammonia from manure or factory, chlorin, strong sulphur fumes, smoke, and other products of combustion, etc.) may start the inflammation. The eyelids often undergo extreme inflammatory and dropsical swelling in urticaria (nettle-rash, surfeit) and in the general inflammatory dropsy known as purpura hemorrhagica.

The affection will, therefore, readily divide itself into (1) inflammations due to constitutional causes; (2) those due to direct injury, mechanical or chemical; and (3) such as are due to inoculation with infecting material.

(1) Inflammations due to constitutional causes are distinguished by the absence of any local wound, and the history of a low, damp pasture, exposure, indigestion from unwholesome feed, or the presence elsewhere on the limbs or body of the general, doughy swellings of purpura hemorrhagica. The lids are swollen and thickened; it may be slightly or it may be so extremely that the eyeball can not be seen. If the lid can be everted to show its mucous membrane, that is seen to be of a deep-red color, especially along the branching lines of the blood vessels. The part is hot and painful, and a profuse flow of tears and mucus escapes on the side of the face, causing irritation

and loss of the hair. If improvement follows, this discharge becomes more tenacious, and tends to cause adhesion to the edges of the upper and lower lids and to mat together the eyelashes in bundles. This gradually decreases to the natural amount, and the redness and congested appearance of the eye disappears, but swelling, thickening, and stiffness of the lids may continue for a time. There may be more or less fever according to the violence of the inflammation, but so long as there is no serious disease of the interior of the eye or of other vital organ, it is usually moderate.

The local treatment consists in astringent, soothing lotions (sugar of lead 30 grains, atropin sulphate 30 grains, rain water—boiled and cooled—1 pint), applied with a soft cloth kept wet with the lotion, and hung over the eye by tying it to the headstall of the bridle on the two sides. If the mucous membrane lining of the lids is the seat of little red granular elevations, a drop of solution of 2 grains of nitrate of silver in an ounce of distilled water should be applied with the soft end of a clean feather to the inside of the lid twice a day. The patient should be removed from all such conditions (pasture, faulty feed, exposure, etc.) as may have caused or aggravated the disease, and from dust and irritant fumes and gases. He should be fed from a manger high enough to favor the return of blood from the head, and should be kept from work, especially in a tight collar which would prevent the descent of blood by the jugular veins. The diet should be laxative and nonstimulating (grass, bran mashes, carrots, turnips, beets, potatoes, or steamed hay), and any costiveness should be corrected by a mild dose of raw linseed oil (1 to 1½ pints). In cold weather warm blanketing may be needful, and even loose flannel bandages to the limbs, but heat should never be sought at the expense of pure air.

(2) In inflammations due to local irritants of a noninfective kind a careful examination will usually reveal their presence, and the first step must be their removal with a pair of blunt forceps or the point of a lead pencil. Subsequent treatment will be in the main the local treatment advised above.

(3) In case of infective inflammation there will often be found a prick or tear by which the septic matter has entered, and in such case the inflammation will for a time be concentrated at that point. A round or conical swelling around an insect bite is especially characteristic. A snake bite is marked by the double prick made by the two teeth and by the violent and rapidly spreading inflammation. Erysipelas is attended with much swelling, extending beyond the lids and causing the mucous membrane to protrude beyond the edge of the eyelid (chemosis). This is characterized by a bright, uniform, rosy red, disappearing on pressure, or later by a dark, livid hue, but with less branching redness than in noninfecting inflammation and

less of the dark, dusky, brownish or yellowish tint of anthrax. Little vesicles may appear on the skin, and pus may be found without any distinct limiting membrane, as in abscess. It is early attended with high fever and marked general weakness and inappetence. Anthrax of the lids is marked by a firm swelling, surmounted by a blister, with bloody serous contents, which tends to burst and dry up into a slough, while the surrounding parts become involved in the same way. Or it may show as a diffuse, dropsical swelling, with less of the hard, central sloughing nodule, but, like that, tending to spread quickly. In both cases alike the mucous membrane and the skin, if white, assume a dusky-brown or yellowish-brown hue, which is largely characteristic. This may pass into a black color by reason of extravasation of blood. Great constitutional disturbance appears early, with much prostration and weakness and generalized anthrax symptoms.

Treatment.—The treatment will vary according to the severity. Insect bites may be touched with a solution of equal parts of glycerin and aqua ammonia, or a 10 per cent solution of carbolic acid in water. Snake bites may be bathed with aqua ammonia, and the same agent given in doses of 2 teaspoonfuls in a quart of water, or tincture of nux vomica in teaspoonful doses may be given every four hours. In erysipelas the skin may be painted with tincture of chlorid of iron, or with a solution of 20 grains of iodin in an ounce of carbolic acid, and one-half an ounce of tincture of chlorid of iron may be given thrice daily in a bottle of water. In anthrax the swelling should be painted with tincture of iodin, or of the mixture of iodin and carbolic acid, and if very threatening it may have the tincture of iodin injected into the swelling with a hypodermic syringe, or the hard mass may be freely incised to its depth with a sharp lancet and the lotion applied to the exposed tissues. Internally, iodid of potassium may be given in doses of 2 drams thrice a day, or tincture of the chlorid of iron every four hours.

If anthrax infection is suspected, immediate assistance of a veterinarian should be obtained. In the early stages of anthrax infection the subcutaneous and intravenous injection of large doses of antianthrax serum (50 to 100 c. c.) is indicated. Prevent spreading the disease to other animals and man by isolation of the affected animals, rigid sanitary precautions, and disinfection of infected quarters.

STY, OR FURUNCLE (BOIL) OF THE EYELID.

This is an inflammation of limited extent, advancing to the formation of matter and the sloughing out of a small mass of the natural tissue of the eyelid. It forms a firm, rounded swelling, usually near the margin of the lid, which suppurates and bursts in four or five days. Its course may be hastened by a poultice of camomile flowers, to which have been added a few drops of carbolic acid, the whole applied in a very thin muslin bag. If the swelling is slow to open after having become yellowish white, it may be opened by a lancet, the incision being made at right angles to the margin of the lid.

ENTROPION AND ECTROPION, OR INVERSION AND EVERSION OF THE EYELID.

These are respectively caused by wounds, sloughs, ulcers, or other causes of loss of substance of the mucous membrane on the inside of the lid and of the skin on the outside; also of tumors, skin diseases, or paralysis which leads to displacement of the margin of the eyelid. As a rule, they require a surgical operation, with removal of an elliptical portion of the mucous membrane or skin, as the case may be, but which requires the skilled and delicate hand of the surgeon.

TRICHIASIS.

This consists in the turning in of the eyelashes so as to irritate the front of the eye. If a single eyelash, it may be snipped off with scissors close to the margin of the eyelid or pulled out by the root with a pair of flat-bladed forceps. If the divergent lashes are more numerous, the treatment may be as for entropion, by excising an elliptical portion of skin opposite the offending lashes and stitching the edges together, so as to draw outward the margin of the lid at that point.

WARTS AND OTHER TUMORS OF THE EYELIDS.

The eyelids form a favorite site for tumors, and above all, warts, which consist in a simple diseased overgrowth (hypertrophy) of the surface layers of the skin. If small, they may be snipped off with scissors or tied around the neck with a stout, waxed thread and left to drop off, the destruction being completed, if necessary, by the daily application of a piece of sulphate of copper (blue vitriol), until any unhealthy material has been removed. If more widely spread, the wart may still be clipped off with curved scissors or knife, and the caustic thoroughly applied day by day.

A bleeding wart, or erectile tumor, is more liable to bleed, and is best removed by constricting its neck with the waxed cord or rubber band, or if too broad it may be transfixed through its base by a needle armed with a double thread, which is then to be cut in two and tied around the two portions of the neck of the tumor. If still broader, the armed needle may be carried through the base of the tumor at regular intervals, so that the whole may be tied in moderately sized sections.

In gray and in white horses black, pigmentary tumors (melanoma) are common on the black portions of skin, such as the eyelids, and are to be removed by scissors or knife, according to their size. In the horse they do not usually tend to recur when thoroughly removed, but at times they prove cancerous (as is the rule in man), and then they tend to reappear in the same site or in internal organs with, it may be, fatal effect.

Encysted, honeylike (melicerous), sebaceous, and fibrous tumors of the lids all require removal with the knife.

TORN EYELIDS OR WOUNDS OF EYELIDS.

The eyelids are torn by attacks with horns of cattle, or with the teeth, or by getting caught on nails in stall, rack, or manger, on the point of stumps, fences, or fence rails, on the barbs of wire fences, and on other pointed bodies. The edges should be brought together as promptly as possible, so as to effect union without the formation of matter, puckering of the skin, and unsightly distortions. Great care is necessary to bring the two edges together evenly without twisting or puckering. The simplest mode of holding them together is by a series of sharp pins passed through the lips of the wound at intervals of not more than a third of an inch, and held together by a thread twisted around each pin in the form of the figure 8, and carried obliquely from pin to pin in two directions, so as to prevent gaping of the wound in the intervals. The points of the pins may then be cut off with scissors, and the wound may be wet twice a day with a weak solution of carbolic acid.

TUMOR OF THE HAW, OR CARIES OF THE CARTILAGE.

Though cruelly excised for alleged " hooks," when itself perfectly healthy, in the various diseases which lead to retraction of the eye into its socket, the haw may, like other bodily structures, be itself the seat of actual disease. The pigmentary, black tumors of white horses and soft (encephaloid) cancer may attack this part primarily or extend to it from the eyeball or eyelids; hairs have been found growing from its surface, and the mucous membrane covering it becomes inflamed in common with that covering the front of the eye. These inflammations are but a phase of the inflammation of the external structures of the eye, and demand no particular notice nor special treatment. The tumors lead to such irregular enlargement and distortion of the haw that the condition is not to be confounded with the simple projection of the healthy structure over the eye when the lids are pushed apart with the finger and thumb, and the same remark applies to the ulceration, or caries, of the cartilage. In the latter case, besides the swelling and distortion of the haw, there is this peculiarity, that in the midst of the red inflamed mass there appears a white line or mass formed by the exposed edge of the ulcerating cartilage. The animal having been thrown and properly fixed, an assistant holds the eyelids apart while the operator seizes the haw with forceps or hook and carefully dissects it out with blunt-pointed scissors. The eye is then covered with a cloth, kept wet with an eyewash, as for external ophthalmia.

OBSTRUCTION OF THE LACRIMAL APPARATUS, OR WATERING EYE.

The escape of tears on the side of the cheek is a symptom of external inflammation of the eye, but it may also occur from any disease of the lacrimal apparatus which interferes with the normal progress of the tears to the nose; hence, in all cases when this symptom is not attended with special redness or swelling of the eyelids, it is well to examine the lacrimal apparatus. In some instances the orifice of the lacrimal duct on the floor of the nasal chamber and close to its anterior outlet will be found blocked by a portion of dry mucopurulent matter, on the removal of which tears may begin to escape. This implies an inflammation of the canal, which may be helped by occasional sponging out of the nose with warm water, and the application of the same on the face. Another remedy is to feed warm mashes of wheat bran from a nosebag, so that the relaxing effects of the water vapor may be secured.

The two lacrimal openings, situated at the inner angle of the eye, may fail to admit the tears by reason of their deviation outward in connection with the eversion of the lower lid or by reason of their constriction in inflammation of the mucous membrane. The lacrimal sac, into which the lacrimal ducts open, may fail to discharge its contents by reason of constriction or closure of the duct leading to the nose, and it then forms a rounded swelling beneath the inner angle of the eye. The duct leading from the sac to the nose may be compressed or obliterated by fractures of the bones of the face, and in disease of these bones (osteosarcoma, so-called osteoporosis, diseased teeth, glanders of the nasal sinuses, abscess of the same cavities).

The narrowed or obstructed ducts may be made pervious by a fine, silver probe passed down to the lacrimal sac, and any existing inflammation of the passages may be counteracted by the use of steaming mashes of wheat bran, by fomentations or wet cloths over the face, and even by the use of astringent eyewashes and the injection of similar liquids into the lacrimal canal from its nasal opening. The ordinary eyewash may be used for this purpose, or it may be injected after dilution to half its strength. The fractures and diseases of the bones and teeth must be treated according to their special demands when, if the canal is still left pervious, it may be again rendered useful.

EXTERNAL OPHTHALMIA, OR CONJUNCTIVITIS.

In inflammation of the outer parts of the eyeball the exposed vascular and sensitive mucous membrane (conjunctiva) which covers the ball, the eyelids, the haw, and the lacrimal apparatus, is usually the most deeply involved, yet adjacent parts are more or less implicated, and when disease is concentrated on these contiguous parts it constitutes a phase of external opththalmia which demands a special notice. These have accordingly been already treated of.

Causes.—The causes of external opththalmia are mainly those that act locally—blows with whips, clubs, and twigs, the presence of foreign bodies, like hayseed, chaff, dust, lime, sand, snuff, pollen of plants, flies attracted by the brilliancy of the eye, wounds of the bridle, the migration of the scabies (mange) insect into the eye, smoke, ammonia arising from the excretions, irritant emanations from drying marshes, etc. Road dust containing infecting microbes is a common factor. A very dry air is alleged to act injuriously by drying the eye as well as by favoring the production of irritant dust; the undue exposure to bright sunshine through a window in front of the stall, or to the reflection from snow or water, also is undoubtedly injurious. The unprotected exposure of the eyes to sunshine through the use of a very short overdraw check is to be condemned, and the keeping of the horse in a very dark stall, from which it is habitually led into the glare of full sunlight, intensified by reflection from snow or white limestone, must be set down among the locally acting causes. Exposure to cold and wet, to wet and snow storms, to cold drafts and wet lairs must also be accepted as causes of conjunctivitis, the general disorder which they produce affecting the eye, if that happens to be the weakest and most susceptible organ of the body, or if it has been subjected to any special local injury, like dust, irritant gases, or excess of light. Again, external opththalmia is a constant concomitant of inflammation of the contiguous and continuous mucous membranes, as those of the nose and throat—hence the red, watery eyes that attend on nasal catarrh, sore throat, influenza, strangles, nasal glanders, and the like. In such cases, however, the affection of the eye is subsidiary and is manifestly overshadowed by the primary and predominating disease.

Symptoms.—The symptoms are watering of the eye, swollen lids, redness of the mucous membrane exposed by the separation of the lids—it may be a mere pink blush with more or less branching redness, or it may be a deep, dark red, as from effusion of blood—and a bluish opacity of the cornea, which is normally clear and translucent. Except when resulting from wounds and actual extravasation of blood, however, the redness is seen to be superficial, and if the opacity is confined to the edges, and does not involve the entire cornea, the aqueous humor behind is seen to be still clear and limpid. The fever is always less severe than in internal ophthalmia, and runs high only in the worst cases. The eyelids may be kept closed, the eyeball retracted, and the haw protruded over one-third or one-half of the ball, but this is due to the pain only and not to any excessive sensibility to light, as shown by the comparatively widely dilated pupil. In internal ophthalmia, on the contrary, the narrow, contracted pupil is the measure of the pain caused by the falling of light on the inflamed and sensitive optic nerve (retina) and choroid.

If the affection has resulted from a wound of the cornea, not only is that the point of greatest opacity, forming a white speck or fleecy cloud, but too often blood vessels begin to extend from the adjacent vascular covering of the eye (sclera) to the white spot, and that portion of the cornea is rendered permanently opaque. Again, if the wound has been severe, though still short of cutting into the anterior layers of the cornea, the injury may lead to ulceration that may penetrate more or less deeply and leave a breach in the tissue which, if filled up at all, is repaired by opaque fibrous tissue in place of the transparent cellular structure. Pus may form, and the cornea assumes a yellowish tinge and bursts, giving rise to a deep sore which is liable to extend as an ulcer, and may be in its turn followed by bulging of the cornea at that point (staphyloma). This inflammation of the conjunctiva may be simply catarrhal, with profuse mucopurulent discharge; it may be granular, the surface being covered with minute reddish elevations, or it may become the seat of a false membrane (diphtheria).

Treatment.—In treating external ophthalmia the first object is the removal of the cause. Remove any dust, chaff, thorn, or other foreign body from the conjunctiva, purify the stable from all sources of ammoniacal or other irritant gas; keep the horse from dusty roads, and, above all, from the proximity of a leading wagon and its attendant cloud of dust; remove from pasture and feed from a rack which is neither so high as to drop seeds, etc., into the eyes nor so low as to favor the accumulation of blood in the head; avoid equally excess of light from a sunny window in front of the stall and excess of darkness from the absence of windows; preserve from cold drafts and rains and wet bedding, and apply curative measures for inflammation of the adjacent mucous membranes or skin. If the irritant has been of a caustic nature, remove any remnant of it by persistent bathing with tepid water and a soft sponge, or with water mixed with white of egg, or a glass filled with the liquid may be inverted over the eye so that its contents may dilute and remove the irritant. If the suffering is very severe, a lotion with a few grains of extract of belladonna in an ounce of water may be applied.

In strong, vigorous patients benefit will usually be obtained from a laxative, such as 2 tablespoonfuls of Glauber's salt daily, and if the fever runs high from a daily dose of half an ounce of saltpeter. As local applications, astringent solutions are usually the best, as 30 grains of borax or of sulphate of zinc in a quart of water, to be applied constantly on a cloth, as advised under "Inflammation of the eyelids." In the absence of anything better, cold water may serve every purpose. Above all, adhesive and oily agents (molasses, sugar, fats) are to be avoided, as only adding to the irritation. By way of suggesting agents that may be used with good effect, salt and sulphate of soda may be named, in solutions double the strength of sulphate of zinc, or 7 grains of nitrate of silver may be added to a quart of distilled water, and will be found especially applicable in granular conjunctivitis, diphtheria, or commencing ulceration. A cantharides blister (1 part of Spanish fly to 4 parts lard) may be rubbed on the side of the face 3 inches below the eye, and washed off next morning with soapsuds and oiled daily till the scabs are dropped.

WHITE SPECKS AND CLOUDINESS OF THE CORNEA.

As a result of external ophthalmia, opaque specks, clouds, or haziness are too often left on the cornea and require for their removal that they be daily touched with a soft feather dipped in a solution of 3 grains nitrate of silver in 1 ounce distilled water. This should be applied until all inflammation has subsided, and until its contact is comparatively painless. It is rarely successful with an old, thick scar following an ulcer, nor with an opacity having red blood vessels running across it.

ULCERS OF THE CORNEA.

These may be treated with nitrate of silver lotion of twice the strength used for opacities. Powdered gentian, one-half ounce, and sulphate of iron, one-fourth ounce, daily, may improve the general health and increase the reparatory power.

INTERNAL OPHTHALMIA (IRITIS, CHOROIDITIS, AND RETINITIS).

Although inflammations of the iris, choroid, and retina—the inner, vascular, and nervous coats of the eye—occur to a certain extent independently of each other, yet one usually supervenes upon the other, and, as the symptoms are thus made to coincide, it will be best for our present purposes to treat the three as one disease.

Causes.—The causes of internal ophthalmia are largely those of the external form only, acting with greater intensity or on a more susceptible eye. Severe blows, bruises, punctures, etc., of the eye, the penetration of foreign bodies into the eye (thorns, splinters of iron, etc.), sudden transition from a dark stall to bright sunshine, to the glare of snow or water, constant glare from a sunny window, abuse of the overdraw checkrein, vivid lightning flashes, drafts of cold, damp air; above all, when the animal is perspiring, exposure in cold rain or snowstorms, swimming cold rivers; also certain general diseases like rheumatism, arthritis, influenza, and disorders of the digestive organs, may become complicated by this affection. From the close relation between the brain and eye—alike in the blood vessels and nerves—disorders of the first lead to affection of the second, and the same remark applies to the persistent irritation to which the jaws are subjected in the course of dentition. So potent is the last agency that we dread a recurrence of ophthalmia so long as dentition is incomplete, and hope for immunity if the animal completes its dentition without any permanent structural change in the eye.

Symptoms.—The symptoms will vary according to the cause. If the attack is due to direct physical injury, the inflammation of the eyelids and superficial structures may be quite as marked as that of the interior of the eye. If, on the other hand, from general causes, or as a complication of some distant disease, the affection may be largely confined to the deeper structures, and the swelling, redness, and tenderness of the superficial structures will be less marked. When the external coats thus comparatively escape, the extreme anterior edge of the white or sclerotic coat, where it overlaps the border of the transparent cornea, is in a measure free from congestion, and, in the absence of the obscuring dark pigment, forms a whitish ring around the cornea. This is partly due to the fact that a series of arteries (ciliary) passing to the inflamed iris penetrate the sclerotic coat a short distance behind its anterior border, and there is therefore a marked difference in color between the general sclera occupied between these congested vessels and the anterior rim from which they are absent. Unfortunately, the pigment is often so abundant in the anterior part of the sclera as to hide this symptom. In internal ophthalmia the opacity of the cornea may be confined to a zone around the outer margin of the cornea, and even this may be a bluish haze rather than a deep, fleecy white. In consequence it becomes impossible to see the interior of the chamber for the aqueous humor and the condition of the iris and pupil. The aqueous humor is usually turbid, and has numerous yellowish-white flakes floating on its substance or deposited in the lower part of the chamber, so as to cut off the view of the lower portion of the iris. The still visible portion of the iris has lost its natural, clear, dark luster, which is replaced by a brownish or yellowish sere-leaf color. This is more marked in proportion as the iris is inflamed, and less so as the inflammation is confined to the choroid. The quantity of flocculent deposit in the chamber of the aqueous humor is also in direct ratio to the inflammation of the iris. Perhaps the most marked feature of internal ophthalmia is the extreme and painful sensitiveness to light. On this account the lids are usually closed, but when opened the pupil is seen to be narrowly closed, even if the animal has been kept in a darkened stall. Exceptions to this are seen when inflammatory effusion has overfilled the globe of the eye, and by pressure on the retina has paralyzed it, or when the exudation into the substance of the retina itself has similarly led to its paralysis. Then the pupil may be dilated, and frequently its margin loses its regular, ovoid outline and becomes uneven by reason of the adhesions which it has contracted with the capsule of the lens, through its inflammatory exudations. In the case of excessive effusion into the globe of the eye that is found to have become tense and hard so that it can not be indented with the tip of the finger, paralysis of the retina is liable to result. With such paralysis of the retina, vision is heavily clouded or entirely lost; hence, in spite of the open pupil, the finger may be approached to the eye without the animal's becoming conscious of it until it touches the surface, and if the nose on the affected side is gently struck and a feint made to repeat the blow the patient makes no effort to evade it. Sometimes the edges of the contracted pupil become adherent to each other by an intervening plastic exudation, and the opening becomes virtually abolished. In severe inflammations pus may form in the choroid or iris, and escaping into the cavity of the aqueous humor show as a yellowish-white stratum below. In nearly all cases there is resulting exudation into the lens or its capsule, constituting a cloudiness or opacity (cataract), which in severe and old-standing cases appears as a white, fleecy mass behind a widely dilated pupil. In the slighter cases cataract is to be recognized by examination of the eye in a dark chamber, with an oblique side light, as described in the introduction to this article. Cataracts that appear as a simple haze or indefinite, fleecy cloud are usually on the capsule (capsular), while those that show a radiating arrangement are in the lens (lenticular), the radiating fibers of which the exudate follows. Black cataracts are formed by the adhesion of the pigment on the back of the iris to the front of the lens, and by the subsequent tearing loose of the iris, leaving a portion of its pigment adherent to the capsule of the lens. If the pupil is so contracted that it is impossible to see the lens, it may be dilated by applying to the front of the eye with a feather some drops of a solution of 4 grains of atropin sulphate in an ounce of water.

Treatment.—The treatment of internal ophthalmia should embrace, first, the removal of all existing causes or sources of aggravation of the disease, which need not be repeated here. Special care to protect the patient against strong light, cold, wet weather, and active exertion must, however, be insisted on. A dark stall and a cloth hung over the eye are important, while cleanliness, warmth, dryness, and rest are equally demanded. If the patient is strong and vigorous, a dose of 4 drams of Barbados aloes may be given, and if there is any reason to suspect a rheumatic origin one-half a dram powdered colchicum and one-half ounce salicylate of soda may be given daily.

Locally the astringent lotions advised for external ophthalmia may be resorted to, especially when the superficial inflammation is well marked. More important, however, is to instill into the eye, a few drops at a time, a solution of 4 grains of atropin sulphate in 1 ounce of distilled water. This may be effected with the aid of a soft feather, and may be repeated at intervals of 10 minutes until the pupil is widely dilated. As the horse is to be kept in a dark stall, the consequent admission of light will be harmless, and the dilation of the pupil prevents adhesion between the iris and lens, relieves the constant tension of the eye in the effort to adapt the pupil to the light, and solicits the contraction of the blood vessels of the eye and the lessening of congestion, exudation, and intraocular pressure. Another local measure is a blister, which can usually be applied to advantage on the side of the nose or beneath the ear. Spanish flies may be used as for external ophthalmia. In very severe cases the parts beneath the eye may be shaved and three or four leeches applied. Setons are sometimes beneficial, and even puncture of the eyeball, but these should be reserved for professional hands.

The diet throughout should be easily digestible and moderate in quantity—bran mash, middlings, grass, steamed hay, etc.

Even after the active inflammation has subsided the atropin sulphate lotion should be continued for several weeks to keep the eye in a state of rest in its still weak and irritable condition, and during this period the patient should be kept in semidarkness, or taken out only with a dark shade over the eye. For the same reason heavy drafts and rapid paces, which would cause congestion of the head, should be carefully avoided.

RECURRENT OPHTHALMIA (PERIODIC OPHTHALMIA, OR MOON-BLINDNESS).

This is an inflammatory affection of the interior of the eye, intimately related to certain soils, climates, and systems, showing a strong tendency to recur again and again, and usually ending in blindness from cataract or other serious injury.

Causes.—Its causes may be fundamentally attributed to soil. On damp clays and marshy grounds, on the frequently overflowed river bottoms and deltas, on the coasts of seas and lakes alternately submerged and exposed, this disease prevails extensively, and in many instances in France (Reynal), Belgium, Alsace (Zundel, Miltenberger), Germany, and England it has very largely decreased under land drainage and improved methods of culture. Other influences, more or less associated with such soil, are potent causative factors. Thus damp air and a cloudy, wet climate, so constantly associated with wet lands, are universally charged with causing the disease. These act on the animal body to produce a lymphatic constitution with an excess of connective tissue, bones, and muscles of coarse, open texture, thick skins, and gummy legs covered with a profusion of long hair. Hence the heavy horses of Belgium and southwestern France have suffered severely from the affection, while high, dry lands adjacent, like Catalonia, in Spain, and Dauphiny, Provence, and Languedoc, in France, have in the main escaped.

The rank, aqueous fodders grown on such soils are other causes, but these again are calculated to undermine the character of the nervous and sanguineous temperament and to superinduce the lymphatic. Other feeds act by leading to constipation and other disorders of the digestive organs, thus impairing the general health. Hence in any animal predisposed to this disease, heating, starchy feeds, such as maize, wheat, and buckwheat, are to be carefully avoided. It has been widely charged that beans, peas, vetches, and other Leguminosæ are dangerous, but a fuller inquiry contradicts the statement. If these feeds are well grown, they invigorate and fortify the system, while, like any other fodder, if grown rank, aqueous, and deficient in assimilable principles, they tend to lower the health and open the way for the disease.

The period of dentition and training is a fertile exciting cause, for though the malady may appear at any time from birth to old age, yet the great majority of victims are from 2 to 6 years old, and if a horse escapes the affection till after 6 there is a reasonable hope that he will continue to resist it. The irritation about the head during the eruption of the teeth, and while fretting in the unwonted bridle and collar, the stimulating grain diet and the close air of the stable all combine to rouse the latent tendency to disease in the eye, while direct injuries by bridle, whip, or hay seeds are not without their influence. In the same way local irritants, like dust, severe rain and snow storms, smoke, and acrid vapors are contributing causes.

It is evident, however, that no one of these is sufficient of itself to produce the disease, and it has been alleged that the true cause is a microbe, or the irritant products of a microbe, which is harbored in the marshy soil. The prevalence of the disease on the same damp soils which produce ague in man and anthrax in cattle has been quoted in support of this doctrine, as also the fact that, other things being equal, the malady is always more prevalent in basins surrounded by hills where the air is still and such products are concentrated, and that a forest or simple belt of trees will, as in ague, at times limit the area of its prevalence. Another argument for the same view is found in the fact that on certain farms irrigated by town sewage this malady has become extremely prevalent, the sewage being assumed to form a suitable nidus for the growth of the germ.

But on these sewage farms a fresh crop may be cut every fortnight, and the product is precisely that aqueous material which contributes to a lymphatic structure and a low tone of health. The presence of a definite germ in the system has not yet been proved, and in the present state of our knowledge we are only warranted in charging the disease to the deleterious emanations from the marshy soil in which bacterial ferments are constantly producing them.

Heredity is one of the most potent causes. The lymphatic constitution is of course transmitted and with it the proclivity to recurring ophthalmia. This is notorious in the case of both parents, male and female. The tendency appears to be stronger, however, if either parent has already suffered. Thus a mare may have borne a number of sound foals, and then fallen a victim to the malady, and all foals subsequently borne have likewise suffered. So it is in the case of the stallion. Reynal even quotes the appearance of the disease in alternate generations, the stallion offspring of blind parents remaining sound through life and yet producing foals which furnish numerous victims of recurrent ophthalmia. On the contrary, the offspring of diseased parents removed to high, dry regions and furnished with wholesome, nourishing rations will nearly all escape. Hence the dealers take colts that are still sound or have had but one attack from the affected low Pyrenees (France) to the unaffected Catalonia (Spain), with confidence that they will escape, and from the Jura Valley to Dauphiny with the same result.

Yet the hereditary taint is so strong and pernicious that intelligent horsemen everywhere refuse to breed from either horse or mare that has once suffered from recurrent ophthalmia, and the French Government studs not only reject all unsound stallions, but refuse service to any mare which has suffered with her eyes. It is this avoidance of the hereditary predisposition more than anything else that has reduced the formerly wide prevalence of this disease in the European countries generally. A consideration for the future of our horses would demand the disuse of all sires that are unlicensed, and the refusal of a license to any sire which has suffered from this or any other communicable constitutional disease.

Other contributing causes deserve passing mention. Unwholesome feed and a faulty method of feeding undoubtedly predisposes to the disease, and in the same district the carefully fed will escape in far larger proportion than the badly fed; it is so also with every other condition which undermines the general health. The presence of worms in the intestines, overwork, and debilitating diseases and causes of every kind weaken the vitality and lay the system more open to attack. Thierry long ago showed that the improvement of close, low, dark, damp stables, where the disease had previously prevailed, practically banished the affection. Whatever contributes to strength and vigor is protective; whatever contributes to weakness and poor health is provocative of the disease in the predisposed subject.

Symptoms.—The symptoms vary according to the severity of the attack. In some cases there is marked fever, and in some slighter cases it may be almost altogether wanting, but there is always a lack of vigor and energy, bespeaking general disorder. The local symptoms are in the main those of internal ophthalmia, in many cases with an increased hardness of the eyeball from effusion into its cavity. The contracted pupil does not expand much in darkness, nor even under the action of belladonna. Opacity advances from the margin, over a part or whole of the cornea, but so long as it is transparent there may be seen the turbid, aqueous humor with or without flocculi, the dingy iris robbed of its clear, black aspect, the slightly clouded lens, and a greenish-yellow reflection from the depth of the eye. From the fifth to the seventh day the flocculi precipitate in the lower part of the chamber, exposing more clearly the iris and lens, and absorption commences, so that the eye may be cleared up in ten or fifteen days.

The characteristic of the disease is, however, its recurrence again and again in the same eye until blindness results. The attacks may follow one another after intervals of a month, more or less, but they show no relation to any particular phase of the moon, as might be inferred from the familiar name, but are determined rather by the weather, the health, the feed, or by some periodicity of the system. From five to seven attacks usually result in blindness, and then the second eye is liable to be attacked until it also is ruined.

In the intervals between the attacks some remaining symptoms betray the condition, and they become more marked after each successive access of disease. Even after the first attack there is a bluish ring around the margin of the transparent cornea. The eye seems smaller than the other, at first because it is retracted in its socket, and often after several attacks because of actual shrinkage (atrophy). The upper eyelid, in place of presenting a uniform, continuous arch, has, about one-third from its inner angle, an abrupt bend, caused by the contraction of the levator muscle. The front of the iris has exchanged some of its dark, clear brilliancy for a lusterless yellow, and the depth of the eye presents more or less of the greenish-yellow shade. The pupil remains a little contracted, except in advanced and aggravated cases, when, with opaque lens, it is widely dilated. If, as is common, one eye only has suffered, the contrast in these respects with the sound eye is all the more characteristic. Another feature is the erect, attentive carriage of the ear, to compensate to some extent for the waning vision.

The attacks vary greatly in severity in different cases, but the recurrence is characteristic, and all alike lead to cataract and intraocular effusion, with pressure on the retina and abolition of sight.

Prevention.—The prevention of this disease is the great object to be aimed at, and this demands the most careful breeding, feeding, housing, and general management, as indicated under " Causes." Much can also be done by migration to a high, dry location, but for this and malarious affections the improvement of the land by drainage and good cultivation should be the final aim.

Treatment is not satisfactory, but is largely the same as for common internal ophthalmia. Some cases, like rheumatism, are benefited by 1-scruple doses of powdered colchicum and 2-dram doses of salicylate of soda twice a day. In other cases, with marked hardness of the globe of the eye from intraocular effusion, aseptic puncture of the eye, or even the excision of a portion of the iris, has helped. During recovery a course of tonics (2 drams oxid of iron, 10 grains nux vomica, and 1 ounce sulphate of soda daily) is desirable to invigorate the system and help to ward off another attack. The vulgar resort to knocking out the wolf teeth and cutting out the haw can only be condemned. The temporary recovery would take place in one or two weeks, though no such thing had been done, and the breaking of a small tooth, leaving its fang in the jaw, only increases the irritation.

CATARACT.

The common result of internal ophthalmia, as of the recurrent type, may be recognized as described under the first of these diseases. Its offensive appearance may be obviated by extraction or depression of the lens, but as the rays of light would no longer be properly refracted, perfect vision would not be restored, and the animal would be liable to prove an inveterate shyer. If perfect blindness continued by reason of pressure on the nerve of sight, no shying would result.

PALSY OF THE NERVE OF SIGHT, OR AMAUROSIS.

Causes.—The causes of this affection are tumors or other disease of the brain implicating the roots of the optic nerve, injury to the nerve between the brain and eye, and inflammation of the optic nerve within the eye (retina), or undue pressure on the same from dropsical or inflammatory effusion. It may also occur from overloaded stomach, from a profuse bleeding, and even from the pressure of the gravid womb in gestation.

Symptoms.—The symptoms are wide dilatation of the pupils, so as to expose fully the interior of the globe, the expansion remaining the same in light and darkness. Ordinary eyes when brought to the light have the pupils suddenly contract and then dilate and contract alternately until they adapt themselves to the light. The horse does not swerve when a feint to strike is made unless the hand causes a current of air. The ears are held erect, turn quickly toward any noise, and the horse steps high to avoid stumbling over objects which it can not see.

Treatment is only useful when the disease is symptomatic of some removable cause, like congested brain, overloaded stomach, or gravid womb. When recovery does not follow the termination of these conditions, apply a blister behind the ear and give one-half dram doses of nux vomica daily.

TUMORS OF THE EYEBALL.

A variety of tumors attack the eyeball—dermoid, papillary, fatty, cystic, and melanotic—but perhaps the most frequent in the horse is encephaloid cancer. This may grow in or on the globe, the haw, the eyelid, or the bones of the orbit, and can be remedied, if at all, only by early and thorough excision. It may be distinguished from the less dangerous tumors by its softness, friability, and great vascularity, bleeding on the slightest touch, as well as by its anatomical structure.

STAPHYLOMA.

This consists in a bulging forward of the cornea at a given point by the sacculate yielding and distention of its coats, and it may be either transparent or opaque and vascular. In the last form the iris has become adherent to the back of the cornea, and the whole structure is filled with blood vessels. In the first form the bulging cornea is attenuated; in the last it may be thickened. The best treatment is by excision of a portion of the rise so as to relieve the intraocular pressure.

PARASITES IN THE EYE.

Acari in the eye have been incidentally alluded to under inflammation of the lids.

Thelaziella lacrymalis is a white worm, one-third to 1 inch long, which inhabits the lacrimal duct and the underside of the eyelids and haw in the horse, producing a verminous conjunctivitis, sometimes with corneal ulcers. The first step in treatment in such cases is to remove the worm with forceps, then treat as for external inflammation. This worm occurs in Brazil, Europe, and India.

Setaria equina is a delicate, white, silvery-looking worm, which I have repeatedly found 2 inches in length (a length as great as 5 inches has been reported). It invades the aqueous humor, where its constant active movements make it an object of great interest, and it is frequently exhibited as a "snake in the eye."[1] When present in the eye it causes inflammation and has to be removed through an incision made with the lancet in the upper border of the cornea close to the sclera, the point of the instrument being directed slightly forward to avoid injury to the iris. Then cold water or astringent antiseptic lotions should be applied.

Filaria conjunctivæ, resembling *Setaria equina* very much in size and general appearance, is another roundworm which has been found in the eye of the horse in Europe.

The echinococcus, the cystic or larval stage of the echinococcus tapeworm of the dog, has been found in the eye of the horse, and a cysticercus is also reported.

---

[1] This worm is normally a parasite of the peritoneal cavity, and is probably transmitted from one horse to another by some biting insect which becomes infected by larvæ in the blood.—M. C. HALL.

LAMENESS: ITS CAUSES AND TREATMENT.

By A. LIAUTARD, M. D., V. M.,

Formerly principal of the American Veterinary College, New York.

[Revised by John R. Mohler, A. M., V. M. D.]

It is as living, organized, locomotive machines that the horse, camel, ox, and their burden-bearing companions are of practical value to man. Hence the consideration of their usefulness and consequent value to their human masters ultimately and naturally resolves itself into an inquiry concerning the condition of that special portion of their organism which controls their function of locomotion. This is especially true in regard to the members of the equine family, the most numerous and valuable of all the beasts of burden, and it naturally follows that with the horse for a subject of discussion the special topic and leading theme of inquiry, by an easy lapse, will become an inquest into the condition and efficiency of his power for usefulness as a carrier or traveler. There is a great deal of abstract interest in the study of that endowment of the animal economy which enables its possessor to change his place at will and convey himself whithersoever his needs or his moods may incline him; how much greater, however, the interest that attaches to the subject when it becomes a practical and economic question and includes within its purview the various related topics which belong to the domains of physiology, pathology, therapeutics, and the entire round of scientific investigation into which it is finally merged as a subject for medical and surgical consideration—in a word, of actual disease and its treatment. It is not surprising that the intricate and complicated apparatus of locomotion, with its symmetry and harmony of movement and the perfection and beauty of its details and adjuncts, by students of creative design and attentive observers of nature and her marvelous contrivances and adaptations, should be admiringly denominated a living machine.

Of all the animal tribe the horse, in a state of domesticity, is the largest sharer with his master in his liability to the accidents and dangers which are among the incidents of civilized life. From his exposure to the missiles of war on the battlefield to his chance of picking up a nail from the city pavement there is no hour when he is not in danger of incurring injuries which for their repair may demand the best skill of the veterinary practitioner. This is true not alone of casualties which belong to the class of external and traumatic cases, but includes as well those of a kind perhaps more numerous, which may result in lesions of internal parts, frequently the most serious and obscure of all in their nature and effects.

The horse is too important a factor in the practical details of human life and fills too large a place in the business and pleasure of the world to justify any indifference to his needs and physical comfort or neglect in respect to the preservation of his peculiar powers for usefulness. In entering somewhat largely, therefore, upon a review of the subject, and treating in detail of the causes, the symptoms, the progress, the treatment, the results, and the consequences of lameness in the horse, we are performing a duty which needs no word of apology or justification. The subject explains and justifies itself, and is its own vindication and illustration, if any are needed.

The function of locomotion is performed by the action of two principal systems of organs, known in anatomical and physiological terminology as passive and active, the muscles performing the active and the bones the passive portion of the movement. The necessary connection between the cooperating parts of the organism is effected by means of a vital contact by which the muscle is attached to the bone at certain determinate points on the surface of the latter. These points of attachment appear sometimes as an eminence, sometimes as a depression, sometimes a border or an angle, or again as a mere roughness, but each perfectly fulfilling its purpose, while the necessary motion is provided for by the formation of the ends of the long bones into the requisite articulations, joints, or hinges. Every motion is the product of the contraction of one or more of the muscles, which, as it acts upon the bony levers, gives rise to a movement of extension or flexion, abduction or adduction, rotation or circumduction. The movement of abduction is that which passes from and that of adduction that which passes toward the median line, or the center of the body. The movements of flexion and extension are too well understood to need defining. It is the combination and rapid alterations of these movements which produce the different postures and various gaits of the animal, and it is their interruption and derangement, from whatever causes, which constitute the pathological condition known as lameness.

A concise examination of the general anatomy of these organs, however, must precede the consideration of the pathological questions pertaining to the subject. A statement, such as we have just given, containing only the briefest hint of matters which, though not necessarily in their ultimate scientific minutiæ, must be clearly comprehended in order to acquire a symmetrical and satisfactory view of the theme as a practical collation of facts to be remembered, analyzed, applied, and utilized.

It was the great Bacon who wrote: "The human body may be compared, from its complex and delicate organization, to a musical instrument of the most perfect construction, but exceedingly liable to derangement." In its degree the remark is equally applicable to the equine body, and if we would keep it in tune and profit by its harmonious action we must at least acquaint ourselves with the relations of its parts and the mode of their cooperation.

ANATOMY.

The bones, then, are the hard organs which in their connection and totality constitute the skeleton of an animal (see Plate XXIII). They are of various forms, three of which—the long, the flat, and the small—are recognized in the extremities. These are more or less regular in their form, but present upon their surfaces a variety of aspects, exhibiting in turn, according to the requirement of each case, a roughened or smooth surface, variously marked with grooves, crests, eminences, and depressions, for the necessary muscular attachments, and, as before mentioned, are connected by articulations and joints, of which some are immovable and others movable.

The substance of the bone is composed of a mass of combined earthy and animal matter surrounded by a fine, fibrous enveloping membrane (the periosteum) which is intimately adherent to the external surface of the bone, and is, in fact, the secreting membrane of the bony structure. The bony tissue proper is of two consistencies, the external portion being hard and " compact," and called by the latter term, while the internal, known as the " spongy " or " areolar tissue," corresponds to the descriptive terms. Those of the bones that possess this latter consistency contain also, in their spongy portion, the medullary substance known as marrow, which is deposited in large quantities in the interior of the long bones, and especially where a central cavity exists, called, for that reason, the medullary cavity. The nourishment of the bones is effected by means of what is known as the nutrient foramen, an opening established for the passage of the blood vessels which convey the nourishment necessary to the interior of the organ. Concerning the nourishment of the skeleton, there are other minutiæ, such as the venous arrangement and the classification of their arterial vessels into several orders, which, though of interest as an abstract study, are not of sufficient practical value to refer to here.

The active organs of locomotion, the muscles (see Plate XXIII), speaking generally, form the fleshy covering of the external part of the skeleton and surround the bones of the extremities. They vary greatly in shape and size, being flat, triangular, long, short, or broad, and are variously and capriciously named, some from their shape, some from their situation, others from their use; and thus we have abductors and adductors—the pyramidal, orbicular, the digastricus, the vastus, and so on. Those which are under the control of the will, known as the voluntary muscles, appear in the form of fleshy structures, red in color, and with fibers of various degrees of fineness, and are composed of fasciculi, or bundles of fibers, united by connective or cellular tissue, each fasciculus being composed of smaller ones but united in a similar manner to compose the larger formations, each of which is enveloped by a structure of similar nature known as the sarcolemma. Many of the muscles are united to the bones by the direct contact of their fleshy fibers, but in other instances the body of the muscle is more or less gradually transformed into a cordy or membranous structure known as the tendon or sinew, and the attachment is made by the very short fibrous threads through the medium of a long tendinous band, which, passing from a single one to several others of the bones, effects its object at a point far distant from its original attachment. In thus carrying its action from one bone to another, or from one region of a limb to another, these tendons must necessarily have smooth surfaces over which to glide, either upon the bones themselves or formed at their articulations, and this need is supplied by the secretion of the synovial fluid, a yellowish, unctuous substance, furnished by a peculiar tendinous synovial sac designed for the purpose.

Illustrations in point of the agency of the synovial fluid in assisting the sliding movements of the tendons may be found under their various forms at the shoulder joint, at the upper part of the bone of the arm, at the posterior part of the knee joint, and also at the fetlocks, on their posterior part.

As the tendons, whether singly or in company with others, pass over these natural pulleys they are retained in place by strong, fibrous bands or sheaths, which are by no means exempt from danger of injury, as will be readily inferred from a consideration of their important special use as supports and reenforcements of the tendons themselves, with which they must necessarily share the stress of whatever force or strain is brought to bear upon both or either.

We have referred to that special formation of the external surface of a bone by which it is adapted to form a joint or articulation, either movable or fixed, and a concise examination of the formation and structure of the movable articulations will here be in place. These are formed generally by the extremities of the long bones, or may exist on the surfaces of the short ones. The points or regions where the contact occurs are denominated the articular surface, which assumes from this circumstance a considerable variety of aspect and form, being in one case comparatively flat and another elevated; or as forming a protruding head or knob, with a distinct convexity; and again presenting a corresponding depression or cavity, accurately adapted to complete, by their coaptation, the ball-and-socket joint. The articulation of the arm and shoulder is an example of the first kind, while that of the hip with the thigh bone is a perfect exhibition of the latter.

The structure whose office it is to retain the articulating surfaces in place is the ligament. This is usually a white, fibrous, inelastic tissue; sometimes, however, it is elastic in character and yellowish. In some instances it is funicular shaped or corded, serving to bind more firmly together the bones to which its extremities are attached; in others it consists of a broad membrane, wholly or partially surrounding the broad articulations, and calculated rather for the protection of the cavity from intrusion by the air than for other security. This latter form, known as capsular, is usually found in connection with joints which possess a free and extended movement. The capsular and funicular ligaments are sometimes associated, the capsular appearing as a membranous sac wholly or partially inclosing the joint, the funicular, here known as an interarticular ligament, occupying the interior, and thus securing the union of the several bones more firmly and effectively than would be possible for the capsular ligament unassisted.

The universal need which pertains to all mechanical contrivances of motion has not been forgotten while providing for the perfect working of the interesting piece of living machinery which performs the function of locomotion, as we are contemplating it, and nature has consequently provided for obviating the evils of attrition and friction and insuring the easy play and smooth movement of its parts by the establishment of the secretion of the synovia, the vital lubricant of which we have before spoken, as a yellow, oily, or rather glairy secretion, which performs the indispensable office of facilitating the play of the tendons over the joints and certain given points of the bones. This fluid is deposited in a containing sac, the lining (serous) membrane of which forms the secreting organ. This membrane is of an excessively sensitive nature, and while it lines the inner face of the ligaments, both capsular and fascicular, it is attached only upon the edges of the bones, without extending upon their length, or between the layers of cartilage which lie between the bones and their articular surfaces.

Our object in thus partially and concisely reviewing the structure and condition of the essential organs of locomotion has been rather to outline a sketch which may serve as a reference chart of the general features of the subject than to offer a minute description of the parts referred to. Other points of interest will receive proper attention as we proceed with the illustration of our subject and examine the matters which it most concerns us to bring under consideration. The foundation of facts which we have thus far prepared will be found sufficiently broad, we trust, to include whatever may be necessary to insure a ready comprehension of the essential matters which are to follow as our review is carried forward to completion. What we have said touching these elementary truths will probably be sufficient to facilitate a clear understanding of the requirements essential to the perfection and regularity which characterize the normal performance of the various movements that result in the accomplishment of the action of locomotion. So long as the bones, the muscles and their tendons, the joints with their cartilages, their ligaments, and their synovial structure, the nerves and the controlling influences which they exercise over all, with the blood vessels which distribute to every part, however minute, the vitalizing fluid which sustains the whole fabric in being and activity—so long as these various constituents and adjuncts of animal life preserve their normal exemption from disease, traumatism, and pathological change, the function of locomotion will continue to be performed with perfection and efficiency.

On the other hand, let any element of disease become implanted in one or several of the parts destined for combined action, any change or irregularity of form, dimensions, location, or action occur in any portion of the apparatus—any obstruction or misdirection of vital power take place, any interference with the order of the phenomena of normal nature, any loss of harmony and lack of balance be betrayed—and we have in the result the condition of lameness.

DEFINITION OF LAMENESS.

Physiology.—Comprehensively and universally considered, then, the term lameness signifies any irregularity or derangement of the function of locomotion, irrespective of the cause which produced it or the degree of its manifestation. However slightly or severely it may be exhibited, it is all the same. The nicest observation may be demanded for its detection, and it may need the most thoroughly trained powers of discernment to identify and locate it, as in cases in which the animal is said to be fainting, tender, or to go sore. On the contrary, the patient may be so far affected as to refuse utterly to use an injured leg, and under compulsory motion keep it raised from the ground, and prefer to travel on three legs rather than to bear any portion of his weight upon the afflicted member. In these two extremes, and in all the intermediate degrees, the patient is simply lame— pathognomonic minutiæ being considered and settled in a place of their own.

This last condition of disabled function—lameness on three legs—and many of the lower degrees of simple lameness are very easy of detection, but the first, or mere tenderness or soreness, may be very difficult to identify, and at times very serious results have followed from the obscurity which has enveloped the early stages of the malady. For it may easily occur that in the absence of the treatment which an early correct diagnosis would have indicated, an insidious ailment may so take advantage of the lapse of time as to root itself too deeply into the economy to be subverted, and become transformed into a disabling chronic case, or possibly one that is incurable and fatal. Hence the impolicy of depreciating early symptoms because they are not accompanied with distinct and pronounced characteristics, and from a lack of threatening appearances inferring the absence of danger. The possibilities of an ambush can never be safely ignored. An extra caution costs nothing, even if wasted. The fulfillment of the first duty of a practitioner, when introduced to a case, is not always an easy task, though it is too frequently expected that the diagnosis, or "what is the matter" verdict, will be reached by the quickest and surest kind of an "instantaneous process" and a sure prognosis, or "how will it end," guessed at instanter.

Usually the discovery that the animal is becoming lame is comparatively an easy matter to a careful observer. Such a person will readily note the changes of movements which will have taken place in the animal he has been accustomed to drive or ride, unless they are indeed slight and limited to the last degree. But what is not always easy is the detection, after discovering the fact of an existing irregularity, of the locality of its point of origin, and whether its seat be in the near or off leg, or in the fore or the hind part of the body. These are questions too often wrongly answered, notwithstanding the fact that with a little careful scrutiny the point may be easily settled. The error, which is too often committed, of pronouncing the leg upon which the animal travels soundly as the seat of the lameness, is the result of a misinterpretation of the physiology of locomotion in the crippled animal. Much depends upon the gait with which the animal moves while under examination. The act of walking is unfavorable for accurate observation, though, if the animal walks on three legs, the decision is easy to reach. The action of galloping will often, by the rapidity of the muscular movements and their quick succession, interfere with a nice study of their rhythm, and it is only under some peculiar circumstances that the examination can be safely conducted while the animal is moving with that gait. It is while the animal is trotting that the investigation is made with the best chances of an intelligent decision, and it is while moving with that gait, therefore, that the points should be looked for which must form the elements of the diagnosis.

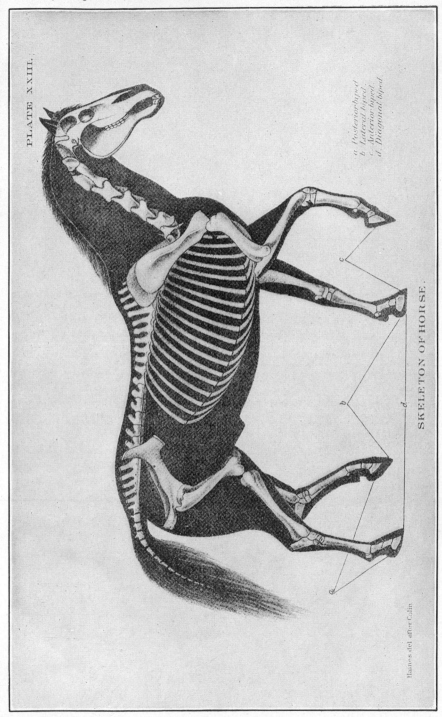

PLATE XXIII.

a. Posterior biped.
b. Lateral biped.
c. Anterior biped.
d. Diagonal biped.

SKELETON OF HORSE.

Hanes del after Colin

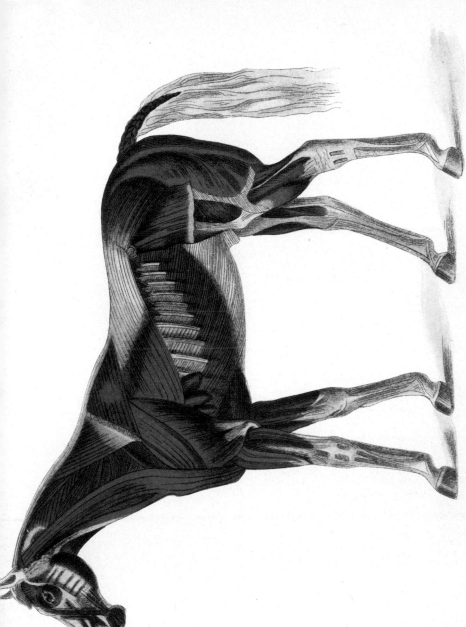

SUPERFICIAL LAYER OF MUSCLES.

Haines, after Mégnin.

Our first consideration should be the physiology of normal or healthy locomotion, that thence we may the more easily reach our conclusions touching lameness, or that which is abnormal, and by this process we ought to succeed in obtaining a clew to the solution of the first problem, to wit, in which leg is the seat of the lameness?

A word of definition is here necessary, in order to render that which follows more easily intelligible. In veterinary nomenclature each two of the legs, as referred to in pairs, is denominated a biped. Of the four points occupied by the feet of the animal while standing at rest, forming a square, the two fore legs are known as the anterior biped; the two hinder, the posterior; the two on one side, the lateral; and one of either the front or hind biped with the opposite leg of the hind or front biped will form the diagonal biped.

Considering, as it is proper to do, that in a condition of health each separate biped and each individual leg is required to perform an equal and uniform function and to carry an even or equal portion of the weight of the body, it will be readily appreciated that the result of this distribution will be a regular, evenly balanced, and smooth displacement of the body thus supported by the four legs, and that therefore, according to the rapidity of the motion in different gaits, each single leg will be required at certain successive moments to bear the weight which had rested upon its congener while it was itself in the air, in the act of moving; or, again, two different legs of a biped may be called upon to bear the weight of the two legs of the opposite biped while also in the air in the act of moving.

To simplify the matter by an illustration, the weight of an animal may be placed at 1,000 pounds, of which each leg, in a normal and healthy condition, supports while at rest 250 pounds. When one of the fore legs is in action, or in the air, and carrying no weight, its 250 pounds share of the weight will be thrown upon its congener, or partner, to sustain. If the two legs of a biped are both in action and raised from the ground, their congeners, still resting in inaction, will carry the total weight of the other two, or 500 pounds. And as the succession of movements continues, and the change from one leg to another or from one biped to another, as may be required by the gait, proceeds, there will result a smooth, even, and equal balancing of active movements, shifting the weight from one leg or one biped to another, with symmetrical precision, and we shall be presented with an interesting example of the play of vital machanics in a healthy organization.

Much may be learned from the accurate study of the action of a single leg. Normally, its movements will be without variation or failure. When at rest it will easily sustain the weight assigned to it without showing hesitancy or betraying pain, and when it is raised from the ground in order to transfer the weight to its mate it will perform the act in such manner that when it is again placed upon the ground to rest it will be with a firm tread, indicative of its ability to receive again the burden to be thrown back upon it. In planting it upon the ground or raising it again for the forward movement while in action, and again replanting it upon the earth, each movement will be the same for each leg and for each biped, whether the act is that of walking or trotting, or even of galloping. In short, the regular play of every part of the apparatus will testify to the existence of that condition of orderly soundness and efficient activity eloquently suggestive of the condition of vital integrity which is simply but comprehensively expressed by the terms health and soundness.

But let some change, though slight and obscure, occur among the elements of the case; some invisible agency of evil intrude among the harmonizing processes going forward; any disorder occur in the relations of cooperating parts; anything appear to neutralize the efficiency of vitalizing forces; any disability of a limb to accept and to throw back upon its mate the portion of the weight which belongs to it to sustain—present itself, whether as the effect of accident or otherwise; in short, let anything develop which tends to defeat the purpose of nature in organizing the locomotive apparatus and we are confronted at once by that which may be looked upon as a cause of lameness.

Not the least of the facts which it is important to remember is that it is not sufficient to look for the manifestation of an existing discordance in the action of the affected limb alone, but that it is shared by the sound one and must be searched for in that as well as the halting member, if the hazard of an error is to be avoided. The mode of action of the leg which is the seat of the lameness will vary greatly from that which it exhibited when in a healthy condition, and the sound leg will also offer important modifications in the same three particulars before alluded to, to wit, that of resting on the ground, that of its elevation and forward motion, and that of striking the ground again when the full action of stepping is accomplished. Inability in the lame leg to sustain weight will imply excessive exertion by the sound one, and lack of facility or disposition to rest the lame member on the ground will necessitate a longer continuance of that action on the sound side. Changes in the act of elevating the leg, or of carrying it forward, or in both, will present entirely opposite conditions between the two. The lame member will be elevated rapidly, moved carefully forward, and returned to the ground with caution and hesitancy, and the contact with the earth will be effected as lightly as possible, while the sound limb will rest longer on the ground, move boldly and rapidly forward, and strike the ground promptly and forcibly. All this is due to the fact that the sound member carries more than its normal, healthy share of the weight of the body, a share which may be in excess from 1 to 250 pounds, and thus bring its burden to a figure varying from 251 to 500 pounds, all depending upon the degree of the existing lameness, whether it is simply a slight tenderness or soreness, or whether the trouble has reached a stage which compels the patient to the awkwardness of traveling on three legs.

That all this is not mere theory, but rests on a foundation of fact may be established by observing the manifestations attending a single alteration in the balancing of the body. In health the support and equilibrium of that mass of the body which is borne by the fore legs is equalized and passes by regular alternations from the right to the left side and vice versa. But if the left leg, becoming disabled, relieves itself by leaning, as it were, on the right, the latter becomes, consequently, practically heavier and the mass of the body will incline or settle upon that side. Lameness of the left side, therefore, means dropping or settling on the right and vice versa. We emphasize this statement and insist upon it, the more from the frequency of the instances of error which have come under our notice, in which persons have insisted upon their view that the leg which is the seat of the lameness is that upon which he drops and which the animal is usually supposed to favor.

HOW TO DETECT THE SEAT OF LAMENESS.

Properly appreciating the remarks which have preceded, and fully comprehending the modus operandi and the true pathology of lameness, but little remains to be done in order to reach an answer to the question as to which side of the animal is the seat of the lameness, except to examine the patient while in action. We have already stated our reasons for preferring the movement of trotting for this purpose. In conducting such an examination the animal should be unblanketed, and held by a plain halter in the hands of a man who knows how to manage his paces, and the trial should always be made over a firm, hard road whenever it is available. He is to be examined from various positions—from before, from behind, and from each side. Watching him as he approaches, as he passes by, and as he recedes, the observer should carefully study that important action which we have spoken of as the dropping of the body upon one extremity or the other, and this can readily be detected by attending closely to the motions of the head and of the hip. The head drops on the same side on which the mass of the body will fall, dropping toward the right when the lameness is in the left fore leg, and the hip dropping in posterior lameness, also on the sound leg, the reversal of the conditions, of course, producing reversed effects. In other words, when the animal in trotting exhibits signs of irregularity of action, or lameness, and this irregularity is accompanied with dropping or nodding the head, or depressing the hip on the right side of the body, at the time the feet of the right side strike the ground, the horse is lame on the left side. If the dropping and nodding are on the near side the lameness is on the off side.

In a majority of cases, however, the answer to the first question relating to the lameness of a horse is, after all, not a very difficult task. There are two other problems in the case more difficult of solution and which often require the exercise of a closer scrutiny, and draw upon all the resources of the experienced practitioner to settle satisfactorily. That a horse is lame in a given leg may be easily determined, but when it becomes necessary to pronounce upon the query as to what part, what region, what structure is affected, the easy part of the task is over, and the more difficult and important, because more obscure, portion of the investigation has commenced—except, of course, in cases of which the features are too distinctly evident to the senses to admit of error. It is true that by carefully noting the manner in which a lame leg is performing its functions, and closely scrutinizing the motions of the whole extremity, and especially of the various joints which enter into its structure; by minutely examining every part of the limb; by observing the outlines; by testing the change, if any, in temperature and the state of the sensibility—all these investigations may guide the surgeon to a correct localization of the seat of trouble, but he must carefully refrain from the adoption of a hasty conclusion, and, above all, assure himself that he has not failed to make the foot, of all the organs of the horse the most liable to injury and lesion, the subject of the most thorough and minute examination of all the parts which compose the suffering extremity.

The greater liability of the foot than of any other part of the extremities to injury from casualties, natural to its situation and use, should always suggest the beginning of an inquiry, especially in an obscure case of lameness at that point. Indeed the lameness may have an apparent location elsewhere when that is the true seat of the trouble, and the surgeon who, while examining his lame patient, discovers a ringbone, and convincing himself that he has encountered the cause of the disordered action suspends his investigation without subjecting the foot to a close scrutiny, at a later day when regrets will avail nothing, may deeply regret his neglect and inadvertence. As in human pathological experience, however, there are instances when inscrutable diseases will deliver their fatal messages, while leaving no mark and making no sign by which they might be identified and classified, so it will happen that in the humbler animals the onset and progress of mysterious and unrecognizable ailments will at times baffle the most skilled veterinarian, and leave our burden-bearing servants to succumb to the inevitable, and suffer and perish in unrelieved distress.

DISEASES OF BONES.

PERIOSTITIS, OSTITIS, AND EXOSTOSIS.

From the closeness and intimacy of the connection existing between the two principal elements of the bony structure while in health, it frequently becomes exceedingly difficult, when a state of disease has supervened, to discriminate accurately as to the part primarly affected and to determine positively whether the periosteum or the body of the bone is originally implicated. Yet a knowledge of the fact is often of the first importance, in order to obtain a favorable result from the treatment to be instituted. It is, however, quite evident that in a majority of instances the bony growths which so frequently appear on the surface of their structure, to which the general term of exostosis is applied, have had their origin in an inflammation of the periosteum, or enveloping membrane, and known as periostitis. However this may be, we have as a frequent result, sometimes on the body of the bone, sometimes at the extremities, and sometimes involving the articulation itself, certain bony growths, or exostoses, known otherwise by the term of splint, ringbone, and spavin, all of which, in an important sense, may be finally referred to the periosteum as their nutrient source and support, at least after their formation, if not for their incipient existence.

Cause.—It is certain that inflammation of the periosteum is frequently referable to wounds and bruises caused by external agencies, and it is also true that it may possibly result from the spreading inflammation of surrounding diseased tissues, but in any case the result is uniformly seen in the deposit of a bony growth, more or less diffuse, sometimes of irregular outline, and at others projecting distinctly from the surface from which it springs, as so commonly presented in the ringbone and the spavin.

Symptoms.—This condition of periostitis is often difficult to determine. The signs of inflammation are so obscure, the swelling of the parts so insignificant, any increase of heat so imperceptible, and the soreness so slight, that even the most acute observer may fail to find the point of its existence, and it is often long after the discovery of the disease itself that its location is positively revealed by the visible presence of the exostosis. Yet the first question had been resolved, in discovering the fact of the lameness, while the second and third remained unanswered, and the identification of the affected limb and the point of origin of the trouble remained unknown until their palpable revelation to the senses.

Treatment.—When, by careful scrutiny, the ailment has been located, a resort to treatment must be had at once, in order to prevent, if possible, any further deposit of the calcareous structure and increase of the exostotic growth. With this view the application of water, either warm or cold, rendered astringent by the addition of alum or sugar of lead, will be beneficial. The tendency to the formation of the bony growth, and the increase of its development after its actual formation, may often be checked by the application of a severe blister of Spanish fly. The failure of these means and the establishment of the diseased process in the form of chronic periostitis cause various changes in the bone covered by the disordered membrane, and the result may be softening, degeneration, or necrosis, but more usually it is followed by the formation of the bony growths referred to, on the cannon bone, the coronet, the hock, etc.

SPLINTS.

We first turn our attention to the splint, as certain bony enlargements that are developed on the cannon bone, between the knee or the hock and the fetlock joint, are called. (See Plate XXV.) They are found on the inside of the leg, from the knee, near which they are frequently found, downward to about the lower third of the principal cannon bone. They are of various dimensions, and are readily perceptible both to the eye and to the touch. They vary considerably in size, ranging from that of a large nut downward to very small proportions. In searching for them they may be readily detected by the hand if they have attained sufficient development in their usual situation, but must be distinguished from a small, bony enlargement that may be felt at the lower third of the cannon bone, which is neither a splint nor a pathological formation of any kind, but merely the buttonlike enlargement at the lower extremity of the small metacarpal or splint bone.

We have said that splints are to be found on the inside of the leg. This is true as a general statement, but it is not invariably so, for they occasionally appear on the outside. It is also true that they appear most commonly on the fore legs, but this is not exclusively the case, because they may at times be found on both the inside and outside of the hind leg. Usually a splint forms only a true exostosis, or a single bony growth, with a somewhat diffuse base, but neither is this invariably the case. In some instances they assume more important dimensions, and pass from the inside to the outside of the bone, on its posterior face, between that and the suspensory ligament. This form is termed the pegged splint, and constitutes a serious and permanent deformity, in consequence of its interference with the play of the fibrous cord which passes behind it, becoming thus a source of continual irritation and consequently of permanent lameness.

Symptoms.—A splint may thus frequently become a cause of lameness though not necessarily in every instance, but it is a lameness possessing features peculiar to itself. It is not always continuous, but at times assumes an intermittent character, and is more marked when the animal is warm than when cool. If the lameness is near the kneejoint, it is very liable to become aggravated when the animal is put to work, and the gait acquires then a peculiar character, arising from the manner in which the limb is carried outward from the knees downward, which is done by a kind of abduction of the lower part of the leg. Other symptoms, however, than the lameness and the presence of the splint, which is its cause, may be looked for in the same connection as those which have been mentioned as pertaining to certain evidences of periostitis, in the increase of the temperature of the part, with swelling and probably pain on pressure. This last symptom is of no little importance, since its presence or absence has in many cases formed the determining point in deciding a question of difficult diagnosis.

Cause.—A splint being one of the results of periostitis, and the latter one of the effects of external hurts, it naturally follows that the parts which are most exposed to blows and collisions will be those on which the splint will most commonly be found, and it may not be improper, therefore, to refer to hurts from without as among the common causes of the lesion. But other causes may also be productive of the evil, and among these may be mentioned the overstraining of an immature organism by the imposition of excessive labor upon a young animal at a too early period of his life. The bones which enter into the formation of the cannon are three in number, one large and two smaller, which, during the youth of the animal, are more or less articulated, with a limited amount of mobility, but which become in maturity firmly joined by a rigid union and ossification of their interarticular surface. If the immature animal is compelled, then, to perform exacting tasks beyond his strength, the inevitable result will follow in the muscular straining, and perhaps tearing asunder of the fibers which unite the bones at their points of juncture, and it is difficult to understand how inflammation or periostitis can fail to develop as the natural consequence of such local irritation. If the result were deliberately and intelligently designed, it could hardly be more effectually accomplished.

The splint is an object of the commonest occurrence—so common, indeed, that in large cities a horse which can not exhibit one or more specimens upon some portion of his extremities is one of the rarest of spectacles. Though it is in some instances a cause of lameness, and its discovery and cure are sometimes beyond the ability of the shrewdest and most experienced veterinarians, yet as a source of vital danger to the general equine organization, or even of functional disturbance, or of practical inconvenience, aside from the rare exceptional cases which exist as mere samples of possibility, it can not be considered to belong to the category of serious lesions. The worst stigma that attaches to it is that in general estimation it is ranked among eyesores and continues indefinitely to be that and nothing different. The inflammation in which they originated, acute at first, either subsides or assumes the chronic form, and the bony growth becomes a permanence—more or less established, it is true, but doing no positive harm and not hindering the animal from continuing his daily routine of labor. All this, however, requires a proviso against the occurrence of a subsequent acute attack, when, as with other exostoses, a fresh access of acute symptoms may be followed by a new pathological activity, which shall again develop, as a natural result, a reappearance of the lameness.

Treatment.—It is, of course, the consideration of the comparative harmlessness of splints that suggests and justifies the policy of noninterference, except as they become a positive cause of lameness. And a more positive argument for such noninterference consists in the fact that any active and irritating treatment may so excite the parts as to bring about a renewed pathological activity, which may result in a reduplication of the phenomena, with a second edition, if not a second and enlarged volume, of the whole story. For our part, our faith is firm in the impolicy of interference, and this faith is founded on an experience of many years, during which our practice has been that of abstention.

Of course, there will be exceptional conditions which will at times indicate a different course. These will become evident when the occasions present themselves, and extraordinary forms and effects of inflammation and growth in the tumors offer special indications. But our conviction remains unshaken that surgical treatment of the operative kind is usually useless, if not dangerous. We have little faith in the method of extirpation except under very special conditions, among which that of diminutive size has been named; this seems in itself to constitute a sufficient negative argument. Even in such a case a resort to the knife or the gouge could scarcely find a justification, since no operative procedure is ever without a degree of hazard, to say nothing of the considerations which are always forcibly negative in any question of the infliction of pain and the unnecessary use of the knife.

If an acute periostitis of the cannon bone has been readily discovered, the treatment we have already suggested for that ailment is at once indicated, and the astringent lotions may be relied upon to bring about beneficial results. Sometimes, however, preference may be given to a lotion possessing a somewhat different quality, the alterative consisting of tincture of iodin applied to the inflamed spot

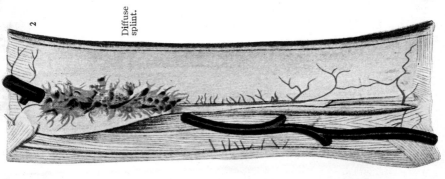

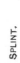

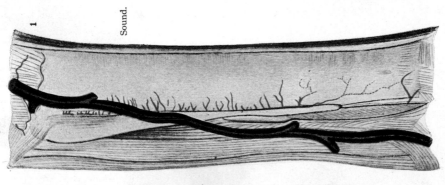

4

Simple
splint.

ZEESE-WILKINSON CO., INC., N.Y.

3

Simple
splint.

2

Diffuse
splint.

1

Sound.

SPLINT.

Haines, Nos. 1, 2 and 3, from Auzoux model. No. 4, Original.

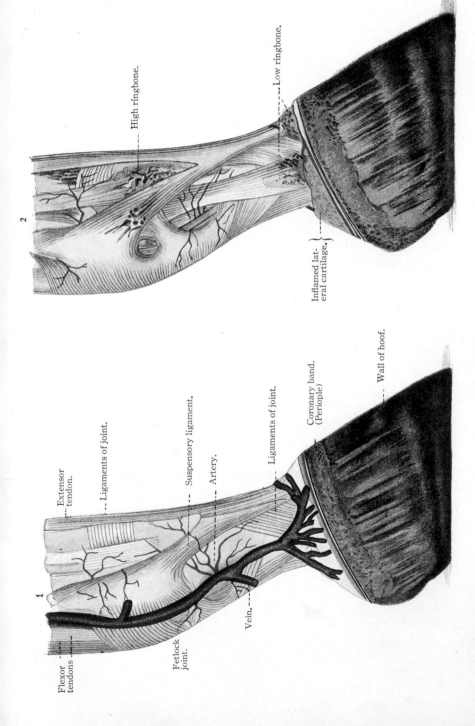

ZEESE-WILKINSON CO., INC., N.Y

RINGBONE.

High ringbone.

Low ringbone.

Inflamed lateral cartilage.

Extensor tendon.

Ligaments of joint.

Suspensory ligament.

Artery.

Ligaments of joint.

Coronary band. (Periople)

Wall of hoof.

Flexor tendons

Fetlock joint.

Vein.

SOUND FOOT.

Haines, from Auzoux Model.

PLATE XXVII.

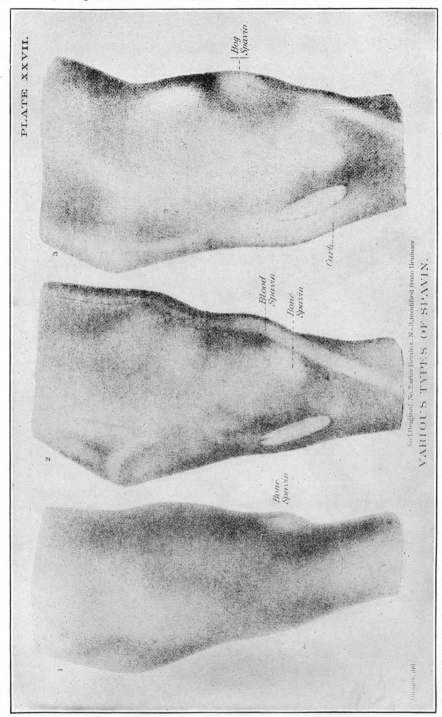

Bog
Spavin.

Blood
Spavin.

Bone
Spavin.

Curb.

Bone
Spavin.

No. 1 Original. No. 2 after Berdez. No. 3, modified from Reubner.

VARIOUS TYPES OF SPAVIN.

Haues, del.

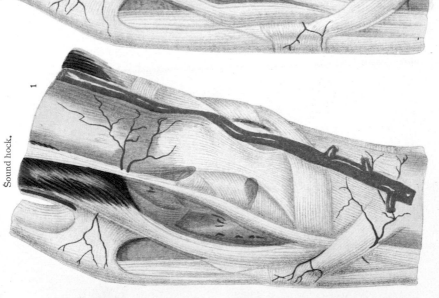

3

Badly spavined hock.

Spavin.

Haines.

ZEESE-WILKINSON CO., INC., N.Y.

2

Spavined hock.

Blood spavin.

Spavin.

BONE SPAVIN. HOCKS, WITH SKIN REMOVED.

1

Sound hock.

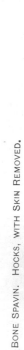

Haines, from Auzoux model.

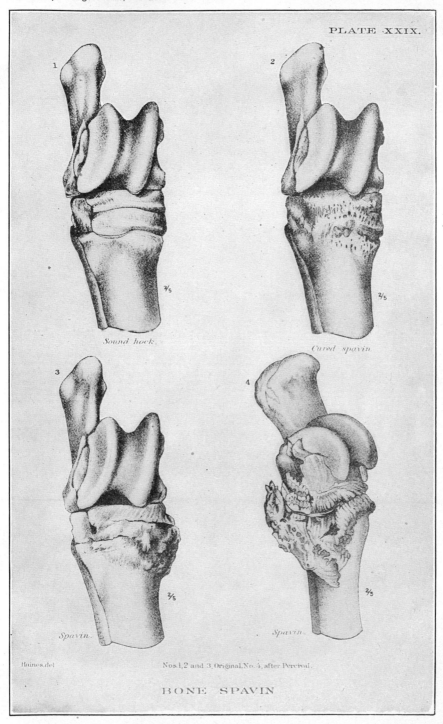

PLATE XXIX.

Sound hock.

Cured spavin.

Spavin.

Spavin.

Haines.del

Nos. 1, 2 and 3, Original, No. 4, after Percival.

BONE SPAVIN

several times daily. If the lameness persists under this mild course of treatment, it must, of course, be attacked by other methods, and we must resort to the cantharides ointment or Spanish-fly blister, as we have before recommended. Besides this, and producing an analogous effect, the compounds of biniodid of mercury are favored by some. It is prepared in the form of an ointment, consisting of 1 dram of the biniodid to 1 ounce of either lard or vaseline. It forms an excellent blistering and alterative application, and is of special advantage in newly formed or recently discovered exostosis.

It remains a pertinent query, however, and one which seems to be easily answered, whether a tumor so diminutive in size that it can be detected only by diligent search, and which is neither a disfigurement nor an obstruction to the motion of the limb, need receive any recognition whatever. Other modes of treatment for splints are recommended and practiced which belong strictly to the domain of operative veterinary surgery; among these are to be reckoned actual cauterization, or the application of the fire iron and the operation of periosteotomy. These are frequently indicated in the treatment of splints which have resisted milder means.

The mode of the development of their growth; their intimacy, greater or less, with both the large and the small cannon bones; the possibility of their extending to the back of these bones under the suspensory ligament; the dangerous complications which may follow the rough handling of the parts, with also a possibility, and, indeed, a probability, of their return after removal—these are the considerations which have influenced our judgment in discarding from our practice and our approval the method of removal by the saw or the chisel, as recommended by certain European veterinarians.

RINGBONES.

Ringbone is the designation of the exostosis which is found on the coronet and in the digital and phalangeal regions. (See Plate XXVI.) The name is appropriate, because the growth extends quite around the coronet, which it encircles in the manner of a ring, or perhaps because it often forms upon the back of that bone a regular osseous arch, through which the back tendons obtain a passage. The places where these growths are usually developed have caused their subdivision and classification into three varieties, with the designations of high, middle, and low, though much can be said as to the importance of the distinction. It is true that the ringbone or phalangeal exostosis may be found at various points on the foot, in one case forming a large bunch on the upper part and quite close to the fetlock joint; in another around the upper border of the hoof, or perhaps on the extreme front or on the very back of the coronet. The shape in which they commonly appear is favorable to their easy discovery, their form when near the fetlock usually varying too much from the natural outlines of the part when compared with those of the opposite side to admit of error in the matter. (See also page 439.)

A ringbone, when on the front of the foot, even when not very largely developed, assumes the form of a diffused convex swelling. If situated on the lower part, it will form a thick ring, encircling that portion of the foot immediately above the hoof; when found on the posterior part, a small, sharp osseous growth somewhat project-ing, sometimes on the inside and sometimes on the outside of the coronet, may comprise the entire manifestation.

Cause.—As with splints, ringbones may result from severe labor in early life, before the process of ossification has been fully perfected; or they may be referred to bruises, blows, sprains, or other violence; injuries of tendons, ligaments, or joints also may be among the accountable causes.

It is certain that they may commonly be traced to diseases and traumatic lesions of the foot, and their appearance may be reason-ably expected among the sequalæ of an abscess of the coronet; or the cause may be a severe contusion resulting from calking, or a deep-punctured wound from picking up a nail or stepping upon any hard object of sufficiently irregular form to penetrate the sole.

Moreover, a ringbone may originate in heredity. This is a fact of no little importance in its relation to questions connected with the extensive interests of the stock breeder and purchaser.

That the hereditary transmission of constitutional idiosyncrasies is an active cause with regard to diseases in general, it would be absurd to assert, but we do say that a predisposition to contract ringbone through faulty conformation, such as long, thin pasterns with narrow joints and steep fetlocks, may be inherited in many cases, and in a smaller proportion of cases this predisposition may act as a secondary cause in the formation of ringbone.

The importance of this point when considered in reference to the policy which should be observed in the selection of breeding stock is obvious, and, as the whole matter is within the control of the owners and breeders, it will be their own fault if the unchecked transmission of ringbones from one equine generation to another is allowed to continue. It is our belief that among the diseases which are known for their tendency to perpetuate and repeat themselves by individual succession, those of the bony structures stand first, and the inference from such fact which would exclude every ani-mal of doubtful soundness in its osseous apparatus from the stud list and the brood farm is too plain for argument.

Symptoms.—Periostitis of the phalanges is an ailment requiring careful exploration and minute inspection for its discovery, and is very liable to result in a ringbone of which lameness is the result.

The mode of its manifestation varies according to the state of development of the diseased growth as affected by the circumstances of its location and dimensions. It is commonly of the kind which, in consequence of its intermittent character, is termed lameness when cool, having the peculiarity of exhibiting itself when the animal starts from the stable and of diminishing, if not entirely disappearing after some distance of travel, to return to its original degree, if not indeed a severer one, when he has again cooled off in his stable. The size of the ringbone does not indicate the degree to which it cripples the patient, but the position may, especially when it interferes with the free movement of the tendons which pass behind and in front of the foot. While a large ringbone will often interfere but little with the motion of the limb, a smaller growth, if situated under the tendon, may become the cause of considerable and continued pain.

A ringbone is doubtless a worse evil than a splint. Its growth, its location, its tendency to increased development, its exposure to the influence of causes of renewed danger, all tend to impart an unfavorable cast to the prognosis of a case and to emphasize the importance and the value of an early discovery of its presence and possible growth. Even when the discovery has been made, it is often the case that the truth has come to light too late for effectual treatment. Months may have elapsed after the first manifestation of the lameness before a discovery has been made of the lesion from which it has originated, and there is no recall for the lapsed time. And by the uncompromising seriousness of the discouraging prognosis must the energy and severity of the treatment and the promptness of its administration be measured. The periostitis has been overlooked; any chance that might have existed for preventing its advance to the chronic stage has been lost; the osseous formation is established; the ringbone is a fixed fact, and the indications are urgent and pressing.

Treatment.—The preventive treatment consists in keeping colts well nourished and in trimming the hoof and shoeing to balance the foot properly and thus prevent an abnormal strain on the ligaments. Even after the ringbone has developed, a cure may sometimes be occasioned by proper shoeing directed toward straightening the axis of the foot as viewed from the side by making the wall of the hoof from the coronet to the toe continuous with the line formed by the front of the pastern. So long as inflammation of the periosteum and ligaments remains, a sharp blister of biniodid of mercury and cantharides may do good if the animal is allowed to rest for four or five weeks. If this fails, some success may be accomplished by point firing in two or three lines over the ringbone. It is necessary to touch the hot iron well into the bone, as superficial firing does little good. When all these measures have failed to remove the lameness, or when the animal is not worth a long and uncertain treatment, a competent veterinarian should be engaged to perform double neurectomy, high or low, of the plantar nerves, or neurectomy of the median nerve as indicated by the seat of the lesion.

SIDEBONES.

On each side of the bone of the hoof—the coffinbone—there are normally two supplementary organs which are called the cartilages of the foot. They are soft, and though in a degree elastic, yet somewhat resisting, and are implanted on the lateral wings of the coffinbone. Evidently their office is to assist in the elastic expansion and contraction of the posterior part of the hoof, and their healthy and normal action doubtless contributes in an important degree to the perfect performance of the functions of that part of the leg. These organs are, however, liable to undergo a process of disease which results in an entire change in their properties, if not in their shape, by which they acquire a character of hardness resulting from the deposit of earthy substance in the intimate structure of the cartilage, and it is this change, when its consummation has been effected, that brings to our cognizance the diseased growth which has received the designation of sidebones. They are situated on one or both sides of the leg, bulging above the superior border of the hoof in the form of two hard bodies composed of ossified cartilage, irregularly square in shape and unyielding under the pressure of the fingers.

Cause.—Sidebones may be the result of a low inflammatory condition or of an acute attack as well, or may be caused by sprains, bruises, or blows; or they may have their rise in certain diseases affecting the foot proper, such as corns, quarter cracks, or quittor. The deposit of calcareous matter in the cartilage is not always uniform, the base of that organ near its line of union with the coffinbone being in some cases its limit, while at other times it is diffused throughout its substance, the size and prominence of the growth varying much in consequence.

Symptoms.—It would naturally be inferred that the degree of interference with the proper functions of the hoof which must result from such a pathological change would be proportioned to the size of the tumor, and that as the dimensions increase the resulting lameness would be the greater in degree. This, however, is not the fact. A small tumor while in a condition of acute inflammation during the formative stage may cripple a patient more severely than a much larger one in a later stage of the disease. In any case the lameness is never wanting, and with its intermittent character may usually be detected when the animal is cooled off after labor or exercise. The class of animals in which this feature of the disease is most frequently seen is that of the heavy draft horse and others similarly employed. There is a wide margin of difference in respect to the degrees of severity which may characterize different cases of side-bone. While one may be so slight as to cause no inconvenience, another may develop elements of danger which may involve the necessity of severe surgical interference.

Treatment.—The curative treatment should be similar to the pro-phylactic, and such means should be used as would tend to prevent the deposit of bony matters by checking the acute inflammation which causes it. The means recommended are the free use of the cold bath; frequent soaking of the feet, and at a later period treat-ment with iodin, either by painting the surface with the tincture several times daily or by applying an ointment made by mixing 1 dram of the crystals with 2 ounces of vaseline, rubbed in once a day for several days. If this proves to be ineffective, a Spanish-fly blister to which a few grains of biniodid of mercury have been added will effect in a majority of cases the desired result and remove the lameness. If finally this treatment is ineffectual the case must be relegated to the surgeon for the operation of neurectomy, or the free and deep application of the firing iron.

SPAVIN.

(Pls. XXVII–XXIX.)

This affection, popularly termed bone spavin, is an exostosis of the hock joint. The general impression is that in a spavined hock the bony growth should be seated on the anterior and internal part of the joint, and this is partially correct, as such a growth will con-stitute a spavin in the most nearly correct sense of the term. But an enlargement may appear on the upper part of the hock also, or possibly a little below the inner side of the lower extremity of the shank bone, forming what is known as a high spavin; or, again, the growth may form just on the outside of the hock and become an out-side or external spavin. And, finally, the entire under surface may become the seat of the osseous deposit, and involve the articular face of all the bones of the hock, which again is a bone spavin. There would seem, then, to be but little difficulty in comprehending the nature of a bone spavin, and there would be none but for the fact that there are similar affections which may confuse one if the diag-nosis is not very carefully made.

But the hock may be "spavined," while to all outward observation it still retains its perfect form. With no enlargement perceptible to sight or touch the animal may yet be disabled by an occult spavin, an anchylosis in fact, which has resulted from a union of several of the bones of the joint, and it is only those who are able to realize the importance of its action to the perfect fulfillment of the function of locomotion by the hind leg who can comprehend the gravity of the only prognosis which can be justified by the facts of the case—a prognosis which is essentially a sentence of serious import in respect to the future usefulness and value of the animal. For no disease, if we except those acute inflammatory attacks upon vital organs to which the patient succumbs at once, is more destructive to the usefulness and value of a horse than a confirmed spavin. Serious in its inception, serious in its progress, it is an ailment which, when once established, becomes a fixed condition which there is no known means of dislodging.

Cause.—The periostitis, of which it is nearly always a termination, is usually the effect of a traumatic cause operating upon the complicated structure of the hock, such as a sprain which has torn a ligamentous insertion and lacerated some of its fibers, or a violent effort in jumping, galloping, or trotting, to which the victim has been compelled by the torture of whip and spur while in use as a gambling implement by a sporting owner, under the pretext of " improving his breed "; the extra exertion of starting an inordinately heavy load, or an effort to recover his balance from a misstep, slipping upon an icy surface, or sliding with worn shoes upon a bad pavement, and other kindred causes. We can repeat here what we have before said concerning bones, in respect to heredity as a cause. From our own experience we know of equine families in which this condition has been transmitted from generation to generation, and animals otherwise of excellent conformation have been rendered valueless by the misfortune of a congenital spavin.

Symptoms.—The evil is one of the most serious character for other reasons, among which may be specified the slowness of its development and the insidiousness of its growth. Certain indefinite phenomena and alarming changes and incidents furnish usually the only portents of approaching trouble. Among these signs may be mentioned a peculiar posture assumed by the patient while at rest, and becoming at length so habitual that it can not fail to suggest the action of some hidden disorder. The posture is due to the action of the adductor muscles, the lower part of the leg being carried inward, and the heel of the shoe resting on the toe of the opposite foot. Then an unwillingness may be noticed in the animal to move from one side of the stall to the other. When driven he will travel, but stiffly, with a sort of sidelong gait between the shafts, and after finishing his task and resting again in his stall will pose with the toe pointing forward, the heel raised, and the hock flexed. Considerable heat and inflammation soon appear. The slight lameness which appears when backing out of the stall ceases to be noticeable after a short distance of travel.

A minute examination of the hock may then reveal the existence of a bony enlargement which may be detected just at the junction of the hock and the cannon bone, on the inside and a little in front, and tangible both to sight and touch. This enlargement, or bone spavin, grows rapidly and persistently and soon acquires dimensions which renders it impossible to doubt any longer its existence or its nature. Once established, its development continues under conditions of progress similar to those to which we have before alluded in speaking of other like affections. The argument advanced by some that because these bony deposits are frequently found on both hocks they are not spavins is fallacious. If they are discovered on both hocks, it proves merely that they are not confined to a single joint.

The characteristic lameness of bone spavin, as it affects the motion of the hock joint, presents two aspects. In one class of cases it is most pronounced when the horse is cool, in the other when he is at work. The first is characterized by the fact that when the animal travels the toe first touches the ground, and the heel descends more slowly, the motion of flexion at the hock taking place stiffly, and accompanied with a dropping of the hip on the opposite side. In the other case the peculiarity is that the lameness increases as the horse travels; that when he stops he seeks to favor the lame leg, and when he resumes his work soon after he steps much on his toe, as in the first variety.

As with sidebones, though for a somewhat different reason, the dimensions of the spavin and the degree of the lameness do not seem to bear any determinate relation, the most pronounced symptoms at times accompanying a very diminutive growth. The distinction between the two varieties of cool and warm, however, may easily be determined by remembering the fact that in most cases the first, or cool, is due to a simple exostosis, while the second is generally connected with disease of the articulation, such as ulceration of the articular surface—a condition which, as we proceed further, will receive our attention when we reach the subject of stringhalt.

An excellent test for spavin lameness, which may be readily applied, consists in lifting the affected leg from the ground for one or two minutes and holding the foot high so as to flex all the joints. An assistant, with the halter strap in his hand, quickly starts the animal off in a trot, when, if the hock joint is affected, the lameness will be so greatly intensified as to lead readily to a diagnosis.

Prognosis.—Having thus fully considered the history of bone spavin, we are prepared to give due weight to the reasons that exist for the adverse prognosis which we must usually feel compelled to pronounce when encountering it in practice, as well as to realize the importance of early discovery. It is but seldom, however, that the necessary advantage of this early knowledge can be obtained, and when the true nature of the trouble has become apparent it is usually too late to resort to the remedial measures which, if duly forewarned, a skillful practitioner might have employed. We are fully persuaded that but for the loss of the time wasted in the treatment of purely imaginary ailments very many cases of bone spavin might be arrested in their incipiency and their victims preserved for years of comfort for themselves and valuable labor to their owners.

Treatment.—To consider a hypothetical case: An early discovery of lameness has been made; that is, the existence of an acute inflammation—of periostitis—has been detected. The increased temperature of the parts has been observed, with the stiffened gait and the characteristic pose of the limb, and the question is proposed for solution, What is to be done? Even with only these comparatively doubtful symptoms—doubtful with the nonexpert—we should direct our treatment to the hock in preference to any other joint, since of all the joints of the hind leg it is this which is most liable to be attacked, a natural result from its peculiarities of structure and function. And in answer to the query, What is the first treatment indicated? We should answer *rest*—emphatically, and as an essential condition, *rest*. Whether only threatened, suspected, or positively diseased, the animal must be wholly released from labor, and it must be no partial or temporary quiet of a few days. In all stages and conditions of the disease, whether the spavin is nothing more than a simple exostosis, or whether accompanied with the complication of arthritis, there must be a total suspension of effort until the danger is over. Less than a month's quiet ought not to be thought of—the longer the better.

Good results may also be expected from local applications. The various lotions which cool the parts, the astringents which lower the tension of the blood vessels, the tepid fomentations which accelerate the circulation in the engorged capillaries, the liniments of various composition, the stimulants, the opiate anodynes, the sedative preparations of aconite, the alterative frictions of iodin—all these are recommended and prescribed by one or another. We prefer counter-irritants, for the reason, among many others, that by the promptness of their action they tend to prevent the formation of the bony deposits. The lameness will often yield to the blistering action of cantharides, in the form of ointment or liniment, and to the alterative preparations of iodin or mercury. If the owner of a "spavined" horse really succeeds in removing the lameness, he has accomplished all that he is justified in hoping for; beyond this let him be well persuaded that a "cure" is impossible.

For this reason, moreover, he will do well to be on his guard against the patented "cures" which the traveling horse doctor may urge upon him, and withhold his faith from the circular of the agent who will deluge him with references and certificates. It is possible that nostrums may in some exceptional instances prove serviceable, but the greater number of them are capable of producing only injurious effects. The removal of the bony tumor can not be accomplished by any such means, and if a trial of these unknown compounds should be followed by complications no worse than the establishment of one or more ugly, hairless cicatrices, it will be well for both the horse and his owner.

Rest and counterirritation, with the proper medicaments, constitute, then, the prominent points in the treatment designed for the relief of bone spavin. Yet there are cases in which all the agencies and methods referred to seem to lack effectiveness and fail to produce satisfactory results. Either the rest has been prematurely interrupted or the blisters have failed to modify the serous infiltration, or the case in hand has some undiscernible characteristics which seem to have rendered the disease neutral to the agencies used against it. An indication of more energetic means is then presented, and free cauterization with the firing iron becomes necessary.

At this point a word of explanation in reference to this operation of firing may be appropriate for the satisfaction of any among our readers who may entertain an exaggerated idea of its severity and possible cruelty.

The operation is one of simplicity, but is nevertheless one which, in order to secure its benefits, must be reserved for times and occasions of which only the best knowledge and highest discretion should be allowed to judge. It is not the mere application of a hot iron to a given part of the body which constitutes the operation of firing. It is the methodical and scientific introduction of heat into the structure with a view to a given effect upon a diseased organ or tissue by an expert surgeon. The first is one of the degrees of mere burning. The other is scientific cauterization, and is a surgical manipulation which should be committed exclusively to the practiced hand of the veterinary surgeon.

Either firing alone or stimulation with blisters is of great efficacy for the relief of lameness from bone spavin. Failure to produce relief after a few applications and after allowing a sufficient interval of rest should be followed by a second or, if needed, a third firing.

In case of further failure there is a reserve of certain special operations which have been tried and recommended, among which those of cunean tenotomy, periosteotomy, the division of nervous branches, etc., may be mentioned. These, however, belong to the peculiar domain of the veterinary practitioner, and need not now engage our attention.

FRACTURES.

In technical language a fracture is a " solution of continuity in the structure or substance of a bone." It ranks among the most serious of the lesions to which the horse—or any animal—can be subject. It is a subject of special interest to veterinarians and horse owners in view of the fact that it occurs in such a variety of forms and subjects the patient to much loss of time, resulting in the suspension of his earning capacity. Though of less serious consequence in the horse than in man, it is always a matter of grave import. It is always slow and tedious in healing and is frequently of doubtful and unsatisfactory result.

This solution of continuity may take place in two principal ways. In the most numerous instances it includes the total thickness of the bone and is a complete fracture. In other cases it involves only a portion of the thickness of the bone, and for that reason is described as incomplete. If the bone is divided into two separate portions and the soft parts have received no injury, the fracture is a simple one, or it becomes compound if the soft parts have suffered laceration, and comminuted if the bones have been crushed or ground into fragments, many or few. The direction of the break also determines its further classification. Broken at a right angle, it is transverse; at a different angle it becomes oblique, and it may be longitudinal or lengthwise. In a complete fracture, especially of the oblique kind, there is a condition of great importance in respect to its effect upon the ultimate result of the treatment in the fact that from various causes, such as muscular contractions or excessive motion, the bony fragments do not maintain their mutual coaptation, but become separated at the ends, which makes it necessary to add another descriptive term—with displacement. These words again suggest the negative and introduce the term without displacement, when the facts justify that description. Furthermore, a fracture may be intra-articular or extra-articular, as it extends into a joint or otherwise, and, once more, intra-periosteal when the periosteum remains intact. Finally, there is no absolute limit to the use of descriptive terminology in the case.

The condition of displacement is largely influential in determining the question of treatment and as affecting the final result of a case of fracture. This, however, is dependent upon its location or whether its seat is in one or more of the axes of the bone, in its length, its breadth, its thickness, or its circumference. An incomplete fracture may also be either simple or comminuted. In the latter case the fragments are held together by the periosteum when it is intact; in that case the fracture belongs to the intraperiosteal class. At times, also, there is only a simple fissure or split in the bone, making a condition of much difficulty of diagnosis.

Causes.—Two varieties of originating cause may be recognized in cases of fracture. They are the predisposing and the occasional. As to the first, different species of animals differ in the degree of their liability. That of the dog is greater than that of the horse, and in horses the various questions of age, the mode of labor, the season of the year, the portion of the body most exposed, and the existence of ailments, local and general, are all to be taken into account.

Among horses, those employed in heavy draft work or that are driven over bad roads are more exposed than light-draft or saddle horses, and animals of different ages are not equally liable. Dogs and young horses, with those which have become sufficiently aged for their bones to have acquired an enhanced degree of frangibility, are more liable than those which have not exceeded the time of their prime. The season of the year is undoubtedly, though in an incidental way, an important factor in the problem of the etiology of these accidents, for though they may be observed at all times, it is during the months when the slippery condition of the icy roads renders it difficult for both men and beasts to keep their feet that they occur most frequently. The long bones, those especially which belong to the extremities, are most frequently the seat of fractures, from the circumstance of their superficial position, their exposure to contact and collision, and the violent muscular efforts involved both in their constant, rapid movement and their labor in the shafts or at the pole of heavy and heavily laden carriages.

The relation between sundry idiosyncrasies and diathesis and a liability to fractures is too constant and well-established a pathological fact to need more than a passing reference. The history of rachitis, of melanosis, and of osteoporosis, as related to an abnormal frangibility of the bones, is a part of our common medical knowledge. There are few persons who have not known of cases among their friends of frequent and almost spontaneous fractures, or at least of such as seem to be produced by the slightest and most inadequate violence, and there is no tangible reason for doubting an analogous condition in dividuals of the equine race. Among local predisposing causes mention must not be omitted of such bony diseases as caries, tuberculosis, and others of the same class.

Exciting, occasional, or " efficient " causes of fracture are in most instances external traumatisms, as violent contacts, collisions, falls, etc., or sudden muscular contractions. These external accidents are various in their character, and are usually associated with quick muscular exertion. A violent, ineffectual effort to move too heavy a load; a semispasmodic bracing of the frame to avoid a fall or resist a pressure; a quick jump to escape a blow; stopping too suddenly after speeding; struggling to liberate a foot from a rail, perhaps to be thrown in the effort—all these are familiar and easy examples of accidents happening hourly by which our equine servants become sufferers. We may add to these the fracture of the bones of the vertebræ, occurring when casting a patient for the purpose of undergoing a surgical operation, quite as much as the result of muscular contraction as of a preexisting diseased condition of the bones. A fracture occurring under these circumstances may be called with propriety indirect, while one which has resulted from a blow or a fall differently caused is of the direct kind.

Symptoms.—We now return to the first items in our classification of the varieties of fractures for the purpose of bringing them in turn under an orderly review, and our first examination will include those which belong to the first category, or the complete kind. Irregularity in the performance of the functions of the apparatus to which the fractured bone belongs is a necessary consequence of the existing lesion, and this is lameness. If the broken bone belongs to one of the extremities, the impossibility of the performance of its natural function in sustaining the weight of the body and contributing to the act of locomotion is usually complete, though the degree of disability will vary according to the kind of fracture and the bone which is injured. For example, a fracture of the cannon bone without displacement, or of one of the phalanges, which are surrounded and sustained by a complex fibrous structure, is, in a certain degree, not incompatible with some amount of resting on the foot. On the contrary, if the shank bone, or that of the forearm is the implicated member, it would be very difficult for the leg to exercise any agency whatever in the support of the body, and in a fracture of the lower jaw it would be obviously unreasonable to expect it to contribute materially to the mastication of feed.

It seldom happens that a fracture is not accompanied with a degree of deformity, greater or less, of the region or the leg affected. This is due to the exudation of the blood into the meshes of the surrounding tissues and to the displacement which occurs between the fragments of the bones, with subsequently the swelling which follows the inflammation of the surrounding tissues. The character of the deformity will mainly depend upon the manner in which the displacement occurs.

In a normal state of things the legs perform their movements with the joints as their only centers or bases of action, with no participation of intermediate points, while with a fracture the flexibility and motion which will be observed at unnatural points are among the most strongly characteristic signs of the lesion. No one need be told that, when the shaft of a limb is seen to bend midway between the joints, with the lower portion swinging freely, the leg is broken. There are still some conditions, however, in which the excessive mobility is not easy to detect. Such are the cases in which the fracture exists in a short bone, near a movable joint, or in a bone of a region where several short and small bones are united in a group, or even in a long bone the situation of which is such that the muscular covering prevents the visible manifestation of the symptom.

If the situation of a fracture precludes its discovery by means of this abnormal flexibility, other modes of detection remain. There is one method which is absolute and positive and which can be applied in by far the most, though not in all cases. This is crepitation, or the peculiar effect which is produced by the friction of the fractured surfaces one against another. Though discerned by the organs of hearing it can scarcely be called a sound, for the grating of the parts as the rubbing takes place is more felt than heard; however, there is no mistaking its import in cases favorable for the application of the test. The conditions in which it is not available are those of incomplete fracture, in which the mobility of the part is lacking, and those in which the whole array of phenomena are usually obscure. To obtain the benefit of this pathognomonic sign requires deliberate, careful, and gentle manipulation. Sometimes the slightest of movements will be sufficient for its development, after much rougher handling has failed to discover it. Perhaps the failure in the latter case is due to a sort of defensive spasmodic rigidity caused by the pain resulting from the rude interference.

More or less reactive fever is a usual accompaniment of a fracture. Ecchymosis in the parts is but a natural occurrence, and is more easily discovered in animals possessing a light-colored and delicate skin than in those of any other character.

There are difficulties in the way of the diagnosis of an incomplete fracture, even sometimes when there is a degree of impairment in the function of locomotion, with evidences of pain and swelling at the seat of lesion. There should then be a careful examination for evidences of a blow or other violence sufficient to account for the fracture, though very often a suspicion of its existence can be converted into a certainty only by a minute history of the patient if it can be obtained up to the moment of the occurrence of the injury. A diagnosis ought not to be hastily pronounced, and where good ground for suspicion exists it ought not to be rejected upon any evidence less than the best. We too often read of serious and fatal complications following careless conclusions in similar cases, among which we may refer to one instance of a complete fracture manifesting itself in an animal during the act of rising in his stall after a decision had been pronounced that he had no fracture at all.

Fractures are, of course, liable to complications, especially those which are of a traumatic character, such as extensive lacerations, tearing of tissues, punctures, contusions, etc. Unless these are in communication with the fracture itself the indication is to treat them simply as independent lesions upon other parts of the body. A traumatic emphysema at times causes trouble, and abscesses, more or less deep and diffused, may follow. In some cases small, bony fragments from a comminuted fracture, becoming loose and acting as foreign bodies, give rise to troublesome fistulous tracts. A frequent complication is hemorrhage, which often becomes of serious consequence. A fracture in close proximity to a joint may be accompanied with dangerous inflammations of important organs, and induce an attack of pneumonia, pleurisy, arthritis, etc., especially if near the chest; it may also cause luxations, or dislocations. Gangrene, as a consequence of contusions or of hemorrhage or of an impediment to the circulation, caused by unskillfully applied apparatus, must not be overlooked among the occasional incidents; nor must lockjaw, which is not an uncommon occurrence. Even founder, or laminitis, has been met with as the result of forced and long-continued immobility of the feet in the standing posture, as one of the involvements of unavoidably protracted treatment.

When a simple fracture has been properly treated and the broken ends of the bone have been securely held in coaptation, one of two things will occur. Either—and this is the more common event— there will be a union of the two ends by a solid cicatrix, the callus, or the ends will continue separated or become only partially united by an intermediate fibrous structure. In the first instance the fracture is consolidated or united; in the second there is a false articulation, or pseudarthrosis.

The time required for a firm union or true consolidation of a fracture varies with the character of the bone affected, the age and constitution of the patient, and the general conditions of the case. The union will be perfected earlier in a young than in an adult animal, and sooner in the latter than in the aged, and a general healthy condition is, of course, in every respect, an advantage.

The mode of cicatrization, or method of repair in lesions of the bones, has been a subject of much study among investigators in pathology, and has elicited various expressions of opinion from those high in authority. The weight of evidence and preponderance of opinion are about settled in favor of the theory that the law of reparation is the same for both the hard and the soft tissues. In one case a simple exudation of material, with the proper organization of newly formed tissue, will bring about a union by the first intention, and in another the work will be accompanied with suppuration, or union by the second intention, a process so familiar in the repair of the soft structures by granulation.

Considering the process in its simplest form, in a case in which it advances without interruption or complication to a favorable result, it may probably be correctly described in this wise:

On the occurrence of the injury an effusion of blood takes place between the ends of the bone. The coagulation of the fluid soon follows, and this, after a few days, undergoes absorption. There is then an excess of inflammation in the surrounding structure, which soon spreads to the bony tissue, when a true ostitis is established, and the compact tissue of the bone becomes the seat of a new vascular organization, and of a certain exudation of plastic lymph, appearing between the periosteum and the external surface of the bone, as well as on the inner side of the medullary cavity. After a few days the ends of the bone thus surrounded by this exudate become involved in it, and the lymph, becoming vascular, is soon transformed into cartilaginous, and in due time into bony, tissue.

Thus the time required for the consolidation of the fractured segments is divisible into two distinct periods. In the first they are surrounded by an external bony ring, and the medullary cavity is closed by a bony plug or stopper, constituting the period of the provisional callus. This is followed by the period of permanent callus, during which the process of converting the cartilaginous into the osseous form is going forward.

The restorative process is sooner completed in the carnivorous than in the herbivorous tribes. In the former the temporary callus may attain sufficient fineness of consistency for the careful use of the limb within four weeks, but with the latter a period of from six weeks to two months is not too long to allow before removing the supporting apparatus from the limb.

This, in general terms, represents the fact when the resources of nature have not been thwarted by untoward accidents, such as a want of vigor in the constitution of the patient or a lack of skill on the part of the practitioner, and especially when, from any cause, the bony fragments have not been kept in a state of perfect immobility and the constant friction has prevented the osseous union of the two portions. Failures and misfortunes are always more than possible, and instead of a solid and practicable bony union the sequel of the accident is sometimes a false joint, composed of mere flexible cartilage, a poor pseudarthrosis. The explanation of this appears to be that, first, the sharp edges of the ends of the bone disappear by becoming rounded at their extremities by friction and polishing against each other. Then follows an exudation of a plastic nature which becomes transformed into a cartilaginous layer of a rough, articular aspect. In this bony nuclei soon appear, and the lymph secreted between the segments thus transformed, instead of becoming truly ossified, is changed into a sort of fibrocartilaginous pouch, or capsular sac, in which a somewhat albuminous secretion, or pseudo-synovia, permits the movement to take place. Most commonly, however, in our animals, the union of the bony fragments is obtained wholly through the medium of a layer of fibrous tissue, and it is because the union has been accomplished by a ligamentous formation only that motion becomes practicable.

Prognosis.—The prognosis in a case of fracture in an animal is one of the gravest vital import to the patient, and therefore of serious pecuniary concern to his owner. The period has not long elapsed when to have received such a hurt was quite equivalent to undergoing a sentence of death for the suffering animal, and perhaps to-day a similar verdict is pronounced in many cases in which the exercise of a little mechanical ingenuity, with a due amount of careful nursing, might secure a contrary result and insure the return of the patient to his former condition of soundness and usefulness.

Treatment.—Considered per se, a fracture in an animal is in fact no less amenable to treatment than the same description of injury in any other living being. But the question of the propriety and expediency of treatment is dependent upon certain specific points of collateral consideration.

(1) The nature of the lesion is a point of paramount importance. A simple fracture occurring in a bone where the ends can be firmly secured in coaptation presents the most favorable condition for successful treatment. If it is that of a long bone, it will be the less serious if situated at or near the middle of its length than if it were in close proximity to a joint, from the fact that perfect immobility can rarely, in the latter case, be secured without incurring the risk of subsequent rigidity of the joint.

A simple is always less serious than a compound fracture. A comminuted is always more dangerous than a simple, and a transverse break is easier to treat than one which is oblique. The most serious are those which are situated on parts of the body in which it is difficult to obtain perfect immobility, and especially those which are accompanied with severe contusions and lacerations in the soft parts; the protrusion of fragments through the skin; the division of blood vessels by the broken ends of the bone; the existence of an articulation near the point to which inflammation is liable to extend; the luxation of a fragment of the bone; laceration of the periosteum; the presence of a large number of bony particles, the result of the crushing of the bone—all these are circumstances which discourage a favorable prognosis, and weigh against the hope of saving the patient for future usefulness.

Fractures which may be accounted curable are those which are not conspicuously visible, as those of the ribs, where displacements are either very limited or do not occur, the parts being kept in situ by the nature of their position, the shape of the bones, the articulations they form with the vertebra, the sternum, or their cartilages of prolongation; those of transverse processes of the lumbar vertebra; those of the bones of the face; those of the ilium; and that of the coffinbones. To continue the category, the following are evidently curable when their position and the character of the patient contribute to aid the treatment: Those of the cranium, in the absence of cerebral lesions; those of the jaws; of the ribs, with displacement; of the hip; and those of the bones of the leg in movable regions, but where their vertical position admits of perfect coaptation.

On the contrary, a compound, complicated, or comminuted fracture, in whatever region it may be situated, may be counted incurable.

In treating fractures time is an important element and "delays are dangerous." Those of recent occurrence unite more easily and more regularly than older ones.

(2) As a general rule, fractures are less serious in animals of the smaller species than in those of more bulky dimensions. This influence of species will be readily appreciated when we realize that the difficulties involved in the treatment of the latter class have hardly any existence in connection with the former. The difference in weight and size, and consequent facility in handling and making the necessary applications of dressings and other appliances for the purpose of securing the indispensable immobility of the parts, and usually a less degree of uneasiness in the deportment of the patients are considerations in this connection of great weight.

(3) In respect to the utilization of the animal, the most obvious point in estimating the gravity of the case in a fracture accident is the certainty of the total loss of the services of the patient during treatment—certainly for a considerable period of time; perhaps permanently. For example, the fracture of the jaw of a steer just fattening for the shambles will involve a heavier loss than a similar accident to a horse. Usually the fracture of the bones of the extremities in a horse is a very serious casualty, the more so proportionately as the higher region of the limb is affected. In working animals it is exceedingly difficult to treat a fracture in such manner as to restore a limb to its original perfection of movement. A fracture of a single bone of an extremity in a breeding stallion or mare will not necessarily impair the value of the animal as a breeder. Other specifications under this head, though pertinent and more or less interesting, may be omitted.

(4) Age and temper are important factors of cure. A young, growing, robust patient whose vis vitæ is active is amenable to treatment which one with a waning constitution and past mature energies would be unable to endure, and a docile, quiet disposition will act cooperatively with remedial measures which would be neutralized by the fractious opposition of a peevish and intractable sufferer.

The fulfillment of three indications is indispensable in all fractures. The first is the reduction, or the replacement, of the parts as nearly

as possible in their normal position. The second is their retention in
that position for a period sufficient for the formation of the provisional callus, and the third, which, in fact, is but an incident of the
second, the careful avoidance of any accidents or causes of miscarriage which might disturb the curative process.

In reference to the first consideration, it must be remembered that
the accident may befall the patient at a distance from his home, and
his removal becomes the first duty to be attended to. Of course, this
must be done as carefully as possible. If he can be treated on the
spot, so much the better, though this is seldom practicable, and the
method of removal becomes the question calling for settlement. But
two ways present themselves—he must either walk or be carried. If
the first, it is needless to say that every caution must be observed in
order to obviate additional pain and to avoid any aggravation of the
injury. Led slowly, and with partial support, if practicable, the
journey will not always involve untoward results. If he is carried,
it must be by means of a wagon, a truck, or an ambulance; the last
being designed and adapted to the purpose, would, of course, be
the most suitable vehicle. As a precaution which should never be
overlooked, a temporary dressing should first be applied. This
may be so done as for the time to answer all the purposes of the permanent adjustment and bandaging. Without thus securing the
patient, a fracture of an inferior degree may be transformed to one of
the severest kind, and, indeed, a curable changed to an incurable
injury. We recall a case in which a fast-trotting horse, after running away in a fright caused by the whistle of a locomotive, was
found on the road limping with excessive lameness in the off fore
leg, and walked with comparative ease some 2 miles to a stable before
being seen by a surgeon. His immediate removal in an ambulance
was advised, but before that vehicle could be procured the horse lay
down, and upon being made to get upon his feet was found with a
well-marked comminuted fracture of the os suffraginis, with considerable displacement. The patient, however, after long treatment, made a comparatively good recovery and though with a large,
bony deposit, a ringbone, was able to trot in the forties.

The two obvious indications in cases of fracture are reduction, or
replacement, and retention.

In an incomplete fracture, where there is no displacement, the
necessity of reduction does not exist. With the bone kept in place
by an intact periosteum, and the fragments secured by the uninjured fibrous and ligamentous structure which surrounds them, there
is no dislocation to correct. Reduction is also at times rendered
impossible by the seat of the fracture itself, by its dimensions, alone,
or by the resistance arising from muscular contraction. That is
illustrated even in small animals, as in dogs, by the exceeding diffi-

culty encountered in bringing together the ends of a broken femur or humerus, the muscular contractions being even in these animals sufficiently forcible to renew the displacement.

It is generally, therefore, only fractures of the long bones, and then at points not in close proximity to the trunk, that may be considered to be amenable to reduction. It is true that some of the more superficial bones, as those of the head, of the pelvis, and of the thoracic walls, may in some cases require special manipulations and appliances for their retention in their normal positions; hence the treatment of these and of a fractured leg can not be the same.

The methods of accomplishing reduction vary with the features of each case, the manipulations being necessarily modified to meet different circumstances. If the displacement is in the thickness of the bone, as in transverse fracture, the manipulation of reduction consists in applying constant pressure upon one of the fragments, while the other is kept steady in its place, the object of the pressure being the reestablishment of the exact coincidence of the two bony surfaces. If the displacement has taken place at an angle it will be sufficient in order to effect the reduction to press upon the summit, or apex, of the angle until its disappearance indicates that the parts have been brought into coaptation. This method is often practiced in the treatment of a fractured rib. In a longitudinal fracture, or when the fragments are pressed together by the contraction of the muscles to which they give insertion until they so overlap as to correspond by certain points of their circumference, the reduction is to be accomplished by effecting the movements of extension, counter extension, and coaptation. Extension is accomplished by making traction upon the lower portion of the limb. Counter extension consists in firmly holding or confining the upper or body portion in such manner that it shall not be affected by the traction applied to the lower part. In other words, the operator, grasping the limb below the fracture, draws it down or away from the trunk, while he seeks not to draw away, but simply to hold the upper portion still until the broken ends of bone are brought to their natural relative positions, when the coaptation, which is thus effected, has only to be made permanent by the proper dressings to perfect the reduction.

In treating fractures in small animals the strength of the hand is usually sufficient for the required manipulations. In the fracture of the forearm of a dog, for example, while the upper segment is firmly held by one hand the lower may be grasped by the other and the bone itself made to serve the purpose of a lever to bring about the desired coaptation. In such case that is sufficient to overcome the muscular contraction and correct the overlapping or other malposition of the bones. If, however, the resistance can not be overcome in this way, the upper segment may be committed to an assistant for the management of the counter extension, leaving to the operator the free use of both hands for the further manipulation of the case.

If the reduction of fractures in small animals is an easy task, however, it is far from being so when the patient is a large animal whose muscular force is largely greater than that of several men combined. In such case resort must be had not only to superior numbers for the necessary force, but in many cases to mechanical aids. A reference to the manner of proceeding in a case of fracture with displacement of the forearm of a horse will illustrate the matter. The patient is first to be carefully cast, on the uninjured side, with ropes or a broad, leather strap about 18 feet long passed under and around his body and under the axilla of the fractured limb and secured at a point opposite to the animal and toward his back. This will form the mechanical means of counter extension. Another rope will then be placed around the inferior part of the leg below the point of fracture, with which to produce extension, and this will sometimes be furnished with a block and pulleys, in order to augment the power when necessary; there is, in fact, always an advantage in their use, on the side of steadiness and uniformity, as well as of increased power. It is secured around the fetlock or the coronet or, what is better, above the knee and nearer the point of fracture, and is committed to assistants. The traction on this should be firm, uniform, and slow, without relaxing or jerking, while the operator carefully watches the process. If the bone is superficially situated he is able, by the eye, to judge of any changes that may occur in the form or length of the parts under traction, and discovering, at the moment of its happening, the restoration of symmetry in the disturbed region he gently but firmly manipulates the place until all appearance of severed continuity has vanished. Sometimes the fact and the instant of restoration are indicated by a peculiar sound or "click" as the ends of the bones slip into contact, to await the next step of the restorative procedure.

The process is the same when the bones are covered with thick muscular masses except that it is attended with greater difficulties from the fact that the finger must be substituted for the eye and taxis must take the place of sight.

It frequently happens that perfect coaptation is prevented by the interposition, between the bony surfaces, of such substances as a small fragment of detached bone or a clot of blood; sometimes the extreme obliquity of the fracture, by permitting the bones to slip out of place, is the opposing cause. These are difficulties which can not always be overcome, even in small-sized animals, and still it is only when they are mastered that a correct consolidation can be looked for. Without it the continuity between the fragments will be by a deformed callus, the union will leave a shortened, crooked, or angular limb, and the animal will be disabled.

If timely assistance can be obtained, and the reduction accomplished immediately after the occurrence of the accident, that is the best time for it, but if it can not be attended to until inflammation has become established and the parts have become swollen and painful, time must be allowed for the subsidence of these symptoms before attempting the operation. A spasmodic, muscular contraction which sometimes interposes a difficulty may be easily overcome by subjecting the patient to general anesthesia, and need not, therefore, cause any loss of time. A tendency to this may also be overcome by the use of sedatives and antiphlogistic remedies.

The reduction of the fracture having been accomplished, the problem which follows is that of retention. The parts which have been restored to their natural position must be kept there, without disturbance or agitation, until the perfect formation of a callus, and it is here that ample latitude exists for the exercise of ingenuity and skill by the surgeon in the contrivance of the necessary apparatus. One of the most important of the conditions which are available by the surgeon in treating human patients is denied to the veterinarian in the management of those which belong to the animal tribes. This is position. The intelligence of the human patient cooperates with the instructions of the surgeon, in the case of the animal sufferer there is a continual antagonism between the parties, and the forced extension and fatiguing position which must for a considerable period be maintained as a condition of restoration require special and effective appliances to insure successful results. To obtain complete immobility is scarcely possible, and the surgeon must be content to reach a point as near as possible to that which is unattainable. For this reason, as will subsequently be seen, the use of slings and the restraint of patients in very narrow stalls is much to be preferred to the practice sometimes recommended of allowing entire freedom of motion by turning them loose in box stalls. Temporary and movable apparatus are not usually of difficult use in veterinary practice, but the restlessness of the patients and their unwillingness to submit quietly to the changing of the dressings render it obligatory to have recourse to permanent and immovable bandages, which should be retained without disturbance until the process of consolidation is complete.

The materials composing the retaining apparatus consist of oakum, bandages, and splints, with an agglutinating compound which forms a species of cement by which the different constituents are blended into a consistent mass to be spread upon the surface covering the locality of the fracture. Its components are black pitch, rosin, and Venice turpentine, blended by heat. The dressing may be applied directly to the skin, or a covering of thin linen may be interposed. A putty made with powdered chalk and the white of egg is recommended for small animals, though a mixture of sugar of lead and burnt alum with the albumen is preferred by others. Another formula is spirits of camphor, Goulard's extract, and albumen. Another recommendation is to saturate the oakum and bandages with an adhesive solution formed with gum arabic, dextrin, flour paste, or starch. This is advised particularly for small animals, as is also the silicate of soda. Dextrin mixed while warm with burnt alum and alcohol cools and solidifies into a stony consistency, and is preferable to plaster of Paris, which is less friable and has less solidity, besides being heavier and requiring constant additions as it becomes older. Starch and plaster of Paris form another good compound.

In applying the dressing the leg is usually padded with a cushion of oakum thick and soft enough to equalize the irregularities of the surface and to form a bedding for the protection of the skin from chafing. Over this the splints are placed. The material for these is, variously, pasteboard, thin wood, bark, laths, gutta-percha, strips of thin metal, as tin or perhaps sheet iron. They should be of sufficient length not only to cover the region of the fracture but to extend sufficiently above and below to render the immobility more nearly complete than in the surrounding joints. The splints, again, are covered with cloth bandages—linen preferably—soaked in a glutinous mixture. These bandages are to be carefully applied, with a perfect condition of lightness. They are usually made to embrace the entire length of the leg in order to avoid the possibility of interference with the circulation of the extremity as well as for the prevention of chafing. They should be rolled from the lower part of the leg upward and carefully secured against loosening. In some instances suspensory bandages are recommended, but except for small animals our experience does not justify a concurrence in the recommendation.

These permanent dressings always need careful watching with reference to their immediate effect upon the region they cover, especially during the first days succeeding that of their application. Any manifestation of pain, or any appearance of swelling above or below, or any odor suggestive of suppuration should excite suspicion, and a thorough investigation should follow without delay. The removal of the dressing should be performed with great care, and especially so if time enough has elapsed since its application to allow of a probability of a commencement of the healing process or the existence of any points of consolidation. With the original dressing properly applied in its entirety in the first instance, the entire extremity will have lost all chance of mobility, and the repairing process may be permitted to proceed without interference. There will be no necessity and there need be no haste for removal or change except under such special conditions as have just been mentioned, or when there is reason to judge that solidification has become perfect, or for the comfort of the animal, or for its readaptation in consequence of the atrophy of the limb from want of use. Owners of animals are often tempted to remove a splint or bandage prematurely at the risk of producing a second fracture in consequence of the failure of the callus properly to consolidate.

The method of applying the splints which we have described refers to the simple variety only. In a compound case the same rules must be observed, with the modification of leaving openings through the thickness of the dressing, opposite the wound, in order to permit the escape of pus and to secure access to the points requiring the application of treatment.

FRACTURE OF CRANIAL BONES.

Fractures of the cranial bones in large animals are comparatively rare, though the records are not destitute of cases. When they occur, it is as the result of external violence, the sufferers being usually runaways which have come in collision with a wall or a tree or other obstruction, or it may occur in those which in pulling upon the halter have broken it with a jerk and been thrown backward, as may occur in rearing too violently. Under these conditions we have witnessed fractures of the parietal, of the frontal, and of the sphenoid bones. These fractures may be of both the complete and the incomplete kinds, which indeed is usually the case with those of the flat bones, and they are liable to be complicated with lacerations of the skin, in consequence of which they are easily brought under observation. When the fact is otherwise and the skin is intact, however, the diagnosis becomes difficult.

Symptoms.—The incomplete variety may be unaccompanied with any special symptoms, but in the complete kind one of the bony plates may be so far detached as to press upon the cerebral substance with sufficient force to produce serious nervous complications. When the injury occurs at the base of the cranium hemorrhage may be looked for, with paralytic symptoms, and when these are present the usual termination is death. It may happen, however, that the symptoms of an apparently very severe concussion may disappear, resulting in an early and complete recovery, and the surgeon will therefore do well to avoid undue haste in venturing upon a prognosis. In fractures of the orbital or the zygomatic bones the danger is less pressing than with injuries otherwise located about the head.

Treatment.—The treatment of cranial fractures is simple, though involving the best skill of an experienced surgeon. When incomplete hardly any interference is needed; even plain bandaging may usually be dispensed with. In the complete variety the danger to be combated is compression of the brain, and attention to this indication must not be delayed. The means to be employed are the trephining of the skull over the seat of the fracture and the elevation of the depressed bone or the removal of the portion which is causing the trouble. Fragments of bone in comminuted cases, bony exfoliations, collections of fluid, or even protruding portions of the brain substance must be carefully cleansed away and a simple bandage so applied as to facilitate the application of subsequent dressings.

FRACTURES OF THE BONES OF THE FACE.

In respect to their origin—usually traumatic—these injuries rank with the preceding, and are commonly of the incomplete variety. They may easily be overlooked, and may even sometimes escape recognition until the reparative process has been well established and the wound is discovered owing to the prominence caused by the presence of the provisional callus which marks its cure. When the fracture is complete it will be marked by local deformity, mobility of the fragments, and crepitation. Nasal hemorrhage, roaring, frequent sneezing, loosening or loss of teeth, difficulty of mastication, and inflammation of the cavities of the sinuses are varying complications of these accidents. The object of the treatment should be the restoration of the depressed bones as nearly as possible to their normal position and their retention in place by protecting splints, which should cover the entire facial region. Special precautions should be observed to prevent the patient from disturbing the dressing by rubbing his head against surrounding objects, such as the stall, manger, rack, etc. Clots of blood in the nasal passages must be washed out, collections of pus removed from the sinuses, and, if the teeth are loosened and liable to fall out, they should be removed. If roaring is threatened, tracheotomy is indicated.

FRACTURES OF THE PREMAXILLARY BONE.

These are mentioned by continental authors and are usually encountered in connection with fractures of the nasal bone, and may take place either in the width or the length of the bone.

The deformity of the upper lip, which is drawn sidewise in this lesion, renders it easy of diagnosis. The abnormal mobility and the crepitation, with the pain manifested by the patient when undergoing examination, are concurrent symptoms. Looseness of the teeth, abundant salivation, and entire inability to grasp the feed complete the symptomatology of these accidents. In the treatment splints of gutta-percha or leather are sometimes used, but they are of difficult application. Our own judgment and practice are in favor of the union of the bones by means of metallic sutures.

FRACTURES OF THE LOWER JAW.

A fracture here is not an injury of infrequent occurrence. It involves the body of the bone, at its symphysis, or back of it, and includes one or both of its branches, either more or less forward, or at the posterior part near the temporomaxillary articulation, at the coronoid process.

Falls, blows, or other external violence, or powerful muscular contractions during the use of the speculum, may be mentioned among the causes of this lesion. The fracture of the neck, or that portion formed by the juncture of the two opposite sides, and of the branches in front of the cheeks, causes the lower jaw, the true dental arch, to drop, without the ability to raise it again to the upper, and the result is a peculiar and characteristic physiognomy. The prehension and mastication of feed become impossible; there is an abundant escape of fetid and sometimes bloody saliva, especially if the gums have been wounded; there is excessive mobility of the lower end of the jawbone; and there is crepitation, and frequently paralysis of the under lip. Although an animal suffering with a complete and often compound and comminuted fracture of the submaxilla presents at times a serious aspect, the prognosis of the case is comparatively favorable, and recovery is usually only a question of time. The severity of the lesion corresponds in degree to that of the violence to which it is due, also to the resulting complications and the situation of the wound. It is simple when at the symphysis, but becomes more serious when it affects one of the branches, and most aggravated when both are involved. Fracture of the coronoid process becomes important principally as an evidence of the existence of a morbid diathesis, such as osteoporosis, or the like.

The particular seat of the injury, with its special features, will, of course, determine the treatment. For a simple fracture, without displacement, provided there is no laceration of the periosteum, an ordinary supporting bandage will usually be sufficient, but when there is displacement the reduction of the fracture must first be accomplished, and for this special splints are necessary. In a fracture of the symphysis or of the branches the adjustment of the fragments by securing them with metallic sutures is the first step necessary, to be followed by the application of supports, consisting of splints of leather or sheets of metal, the entire front of the head being then covered with bandages prepared with adhesive mixtures. During the entire course of treatment a special method of feeding becomes necessary. The inability of the patient to appreciate the situation, of course, necessitates a resort to an artificial mode of introducing the necessary feed into his stomach; this is accomplished by forcing between the commissures of the lips, in a liquid form, by means of a syringe, the milk or nutritive gruels selected for his sustenance until the consolidation is sufficiently advanced to permit the ingestion of feed of a more solid consistency. The callus will usually be sufficiently hardened in two or three weeks to allow of a change of diet to mashes of cut hay and scalded grain, until the removal of the dressing restores the animal to its old habit of mastication.

FRACTURES OF VERTEBRÆ.

These are not very common, but when they do occur the bones most frequently injured are those of the back and loins.

Causes.—The ordinary causes of fracture are responsible here as elsewhere, such as heavy blows on the spinal column, severe falls while conveying heavy loads, and especially violent efforts in resisting the process of casting. Although occurring more or less frequently under the latter circumstances, the accident is not always attributable to carelessness or error in the management. It may, of course, sometimes result from such a cause as a badly prepared bed, or the accidental presence of a hard body concealed in the straw, or to a heavy fall when the movements of the patient have not been sufficiently controlled by an effective apparatus and its skillful adaptation, but it is quite as liable to be caused by the violent resistance and the consequent powerful muscular contraction by the frightened patient. The simple fact of the overarching of the vertebral column, with excessive pressure against it from the intestinal mass, owing to the spasmodic action of the abdominal muscles, may account for it, and so also may the struggles of the animal to escape from the restraint of the hobbles while frantic under the pain of an operation without anesthesia. In these cases the fracture usually occurs in the body or the annular part, or both, of the posterior dorsal or the anterior lumbar vertebra. When the transverse processes of the last-named bones are injured, it is probably in consequence of the heavy concussion incident to striking the ground when cast. The diagnosis of a fracture of the body of a vertebra is not always easy, especially when quite recent, and more especially when there is no accompanying displacement.

Symptoms.—There are certain peculiar signs accompanying the occurrence of the accident while an operation is in progress which should at once excite the suspicion of the surgeon. In the midst of a violent struggle the patient becomes suddenly quiet; the movement of a sharp instrument, which at first excited his resistance, fails to give rise to any further evidence of sensation; perhaps a general trembling, lasting for a few minutes, will follow, succeeded by a cold, profuse perspiration, particularly between the hind legs, and frequently there will be micturition and defecation. Careful examination of the vertebral column may then detect a slight depression or irregularity in the direction of the spine, and there may be a diminution or loss of sensation in the posterior part of the trunk, while the anterior portion continues to be as sensitive as before. In making an attempt to get upon his feet, however, upon the removal of the hobbles, only the fore part of the body will respond to the effort, a degree of paraplegia being present, and while the head, neck, and fore part of the body will be raised, the hind quarters and hind legs will remain inert. The animal may perhaps succeed in rising and probably may be removed to his stall, but the displacement of the bone will follow, converting the fracture into one of the complete kind, either through the exertion of walking or by a renewed attempt to rise after another fall before reaching his stall. By this time the paralysis is complete, and the extension of the meningitis, which has become established, is a consummation soon reached.

To say that the prognosis of fracture of the body of the vertebra is always serious is to speak very mildly. It would be better, perhaps, to say that *occasionally* a case *may* recover. Fractures of the transverse processes are less serious.

Treatment.—Instead of stating the indication in this class of cases as if assuming them to be amenable to treatment, the question naturally would be: Can any treatment be recommended in a fracture of the body of a vertebra? The only indication in such a case, in our opinion, is to reach the true diagnosis in the shortest possible time and to act accordingly. If there is displacement, and the existence of serious lesions may be inferred from the nervous symptoms, the destruction of the suffering animal appears to suggest itself as the one conclusion in which considerations of policy, humanity, and science at once unite.

If, however, it is fairly evident that no displacement exists; that pressure upon the spinal cord is not yet present; that the animal with a little assistance is able to rise upon his feet and to walk a short distance—it may be well to experiment upon the case to the extent of placing the patient in the most favorable circumstances for recovery and allow nature to operate without further interference. This may be accomplished by obtaining immobility of the whole body as much as possible, and especially of the suspected region, by placing the patient in slings, in a stall sufficiently narrow to preclude lateral motion, and covering the loins with a thick coat of agglutinative mixture. Developments should be watched and awaited.

FRACTURE OF THE RIBS.

The different regions of the chest are not equally exposed to the violence that causes fractures of the ribs, and they are therefore either more common or more easily discovered during life at some points than at others. The more exposed regions are the middle and the posterior, while the front is largely covered and defended by the shoulder. A single rib may be the seat of fracture, or a number may be involved, and there may be injuries on both sides of the chest at the same time. It may take place lengthwise, in any part of the bone, though the middle, being the most exposed, is the most frequently hurt. Incomplete fractures are usually lengthwise, involving a portion only of the thickness of one or other of the surfaces. The complete kind may be either transverse or oblique, and are most commonly denticulated. The fracture may be comminuted, and a single bone may show one of the complete and one of the incomplete kind at different points. The extent of surface presented by the thoracic region, with its complete exposure at all points, explains the liability of the ribs to suffer from all the forms of external violence.

Symptoms.—In many instances fractures, especially the incomplete variety, of these bones continue undiscovered, without displacement, though the evidences of local pain, a certain amount of swelling, and a degree of disturbance of the respiration, if noticed during the examination of a patient, may suggest a suspicion of their existence. Abnormal mobility and crepitation are difficult of detection, even when present, and they are not always present. When there is displacement the deformity which it occasions will betray the fact, and when such an injury exists the surgeon, in view of possible and probable complications of thoracic trouble, of course will become vigilant and prepare himself for an encounter with a case of traumatic pleuritis or pneumonia. Fatal injuries of the heart are recorded. Subcutaneous emphysema is a common accompaniment of broken ribs, and I recall the death, from this cause, of a patient of my own which had suffered a fracture of two ribs in the region of the withers, under the cartilages of the shoulder, and of which the diagnosis was made only after the fatal ending of the case.

These hurts are not often of a very serious character, though the union is never so solid and complete as in other fractures, the callus being usually imperfect and of a fibrous character, with an amphiarthrosis formation. Still, complications occur which may impart gravity to the prognosis.

Treatment.—Fractures with but a slight or no displacement need no reduction. All that is necessary is a simple application of a blistering nature as a preventive of inflammation or for its subjugation when present, and in order to excite an exudation which will tend to aid in the support and immobilization of the parts. At times, however, a better effect is obtained by the application of a bandage placed firmly around the chest, although, while this limits the motion of the ribs, it is liable to render the respiration more labored.

If there is displacement, with much accompanying pain and evident irritation of the lungs, the fracture must be reduced without delay. The means of effecting this vary according to whether the displacement is outward or inward. In the first case the bone may be straightened by pressure from without, while in the second the end of it must be raised by a lever, for the introduction of which a small incision through the skin and intercostal spaces will be necessary. When coaptation has been effected it must be retained by the external application of an adhesive mixture, with splints and bandages around the chest.

FRACTURES OF THE BONES OF THE PELVIS.

These fractures will be considered under their separate denominations, as those of the sacrum and the os innominatum, or hip, which includes the subdivisions of the ilium, the pubes, and the ischium.

The sacrum.—Fractures of this bone are rarely met with among solipeds. Among cattle, however, it is of common occurrence, being attributed not only to the usual varieties of violence, as blows and other external hurts, but to the act of coition and violent efforts in parturition. It is generally of the transverse kind and may be recognized by the deformity which it occasions. This is due to the dropping of the bone, with a change in its direction and a lower attachment of the tail, which also becomes more or less paralyzed. The natural and spontaneous relief which usually interposes in these cases has doubtless been observed by the extensive cattle breeders of the West, and their practice and example fully establish the inutility of interference. Still, cases may occur in which reduction may be indicated, and it then becomes a matter of no difficulty. It is effected by the introduction of a round, smooth piece of wood into the rectum as far as the fragment of bone and using it as a lever, resting upon another as a fulcrum placed under it outside. The bone, having been thus returned, may be kept in place by the ordinary external means in use.

The os innominatum.—Fracture of the ilium may be observed either at the angle of the hip or at the neck of the bone; those of the pubes may take place at the symphysis, or in the body of the bone; those of the ischium on the floor of the bone, or at its posterior external angle. Or, again, the fracture may involve all three of these constituent parts of the hip bone by having its situation in the articular cavity—the acetabulum by which it joins the femur or thigh bone.

Symptoms.—Some of these fractures are easily recognized, while others are difficult to identify. The ordinary deformity which characterizes a fracture of the external angle of the ilium, its dropping and the diminution of that side of the hip in width, unite in indicating the existence of the condition expressed by the term "hipped." An incomplete fracture, however, or one that is complete without displacement, or even one with displacement, often demands the closest scrutiny for its discovery. The lameness may be well marked, and an animal may show it but little while walking, though upon being urged into a trot will manifest it more and more, until presently it will cease to use the crippled limb altogether, and travel entirely on three legs. The acute character of the lameness will vary in degree as the seat of the lesion approximates the acetabulum. In walking, the motion at the hip is very limited, and the leg is dragged; while at rest it is relieved from bearing its share in sustaining the body. An intelligent opinion and correct conclusion will depend largely upon a knowledge of the history of the case, and while in some instances that will be but a report of the common etiology of fractures, such as blows, hurts, and other external violence, the simple fact of a fall may furnish in a single word a satisfactory solution of the whole matter.

With the exception of the deformity of the ilium in a fracture of its external angle, and unless there has been a serious laceration of tissues and infiltration of blood, or excessive displacement, there are no very definite external symptoms in a case of a fracture of the hip bone. There is one, however, which, in a majority of cases, will not fail—it is crepitation. This evidence is attainable by both external and internal examination—by manipulation of the gluteal surface and by rectal taxis. Very often a lateral motion, or balancing of the hinder parts by pressing the body from one side to the other, will be sufficient to render the crepitation more distinct—a slight sensation of grating, which may be perceived even through the thick coating of muscle which covers the bone—and the sensation may not only be felt, but to the expert may even become audible. This external manifestation is, however, not always sufficient in itself, and should invariably be associated with the rectal taxis for corroboration. It is true that this may fail to add to the evidence of fracture, but till then the simple testimony afforded by the detection of crepitation from the surface, though a strong confirmatory point, is scarcely sufficiently absolute to establish more than a reasonable probability or strong suspicion in the case.

In addition to the fact that the rectal examination brings the exploring hand of the surgeon into near proximity to the desired point of search, and to an accurate knowledge of the situation of parts, both pro and con as respects his own views, there is another advantage attendant upon it which is well entitled to appreciation. This is the facility with which he can avail himself of the help of an assistant, who can aid him by manipulating the implicated limb and placing it in various positions, so far as the patient will permit, while the surgeon himself is making explorations and studying the effect from within. By this method he can hardly fail to ascertain the character of the fracture and the condition of the bony ends. By the rectal taxis, as if with eyes in the finger ends, he will " see " what is the extent of the fracture of the ilium or of the neck of that bone; to what part of the central portion of the bone (the acetabulum) it reaches; whether this is free from disease or not, and in what location on the floor of the pelvis the lesion is situated. By this method we have frequently been able to detect a fracture at the symphysis, which, from its history and symptoms and an external examination, could only have been guessed at. Yet, with all its advantages, the rectal examination is not always necessary, as, for example, when the fracture is at the posterior and external angle of the ischium, when by friction of the bony ends the surgeon may discern the crepitation without it.

Every variety of complication, including muscular lacerations with the formation of deep abscesses and injuries to the organs of the pelvic cavity, the bladder, the rectum, and the uterus, may be associated with fractures of the hip bone.

Prognosis.—The prognosis of these lesions will necessarily vary considerably. A fracture of the most superficial part of the bone of the ilium or of the ischium, especially if there is little displacement, will unite rapidly, leaving a comparatively sound animal often quite free from subsequent lameness. If there is much displacement, however, only a ligamentous union will take place, with much deformity and more or less irregularity in the gait. Other fractures may be followed by complete disability of the patient, as, for example, when the cotyloid cavity is involved, or when the reparatory process has left bony deposits in the pelvic cavity at the seat of the union, which may, in the case of the female, interfere with the steps of parturition, or induce some local paralysis by pressure upon the nerves which govern the muscles of the hind legs. This is a condition not infrequently observed when the callus has been formed on the floor of the pelvis near the obturator foramen, pressing upon the course or involving the obturator nerve.

Treatment.—In our estimation, the treatment of all fractures of the hip bone should be of the simplest kind. Rendered comparatively immovable by the thickness of the muscles by which the region is enveloped, one essential indication suggests itself, and that is to place the animal in a position which, so far as possible, will be fixed and permanent. For the accomplishment of this purpose the best measure, as we consider it, is to place the horse in a stall of just sufficient width to admit him, and to apply a set of slings, snugly, but comfortably. (See Plate XXXI.) This will fulfill the essential conditions of recovery—rest and immobility. Blistering applications would be injurious, though the adhesive mixture might prove in some degree beneficial.

The minimum period allowable for solid union in a fractured hip is, in our judgment, two months, and we have known cases in which that was too short a time.

As we have said before, there may be cases in which the treatment for fracture at the floor of the pelvis has been followed by symptoms of partial paralysis, the animal, when lying down, being unable to regain his feet, but moving freely when placed in an upright position. This condition is owing to the interference of the callus with the functions of the obturator nerve, which it presses upon or surrounds. By my experience in similar cases I feel warranted in cautioning owners of horses in this condition to exercise due patience, and to avoid a premature sentence of condemnation against their invalid servants; they are not all irrecoverably paralytic. With alternations of moderate exercise, rest in the slings, and the effect of time while the natural process of absorption is taking effect upon the callus, with other elements of change that may be so operating, the horse in due time may become able once more to earn his subsistence and serve his master.

FRACTURE OF THE SCAPULA.

This bone is seldom fractured, its comparative exemption being due to its free mobility and the protection it receives from the superimposed soft tissues. Only direct and powerful causes are sufficient to effect the injury, and when it occurs the large rather than the smaller animals are the subjects.

Cause.—The causes are heavy blows or kicks and violent collisions with unyielding objects. Those which are occasioned by falls are generally at the neck of the bone, and of the transverse and comminuted varieties.

Symptoms.—The diagnosis is not always easy. The symptoms are inability to rest the leg on the ground and to carry weights, and they are present in various degrees from slight to severe. The leg rests upon the toe, seems shortened, and locomotion is performed by jumps. Moving the leg while examining it and raising the foot for inspection seem to produce much pain and cause the animal to rear. Crepitation is readily felt with the hand upon the shoulder when the leg is moved. If the fracture occurs in the upper part of the bone, overlapping of the fragments and displacement will be considerable.

The fracture of this bone is usually classed among the more serious accidents, though cases may occur which are followed by recovery without very serious ultimate results, especially when the seat of the injury is at some of the upper angles of the bone or about the acromion crest. But if the neck and the joint are the parts involved, complications which are likely to disable the animal for life are liable to be present.

Treatment.—If there is no displacement, a simple adhesive dressing to strengthen and immobilize the parts will be sufficient. A coat of black pitch dissolved with wax and Venice turpentine, and kept in place over the region with oakum or linen bands, will be all the treatment required, especially if the animal is kept quiet in the slings.

Displacement can not be remedied, and reduction is next to impossible. Sometimes an iron plate is applied over the parts and retained by bandages, as in the dressing of Bourgelat (Plate XXX); this may be advantageously replaced by a pad of thick leather. In smaller animals the parts are retained by figure-8 bandages, embracing both the normal and the diseased shoulders, crossing each other in the axilla and covered with a coating of adhesive mixture.

FRACTURES OF THE HUMERUS.

These are more common in small than in large animals, and are always the result of external traumatism, such as falls, kicks, and collisions. They are generally very oblique, are often comminuted, and though more usually involving the shaft of the bone will in some cases extend to the upper end and into the articular head.

Symptoms.—There is ordinarily considerable displacement in consequence of the overlapping of the broken ends of the bone, and this of course causes more or less shortening of the limb. There will also be swelling, with difficulty of locomotion, and crepitation will be easy of detection. This fracture is always a serious damage to the patient, leaving him with a permanently shortened limb and an incurable, lifelong lameness.

Treatment.—If treatment is determined on, it will consist in the reduction of the fracture by means of extension and counter extension, to accomplish which the animal must be thrown. If successful in the reduction, then follows the application and adjustment of the apparatus of retention, which must be of the most perfect and efficient kind. Finally, this, however skillfully contrived and carefully adapted, will often fail to effect any good purpose whatever.

FRACTURES OF THE FOREARM.

A fracture in this region may also involve the radius or the ulna, the latter being broken at times in its upper portion above the radio-ulnar arch at the olecranon. If the fracture occurs at any part of the forearm from the radio-ulnar arch down to the knee, it may involve either the radius alone or the radius and the cubitus, which are there intimately united.

Cause.—Besides having the same etiology with most of the fractures, those of the forearm are, nevertheless, more commonly due to kicks from other animals, especially when crowded together in large numbers in insufficient space. It is a matter of observation that under these circumstances fractures of the incomplete kind are those which occur on the inside of the leg, the bone being in that region almost entirely subcutaneous, while those of the complete class are either oblique or transverse. The least common are the longitudinal, in the long axis of the bone.

Symptoms.—This variety of fracture is easily recognized by the appearance of the leg and the different changes it undergoes. There is inability to use the limb; impossibility of locomotion; mobility below the injury; the ready detection of crepitation—in a word, the assemblage of all the signs and symptoms which have been already considered as associated with the history of broken bones.

The fracture of the ulna alone, principally above the radio-ulnar arch, may be ascertained by the aggravated lameness, the excessive soreness on pressure, and perhaps a certain increase of motion, with a very slight crepitation if tested in the usual way. Displacement is not likely to take place except when it is well up toward the olecranon or its tuberosity, the upper segment of the bone being in that case likely to be drawn upward. For a simple fracture of this region there is a fair chance of recovery, but in a case of the compound and comminuted class there is less ground for a favorable prognosis, especially if the elbow joint has suffered injury. A fracture of the ulna alone is not of serious importance, except when the same conditions prevail. A fracture of the olecranon is less amenable to treatment, and promises little better than a ligamentous union.

Treatment.—Considering all the various conditions involving the nature and extent of these lesions, the position and direction of the bones of the forearm are such as to render the chances for recovery from fracture as among the best. The reduction, by extension and counterextension; the maintenance of the coaptation of the segments; the adaptation of the dressing by splints, oakum, and agglutinative mixtures; in fact, all the details of treatment may be here fulfilled with a degree of facility and precision not attainable in any other part of the organism. An important, if not an essential, point, however, must be emphasized in regard to the splints. Whether they are of metal, wood, or other material, they should reach from the elbow joint to the ground, and should be placed on the posterior face and on both sides of the leg. This is then to be so confined in a properly constructed box as to preclude all possibility of motion, while yet it must sustain a certain portion of the weight of the body. The iron splint (represented in Plate XXX) recommended by Bourgelat is designed for fractures of the forearm, of the knee, and of the cannon bone, and will prove to be an appliance of great value. For small animals the preference is for an external covering of gutta-percha, embracing the entire leg. A sheet of this substance of suitable thickness, according to the size of the animal, softened in lukewarm water, is, when sufficiently pliable, molded on the outside of the leg, and when suddenly hardened by the application of cold water forms a complete casing sufficiently rigid to resist all motion. Patients treated in this manner have been able to use the limb freely, without pain, immediately after the application of the dressing. The removal of the splint is easily effected by cutting it away, either wholly or in sections, after softening it by immersing the leg in a warm bath.

FRACTURE OF THE KNEE.

This accident, happily, is of rare occurrence, but when it takes place is of a severe character, and always accompanied with synovitis, with disease of the joint.

Cause.—It may be caused by falling upon a hard surface, and is usually compound and comminuted. Healing seldom occurs, and when it does there is usually a stiffness of the joint from arthritis.

Symptoms.—As a result of this fracture there is inability to bear weight on the foot. The leg is flexed as in complete radial paralysis, or fracture of the ulna. There is abnormal mobility of the bones of the knee, but crepitation is usually absent.

Prognosis.—Healing is hard to effect, as one part of the knee is drawn upward by the two flexor muscles which separate it from the lower part. The callus which forms is largely fibrous, and if the animal is put to work too quickly this callus is liable to rupture. In favorable cases healing takes place in two or three months. Many horses during the treatment develop founder, with consequent drop sole in the sound leg, as a result of pressure due to continuous standing.

Treatment.—Place the animal in the slings, bring the pieces of bone together if possible, and try to keep them in place by a tight plaster-of-Paris dressing about the leg, extending down to the fetlock. Place the animal in a roomy box stall well provided with bedding so that he can lie down, to prevent founder.

FRACTURE OF THE FEMUR.

The protection which this bone receives from the large mass of muscles in which it is enveloped does not suffice to invest it with immunity in regard to fractures.

Cause.—It contributes its share to the list of accidents of this description, sometimes in consequence of external violence and sometimes as the result of muscular contraction; sometimes its takes place at the upper extremity of the bone; sometimes at the lower; sometimes at the head, when the condyles become implicated; but it is principally found in the body or diaphysis. The fracture may be of any of the ordinary forms, simple or compound, complete or incomplete, transverse or oblique, etc. A case of the comminuted variety is recorded in which 85 fragments of bone were counted and removed.

The thickness of the muscular covering sometimes renders the diagnosis difficult by interfering with the manipulation, but the crepitation test is readily available, even when the swelling is considerable, and which is liable to be the case as the result of the interstitial hemorrhage which naturally follows the laceration of the blood vessels of the region involved.

Symptoms.—If the fracture is at the neck of the bone the muscles of that region (the gluteal) are firmly contracted, and the leg seems to be shortened in consequence. Locomotion is impossible. There is intense pain and violent sweating at first. Crepitation may in some cases be discerned by rectal examination, with one hand resting over the coxo-femoral (hip) articulation. Fractures of the tuberosities of the upper end of the bone, the great trochanter, may be identified by the deformity, the swelling, the impossibility of rotation, and the dragging of the leg in walking. Fracture of the body is always accompanied with displacement, and as a consequence a shortening of the leg, which is carried forward. The lameness is excessive, the foot being moved, both when raising it from the ground and when setting it down, very timidly and cautiously. The manipulations for the discovery of crepitation always cause much pain. Lesions of the lower end of the bone are more difficult to diagnosticate with certainty, though the manifestation of pain while making heavy pressure upon the condyles will be so marked that only crepitation will be needed to turn a suspicion into a certainty.

Treatment.—The question as to treatment in fractures of this description resolves itself into the query whether any treatment can be suggested that will avail anything practically as a curative measure; whether, upon the hypothesis of reduction as an accomplished fact, any permanent or efficient device as a means of retention is within the scope of human ingenuity. If the reduction were successfully performed, would it be possible to keep the parts in place by any known means at our disposal? At the best the most favorable result that could be anticipated would be a reunion of the fragments with a considerable shortening of the bone and a helpless, limping, crippled animal to remind us that for human achievement there is a " thus far and no farther."

In small animals, such as dogs and cats, however, attempts at treatment are justifiable, and we are convinced that in many cases of difficulty in the application of splints and bandages a patient may be placed in a condition of undisturbed quiet and left to the processes of nature for " treatment " as safely and with as good an assurance of a favorable result as if he had been subjected to the most heroic secundum artem doctoring known to science. As a case in point, mention may be made of the case of a pregnant bitch which suffered a fracture of the upper end of the femur by being run over by a light wagon. Her "treatment" consisted in being tied up in a large box and let alone. In due time she was delivered of a family of puppies, and in three weeks she was running in the streets, limping very slightly, and nothing the worse for her accident.

FRACTURE OF THE PATELLA.

This, fortunately, is a rare accident, and can result only from direct violence, as a kick or other blow. The lameness which follows it is accompanied with enormous tumefaction of the joint, pain, inabiilty to bear weight upon the foot, and finally disease of the articulation. Crepitation is absent, because the hip muscles draw away the upper part of the bone. The prognosis is unavoidably adverse, destruction being the only termination of this incurable and very painful injury. Most of the reported cases of cures are based upon a wrong diagnosis.

FRACTURES OF THE TIBIA.

Of all fractures these are probably more frequently encountered than any others among the class of accidents we are considering. As with injuries of the forearm of a like character, they may be complete or incomplete; the former when the bone is broken in the middle or at the extremities, and transverse, oblique, or longitudinal. The incomplete kind are more common in this bone than in any other.

Symptoms.—Complete fractures are easy to recognize, either with or without displacement. The animal is very lame, and the leg is either dragged or held clear from the ground by flexion at the stifle, while the lower part hangs down. Carrying weight or moving backward is impossible. There is excessive mobility below the fracture, and well-marked crepitation. If there is much displacement, as in an oblique fracture, there will be considerable shortening of the leg.

While incomplete fractures can not be recognized in the tibia with any greater degree of certainty than in any other bone, there are some facts associated with them by which a diagnosis may be justified. The hypothetical history of a case may serve as an illustration:

An animal has received an injury by a blow or a kick on the inside of the bone, perhaps without showing any mark. Becoming very lame immediately afterwards, he is allowed a few days' rest. If taken out again, he seems to have recovered his soundness, but within a day or two he betrays a little soreness, and this increasing he becomes very lame again, to be furloughed once more, with the result of a temporary improvement, and again a return to labor and again a relapse of the lameness; and this alternation seems to be the rule. The leg being now carefully examined, a local periostitis is readily discovered at the point of the injury, the part being warm, swollen, and painful. What further proof is necessary? Is it not evident that a fracture has occurred, first superficial—a mere split in the bony structure, which, fortunately, has been discovered before some extra exertion or a casual misstep had developed it into one of the complete kind, possibly with complications? What other inference can such a series of symptoms thus repeated establish?

The prognosis of fracture of the tibia, as a rule, must be unfavorable.

Treatment.—The difficulty of obtaining a union without shortening, and consequently without lameness, is proof of the futility of ordinary attempts at treatment, but though this may be true in respect to fractures of the complete kind, it is not necessarily so with the incomplete variety, and with this class the simple treatment of the slings is all that is necessary to obtain consolidation. A few weeks of this confinement will be sufficient.

With dogs and other small animals there are cases which may be successfully treated. If the necessary dressings can be successfully applied and retained, a cure will follow.

FRACTURES OF THE HOCK.

Injuries of the astragalus which had a fatal termination have been recorded. Fractures of the os calcis have also been observed, but never with a favorable prognosis, and attempts to induce recovery, as might have been expected, have proved futile.

FRACTURES OF THE CANNON BONES.

Whether these occur in the fore or hind legs, they appear either in the body or near their extremities. If in the body as a rule the three metacarpal or metatarsal bones are affected, and the fracture is generally transverse and oblique. On account of the absence of soft tissue and tightness of the skin, the broken bones pierce the skin and render the fracture a complicated one. The diagnosis is easy when all the bones are completely broken, but the incomplete fracture can be only suspected.

Symptoms.—There is no displacement, but excessive mobility, crepitation, inability to sustain weight, and the leg is kept off the ground by the flexion of the upper joint.

No region of the body affords better facilities for the application of treatment, and the prognosis on this account is usually favorable. We recall a case, however, which proved fatal, though under exceptional circumstances. The patient was a valuable stallion of highly nervous organization, with a compound fracture of one of the cannon bones, and his unconquerable resistance to treatment, excited by the intense pain of the wound, precluded all chance of recovery, and ultimately caused his death.

Treatment.—The general form of treatment for these lesions will not differ from that which has been already indicated for other fractures. Reduction, sometimes necessitating the casting of the patient; coaptation, comparatively easy by reason of the subcutaneous situation of the bone; retention, by means of splints and bandages—applied on both sides of the region, and reaching to the ground as in fractures of the forearm—these are always indicated. We have obtained excellent results by the use of a mold of thick gutta-percha, composed of two sections and made to surround the entire lower part of the leg as in an inflexible case.

FRACTURE OF THE FIRST PHALANX.

The hind extremity is more liable than the fore to this injury. It is usually the result of a violent effort, or of a sudden misstep or twisting of the leg, and may be transverse, or, as has usually been the case in our experience, longitudinal, extending from the upper articular surface down to the center of the bone, and generally oblique and often comminuted. The symptoms are the swelling and tenderness of the region, possibly crepitation; a certain abnormal mobility; an excessive degree of lameness, and in some instances a dropping back of the fetlock, with perhaps a straightened or upright condition of the pastern.

The difficulty of reduction and coaptation in this accident, and the probability of bony deposits, as of ringbones, resulting in lameness, are circumstances which tend to discourage a favorable prognosis.

The treatment is that which has been recommended for all fractures, so far as it can be applied. The iron splint which has been mentioned gives excellent results in many instances, but if the fracture is incomplete and without displacement, a form of treatment less energetic and severe should be attempted. One case is within our knowledge in which the owner lost his horse by his refusal to subject the animal to treatment, the post-mortem revealing only a simple fracture with very slight displacement.

FRACTURES OF THE SECOND PHALANX (CORONET).

Though these are generally of the comminuted kind, there are often conditions associated with them which justify the surgeon in attempting their treatment. Though crepitation is not always easy to detect, the excessive lameness, the soreness on pressure, the inability to carry weight, the difficulty experienced in raising the foot, all these suggest, as the solution of the question of diagnosis, the fracture of the coronet, with the accompanying realization of the fact that there is yet, by reason of the situation of the member, immobilized as it is by its structure and its surroundings, room left for a not unfavorable prognosis. Only a slight manipulation will be needed in the treatment of this lesion. To render the immobility of the region more fixed, to support the bones in their position by bandaging, and to establish forced immobility of the entire body with the slings is usually all that is required. Ringbone, being a common sequela of the reparative process, must receive due attention subsequently. One of the severest complications liable to be encountered is an immobile joint (anchylosis). Neurectomy of the median nerve may relieve lameness after a fracture of the phalanges.

FRACTURES OF THE THIRD PHALANX (OS PEDIS).

These lesions may result from a penetrating street nail, or follow plantar or median neurectomy. In the latter instance it is caused by the animal setting the foot down carelessly and too violently, and partly due to degeneration of bone tissue which follows nerving.

Though these fractures are not of very rare occurrence, their recognition is not easy, and there is more of speculation than of certainty pertaining to their diagnosis. The animal is very lame and spares the injured foot as much as possible, sometimes resting it upon the toe alone and sometimes holding it from the ground. The foot is very tender, and the exploring pinchers of the examining surgeon cause much pain. During the first 24 hours there is no increased pulsation in the digital and plantar arteries, but on the second day it is apparent.

There is nothing to encourage a favorable prognosis, and a not unusual termination is an anchylosis with either the navicular bone or the coronet.

No method of treatment needs to be suggested here, the hoof performing the office of retention unaided. Local treatment by baths and fomentations will do the rest. It may be months before there is any mitigation of the lameness.

An ultimate recovery depends to a great extent upon whether the other foot can support the weight during the healing process without causing a drop sole in the supporting foot.

FRACTURE OF THE SESAMOID BONES.

This lesion has been considered by veterinarians, erroneously, we think, as one of rare occurrence. We believe it to be more frequent than has been supposed. Many observations and careful dissections have convinced us that fractures of these little bones have been often mistaken for specific lesions of the numerous ligaments that are implanted upon their superior and inferior parts, and which have been described as a "giving way" or "breaking down" of these ligaments. In my post-mortem examinations I have always noted the fact that when the attachments of the ligaments were torn from their bony connections minute fragments of bony structure were also separated, though we have failed to detect any diseased process of the fibrous tissue composing the ligamentous substance.

Cause.—From whatever cause this lesion may arise, it can hardly be considered as of a traumatic nature, no external violence having any apparent agency in producing it, and it is our belief that it is due to a peculiar degeneration or softening of the bones themselves, a theory which acquires plausibility from the consideration of the spongy consistency of the sesamoids. The disease is a peculiar one, and the suddenness with which different feet are successively attacked, at short intervals and without any obvious cause, seems to prove the existence of some latent, morbid cause which has been unsuspectedly incubating. It is not peculiar to any particular class of horses, nor to any special season of the year, having fallen under our observation in each of the four seasons.

Symptoms.—The general fact is reported in the history of most cases that it makes its appearance without premonition in animals which, after enjoying a considerable period of rest, are first exercised or put to work, though in point of fact it may manifest itself while the horse is still idle in his stable. A hypothetical case, in illustration, will explain our theory: An animal which has been at rest in his stable is taken out to work, and it will be presently noticed that there is something unusual in his movement. His gait is changed, and he travels with short, mincing steps, without any of his accustomed ease and freedom. This may continue until his return to the stable, and then, after being placed in his stall, he will be noticed shifting his weight from side to side and from one leg to another, continuing the movement until rupture of the bony structure takes place. But it may happen that the lameness in one or more of the extremities, anterior or posterior, suddenly increases, and it becomes evident that the rupture has taken place in consequence of a misstep or a stumble while the horse is at work. Then, upon coming to a standstill, he will be found with one or more of his toes turned up; he is unable to place the affected foot flat on the ground. The fetlock has dropped and the leg rests upon this part, the skin of which may have remained intact or may have been more or less extensively lacerated. It seldom happens that more than one toe at a time will turn up, yet still the lesion in one will be followed by its occurrence in another. Commonly two feet, either the anterior or posterior, are affected, and we recall one case in which the two fore and one of the hind legs were included at the same time. The accident, however, is quite as liable to happen while the horse is at rest in his stall, and he may be found in the morning standing on his fetlocks. One of the earliest of the cases occurring in my own experience had been under care for several weeks for suspected disease of the fetlocks, the nature of which had not been made out, when, apparently improved by the treatment which he had undergone, the patient was taken out of the stable to be walked a short distance into the country, but had little more than started when he was called to a halt by the fracture of the sesamoids of both fore legs.

While there are no positive premonitory symptoms of these fractures known, we believe that there are signs and symptoms which come but little short of being so, and the appearance of which will always justify a strong suspicion of the truth of the case. These have been indicated when referring to the soreness in standing, the short, mincing gait, and the tenderness betrayed when pressure is made over the sesamoids on the sides of the fetlock, with others less tangible and definable.

Prognosis.—These injuries can never be accounted less than serious, and in our judgment will never be other than fatal. If our theory of their pathology is the correct one, and the cause of the lesions is truly the softening of the sesamoidal bony structure and independent of any changes in the ligamentous fibers, the possibility of a solid osseous union can hardly be considered admissible.

Treatment.—In respect to the treatment to be recommended and instituted it can be employed only with any rational hope of benefit during the incubation, and with the anticipatory purpose of prevention. It must be suggested by a suspicion of the verities of the case, and applied before any rupture has taken place. To prevent this and to antagonize the causes which might precipitate the final catastrophe—the elevation of the toes—resort must be had to the slings and to the application of firm bandages or splints, perhaps of plaster of Paris, with a high shoe, as about the only indications which science and nature are able to offer. When the fracture is an occurred event, and the toes, one or more, are turned up, any further resort to treatment will be futile.

DISEASES OF JOINTS.

Three classes of injury will be considered under this head. These are, affections of the synovial sacs, those of the joint structures, or of the bones and their articular surfaces, and those forms of solution of continuity known as dislocations or luxations.

DISEASES OF THE SYNOVIAL SACS.

Two forms of affection here present themselves, one being the result of an abnormal secretion which induces a dropsical condition of the sac without any acute, inflammatory action, while the other is characterized by excessive inflammatory symptoms, with their modifications, constituting synovitis.

SYNOVIAL DROPSIES.

We have already considered in a general way the presence of these peculiar oil bags in the joints, and in some regions of the legs where the passage of the tendons takes place, and have noticed the similarity of structure and function of both the articular and the tendinous bursæ, as well as the etiology of their injuries and their pathological history, and we will now treat of the affections of both.

WINDGALLS.

This name is given to the dilated bursæ found at the posterior part of the fetlock joint. They have their origin in a dropsical condition of the bursæ of the joint itself, also of the tendon which slides behind it, and are therefore further known by the designations of articular and tendinous windgalls, or puffs. (See also p. 401.)

They appear in the form of soft and somewhat symmetrical tumors, of varying dimensions, and generally well defined in their circumference. They are more or less tense, according to the quantity of secretion they contain, apparently becoming softer as the foot is raised and the fetlock flexed. Usually they are painless and only cause lameness under certain conditions, as when they begin to develop themselves under the stimulus of inflammatory action, or when large enough to interfere with the functions of the tendons, or again when they have undergone certain pathological changes, such as calcification, which is among their tendencies.

Cause.—Windgalls may be attributed to external causes, such as severe labor or strains resulting from heavy pulling, fast driving, or jumping, or they may be among the sequelæ of internal disorders, such as strangles or the resultants of a pleuritic or pneumonic attack.

Unnecessary anxiety is sometimes experienced respecting these growths, with much questioning touching the expediency of their removal, all of which might be spared, for, while they constitute a blemish, their unsightliness will not hinder the usefulness of the animal, and in any case they rarely fail to show themselves easily amenable to treatment.

Treatment.—When in their acute stage, and when the dropsical condition is not excessive, the inflammation may be checked during the day by continuous, cold-water irrigation by means of a hose or soaking tub and at night by applying a moderately tight-roller bandage. Later absorption may be promoted by a Priessnitz bandage,[1] pressure by roller bandages, sweating, the use of liniments, or if necessary by a sharp blister of biniodid of mercury. This treatment should subdue the inflammation, abate the soreness, absorb the excess of secretion, strengthen the walls of the sac, and finally cause the windgalls to disappear, provided the animal is not too quickly returned to labor and exposed to the same factors that occasioned them at first.

If the inflammation has become chronic, however, and the enlargement has been of considerable duration, the negative course will be the wiser one. If any benefit results from treatment it will be of only a transient kind, the dilatation returning when the patient is again subjected to labor, and it will be a fortunate circumstance if inflammation has not supervened.

Notwithstanding the generally benignant nature of the swelling there are exceptional cases, usually when it is probably undergoing certain pathological changes, which may result in lameness and disable the animal, in which case surgical treatment will be indicated, especially if repeated blisters have failed to improve the symptoms. Line firing is then a preeminent suggestion, and many a useful life has received a new lease as the result of this operation timely performed. Another method of firing, which consists in emptying the sac by means of punctures through and through, made with a red-hot needle or wire, and the subsequent injection of certain irritating and alterative compounds into the cavity, designed to effect its closure by exciting adhesive inflammation, such as tincture of iodin, may be commended. But they are all too active and energetic in their effects and require too much special attention and intelligent management to be trusted to any hands other than those of an expert veterinarian.

BLOOD SPAVIN, BOG SPAVIN, AND THOROUGHPIN.

The blood spavin is situated in front and to the inside of the hock and is merely a varicose or dilated condition of the saphena vein. It occurs directly over the point where the bog spavin is found, and has thus been frequently confused with the latter.

The complicated arrangement of the hock joint, and the powerful tendons which pass on the posterior part, are lubricated with the product of secretion from one tendinous synovial and several articular synovial sacs. A large articular sac contributes to the lubrica-

---

[1] This bandage consists of a cloth drenched in warm water or a dripping bandage laid around the diseased part, then covered by several layers of woolen blanket or cloth, which is in turn covered by parchment paper, rubber cloth, or other impervious material. Heat, moisture, and pressure are obtained by such a bandage if water is poured upon it several times daily.

tion of the shank bone (the tibia) and one of the bones of the hock (the astragalus). The tendinous sac lies back of the articulation itself and extends upward and downward in the groove of that joint through which the flexor tendons slide. The dilatation of this articular synovial sac is what is denominated bog spavin, the term thoroughpin being applied to the dilatation of the tendinous capsule.

The bog spavin is a round, smooth, well-defined, fluctuating tumor situated in front and a little inward of the hock. On pressure it disappears at this point to reappear on the outside and just behind the hock. If pressed to the front from the outside it will then appear on the inside of the hock. On its outer surface it presents a vein which is quite prominent, running from below upward, and it is to the preternatural dilatation of this blood vessel that the term blood spavin is applied.

The thoroughpin is found at the back and on the top of the hock in that part known as the " hollows," immediately behind the shank bone. It is round and smooth, but not so regularly formed as the bog spavin, and is most apparent when viewed from behind. The swelling is usually on both sides and a little in front of the so-called hamstring, but may be more noticeable on the inside or on the outside.

In their general characteristics bog spavins and thoroughpins are similar to windgalls, and one description of the origin, symptoms, pathological changes, and treatment will serve for all equally, except that it is possible for a bog spavin to cause lameness, and thus to involve a verdict of unsoundness in the patient, a circumstance which will, of course, justify its classification by itself as a severer form of a single type of disease.

We have already referred to the subject of treatment and the means employed—rest, of course—with liniments, blisters, etc., and what we esteem as the most active and beneficial of any, early, deep, and well-performed cauterization. There are, besides, commendatory reports of a form of treatment by the application of pressure pads and peculiar bandages upon the hocks, and it is asserted that the removal of the tumors has been effected by their use. Our experience with this apparatus, however, has not been accompanied with such favorable results as would justify our indorsement of the flattering representations which have sometimes appeared in its behalf.

OPEN JOINTS, BROKEN KNEES, SYNOVITIS, AND ARTHRITIS.

The close relationship which exists among these several affections, their apparently possible connection as successive developments of a similar, if not an essentially identical, origin, together with the advantage gained by avoiding frequent repetitions in the details of symptoms, treatment, etc., are our reasons for treating under a single head the ailments we have grouped together in the present section.

Cause.—The great, comprehensive, common cause of, sometimes permanent, sometimes only transient, disability of the horse is external traumatism.

Blows, bruises, hurts by nearly every known form of violence, falls, kicks, lacerations, punctures—we may add compulsory speed in racing and cruel overloading of draft animals—cover the entire ground of causation of the diseases and injuries of the joints now receiving our consideration.

In one case, a working horse making a misstep stumbles, and falling on his knees receives a hurt, variously severe, from a mere abrasion of the skin to a laceration, a division of the teguments, a slough, mortification, and the escape of the synovial fluid, with or without exposure of the bones and their articular cartilages.

In another case, an animal, from one cause or another, perhaps an impatient temper, has formed the habit of striking or pawing his manger with his fore feet until inflammation of the knee joint is induced, first as a little swelling, diffused, painless; then as a periostitis of the bones of the knee; later as bony deposits, then lameness, and finally the implication of the joint, with all the various sequelae of chronic inflammation of the knee joint.

In another case, a horse has received a blow with a fork from a careless hostler on or near a joint, or has been kicked by a stable companion, with the result of a punctured wound, at first mild-looking, painless, apparently without inflammation, and not yet causing lameness, but which, in a few hours, or it may be only after a few days, becomes excessively painful, grows worse, the entire joint swells, presently discharges, and at last a case of suppurative synovitis is presented, with perhaps disease of the joint proper, and arthritis as a climax. The symptoms of articular injuries vary not only in the degrees of the hurt but in the nature of the lesion.

Or the condition of broken knees, resulting as we have said, may have for its starting point a mere abrasion of the skin—a scratch, apparently, which disappears without a scar. The injury may, however, have been more severe, the blow heavier, the fall aggravated by occurring upon an irregular surface, or sharp or rough object, with tearing or cutting of the skin, and this laceration may remain. A more serious case than the first is now brought to our notice.

Another time, immediately following the accident, or possibly as a sequel of the traumatism, the tendinous sacs may be opened, with the escape of the synovia, or, worse, the tendons which pass in front of the knee are torn, the inflammation spreads, the joint and leg are swollen, the animal is becoming very lame; synovitis has set in.

With this the danger becomes very great, for soon suppuration will be established, then the external coat of the articulation proper becomes ulcerated, if it is not already in that state, and we find ourselves in the presence of an open joint with suppurative synovitis—that is, with the worst among the conditions of diseased processes, because of the liability of the suppuration to become infiltrated into every part of the joint, macerating the ligaments and irritating the cartilages, soon to be succeeded by their ulceration, with the destruction of the articular surface—or the lesion of ulcerative arthritis, one of the gravest among all the disorders known to the animal economy.

Ulcerative arthritis and suppurative synovitis may be developed otherwise than in connection with open joints; the simplest and apparently most harmless punctures may prove to be sufficient cause. For example, a horse may be kicked, perhaps, on the inside of the hock; there is a mark and a few drops of blood to indicate the spot; he is put to work apparently free from pain or lameness and performs his task with his usual ease and facility. On the following morning, however, the hock is found to be a little swollen and there is some stiffness. A little later on he betrays a degree of uneasiness in the leg, and shrinks from resting his weight upon it, moving it up and down for relief. The swelling has increased and is increasing; the pain is severe; and finally, at the spot where the kick inpinged, there is an oozing of an oily liquid mixed with whitish drops of suppuration. The mischief is done; a simple, harmless, punctured wound has expanded into a case of ulcerative arthritis and suppurative synovitis.

Prognosis.—From ever so brief and succinct description of this traumatism of the articulations, the serious and important character of these lesions, irrespective of which particular joint is affected, will be readily understood. Yet there will be modifications in the prognosis in different cases, in accordance with the peculiarities of structure in the joint specially involved, as, for example, it is obvious that a better result may be expected from treatment when but a single joint, with only its plain articular surfaces, is the place of injury, than in one which is composed of several bones, united in a complex formation, as in the knee or hock. As severe a lesion as suppurative synovitis always is, and as frequently fatal as it proves to be, still cases arise in which, the inflammation assuming a modified character and at length subsiding, the lesion terminates favorably and leaves the animal with a comparatively sound and useful joint. There are cases, however, which terminate in no more favorable a result than the union of the bones and occlusion of the joint, to form an anchylosis, which is scarcely a condition to justify a high degree of satisfaction, as it insures a permanent lameness with very little capacity for usefulness.

Appreciating now the dangers associated with all wounds of articulations, however simple and apparently slight, and how serious and troublesome are the complications which are liable to arise during their progress and treatment, we are prepared to understand and realize the necessity and the value of early and prompt attention upon their discovery and diagnosis.

Treatment.—For simple bruises, like those which appear in the form of broken knees or of carpitis, simple remedies, such as warm fomentations or cold-water applications and compresses of astringent mixtures, suggest themselves at once. Injuries of a more complicated character, as lacerations of the skin or tearing of soft structures, will also be benefited by simple dressings with antiseptic mixtures, as those of the carbolic-acid order. The escape of synovia should suggest the prompt use of collodion dressings to check the flow and prevent the further escape of the fluid. But if the discharge is abundant and heavily suppurative, little can be done more than to put in practice the "expectant" method with warm fomentations, repeatedly applied, and soothing, mucilaginous poultices. Improvement, if any is possible, will be but slow to manifest itself. The most difficult of all things to do, in view of varying interests and opinions—that is, in a practical sense—is to abstain from "doing" entirely, and yet in the cases we are considering we are firmly convinced that noninterference is the best and wisest policy.

In cases which are carried to a successful result the discharge will diminish by degrees, the extreme pain will gradually subside, the convalescent will begin timidly to rest his foot upon the ground, and presently to bear weight upon it, and perhaps, after a long and tediour process of recuperation, he may be returned to his former and normal condition of usefulness. When the discharge has wholly ceased and the wounds are entirely healed, a blister covering the whole of the joint for the purpose of stimulating the absorption of the exudation will be of great service. If, on the contrary, there is no amelioration of symptoms and the progress of the disease resists every attempt to check it; if the discharge continues to flow not only without abatement but in an increased volume, and not alone by a single opening but by a number of fistulous tracts which have successively formed; if it seems evident that this drainage is rapidly and painfully sapping the suffering animal's vitality, and a deficient *vis vitæ* fails to cooperate with the means of cure—all rational hope of recovery may be finally abandoned. Any further waiting for chances, or time lost in experimenting, will be mere cruelty and there need be no hesitation concerning the next step. The poor beast is under sentence of death, and every consideration of interest and of humanity demands an anticipation of nature's evident intent in the quick and easy execution of the sentence.

PLATE XXX.

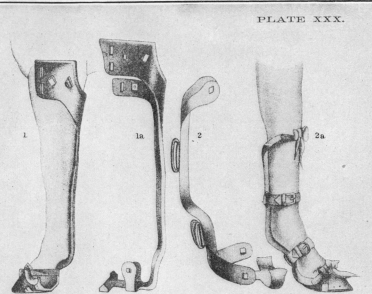

1 Brace for dislocation of the elbow applied to the horse.
1a. The same brace seen alone. 2, Brace for dislocation
of fetlock 2a, The same brace applied to the horse.

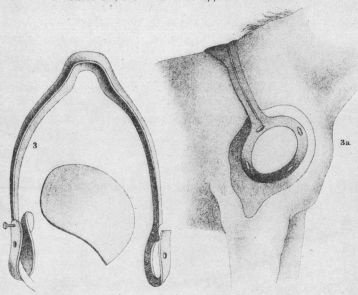

3, Brace for sprained or dislocated shoulder.
3a, The same brace applied to the shoulder.

Haines, del. after Peuch and Toussaint

DISLOCATION OF SHOULDER AND ELBOW
Bourgelat's apparatus

PLATE XXXI.

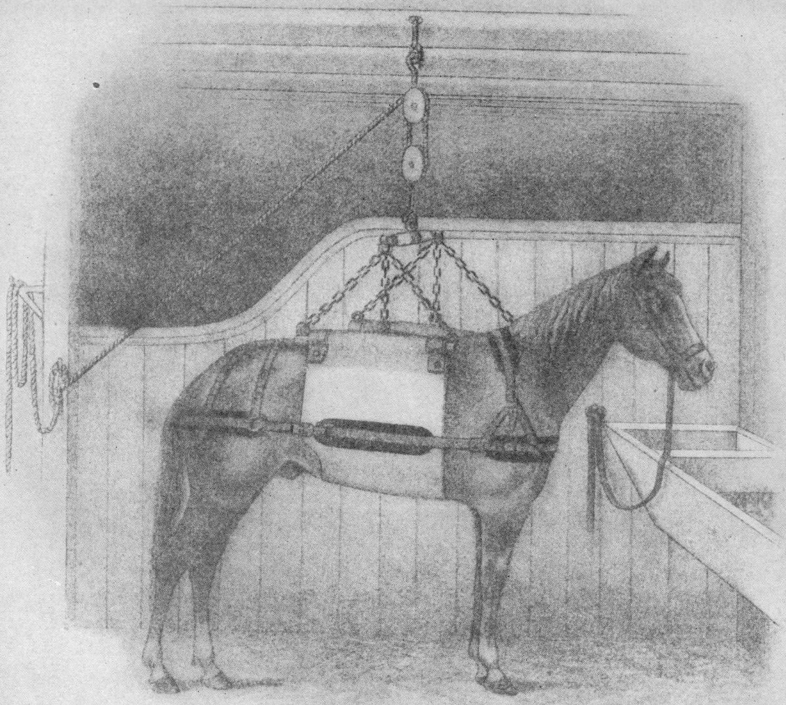

Haines, del after Reynders

THE SLING IN USE

One of the essentials of treatment, and probably an indispensable condition when recovery is in any wise attainable, is the suspension of the patient in slings. He should be continued in them so long as he can be made to submit quietly to their restraint.

DISLOCATIONS.

Dislocations and luxations are interchangeable terms, meaning the separation and displacement of the articulating surfaces of the bones entering into the formation of a joint. This injury is rarely encountered in our large animals on account of the combination of strength and solidity in the formation of their joints. It is met with but seldom in cattle and less so in horses, while dogs and smaller animals are more often the sufferers.

Cause.—The accident of a luxation is less often encountered in the animal races than in man. This is not because the former are less subject to occasional violence involving powerful muscular contractions, or are less often exposed to casualties similar to those which result in luxations in the human skeleton, but because it requires the cooperation of conditions—anatomical, physiological, and perhaps mechanical present in the human race and lacking in the others, which, however, can not in every case be clearly defined. Perhaps the greater relative length of the bony levers in the human formation may constitute a cause of the difference.

Among the predisposing causes in animals may be enumerated caries of articular surfaces, articular abscesses, excessive dropsical conditions, degenerative softening of the ligaments, and any excessive laxity of the soft structures.

Symptoms and diagnosis.—Three signs of dislocation must usually be taken into consideration. They are: (1) An alteration in the shape of the joint and in the normal relationship of the articulating surfaces; (2) an alteration in the length of the limb, either shortening or lengthening; (3) an alteration in the movableness of the joint, usually an unnatural immobility. Only the first, however, can be relied upon as essential. Luxations are not always complete; they may be partial; that is, the articulating surfaces may be displaced but not separated. In such cases several symptoms may not be present. And not only may the third sign be absent, but the mobility of the first be greatly increased when the character of the injury has been such as to produce extensive lacerations of the articular ligaments.

In addition to the above signs, a luxation is usually characterized by pain, swelling, hemorrhage beneath the skin from damaged or ruptured blood vessels, and even paralysis, when important nerves are pressed on by the displaced bones.

Sometimes a bone is fractured in the immediate vicinity of a joint. The knowledge of this fact requires us to be able to diagnose between a dislocation and such a fracture. In this we generally have three points to assist us: (1) The immobility of a dislocated joint as against the apparently remarkable freedom of movement in fracture; (2) in a dislocation there is no true crepitus—that peculiar grating sensation heard as well as felt on rubbing together the rough ends of fractured bones; however, it must be remembered that in a dislocation two or three days old the inflammatory changes around the joint may give rise to a crackling sensation similar to that in fracture; (3) as a rule, in luxations, if the ligamentous and muscular tissues about the joint are not badly torn, the displacement, when reduced, does not recur.

Prognosis.—The prognosis of a luxation is comparatively less serious than that of a fracture, though at time the indications of treatment may prove to be so difficult to apply that complications of a very severe character may arise.

Treatment.—The treatment of luxations must, of course, be similar to that of fractures. Reduction, naturally, will be the first indication in both cases, and the retention of the replaced parts must follow. The reduction involves the same steps of extension and counter extension, performed in the same manner, with the patient subdued by anesthetics.

The difference between the reduction of a dislocation and that of a fracture consists in the fact that in the former the object is simply to restore the bones to their true, normal position, with each articular surface in exact contact with its companion surface, the apparatus necessary afterwards to keep them in situ being similar to that which is employed in fracture cases, and which will usually require to be retained for a period of from 40 to 50 days, if not longer, before the ruptured retaining ligaments are sufficiently firm to be trusted to perform their office unassisted. A variety of manipulations are to be used by the surgeon, consisting in pushing, pulling, pressing, rotating, and, indeed, whatever movement may be necessary, until the bones are forced into such relative positions that the muscular contraction, operating in just the right directions, pulls the opposite matched ends together in true coaptation—a head into a cavity, an articular eminence into a trochlea, as the case may be. The " setting " is accompanied with a peculiar, snapping sound, audible and significant, as well as a visible return of the surface to its normal symmetry.

Special dislocations.—While all the articulations of the body are liable to this form of injury, there are three in the large animals which may claim a special consideration, viz:

THE SHOULDER JOINT.

We mention this displacement without intending to imply the practicability of any ordinary attempt at treatment, which is usually unsuccessful, the animal whose mishap it has been to become a victim to it being disabled for life. The superior head of the arm bone as it is received into the lower cavity of the shoulder blade is so situated as to be liable to be forced out of place in four directions. It may escape from its socket, according to the manner in which the violence affects it—outward, inward, backward, or forward—and the deformity which results and the effects which follow will correspondingly differ. We have said that treatment is generally unsuccessful. It may be added that the difficulties which interpose in the way of reduction are nearly insurmountable, and that the application of means for the retention of the parts after reduction would be next to impossible. The prognosis, from any point of view, is sufficiently grave for the luckless animal with a dislocated shoulder.

THE HIP JOINT.

This joint partakes very much of the characteristics of the humeroscapular articulation, but is more strongly built. The head of the thigh bone is more separated, or prominent and rounder in form, and the cup-like cavity, or socket, into which it fits is much deeper, forming together a deep, true ball-and-socket joint, which is, moreover, reenforced by two strong cords of funicular ligaments, which unite them. It will be easily comprehended, from this hint of the anatomy of the region, that a luxation of the hip joint must be an accident of comparatively rare occurrence; yet cases are recorded in which the head of the bone has been affirmed to slip out of its cavity and assume various positions—inward, outward, forward, or backward.

The indications of treatment are those of all cases of dislocation. When the reduction is accomplished the surgeon will be apprised of the fact by the peculiar, snapping sound usually heard on such occasions.

PSEUDO-LUXATIONS OF THE PATELLA.

This is not a true dislocation. The stifle bone is so peculiarly articulated with the thigh bone that the means of union are of sufficient strength to resist the causes which usually give rise to luxations, yet there is sometimes discovered a peculiar, pathological state in the hind legs of animals, the effect of which is closely to simulate the manifestation of many of the general symptoms of dislocations. This condition originates in muscular cramps, the action of which is seen in a certain change in the coaptation of the articular surfaces of the stifle and thigh bone, resulting in the exhibition of a sudden and alarming series of symptoms which have suggested the phrase of " stifle out " as a descriptive term.

Symptoms.—The animal so affected stands quietly and firmly in his stall, or perhaps with one of his hind legs extended backward, and resists every attempt to move him backward. If urged to move forward he will either refuse or comply with a jump, with the toe of the disabled leg dragging on the ground and brought forward by a second effort. There is no flexion at the hock and no motion at the stifle, while the circular motion of the hip is quite free. The leg appears to be much longer than the other, owing to the straightened position of the thigh bone, which forms almost a straight line with the tibia from the hip joint down. The stifle joint is motionless, and the motions of all the joints below it are more or less interfered with. External examination of the muscles of the hip and thigh reveals a certain degree of rigidity, with perhaps some soreness, and the stifle bone may be seen projecting more or less on the outside and upper part of the joint.

This state of things may continue for some time and until treatment is applied, or it may spontaneously and suddenly terminate, leaving everything in its normal condition, but perhaps to return again.

Cause.—Pseudo-dislocation of the patella is liable to occur under many of the conditions which cause actual dislocation, and yet it may often occur in animals which have not been exposed to the ordinary causes, but which have remained at rest in their stables. Sometimes these cases are assignable to falls in a slippery stall, or perhaps slipping when endeavoring to rise; sometimes to weakness in convalescing patients; sometimes to lack of tonicity of structure and general debility; sometimes to relaxation of tissues from want of exercise or use. A straight leg, sloping croup, and the young are predisposed to this dislocation.

Treatment.—The reduction of these displacements of the patella is not usually attended with difficulty. A sudden jerk or spasmodic action will often be all that is required to spring the patella into place, when the flexion of the leg at the hock ends the trouble for the time. But this is not always sufficient, and a true reduction may still be indicated. To effect this the leg must be drawn well forward by a rope attached to the lower end, and the patella, grasped with the hand, forcibly pushed forward and inward and made to slip over the outside border of the trochlea of the femur. The bone suddenly slips into position, the excessive rigor of the leg ceases with a spasmodic jerk, and the animal may walk or trot away without suspicion of lameness. Though this may end the trouble for the time, and the restoration seem to be perfect and permanent, a repetition of the entire transaction may subsequently take place, and perhaps from the loss of some proportion of tensile power which would naturally follow the original attack in the muscles involved the lesion might become a habitual weakness.

Warm fomentations and douches with cold water will often promote permanent recovery, and liberty in a box stall or in the field will in many cases insure constant relief. The use of a high-heeled shoe is recommended by European veterinarians. The use of stimulating liniments, with frictions, charges, or even severe blisters, may be resorted to in order to prevent the repetition of the difficulty by strengthening and toning up the parts.

DISEASES OF MUSCLES AND TENDONS.

SPRAINS.

This term expresses a more or less complete laceration or yielding of the fibers of the muscles, tendons, or the sheaths surrounding and supporting them. The usual cause of a sprain is external violence, such as a fall or a powerful exertion of strength, with following symptoms of soreness, heat, swelling, and a suspension of function. Their termination varies from simple resolution to suppuration, and commonly fibrinous exudation difficult to remove. None of the muscles or tendons of the body are exempt from liability to this lesion, though naturally from their uses and the exposure of their situation the extremities are more liable than other regions to become their seat. The nature of the prognosis will be determined by a consideration of the seat of the injury and the complications likely to arise.

Treatment.—The treatment will resolve itself into the routine of local applications, including warm fomentations, stimulating liniments, counterirritation by blistering, and in some cases even firing. Rest, in the stable or in a box stall, will be of advantage by promoting the absorption of whatever fibrinous exudation may have formed, or absorption may be stimulated by the careful persevering application of iodin in the form of ointments of various degrees of strength.

There are many conditions in which not only the muscular and tendinous structures proper are affected by a strain, but, by contiguity of parts, the periosteum of neighboring bones may become involved, with a complication of periostitis and its sequelæ.

LAMENESS OF THE SHOULDER.

The frequency of the occurrence of lameness in the shoulder from sprains entitles it to precedence of mention in the present category, for, though so well covered with its muscular envelope, it is often the seat of injuries which, from the complex structure of the region, become difficult to diagnosticate with satisfactory precision and facility. The flat bone which forms the skeleton of that region is articulated in a comparatively loose manner with the bone of the arm, but the joint is, notwithstanding, rather solid, and is powerfully strengthened by tendons passing outside, inside, and in front of it. Still, shoulder lameness or sprain may exist, originating in lacerations of the muscles, the tendons or the ligaments of the joint, or perhaps in diseases of the bones themselves. " Slip of the shoulder " is a phrase frequently applied to such lesions.

The identification of the particular structures involved in these lesions is of much importance, in view of its bearing upon the question of prognosis. For example, while a simple superficial injury of the spinatus muscles, or the muscles by which the leg is attached to the trunk, may not be of serious import and may readily yield to treatment, or even recover spontaneously and without interference, the condition is quite changed in a case of tearing of the flexor brachii, or of its tendons as they pass in front of the articulation, or, what is still more serious, if there is inflammation or ulceration in the groove over which this tendon slides, or upon the articular surfaces or their surroundings, or periostitis at any point adjacent.

Causes.—The frequency of attacks of shoulder lameness is not difficult to account for. The superficial and unprotected position of the part and the numerous movements of which it is capable, and which, in fact, it performs, render it both subjectively and objectively preeminently liable to accident or injury. It would be difficult and would not materially avail to enumerate all the forms of violence by which the shoulder may be crippled. A fall, accompanied with powerful concussion; a violent muscular contraction in starting a heavily loaded vehicle from a standstill; a misstep following a quick muscular effort; a jump accompanied with miscalculated results in alighting; a slip on a smooth, icy road; balling the feet with snow; colliding with another horse or other object—indeed, the list may be indefinitely extended, but without profit or utility.

Symptoms.—Some of the symptoms of shoulder lameness are peculiar to themselves, and yet the trouble is frequently mistaken for other affections—navicular disease more often than any other. The fact that in both affections there are instances when the external symptoms are but imperfectly defined, and that one of them especially is very similar in both, is sufficient to mislead careless or inexperienced observers and to occasion the error which is sometimes committed of applying to one disease the name of the other, erring both ways in the interchange. The true designation of pathological lesions is very far at times from being of certain and easy accomplishment, and, owing to the massive structure of the parts we are considering, this is especially true in the present connection. Still there are many cases in which there is really no reasonable excuse for an error in diagnosis by an average practitioner.

Shoulder lameness will, of course, manifest itself by signs and appearances more or less distinct and pronounced, according to the nature of the degrees and the extent of the originating cause. We summarize some of these signs and appearances:

The lameness is not intermittent, but continued, the disturbance of motion gaging the severity of the lesion and its extent. It is more marked when the bones are diseased than when the muscles alone are affected. When in motion the two upper bony levers—the shoulder blade and the bone of the upper arm—are reduced to nearly complete immobility and the walking is performed by the complete displacement of the entire mass, which is dragged forward without either flexion of extension. The action of the joint below, as a natural consequence, is limited in its flexion. In many instances there is a certain degree of swelling at the point of injury—at the joint, or, more commonly, in front of it, or on the surface of the spinatus muscle. Again, instead of swelling there will be muscular atrophy, though, while this condition of loss of muscular power may interfere with perfect locomotion, it is not in itself usually a cause of shoulder lameness. "Sweenied" shoulders are more often due to disease below the fetlock than to affections above the elbow.

During rest the animal often carries his leg forward, somewhat analogous to the "pointing" position of navicular disease, though in some cases the painful member drops at the elbow in a semiflexed position. The backing is sometimes typical, the animal when performing it, instead of flexing his shoulder, dragging the whole leg without motion in the upper segment of the extremity.

The peculiar manner in which the leg is brought forward in the air for another step in the act of walking or trotting is in some instances characteristic of injuries of the shoulder. The lameness also manifests itself in bringing the leg forward with a circumflex swinging motion and a shortening in the extension of the step. The foot is carried close to the ground and stumbling is frequent, especially on an uneven road.

With the utmost scrutiny and care the vagueness and uncertainty of the symptoms will contribute to perplex and discredit the diagnosis and embarrass the surgeon, and sometimes the expedient is tried of aggravating the symptoms by way of intensifying their significance, and thus rendering them more intelligible. This has been sought by requiring the patient to travel on hard or very soft ground and compelling him to turn on the sound leg as a pivot, with other motions calculated to betray the locality of the pain.

Treatment.—It is our conviction that lameness of the shoulder will in many cases disappear with no other prescription than that of rest. Provided the lesions occasioning it are not too severe, time is all that is required. But the negation of letting alone is seldom accepted as a means of doing good, in the place of the active and the positive forms of treatment. This is in accordance with a trait of human nature which is universal, and is unlimited in its applications; hence something must be done. In mild cases of shoulder lameness, then, the indications are water, either in the cold douche or by showering, or by warm fomentations. Warm, wet blankets are of great service; in addition, or as alternative, anodyne liniments, camphor, belladonna, either in the form of tincture or the oils, are of benefit, and at a later period stimulating friction with suitable mixtures, sweating liniments, blistering compounds, subcutaneous injections over the region of the muscle of 1½ grains of veratrin (the variety insoluble in water) mixed in 2 drams of water, etc., will find their place, and finally, when necessity demands it, the firing iron and the seton.

The duration of the treatment must be determined by its effects and the evidence that may be offered of the results following the action of the reparative process. But the great essential condition of cure, and the one without which the possibility of relapse will always remain as a menace, is, as we have often reiterated in analogous cases, *rest*, imperatively rest, irrespective of any other prescriptions with which it may be associated.

SPRAIN OF THE ELBOW MUSCLES.

Causes.—This injury, which fortunately is not very common, is mostly encountered in cities among heavy draft horses or rapidly driven animals which are obliged to travel, often smooth shod, upon slippery, icy, or greasy pavements, where they are easily liable to lose their foothold. The region of the strain is the posterior part of the shoulder, and the affected muscles are those which occupy the space between the posterior border of the scapula and the posterior face of the arm. It is the muscles of the olecranon which give way.

Symptoms.—The symptoms are easily recognized, especially when the animal is in action. While at rest the attitude may be normal, or by close scrutiny a peculiarity may perhaps be detected. The leg may seem to drop; the elbow may appear to be lower than its fellow, with the knee and lower part of the leg flexed and the foot resting on the toe, with the heel raised. Such an attitude, however, may be occasionally assumed by an animal without having any special significance, but when it becomes more pronounced in motion the fact acquires a symptomatic value, and this is the case in the present instance. A rapid gait becomes quite impossible, and the walk, as in some few other diseases, becomes sufficiently characteristic to warrant a diagnosis even when observed from a distance. An entire dropping of the anterior part of the trunk becomes manifest, and no weight is carried on the disabled side in consequence of the loss of action in the suspensory muscles. There are often heat, pain, and swelling in the muscular mass at the elbow, though at times a hollow, or depression, may be observed near the posterior border of the scapula, which is probably the seat of injury.

These hurts are of various degrees of importance, varying from mere minor casualties of quick recovery to lesions which are of sufficient severity to render an animal useless and valueless for life.

Treatment.—The prime elements of treatment, which should be strictly observed, are rest and quiet. Prescriptions of all kinds, of course, have their advocates. Among them are ether, chloroform, camphor, alcoholic frictions, warm fomentations, blisters, setons, etc. Unless the conclusions of experience are to be ignored, my own judgment is decisive in favor of rest, judiciously applied, however, and my view of what constitutes a judicious application of rest has been more than once presented in these pages. There are degrees of this rest. One contemplates simple immobility in a narrow stall. Another means the enforced mobility of the slings and a narrow stall as well. Another a box stall, with ample latitude as to posture and space, and option to stand or lie down. As wide as this range may appear to be, radical recovery has occurred under all of these modified forms of *letting our patients alone.*

HIP LAMENESS.

The etiology of injuries and diseases of the hip is one and the same with that of the shoulder. The same causes operate and the same results follow. The only essential change, with an important exception, which would be necessary in passing from one region to the other in a description of its anatomy, its physiology, and its pathology would be a substitution of anatomical names in reference to certain bones, articulations, muscles, ligaments, and membranes concerned in the injuries and diseases described. It would be only a useless repetition to cover again the ground over which we have so recently passed in recital of the manner in which certain forms of external violence (falls, blows, kicks, etc.) result in other certain forms of lesion (luxation, fracture, periostitis, ostitis, etc.), and to recapitulate the items of treatment and the names of the medicaments proper to use. The same rules of diagnosis and the same indications and prognosis are applicable equally to every portion of the organism, with only such modifications in applying dressings and apparatus as may be required by differences of conformation and other minor circumstances, which must suggest themselves to the judgment of every experienced observer when the occasion arrives for its exercise.

An exception is to be made, while considering the subject in connection with the region now under advisement, in respect to the formidable affection known as morbus coxarius, or hip-joint disease; and leaving the detail of other lesions to take their place under other heads, that relating to the shoulder, for instance, we turn to the hip joint and its ailments as the chief subject of our present consideration.

Symptoms.—In investigating for morbus coxarius, let the observer first examine the lame animal by scanning critically the outlines of the joint and the region adjacent for any difference of size or disturbance of symmetry in the parts, any prominence or rotundity, and on both sides. The lame side will probably be warmer, more developed, and fuller, both to the touch and to the eye. Let him then grasp the lower part of the leg (as he would in examining a case of shoulder lameness) and endeavor to produce excessive passive motion. This will probably cause pain when the leg is made to assume a given position. Let him push the thigh forcibly against the hip bone, and the contact will again probably cause a manifestation of pain. If the horse is trotted, the limited action of the hip joint proper and the excessive dropping and rising of the hip of the opposite side will be easily recognized. Usually the animal does not extend the foot so far as customarily and picks it up much sooner.

The abductive or circumflex motion observed in shoulder lameness is also present in hip lameness, but under special conditions, and the test of the difficulty, either by traveling on soft ground or in turning the horse in a circle, may here also contribute to the diagnosis, as in testing for lameness in the anterior extremity.

Prognosis.—The prognosis of hip lameness is at times quite serious, not only on account of the long duration of treatment required to effect good results, and because of the character which may be assumed by the disease, but of the permanence of the disability resulting from it. Exostosis and ulcerative arthritis are sequelæ which often resist every form of treatment.

Treatment.—As before intimated, this is little more than a repetition of the remarks upon the lameness of the shoulder, with slight modifications occasioned by the muscular structure of the hip, and we are limited to the same recommendations of treatment. The advantages of rest must be reaffirmed, with local applications, of which, however, it may be said that they are more distinctly indicated and likely to be more effective in their results than in shoulder lameness, and may be more freely employed, whether in the form of liniments, blisters (singly or repeated), firing, or setoning.

SPRAINS OF SUSPENSORY LIGAMENTS AND OF FLEXOR TENDONS OR THEIR SHEATHS.

The fibrous structure situated behind the cannon bones, both in the fore and hind legs, is often the seat of lacerations or sprains resulting from violent efforts or sudden jerks.

Cause.—The injury may be considered serious or trifling, according to the circumstances of each case as judged by its own history. Among the predisposing causes are a long, thin fetlock and a narrow knee or hock as viewed from the side, with the flexor muscles tied in just below the joint. The longer and more oblique the pastern the greater is the strain on the flexor tendons and suspensory ligaments; hence a low quarter, a toe calk, and no heel calks, or a thin calk placed at the tip under the toe, and leaving the quarters long abnormally stretches the back tendons and causes a great strain upon them just before the weight is shifted from the foot in locomotion. In runners and hunters the disease is liable to be periodic. In driving horses it is most common in well-bred animals of nervous temperament. Draft horses suffer most frequently in the hind legs.

Symptoms.—The injury is readily recognized by the changed aspect of the region and the accompanying local symptoms. The parts which in health are well defined, with the outlines of the tendons and ligaments well marked, become the seat of a swelling, more or less developed, from a small spot on the middle of the back of the tendon to a tumefaction reaching from the knee down to and even involving the fetlock itself. It is always characterized by heat, and it is variously sensitive, ranging from a mere tenderness to a degree of soreness which shrinks from the lightest touch. The degree of the lameness varies, and it has a corresponding range with the soreness, sometimes showing only a slight halting and at others the extreme of lameness on three legs, with intermediate degrees.

The lameness is always worse when the weight is thrown on the foot and is most marked toward the end of the phase of contact with the ground. Either passive irritation of the leg or turning the animal in a circle causes pain as in diseases of the joints. Sometimes the horse likes to get the heels on a stone or some elevation so as to relieve the weight from the flexor tendons. Finally, in cases of long standing, a shortening of the tendons occurs, resulting in the abnormal flexion of the foot known by horsemen as " broken down," or a more upright position of the foot may follow, producing perhaps knuckling or the so-called clubfoot.

Prognosis.—It may be safely assumed on general principles that a leg which has received such injuries seldom returns to a perfect condition of efficiency and soundness, and that as a fact a certain absolute amount of thickening and deformity will remain permanent, even when the lameness has entirely disappeared.

Treatment.—The injured member should receive the earliest atten-tion possible, not only when the inflammatory condition is present, but when it is subsiding and there is only the thickening of the liga-ments, the tendons, or the sheath.

The most important remedy is rest, and the shoes should always be removed. During the first three days cold in the form of immersion or continuous irrigation is indicated. Then warm moisture and con-tinuous pressure are advised. The latter is best applied by placing two padded splints about the thickness of the thumb along the two sides of the tendon and binding them in place with even pressure by bandage. Frequent bathing with warm soap suds is also beneficial. The absorption of the exudate may be promoted and the work of restoration effected by frictions with alcohol, tincture of soap, spirits of camphor, mild liniments, strong, sweating liniments, and blisters. An excellent ointment to apply with massage consists of equal parts of blue ointment and green soap, with double the quantity of vaseline. The action of blisters in these cases depends chiefly upon the massage used in applying them and upon the continuous pressure of the swol-len skin on the inflamed tendons. In old cases more beneficial results will follow line firing. In these cases shoeing is very important. Leave the quarters long, shorten the toe, give the shoe rolling motion, and either put short heel calks on the branches or thicken the branches. Although this line of treatment is efficacious in many cases, there are others in which the thickening of the tendons refuses to yield and the changed tissues remain firmly organized, leaving them in the form of a thick mass resting upon the back part of the cannon bone.

KNUCKLING OF FETLOCK.

As a consequence of the last-mentioned lesion of the tendons, a new condition presents itself in the articular disposition, constituting the deformity known as the knuckling fetlock. (See also p. 400.)

By this is meant a deformity of the fetlock joint by which the natural angle is changed from that which pertains to the healthy articulation. The first pastern, or suffraginis, loses its oblique direc-tion and assumes another, which varies from the upright to the oblique, from before backward, and from above downward; in other words, forming an angle with its apex in front.

Causes.—This condition, as we have seen, may be the result of chronic disease producing structural changes in the tendons, and it may also occur as the result of other affections or some peculiarity independent of this and situated below the fetlock, such as ringbones, sidebones, or traumatic disease of the foot proper. Animals are sometimes predisposed to knuckling, such, for example, as are natur-ally straight in their pasterns, or animals which are compelled to labor when too young. The hind legs are more predisposed than the fore to this deformity, in consequence of the greater amount of labor they are required to perform as the propelling levers of the body.

Symptoms.—The symptoms of knuckling are easily recognized. The changes in the direction of the bones vary more or less with the degree of the lesion, sometimes assuming such a direction that it almost becomes a true dislocation of the pastern.

The effect of knuckling upon the gait also varies according to the degree of the deformity. As the different degrees of the shortening of the leg affect the motion of the fetlock, the lameness may be very slight or quite extreme. Another consequence of this shortening is such a change in the position of the foot that the heels cease to come in contact with the ground and assume a greater elevation, and the final result of this is soon witnessed in the development of a clubfoot.

Treatment.—To whatever cause the knuckling may be ascribed, it is always a severe infirmity, and there is but little room for hoping to overcome it unless it be during the very first stages of the trouble, and the hope dwindles to still smaller dimensions when it is secondary to other diseases below the fetlock. If it is caused by overworking the animal, the first indication, of course, will be rest. Line firing has proved very efficacious in these cases. The animal must be turned loose and left unemployed. Careful attention should be given to the condition of his feet and to the manner of shoeing, while time is allowed for the tendons to become restored to their normal state and the irritation caused by excessive stretching has subsided. A shoe with a thick heel will contribute to this. If no improvement can be obtained, however, and the tendons though retracted have yet been relieved of much of their thickening, the case is not a desperate one, and may yet be benefited by the operation of tenotomy, single or double—an operative expedient which must be committed to the experienced surgeon for its performance.

SPRUNG KNEES.

Though not positively the result of diseases of the tendons acting upon the knees, we venture to consider this deformity in connection with that which we have just described. It consists in such an alteration in the direction and articulation of the bones which form the various carpal joints that instead of forming a vertical line from the lower end of the forearm to the cannon bone they are so united that the knee is more or less bent forward, presenting a condition caused by the retraction of two of the principal muscles by which the cannon bone is flexed.

Cause.—This flexion of the knee may be a congenital deformity and have continued from the foaling of the animal; or, like clubfoot, it may be the result of heavy labor which the animal has been compelled to perform when too young. It may also be due to other diseases existing in parts below the knee joint.

Symptoms.—This change of direction largely influences the movement of the animal by detracting from its firmness and practically weakening the entire frame, even to the extent of rendering him insecure on his feet and liable to fall. This condition of weakness is sometimes so pronounced that he is exposed to fall even when standing at rest and unmolested, the knees being unable even to bear their portion of the mere weight of the frame. This results in another trouble—that of being unable to keep permanently upright. He is liable to fall on his knees, and by this act becomes presently a sufferer from the lesion known by the term of " broken knees."

Treatment.—Whatever may be the originating cause of this imperfection, it detracts very largely from the usefulness and value of a horse, disqualifying him for ordinary labor and wholly unfitting him for service under the saddle without jeopardizing the safety of his rider. If, however, the trouble is known from the start, and is not the result of congenital deformity or weakness of the knee joint, or secondary to other diseases, rest, with fortifying frictions, may sometimes aid in strengthening the joints; and the application of blisters on the posterior part of the knee, from a short distance above to a point a little below the joint, may be followed by some satisfactory results; but with this trouble, as with knuckling fetlocks, the danger of relapse must be kept in mind as a contingency always liable to occur.

CURB.

This lesion is the bulging backward of the posterior part of the hock, where in the normal state there should be a straight line, extending from the upper end of the point of the hock down to the fetlock.

Cause.—The cause may be a sprain of the tendon which passes on the posterior part of the hock, or of one of its sheaths, or of the strong ligament situated on the posterior border of the os calcis.

Hocks of a certain conformation seems to possess a greater liability to curb than others. They are overbent, coarse, and thick in appearance, or may be too narrow from front to back across the lower portion. This condition may therefore result as a sequence to congenital malformation, as in the case of horses that are " saber-legged." It often occurs, also, as the result of violent efforts, of heavy pulling, of high jumping, or of slipping; in a word, it may result from any of the causes heretofore considered as instrumental in producing lacerations of muscular, tendinous, or ligamentous structure.

Symptoms.—A hock affected with curb will present at the outset a swelling more or less diffuse on its posterior portion, with varying degrees of heat and soreness, and these will be accompanied with lameness of a permanent character. At a later period, however, the swelling will become better defined, the deformity more characteristic, the prominent, curved line readily detected, and the thickness of the infiltrated tissue easily determined by the fingers. At this time, also, there may be a condition of lameness, varying in degree, while at others, again, the irregularity of action at the hock will be so slight as to escape detection, the animal betraying no appearance of its existence.

A curb constitutes, by a strict construction of the term, an "unsoundness," since the hock thus affected is less able to endure severe labor, and is more liable to give way with the slightest effort. Yet the prognosis of a curb can not be considered to be serious, as it generally yields to treatment, or at least the lameness it may occasion is generally easily relieved, though the loss of contour caused by the bulging will always constitute a blemish.

Treatment.—On the first appearance of a curb, when it exhibits the signs of an acute inflammation, the first indication is to subdue it by the use of cold applications, as intermittent or constant irrigation or an ice poultice; when these have exhausted their effect and the swelling has assumed better defined boundaries, and the infiltration of the tendons or of the ligaments is all that remains of a morbid state, then every effort must be directed to the object of effecting its absorption and reducing its dimensions by pressure and other methods. The medicaments most to be trusted are blisters of cantharides and frictions with ointments of iodin, or, preferably, biniodid of mercury. Mercurial agents alone, by their therapeutic properties or by means of the artificial bandages which they furnish by their incrustations when their vesicatory effects are exhausted, will give good results in some instances by a single application, and often by repeated applications. The use of the firing iron must, however, be frequently resorted to, either to remove the lameness or to stimulate the absorption. We believe that its early application ought to be resorted to in preference to waiting until the exudation is firmly organized. Firing in dull points or in lines will prove as beneficial in curb as in any other disease of a similar nature.

LACERATED TENDONS.

This form of injury, whether of a simple or of a compound character, may become a lesion of a very serious nature, and will usually require long and careful treatment, which may yet prove unavailing in consequence either of the intrinsically fatal character of the wound itself or the complications which have rendered it incurable.

Cause.—Like all similar injuries, they are the result of traumatic violence, such as contact with objects either blunt or sharp; a curbstone in the city; in the country, a tree stump or a fence, especially one of wire. It may easily occur to a runaway horse when he is "whipped" with fragments of harness or "flogged" by fragments of splintered shafts "thrashing" his legs, or by the contact of his legs with the wagon he has overturned and shattered with his heels while disengaging himself from the wreck.

Symptoms.—It is not always necessary that the skin be involved in this form of injury. On the contrary, the tegument is frequently left entirely intact, especially when the injury follows infectious diseases or occurs during light exercise after long periods of rest in the stable. Again, the skin may be cut through and the tendons nearly severed. A point a little above the fetlock is usually the seat of the injury. But irrespective of this, and whether the skin is or is not implicated, the symptoms resemble very much those of a fracture. There is excessive mobility, at least more than in a normal state, with more or less inability to carry weight. There may be swelling of the parts, and on passing the hands carefully along the tendon to the point of division the stumps of the divided structure will be felt more or less separated, perhaps wholly divided. The position of the animal while at rest and standing is peculiar and characteristic. While the heels are well placed on the ground, the toe is correspondingly elevated, with a tendency to turn up— a form of breaking down which was described when speaking of the fracture of the sesamoids. Carrying weight is done only with considerable difficulty, but with comparatively little pain, and the animal will unconsciously continue to move the leg as if in great suffering, notwithstanding the fact that his general condition may be very good and his appetite unimpaired.

The effect upon the general organism of compound lacerated wounds of tendinous structures, or those which are associated with injuries of the skin, are different. The wound becomes in a short time the seat of a high degree of inflammation, with abundant suppuration filling it from the bottom; the tendon, whether as the result of the bruise or of the laceration, or of maceration in the accumulated pus, undergoes a process of softening, and necrosis and sloughing ensue. This complicates the case and probably some form of tendinous synovitis follows, running into suppurative arthritis, to end, if close to a joint, with a fatal result.

Prognosis.—The prognosis of lacerated tendons should be very conservative. Under the most favorable circumstances a period of from six weeks to two months will be necessary for the treatment, before the formation of the cicatricial callus and the establishment of a firm union between the tendinous stumps.

Treatment.—As with fractures, and even in a greater degree, the necessity is imperative, in the treatment of lacerated tendons, to obtain as perfect a state of immobility as can be obtained compatibly with the disposition of the patient; the natural opposition of the animal, sometimes ill-tempered and fractious at best, under the necessary restraint causing at times much embarrassment to the practitioner in applying the necessary treatment. Without the necessary immobility there can be no close connection of the ends of the tendons. To fulfill this necessary condition the posterior part of the foot and the fetlock must be supported and the traction performed by them relieved, an object which can be obtained by the use of the high-heeled and bar shoe, or possibly better accomplished with a shoe of the same kind extending about 2 or 2½ inches back of the heels. The perfect immobility of the legs is obtained in the same way as in the treatment of fracture, with splints, bandages, iron apparatus, plaster of adhesive mixtures, and similar means. So long as the dressings remain in place undisturbed and no chafing or other evidence of pain is present, the dressings may be continued without changing, the patient being kept in the slings for a period sufficient to insure the perfect union of the tendons. For a compound lesion when there is laceration of the skin some special care is necessary. The wound must be carefully watched and the dressings removed at intervals of a few days or as often as may be needful, all of which additional manipulation and extra nursing, however indispensable, still adds to the gravity of the case and renders the prognosis more and more serious. When the tendons have sloughed in threads of various dimensions, or if in the absence of this process of mortification healthy granulations should form and fill up the wound, still very careful attention will be required, the granulating ends of the tendons having a tendency to bulge between the edges of the skin and to assume large dimensions, forming bulky excrescences or growths of a warty or cauliflower appearance, the removal of which becomes a troublesome matter.

The union of the tendons will at times leave a thickening of varying degree near the point of cicatrization, the absorption of which becomes an object of difficult and doubtful accomplishment, but which may be promoted by moderate blistering and the use of alterative and absorbent mixtures or perhaps the fire iron. A shoe with heels somewhat higher than usual will prove a comfort to the animal and aid in moderating and relieving the tension of the tendons.

RUPTURE OF THE FLEXOR METATARSI.

This is a muscle of the anterior part of the shank. It is situated in front of the tibia, and is of peculiar formation, being composed of a muscular portion with a very powerful tendon, which are at first distinct and separate, to be intimately united lower down, and terminating at the lower end by a division into four tendinous bands. It is a powerful muscle of the hinder shank bone, and also acts as a strong means of support for the stifle joint; that is, of the articulation of the thigh and shank bone, in front and outside of which it passes. Its situation and its use cause it to be liable to severe stretching and straining, and a rupture of some of its fibers is sometimes the consequence.

Cause.—This injury may be the result of a violent effort of the animal in leaping over a high obstacle; in missing his foothold and suddenly slipping backward while powerfully grasping the ground with the feet in striving to start a heavily loaded vehicle; in making a violent effort to prevent a probable fall; or in attempting to lift the feet from miry ground.

Symptoms.—The accident is immediately followed by disability which will vary according to the true seat of the injury and the period of its duration. This rupture will not prevent the horse from standing perfectly and firmly on his feet when kept at rest, and while no muscular efforts are required from him there is no appearance of any lesion or unsoundness. An attempt to move him backward, however, will cause him to throw all his weight upon his hindquarters, and he will refuse to raise his foot from the ground. If compelled to do so, or required to move forward, the hock being no longer capable of flexion, the muscle which effects that movement being the injured one, the opposite muscles, the extensors, acting freely, the entire lower part of the leg, from the hock down, will be suddenly, with a jerk, extended on the tibia or shank bone, and simultaneously with this the tendo Achillis, the cord of the hock, the tendons of the extensors of the hock will be put in a wrinkled and relaxed condition. The leg is behind the animal and the toe rests on the ground. Examination of the fore part of the shank from the stifle down to the hock may reveal soreness, and possibly some swelling and heat at the seat of the lesion.

Treatment.—Our experience with injuries of this form convinces us that, generally speaking, they are amenable to treatment. Provided a sufficient time has been allowed for union to take place, very few instances in which radical recovery has not been effected have come to our knowledge. The more flexed the leg can be kept, the quicker will it heal.

In these cases, as in those of simple laceration of tendons, already considered, the indications resemble those which apply in the treatment of fractures, as near as coaptation of the lacerated ends is possible, with immobility, being the necessary conditions to secure. The first is a matter of very difficult accomplishment, by bandaging alone, and some have recommended instead the application of charges or blisters in order to compel the animal to keep more quiet.

To secure the necessary immobility the animal should be placed in slings snugly applied, and kept in a narrow stall. He should also be tied short, and restrained from any backward movement by ropes or boards, and should, moreover, be kept in as quiet a temper as possible by the exclusion of all causes of irritation or excitement. Weeks must then elapse, not less, but frequently more than six, often eight, before he can be considered out of danger and able to return to his labor, which should for a time be light and easy, and gradually, if ever, increased to the measure of a thoroughly sound and strong animal. If he is used too soon the newly formed tissue between the ends of the muscle will be liable to stretch and leave the flexor muscle too long and permanently displaced.

SUNDRY ADDITIONAL AFFECTIONS OF THE EXTREMITIES.

Among these there are three which will principally occupy our attention, and which may be considered as forming a single group. In some parts of the legs may be found certain peculiar little structures of a saclike formation, containing an oily substance designed for the lubrication of the parts upon which they are placed for the purpose of facilitating the movements of the tendons which pass over them. These little sacs or muco-synovial capsules, under peculiar conditions of traumatism, are liable to become subject to a diseased process, which consists principally in a hypersecretion of their contents and an increase in dimensions, and they may undergo peculiar pathological changes of such character as to disable an animal, and in many instances to cause serious blemishes which can but depreciate its value. These growths, which are known as hygromata, may result from external violence, as blows or bruises, and may appear in the form of small, soft tumors, painless and not inflammatory in character, but, by a repetition of the cause or renewal of violence, liable to acquire increased severity. Severe inflammation, with suppuration, may follow, which, filling up the cavity, the walls will become thickened and hard, resulting in the formation of a tumor.

The elbow, the knee, and the hock are the parts of the body where these lesions are ordinarily found, and on account of their peculiar shape and the position they occupy they have received the denomination "capped." They will be considered in their peculiar aspect.

CAPPED ELBOW.

Capped elbow, or "shoe boil," is a term applied to an enlargement often found at the point of the elbow.

Cause.—This lesion is due to injury or pressure of the part while it is resting on the ground. The horse, unlike the cow, does not rest directly on the under surface of the sternum, or breastbone, on account of its sharp, ridge-like formation. He rests more on the side of the breastbone and chest, and consequently the leg which is flexed under the body is subject to considerable pressure. If the leg is flexed under the body so that the hoof or shoe is directly in contact with the elbow, which may occur in horses having an extremely long cannon bone or excessive length in the shoes, the greater part of the weight of the chest is concentrated at this point and the pressure may cause a bruise or an inflammation.

Symptoms.—Under these conditions the point of the elbow may become swollen and tender and exhibit heat and pain. This swelling may not only cover the point of the elbow, but sometimes reaches the axilla and assumes such proportions that there is great difficulty in using the leg, the animal showing signs of lameness even to the extent of the circumflex step, as in shoulder lameness. This edematous condition, however, does not remain stationary. It may by degrees subside or perhaps disappear. In the first instance it will become more distinctly defined, with better marked boundaries, until it is reduced to a soft, round, fluctuating tumor, with or without heat or pain. There is then either a bloody or serous tumor or a purulent collection, and following the puncture of its walls with the knife there will be an escape of blood, serum, or pus, as the case may be, in variable quantities. In either case, but principally in that of the cystic form, the tumor will be found to be subdivided by septa, or bands running in various directions.

Various changes will follow the opening of the tumor and the escape of its contents. In a majority of cases the process of cicatrization will take place, and the cavity fill up by granulation, the discharge, at first abundant, gradually diminishing and the wound closing, usually without leaving any mark. At times, however, and especially if the disease has several times repeated its course, there may remain a pendulous sac, partly obliterated, which a sufficient amount of excitement or irritation may soon restore to its previous dimensions and condition.

In other cases an entirely different process takes place. The walls of the cavity, cyst, or abscess become ulcerated and thickened, the granulations of the sac become fibrous in their structure and fill up the cavity, and it assumes the character of a hard tumor on the back of the elbow, sometimes partly and sometimes entirely covered by the skin. It is fibrous in its nature, painless to the touch, well defined in its contour, and may vary in size from that of a small apple to that of a child's head.

This last form of capped elbow is the most serious of any, resisting all known forms of mild treatment, and removable by the knife only. The other forms, even that with the inflammatory aspect and its large edematous swelling which interferes with the work of the animal, may justify a much milder prognosis, and, aside from their liability to recur, may be ranked with the comparatively harmless affections.

Treatment.—So long as the danger of recurrence is the principal bad feature of capped elbow the most important consideration is that of devising a means for its prevention. To prevent the animal from lying down is evidently the simplest method of keeping the heels and the elbow apart; but the impracticability of this prescription is apparent, since most animals are obliged to lie down when they sleep, though it is true that a few take their sleep on their feet. The question of shoeing here enters into the discussion. The shortening of the inside branch of the shoe, which is the one with which the pressure is made, may be of advantage, and especially if the truncated end of the shoe is smooth and filed over to remove all possibility of pressure and contusion upon the skin. The protection of the skin of the elbow by interposing soft tissues between that and the shoe, or by bandaging the heel with bags or covering it with boots, is considered by many the best of the preventive methods, and the advantage to be obtained by resorting to it can not be overlooked when the number of horses which develop shoe boil whenever the use of the boot is intermitted is considered. In order to prevent the animal from assuming the sternal decubitus, many give preference to the plan of fastening a piece of wood across the stall at some distance from the front wall or manger. It is a simple expedient, primitive, perhaps, but nevertheless practical, and followed by good results.

The therapeutic treatment is also important. The edematous swelling, when recognized by its external appearance and the existing inflammation, should be treated without delay. Warm fomentations, repeated several times daily, are then indicated, the degree of warmth being as high as can be borne comfortably. They are easily applied and often yield decided relief in a few hours. In some cases, however, astringents, in the form of poultices or pastes, are used in preference; these are made to cover the entire swelling and allowed to remain, drying after a short time, it is true, and perhaps falling off, but are easily renewed and reapplied. An excellent astringent for these cases is a putty made of powdered chalk and vinegar (acetate of lime), and the whole swelling is then covered with a thick coating of soft clay made into a mass with water.

These simple remedies are often all that is required. Under their use the swelling passes off by degrees and after a short interval the animal is fit for work again, but not uncommonly instead a swelling develops, puffy, not painful, and perhaps giving a sensation of crepitation when pressure is applied with the finger. It is soft, evidently contains a liquid, and when freely opened with a good-sized incision discharges a certain quantity of blood, partly liquid and partly coagulated, and perhaps a little hemorrhage will follow. The cavity should then be well washed out and a plug of oakum introduced, leaving a small portion protruding through the cut to prevent it from closing prematurely. It may be taken off the next day, and a daily cleansing will then be all that is necessary. In another case the tumor becomes very soft in its whole extent, with evident fluctuation and a well-defined form. The discharge of the fluid is then indicated, and a free incision will be followed by the escape of a quantity of thin yellowish liquid from a single sac. The wound should be kept clean and dressed frequently, in order to insure prompt healing. But if the cavity is found to be subdivided in its interior by numerous bands and the cyst proves to be multilocular the partitions should be torn out with the fingers and the cavity then treated in the same manner as the unilocular sac. In still another case the swelling may be warm and painful with indistinct fluctuation, or fluctuation only at a certain point. This indicates an abscess, and necessitates an incision to drain the pus, followed by the careful cleansing and dressing of the wound.

But cases occur in which all the treatment that has been described fails to effect a full recovery, and instead a fibrous tumor begins to develop. A change of treatment is, of course, then in order. The inflammation being chronic will necessitate stimulating treatment of the part in order to increase the process of absorption. We must again draw upon the resources of experience in the form of blisters, the fomentations, the iodin, and the mercurial ointments, as heretofore mentioned. Good results may always be insured from their judicious and timely administration. In applying the powerful mineral inunctions much patience and wisdom are required. It should be done by carefully and perseveringly rubbing in small quantities daily; it should be done softly and gently, not with force, nor with the expectation of producing an astonishing effect by heavy dosing and main strength in a few hours; it should be after the manner of a siege rather than that of a charge. The object is to induce the drugs to permeate the affected part until the entire mass is penetrated. Of course cases will be encountered which resist all forms of medical treatment. The tumor remains as a fixed fact; it continues to grow; it is large and pendulous at the elbow; its weight is estimated in pounds; it is not an eyesore merely, but an uncomfortable, burdensome mass, excoriating all the surrounding parts and being itself excoriated in turn; mild treatment has failed and is no longer to be relied on.

Resort must now be made to surgical methods, and here again we must choose between the ligature, the cautery, and the knife. Each has its advocates among practitioners. In a case like the present, one of the difficulties arises in connection with the application and retention of bandages and other dressings after the amputation has been performed. It is a somewhat difficult problem, owing to the conformation and proportions of the body of the patient, and involves the exercise of considerable practical ingenuity to adjust and retain the appliances necessary to insure a good final result.

In the long description of the treatment of the varieties of capped elbow I have thus far omitted any mention of one method which is practiced and commended by not a few. I refer to the use of setons, introduced through the tumor. My own experience and the observation of many failures from this method led me to abandon it.

CAPPED KNEE.

The passage of the tendons of the extensor muscle of the cannon, as it glides in front of the knee joint, is assisted by one of the little bursæ before mentioned, and when this becomes the seat of dropsical collection a hygroma is formed and the knee is " capped." Though in its history somewhat analogous to the capped elbow, there are points of difference between them. Their development may prove a source of great annoyance from the fact of the blemish which they constitute.

Cause.—The capped knee presents itself under various conditions. It is sometimes the result of a bruise or contusion, often repeated, inflicted upon himself by a horse addicted to the habit of pawing while in the stable and striking the front of the stall with his knees. Another class of patients is formed of those weak-kneed animals which are subject to falling and bruising the front of the joint against the ground, the results no being always of the same character.

Symptoms.—The lesion may be a simple bruise, or it may be a severe contusion with swelling, edema, heat, and pain. The joint becomes so stiff and rigid that it interferes with locomotion and yet under careful simple treatment the trouble may disappear.

Again, instead of altogether passing off, the edema may diminish in extent, becoming more defined in form and may remain as a swelling on the front part of the knee. Resulting from the crushing of small blood vessels, this is necessarily full of blood. The swelling is somewhat soft, diffuse, not painful, more or less fluctuating, and after a few days becomes crepitant under the pressure of the hand.

Instead of being filled with blood the swelling may be full of serum, as often occurs when violence, though perhaps slight, has been frequently repeated. In that case the swelling is generally well defined, soft, and painless, with more or less fluctuation, and it may even become pendulous. In other cases the swelling may be of an acute, inflammatory nature, with heat and pain, accompanied with stiffness of the joint. This leads to the formation of an abscess. Whatever the nature of these swellings may be, either full of blood, serum, or pus, some blemish usually remains after treatment.

Prognosis.—Though simple bruises of the knee without extensive lesions are usually of trifling account, a different prognosis must be pronounced when the lesion assumes more important dimensions, and though a capped knee may be comparatively of little importance we have seen cases in which not only extensive blemishes were left to disfigure the patient, but the animals had become worthless in consequence of the extension of the diseased process to the various elements composing the joint, and giving rise to the most complicated cases of carpitis.

Treatment.—Usually the first symptom of trouble is the edematous swelling on the front of the " knee." The prevention of the inflammation and consequently of the abscess, is the prime object in view, and it may be realized by the use of warm-water fomentations or compresses applied over the swelling, which may be used either in a simple form or combined with astringents, such as Goulard's extract, alum, or sulphate of zinc. The application of warm poultices of oil meal or ground flaxseed, enveloping the whole joint and kept in place by bandages, is often followed by absorption of the swelling, or, if the abscess is in process of formation, by the active excretion of pus. If an abscess forms in spite of these precautions it may be treated surgically in several ways.

In one it should be done by a careful incision, which will allow the escape of the blood or the serum, or of the pus which is inclosed in the sac; in another it may be by means of a seton, in order that the discharge may be maintained and allowed to escape; for another we may adopt the more cautious manner of emptying the cavity by means of punctures with small trocars or aspirators. The danger attending this last method arises from the possible sloughing of large portions of the skin, while that attending the first is the hazard of the possibility of the extension of the inflammation to the capsular ligament of the knee, with the possibility of an open joint in prospect.

As we have remarked, the cavity after being emptied may rapidly close and leave in a short time but slight traces of its previous existence. But in many, if not in most cases, there will remain, after the cicatrization is complete, a thickening or organized exudation at one time round and well defined, at another spreading by a diffused infiltration, to which it will be necessary to give immediate attention, from the fact of its tendency to form into an organized and permanent body. To stimulate inflammation in this diseased structure, blisters are recommended, but chiefly for the purpose of promoting the process of absorption.

If this treatment fails, the use of iodin and mercurial preparations is recommended.

Plain mercurial or plain iodin ointment, or both in combination as iodid of mercury, are commonly used, and may be applied either moderately and by gentle degrees, as we have suggested, or more freely and vigorously with a view to more immediate effects, which, however, will also be more superficial. The use of the firing iron applied deeply with fine points is then to be strongly recommended, to be followed by blisters and various liniments. This course may generally be relied on as quite sure to be followed by satisfactory results.

While the treatment is in progress it will, of course, be necessary to secure the animal in such manner that a recurrence of the injury will be impossible from similar causes to those which were previously responsible.

CAPPED HOCK.

A bad habit of rubbing or striking the partitions of their stalls with their hocks prevails among some horses, with the result of an injury which shows itself on the upper points of those bones, the summit of the os calcis. From its analogy to the condition of capped elbow the designation of capped hock has been applied to this condition.

Symptoms.—A capped hock is therefore but the development of a bruise at the point of the hock, which if many times repeated may excite an inflammatory process, with all its usual external symptoms of swelling, heat, soreness, and the rest of the now-familiar phenomena. The swelling is at first diffused, extending more or less on the exterior part of the hock, and in a few instances running up along the tendons and muscles of the back of the shank. Soon, however, unless the irritating causes are continued and repeated, the edema diminishes, and, becoming more defined in its external outlines, leaves the hock capped with a hygroma. The hygroma, at the very beginning of the trouble, contains a bloody serosity which soon becomes strictly serum, and this, through the influence of an acute inflammatory action, is liable to undergo a change which converts it into the usual purulent product of suppuration.

The external appearance ought to be sufficient to determine the diagnosis, but there are a few signs which may contribute toward a nicer identification of the lesion. The capped hock, whether under the appearance of an acute, edematous swelling, or as a bloody serous collection, or as a simple serous cyst, does not give rise to any remarkable local manifestation other than such as have already passed under our survey in considering similar cases, nor will it be liable to interfere with the functions which belong to the member in question, unless it assumes very large dimensions and on each side of the tendons, as well as on the summit of the bone. But if the inflammation is quite high, if suppuration is developing, if there is a true abscess, or—and this is a common complication—especially when the kicking or rubbing of the animal is frequently recurring, then, besides the local trouble of the cyst or of the abscess, the bones become diseased and the periosteum inflamed; perhaps the superior ends of the bone and its fibro-cartilage become affected, and a simple lesion or bruise, whatever it may have been, becomes complicated with periostitis and ostitis, and is naturally accompanied with lameness, developed in a greater or less degree, which in some cases may be permanent and in others increased by work. These complications, however, are not common or frequent.

Treatment.—Capped hocks are in many cases amenable to treatment, and yet they often become the opprobrium of the practioner by remaining, as they frequently do, an eyesore on the top of the hock; they do not interfere, it is true, with the work of the horse, but fixing upon him the stigma of what, in human estimation, is a most unreliable and objectionable reputation, to wit, that of being an habitual "kicker," and, worse than all, one that kicks when fed.

The maxim that "an ounce of prevention is worth a pound of cure" fits the present case very neatly. A horse whose hocks have a somewhat puffy look and whose skin on the front of the hock is loose and flabby, justly subjects himself to a suspicion of addictedness to this bad habit, but a little watching will soon establish the truth. If, then, the verdict is one of conviction, precautions should be immediately adopted against a continuance of the evil. The padding of the sides of the stall with straw mats or mattresses and covering the posts with similar material, in such manner as to expose no hard surface with which to come in contact, will reduce the evil to its minimum. The animal may jar his frame when he kicks, but even then there will be less force in the concussion than if it impinged upon the solid plank, and cuts and abrasions can not be inflicted by a properly made cushion. Hobbles are also rightly recommended with a view to the required restraint of motion, so applied as to secure the leg with which the kicking is performed, or even both hind legs, in such manner as not to interfere with the movement of lying down and rising again and yet preventing that of kicking backward. Boots similar in pattern to those which are used for the prevention of shoe boil are also prescribed. These are placed above the hock and retained by straps tightly fastened. We apprehend, however, that the difficulty of retaining them in the proper place without the danger of chafing from the tightness of the straps may form an objection to their use. Notwithstanding all precautions, hocks will be capped in the future as in the past, and the study of their treatment will always be in order.

The mode of dealing with them will, of course, be greatly influenced by the condition of the parts. When the inflammation is excessive and the swelling large, hot, and painful to the touch, the application of warm water will be very painful. The leg should be well fomented several times a day, for from 15 to 20 minutes each time, a strong decoction of marsh-mallow leaves being added to the water, and after each application swathed with flannel bandages soaked in the same warm mixture. A few days of this treatment will usually effect a resolution of the inflammation; if not complete, at least sufficiently so to disclose the correct outlines of the hygroma and exhibit its peculiar and specific symptoms. The expediency of its removal and the method of accomplishing it are then to be considered, with the question of opening it to give exit to its contents. If the fluid is of a purulent character, the indication is in favor of its immediate discharge. No time should be lost, and it should be by means of a small opening made with a narrow bistoury. If, however, the fluid is a serosity, we prefer to remove it by punctures with a very small trocar. Our reason for special caution in these cases is our fear of the possibility of the existence of diseased conditions of a severe character in the pseudo joint. For the same reason we prefer the treatment of those growths by external applications. In the first stages of the disease a severe and stiff blister, such as the cantharide of collodium, entirely covering the cyst, perhaps not yet completely formed, when the inflammation has subsided, will be of great benefit by its stimulating effect, the absorption it may excite, and the pressure which, when dry, it will maintain upon the tumor. If, however, the thickening of the growth fails to diminish, it should be treated with some of the iodin preparations in the form of ointments, pure or in combination with potassium, mercury, etc., of various strengths and in various proportions. My opinion of setons is not favorable, but the actual cautery, by deep and fine firing, in points—needle cauterization—I believe to be the best mode of treatment, and especially when applied early.

A very satisfactory way to treat these cases is to burst the swelling by pressure from without. A strap or strong linen bandage is placed about the hock, pressing on the bursa, while the affected leg is on the ground, the other hind foot being lifted up. When the bandage is in place the leg should be released, and the horse will violently flex the bandaged limb and produce pressure on the bursa, with consequent bursting and discharging of its contents.

Whatever treatment may be adopted for capped hock, patience must be one of the ingredients. In these parts absorption is slow, the skin is very thick, and its return to a soft, pliable, natural condition, if effected at all, will take place only after weeks added to other weeks of medical treatment and patient waiting.

INTERFERING, AND SPEEDY CUTS.

These designations belong to certain special injuries of the extremities, produced by similar causes, giving rise to kindred patho-

logical lesions with allied phenomena, requiring about the same treatment and often followed by the same results, to wit, a blemish which
may not only subject the animal to a suspicion of unsoundness, but
in some special circumstances may interfere with his ability to labor.
It is known as "interfering" when the location of the trouble is the
inside of the fetlock of either the fore or hind leg. It is called
"speedy cut" when it occurs on the inside of the fore leg, a little
below the knee, at the point of contact of that joint with the cannon.
It is always the result of a blow, self-inflicted, of varying severity,
and giving rise to various lesions. (See also p. 399.)

Symptoms.—At times the injury is too slight to be seriously
noticed, the hair being scarcely cut and the skin unmarked. At other
times the skin will be cut through, partly or wholly, and it may for
the time cause sufficient pain to check the motion of the animal and
induce him to suspened his labor through his inability to use the
wounded limb, traveling meanwhile for a short space on three legs
only. Sometimes a single blow will suffice, or again there will be a
repetition of lighter strokes. In the latter case the parts will become
much swollen, hot, and so painful to the touch that the motion of
the knee or the fetlock will be sufficiently disturbed to cause lameness of a degree of severity corresponding to that of the lesion. Following the subsidence of this diffused and edematous swelling is
sometimes the formation of a tumor, either at the knee or the fetlock.
This may be soft at first or become so by degrees, with fluctuation,
its contents being at first extravasted blood, and later a serosity; or,
if there has been a sufficient degree of inflammation, it may become
suppurative. The result of the fault of interfering may thus be
exhibited, whether at the knee or at the fetlock, as characterized by
all the pathological conditions which have appeared as accompaniments of capped knee or capped hock. If, in consequence of the force
of the blow or blows, the inflammation has been usually severe, a
mortification of the skin may become one of the consequences, a slough
taking place, succeeded by a cutaneous ulcer on the inside of the fetlock or when the greater number of the original wounds are inflicted.
If the interfering has been often repeated it may be followed by
another condition, which has been considered in our remarks upon
other affections. It is a plastic exudation or thickening of the parts,
which are commonly said to have become "callous," and the effect
of it is to destroy the regularity of the outlines of the joint to an extent which constitutes a serious blemish, which will be permanent,
and according to the degree of the aberration from the natural and
symmetrical lines will enevitably depreciate the commercial value of
the animal.

An animal in interfering may thus exhibit a range of symptoms
which from the simplest form of a mere "touching," may succes-

sively assume the serious characters of an ugly cicatrix, a hard, plastic swelling, or perhaps, as witnessed at the knee, of periostitis with its sequelæ.

If a single and constantly recurring cause—a blow—is the starting point in interfering, we may now consider the subject of the predisposition which brings such serious results upon the suffering animal, and the conditions which lead to and accompany it. These are numerous, but the first in frequency and importance is peculiarity of conformation in the animals addicted to it. The first class will include horses whose chests are narrow and whose legs do not stand straight and upright, but are crooked and pigeon-toed in and out. The second class includes those whose legs are weak, either from youth or hard labor, or from severe attacks of sickness. Another class is made up of those having abnormally developed feet, or which have been badly shod with unnecessarily wide or heavy shoes. Another class consists of those that are affected with swollen fetlocks or chronic, edematous swelling of the leg. Another is formed of animals with a peculiar action, as those whose knee action is very high, and it is these that furnish most of the cases of speedy cut.

Prognosis.—The prognosis of interfering is never a very serious one. However violent the blow may be it is rarely that subsequent complications of a troublesome nature occur. The principal evil attending it is a liability to be followed by a thickened or callous deposit which is not only an eyesore and a blemish, but constitutes a new and increased predisposition. The remark that " an animal which has interfered once is always liable to interfere," is often confirmed and sanctioned by a recurrence of the trouble.

Treatment.—Another point in which there is a resemblance between this lesion and others which we have considered is in its responsiveness to the same treatment with them. Indeed, the prescription of warm fomentations, soothing applications, and astringent and resolvent mixtures, in a majority of cases, is the first that occurs all through the list. If the swelling assumes the character of a serous collection, pressure, cold water, and bandages will contribute to its removal. If suppuration seems to be established and the swelling assumes the character of a developing abscess, hot poultices of flaxseed or of boiled vegetables and the embrocations of sedative ointments, those of basilicon, or vaseline, impregnated with preparations of opium or belladonna—all these recommend themselves by their general adaptation and the beneficial results which have followed their administration, not less in one case than in another. When an abscess has formed and is fluctuating, it should be carefully but fully opened to evacuate the pus. If it is a serous cyst, some care is necessary in emptying it, and the possibility of the extension of the inflammation to the joint must be taken into consideration. When the cavities have been emptied and have closed by filling up with granulations, or if, not being opened, the contents have been reabsorbed, and there remains in either case a plastic exudation and a tendency to the callous organization that may yet exist, blisters under their various forms, including those of cantharides, of mercury, and of iodin, are then indicated, principally in the early stages, as it is then that their effects will prove most satisfactory. The use of the actual cautery, with fine points, penetrating deeply throughout the enlargement, has in our hands, when used in the very early stages of its formation, nearly always brought on a radical recovery with complete absorption of the thickening.

STRINGHALT.

This is an involuntary movement of one or both hind legs, in which the foot is suddenly and spasmodically lifted from the ground much higher than it is normally carried, with excessive flexion of one bone upon the other. This peculiarity is usually prominent, although it may disappear with work, only to reappear after a short rest. Sometimes it is most apparent at a trot, sometimes at a walk, and other times only when turned around; or it may not be affected by the gait of the horse. It does not seem to be influenced by the horse's age, young and old being alike affected. Its first manifestations are sometimes very slight. It has been noticed as occurring in an animal when backing out of his stable and ceasing immediately after. In some animals it is best seen when the animal is turning around on the affected leg, and it is not noticed when he moves straight forward. That this peculiar action interferes with facility of locomotion and detracts from a horse's claim to soundness can not for a moment be denied.

Cause.—Veterinarians and pathologists are yet in doubt in respect to the cause of this affection, as well as to its essential nature. Whether it results from disease of the hock, of an ulcerative character; whether it springs from a malformation; whether it is a shortening of the ligaments, a chronic inflammation of the sciatic nerve, or a disease of the spinal cord; whether it is purely a muscular or purely a nervous lesion, or a compound of both—it still continues, if an etiologist is bound to possess universal knowledge within the scope of his special studies, to be his reproach and his puzzle.

Treatment.—When there is a known or suspected cause the treatment should be directed toward this factor. If due to local inflammation of the hock or foot, only this local lesion should be treated. If it remains after the local lesion has healed, or if we have no assignable cause, the best results have followed the sectioning of the lateral extensor of the foot. A competent veterinarian alone should undertake this operation.

THROMBOSIS.

There are certain forms of lameness which are very peculiar in their manifestation, and which to the nonprofessional mind must appear to belong to the domain of mystery or theory instead of occupying a well-established position among the subjects of equine pathology. Yet they are no less susceptible of actual demonstration and of positive comprehension than many facts which, plain and familiar to the general understanding now, were once ranked among things occult and unsearchable. A thrombus, considered as a cause of lameness, may find a place among these understood mysteries.

Cause.—Under certain peculiar conditions of inflammation of the blood vessels, and also in aneurisms, clots of blood are sometimes formed in the arteries and find their way in the general circulation. At first, while very small, or sufficiently so to pass from one vessel to another, they move from a small vessel to a larger, and from that to one still larger, constantly increasing in size until at some given point, from their inability to enter smaller vessels, their movement is finally arrested. The artery is thus effectually dammed, and the clot in a short time cuts off completely the supply of blood from the parts beyond. This is thrombosis, and it often gives rise to sudden and excessive lameness of a very painful character.

Symptoms.—Thrombi may form in any of the arteries, and doubtless have been the cause of many cases of lameness which could never be accounted for. If they exist in small arteries their diagnosis will probably fail to be made out with certainty, but when situated in the larger trunks a strong suspicion of their presence may be excited. In some cases they may even be recognized with possitive accuracy, as when the vessels which supply the posterior extremities are affected by the blocking up of the posterior aorta or its ramifications.

The existence of thrombosis of the arteries of the hind leg may always be suspected when the following history is known: The general health of the animal is good, but symptoms of lameness in one of the legs have been developed, becoming more marked as he is worked, and especially when driven at a fast gait. But the disturbance is not permanent, and the lameness disappears almost immediately after a rest. There is an increase of the difficulty, however, and, though the animal may walk normally, he will, when made to trot, very soon begin to slacken his pace and to show signs of the trouble, and if urged to increase his speed will become lamer and lamer; an abundant perspiration will break out; he will refuse to go, and if forced he shows weakness behind, seems ready to fall, and perhaps does fall. While on his feet the leg is kept in constant motion, up and down, and is kept from the ground as if the contact were too painful to bear. If undisturbed this series of symptoms will gradually subside, sometimes very soon, and occasionally after a few hours he will return to an apparently perfect condition. A return to labor will lead to a renewal of the same incidents.

A history like this suggests a strong suspicion of a thrombus in an artery of the hind leg, and this suspicion will be confirmed by the external symptoms exhibited by the animal. The total absence of any other disease which might account for the lameness, and a manifest diminution of heat over a part or the whole of the extremity, when compared with the opposite side or with any other portion of the body; a sensation of cold attendant on the pain, but gradually subsiding as the pain subsides, and the circulation, quickened by the rest, has been reestablished throughout the extremity; all these are confirmatory circumstances. Still, it is thus far only a suspicion, and absolute certainty is yet wanting. To establish the truth of the case the rectal exploration must be resorted to. The hands then, well prepared and carefully introduced into the rectum, must explore for the truth, first feeling for the large blood vessels which, divided at the aorta, separate to supply the right and left legs. These must be compared in respect to the pulsation and other particulars. The artery which is healthy will, of course, exhibit all the proper conditions of that state. On the other hand, if the vessel appears to the feel hard, more or less cordy, and pulseless, or giving a sensation of fluttering, as of a small volume of blood with a trickling motion passing through a confined space, the difference between the sides will make the case plain. The first will be the full flow of the circulation through an unobstructed channel, the other a forced passage of the fluid between the thrombus and the coats of the artery. In such case the prognosis is necessarily a grave one and the disease is more liable to grow worse than better.

Treatment.—No form of treatment can be advised; the suffering of a helpless and useless animal can only be terminated by that which ends all.

Cases occur, however, where this condition of the blood vessels exists in a much less degree, and the diseased condition is not sufficiently pronounced for final condemnation. There may even be a possibility of the absorption of the clot, or that an increase of the collateral circulation may be sufficient to supply the parts with blood. In such cases spontaneous recovery may follow moderate exercise in the pasture, field, or stable, or continuous light work may be given, but too much hope should not be placed in such treatment.

SPRAINS OF THE LOINS.

This is an affection which suggests to the mind the idea of muscular injury, and is difficult to distinguish from many similar cases. If the animal shrinks from the slightest pressure or pinching of the spine in the region of the loins, he is by many pronounced to be "lame in the loins," or "sprained in the loins," or "weak in the kidneys." This is a grave error, as in fact this simple and gentle yielding to such a pressure is not a pathological sign, but is normal and significant of health. Yet there are several conditions to which the definition of "sprains of the loins" may apply which are not strictly normal.

Cause.—The muscles of the back and those of the loins proper, as the psoas, may have been injured, or again there may be trouble of a rheumatic nature, perhaps suggestive of lumbago. Diseases of the bones of the vertebral column, or even those of the organs of circulation, may give rise to an exhibition of similar symptoms.

Symptoms.—The symptoms are characteristic of a loss of rigidity or firmness of the vertebral column, both when the animal is at rest and in action. In the former condition, or when at rest, there is an arched condition of the back and a constrained posture in standing, with the hind legs separated. In the latter there is a lateral, balancing movement at the loins, principally noticeable while the animal is in the act of trotting—a peculiar motion, sometimes referred to as a "crick in the back," or what the French call a "tour de bateau." If, while in action, the animal is suddenly made to halt, the act is accompanied with much pain, the back suddenly arching or bending laterally, and perhaps the hind legs thrown under the body, as if unable to perform their functions in stopping, and sometimes it is only accomplished at the cost of a sudden and severe fall. This manifestation is also exhibited when the animal is called upon to back, when a repetition of the same symptoms will also occur.

If a slight pressure on the back or the loins is followed by a moderate yielding of the animal, it is, as before remarked, a good sign of health. With a sprain of the loins pressure of any kind is painful, and will cause the animal to bend or to crouch under it more or less, according to the weight of the pressure. Heavy loads, and even heavy harnessing, will develop this tenderness. In lying down he seems to suffer much discomfort, and often accompanies the act with groaning, and when compelled to rise does so only with great difficulty and seldom succeeds without repeated efforts.

Sprains of muscles proper, when recent, will always be accompanied with this series of symptoms, and the fact of their exhibition, with an excessive sensibility of the parts, and possibly with a degree of swelling, will always justify a diagnosis of acute muscular lesion, and especially so if accompanied with a history of violent efforts, powerful muscular strains, falls, heavy loading, etc., connected with the case. If the symptoms have been of slow development and gradual increase, it becomes a more difficult task to determine whether the diagnosis points to pathological changes in the structure of the muscles or of the bones, the nervous centers, or the blood vessels of the region. And yet it is important to decide as to which particular structure is affected in reference to the question of prognosis, as the degree of gravity of the lesion will depend largely upon whether the disabled condition of the animal is due to an acute or a chronic disease.

Treatment.—The prescription which will necessarily first of all suggest itself for sprains of the loins is rest. An animal so affected should be immediately placed in slings, and none of his efforts to release himself should be allowed to succeed. Hot compresses, cold-water douches, sweating applications, stimulating frictions, strengthening charges, blistering ointments of cantharides and the actual cautery, all have their advocates, but in no case can the immobility obtained by the slings be dispensed with. In many cases in which the weakness of the hind quarters was caused by disease of the nervous centers electricity has also yielded good results.

DISEASES OF THE FETLOCK, ANKLE, AND FOOT.

By A. A. HOLCOMBE, D. V. S.,

Veterinary Inspector, Bureau of Animal Industry.

ANATOMICAL REVIEW OF THE FOOT.

In a description of the foot of the horse it is customary to include only the hoof and its contents, yet, from a zoological standpoint, the foot includes all the leg from the knee and the hock down.

The foot of the horse is undoubtedly the most important part of the animal, so far as veterinary surgery is concerned, for the reason that it is subject to so many injuries and diseases which in part or in whole render the patient unfit for the labor demanded of him. The old aphorism "no foot no horse" is as true to-day as when first expressed; in fact, domestication, coupled with the multiplied uses to which the animal is put, and the constant reproduction of hereditary defects and tendencies, has largely transformed the ancient "companion of the wind" into a very common piece of machinery which is often out of repair, and at best is but shortlived in its usefulness.

Since the value of the horse depends largely or even entirely upon his ability to labor, it is essential that his organs of locomotion be kept sound. To accomplish this end it is necessary not only to know how to cure all diseases to which these organs are liable but, better still, how to prevent them.

An important prerequisite to the detection and cure of disease is a knowledge of the construction and function of the parts which may be involved in the diseased process. Hence, first of all, the anatomical structures must be understood. (See also p. 583.)

The bones of the fetlock and foot constitute the skeleton on which the other structures are built and comprise the lower end of the cannon bone (the metacarpus in the fore leg, the metatarsus in the hind leg), the two sesamoids, the large pastern or os suffraginis, the small pastern or coronet, the small sesamoid or navicular bone, and the coffin bone or os pedis. (Plate XXXIV, fig. 3.)

The cannon bone extends from the knee or hock to the fetlock, is cylindrical in shape, and stands nearly or quite perpendicular.

The sesamoids occur in pairs, are small, shaped like a three-faced pyramid, and are set behind the fetlock joint, at the upper end of the large pastern, with the base of the pyramid down.

395

The large pastern is a very compact bone, set in an oblique direction downward and forward, and extends from the cannon bone to the coronet.

The coronet is a short, cube-shaped bone, set between the large pastern and coffin bone, in the same oblique direction.

The navicular bone is short, flattened above and below, and is attached to the coffin bone behind.

The coffin bone forms the end of the foot and is shaped like the horny box in which it is inclosed.

All these bones are covered on the surfaces which go to make up the joints with a cartilage of incrustation, while the portions between are covered with a fibrous membrane called the periosteum.

The joints of the legs are of especial importance, since any interference with their function very largely impairs the value of the animal for most purposes. As the joints of the foot and ankle are at the point of greatest concussion they are the ones most subject to injury and disease.

There are three of these joints—the fetlock, pastern, and coffin. They are made by the union of two or more bones, held together by ligaments of fibrous tissue, and are lubricated by a thick, viscid fluid, called synovia, which is secreted by a special membrane inclosing the joints.

The fetlock joint is made by the union of the lower end of the cannon and the upper end of the large pastern bones, supplemented by the two sesamoids, so placed behind the upper end of the pastern that the joint is capable of a very extensive motion. These bones are held together by ligaments, only one of which—the suspensory—demands special mention.

The suspensory ligament of the fetlock starts from the knee, extends down behind the cannon, lying behind the two splint bones, until near the fetlock, where it divides and sends a branch on each side of the joint, downward and forward, to become attached on the sides of the extensor tendon at the lower end of the pastern bone. As it crosses the sesamoids, on the posterior borders of the fetlock, it throws out fibers which hold it fast to these bones. (Plate XXXIV, fig. 2.)

The pastern joint is made by the union of the two pastern bones.

The coffin joint is made by the union of the small pastern, coffin, and small sesamoid, or navicular bones, the latter being set behind and beneath the joint surface of the coffin bone in such way as to receive largely the weight of the small pastern.

Three tendons serve to move the bones of the foot one on another. Two of these flex, or bend, the joints, while the other extends, or straightens, the column of bones. (Plate XXXIII, fig. 5.)

The flexor pedis perforans, or deep flexor of the foot, passes down behind the cannon bone, lying against the suspensory ligament in front, crosses the fetlock joint in the groove made by the union of the two sesamoids, and is attached to the bottom on the coffin bone, after covering the navicular, by a wide expansion of its fibers. It is the function of this tendon to flex the coffin bone and, with it, the horny box.

The flexor pedis perforatus, or superficial flexor of the foot, follows the course of the preceding tendon and is attached to the middle of the ankle. The function of this tendon is to flex the foot at the fetlock.

The extensor pedis runs down in front of the leg, is attached on the most prominent point of the coffin bone, and has for function the straightening of the bones of the ankle and foot.

The bones, ligaments, and tendons are covered by a loose connective tissue, which gives a symmetry to the parts by filling up and rounding off, and all are protected by the skin and hoof.

The skin of the fetlock and ankle is generally characterized by its thickness and the length of its hairs, especially around the hind parts of the fetlock joint in certain breeds of horses. The most important part of this envelope is that known as the coronary band.

The coronary band is that portion of the skin which secretes the horn of which the wall of the hoof is made. This horn much resembles the nail which grows on the fingers and toes of man. It is composed of cylindrical tubes, which are held together by a tenacious, opaque matter. The horn extends from the coronary band to the lower border of the hoof. (Plate XXXII, fig. 1.)

The hoof is a box of horn, consisting of a wall, sole, and frog, and contains, besides the coffin, navicular, and part of the small pastern bones, the sensitive laminæ, plantar cushion, and the lateral cartileges. (Plate XXXIII, fig. 4.)

The sole of the foot incloses the box on the ground surface, is shaped like the circumference of the foot, except that a V-shaped opening is left behind for the reception of the frog, and is concave on the lower surface. The sole is produced by the velvety tissue, a thin membrane covering the plantar cushion and other soft tissues beneath the coffin bone. The horn of the sole differs from the horn of the wall in that its tubes are not straight and from the fact that it scales off in pieces over the whole surface.

The frog is a triangular-shaped body, divided into two equal parts by a deep fissure, extending from its apex in front to the base. It fills the triangular space in the sole, to which it is intimately attached by its borders. The horn of the frog is produced in the same manner as the sole; but it differs from both the wall and sole in that the horn

is soft, moist, and elastic to a remarkable degree. It is the function
of the frog to destroy shock and to prevent slipping.

The sensitive laminæ are thin plates of soft tissue covering the entire anterior surface of the coffin bone. They are present in great
numbers, and by fitting into corresponding grooves on the inner surface of the horn of the wall the union of the soft and horny tissues is
made complete. (Plate XXXII, fig. 1.)

The plantar cushion is a thick pad of fibrous tissue placed behind
and under the navicular and coffin bones and resting on the sole and
frog, for the purpose of receiving the downward pressure of the column of bones and to destroy shock. (Plate XXXII, fig. 4.)

The lateral cartilages are attached, one on each side, to the wings
of the coffin bone by their inferior borders. They are thin plates of
fibro-cartilage, and their function is to assist the frog and adjacent
structures to regain their proper position after having been displaced
by the weight of the body while the foot rested on the ground. (Plate
XXXII, fig. 2.)

FAULTS OF CONFORMATION.

A large percentage of horses have feet which are not perfect in
conformation, and as a consequence they are especially predisposed to
certain injuries and diseases.

Flatfoot is that condition in which the sole has little or no convexity. It is a peculiarity common to some breeds, especially heavy,
lymphatic animals raised on low, marshy soils. It is confined to the
fore feet, which are generally broad, low-heeled, and with a wall less
upright than is seen in the perfect foot.

In flatfoot there can be little or no elasticity in the sole, for the
reason that it has no arch, and the weight of the animal is received on
the entire plantar surface, as it rests upon the ground instead of on
the wall. For these reasons such feet are particularly liable to bruises
of the sole, corns, pumiced sole, and excessive suppuration when the
process is once established. Horses with flatfoot should be shod with a
shoe having a wide web, pressing on the wall only, while the heels and
frog are never to be pared. Flatfoot generally has weak walls, and as
a consequence the nails of the shoe are readily loosened and the shoe
cast.

Clubfoot is a term applied to such feet as have the walls set nearly
perpendicular. When this condition is present the heels are high, the
fetlock joint is thrown forward, or knuckles, and the weight of the
animal is received on the toes. Many mules are clubfooted, especially
behind, where it seems to cause little or no inconvenience. Severe
cases of clubfoot may be cured by cutting the tendons, but as a rule
special shoeing is the only measure of relief that can be adopted. The
toe should not be pared, but the heels are to be lowered as much as

possible and a shoe put on with a long, projecting toe piece, slightly turned up, while the heels of the shoe are to be made thin.

Crookedfoot is that condition in which one side of the wall is higher than the other. If the inside wall is the higher, the ankle is thrown outward, so that the fetlock joints are abnormally wide apart and the toes close together. Animals with this deformity are " pigeon-toed," and are prone to interfere, the inside toe striking the opposite fetlock. If but one foot is affected, the liability to interfere is still greater, for the reason that the fetlock of the perfect leg is nearer the center plane.

When the outside heel is the higher the ankle is thrown in and the toe turns out. Horses with such feet interfere with the heel. If but one foot is so affected, the liability to interfere is less than when both feet are affected, for the reason that the ankle of the perfect leg is not so near to the center plane. Such animals are especially liable to stumbling and to lameness from injury to the ligaments of the fetlock joints. This deformity is to be overcome by such shoeing as will equalize the disparity in length of walls, and by proper boots to protect the fetlocks from interfering.

INTERFERING.

An animal is said to interfere when one foot strikes the opposite leg, as it passes by, during locomotion. The inner surface of the fetlock joint is the part most subject to this injury, although, under certain conditions, it may happen to any part of the ankle. It is seen more often in the hind than in the fore legs. Interfering causes a bruise of the skin and deeper tissues, generally accompanied with an abrasion of the surface. It may cause lameness, dangerous tripping, and thickening of the injured parts. (See also p. 387.)

Causes.—Faulty conformation is the most prolific cause of interfering. When the bones of the leg are so united that the toe of the foot turns in (pigeon-toed), or when the fetlock joints are close together and the toe turns out, when the leg is so deformed that the whole foot and ankle turn either in or out, interfering is almost sure to follow. It may happen, also, when the feet grow too long, from defective shoeing, rough or slippery roads, from the exhaustion of labor or sickness, swelling of the leg, high knee action, fast work, and because the chest or hips are too narrow.

Symptoms.—Generally, the evidences of interfering are easily detected, for the parts are tender, swollen, and the skin broken. But very often, especially in trotters, the flat surface of the hoof strikes the fetlock without evident injury, and attention is directed to these parts only by the occasional tripping and unsteady gait. In such cases proof of the cause may be had by walking and trotting the animal, after first painting the inside toe and quarter of the suspected foot with a thin coating of chalk, charcoal, mud, or paint.

Treatment.—When the trouble is due to deformity or faulty conformation it may not be possible to overcome the defect.

In such cases, and as well in those due to exhaustion or fatigue, the fetlock or ankle boot must be used. In many instances interfering may be prevented by proper shoeing. The outside heel and quarter of the foot on the injured leg should be lowered sufficiently to change the relative position of the fetlock joint by bringing it farther away from the center plane of the body, thereby permitting the other foot to pass by without striking.

A very slight change is often sufficient to effect this result. At the same time the offending foot should be so shod that the shoe may set well under the hoof at the point responsible for the injury. The shoe should be reset every three or four weeks.

When the cause has been removed, cold-water bandages to the injured parts will soon remove the soreness and swelling, especially in recent cases. If, however, the fetlock has become calloused from long-continued bruising, a Spanish-fly blister over the parts, repeated in two or three weeks if necessary, will aid in reducing the leg to its natural condition.

KNUCKLING, OR COCKED ANKLES.

Knuckling is a partial dislocation of the fetlock joint, in which the relative position of the pastern bone to the cannon and coronet bones is changed, the pastern becoming more nearly perpendicular, with the lower end of the cannon bone resting behind the center line of the large pastern, while the lower end of this bone rests behind the center line of the coronet. While knuckling is not always an unsoundness, it nevertheless predisposes to stumbling and to fracture of the pastern.

Causes.—Young foals are quite subject to this condition, but in the great majority of cases it is only temporary. It is largely due to the fact that before birth the legs were flexed; and time is required after birth for the ligaments, tendons, and muscles to adapt themselves to the function of sustaining the weight of the body.

As they grow old, horses with erect pasterns are very prone to knuckle, especially in the hind legs. All kinds of heavy work, particularly in hilly districts, and fast work on hard race tracks or roads are exciting causes of knuckling. It is also commonly seen as an accompaniment of that faulty conformation called clubfoot, in which the toe of the wall is perpendicular and short, and the heels high—a condition most often seen in the mule, especially in the hind feet.

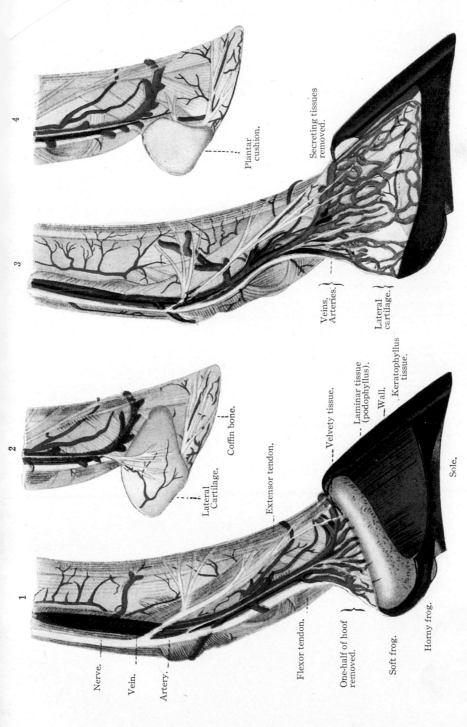

ZEESE-WILKINSON CO., INC., N.Y.

4

3

2

1

Plantar cushion.

Secreting tissues removed.

Veins,
Arteries.

Lateral cartilage.

Keratophyllus tissue.

Wall.

Laminar tissue (podophyllus).

Velvety tissue.

Coffin bone.

Lateral Cartilage.

Extensor tendon.

Nerve.

Vein.

Artery.

Flexor tendon.

One-half of hoof removed.

Soft frog.

Horny frog.

Sole.

ANATOMY OF FOOT.

Haines, from Auzoux Model.

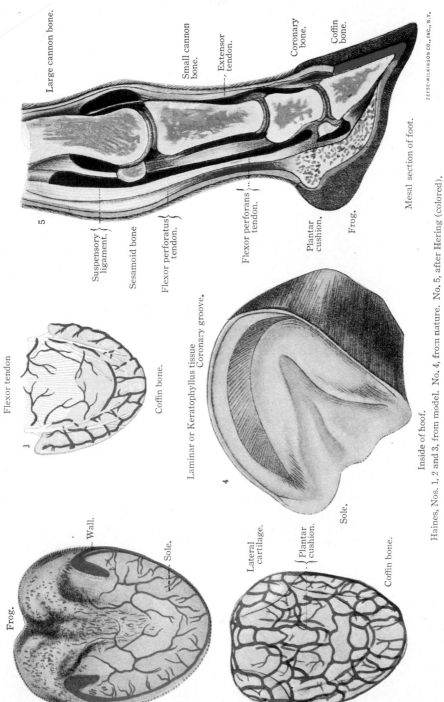

ZEESE-WILKINSON CO., INC., N.Y.

Large cannon bone.

Small cannon bone.

Extensor tendon.

Coronary bone.

Coffin bone.

Suspensory ligament.

Sesamoid bone

Flexor perforatus tendon.

Flexor perforans tendon.

Plantar cushion.

Frog.

Mesal section of foot.

Flexor tendon

Coffin bone.

Laminar or Keratophyllus tissue

Coronary groove.

Inside of hoof.

Sole.

Frog.

Wall.

Sole.

Lateral cartilage.

Plantar cushion.

Coffin bone.

ANATOMY OF FOOT

Haines, Nos. 1, 2 and 3, from model. No. 4, from nature. No. 5, after Hering (colored).

PLATE XXXIV.

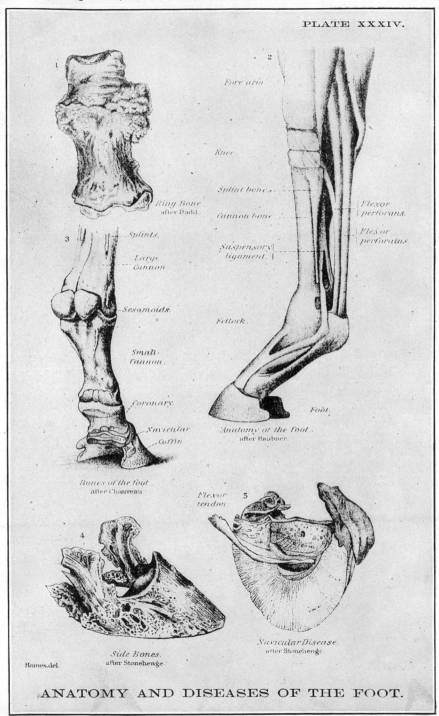

1

Ring Bone.
after Dadd.

2

Fore arm.

Knee.

Splint bone.

Cannon bone.

Suspensory
ligament.

Fellock.

Flexor
perforans.

Flexor
perforatus.

Foot.

Anatomy of the foot.
after Haubner.

3

Splints.

Large
Cannon.

Sesamoids.

Small
Cannon.

Coronary.

Navicular.

Coffin.

Bones of the foot.
after Chauveau

Flexor
tendon.

5

4

Side Bones.
after Stonehenge.

Navicular Disease.
after Stonehenge.

Haines.del.

ANATOMY AND DISEASES OF THE FOOT.

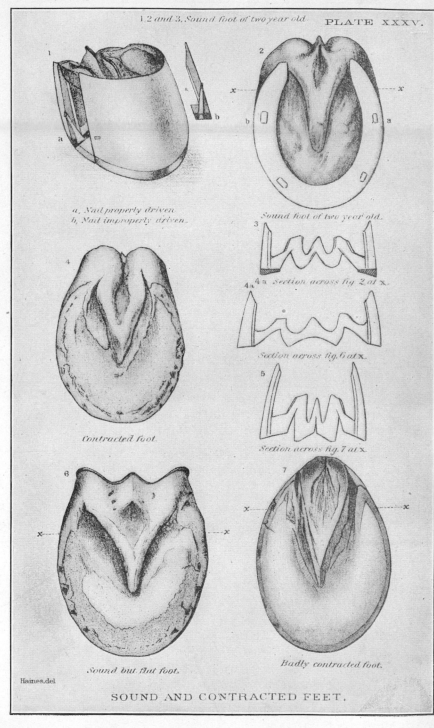

SOUND AND CONTRACTED FEET.

Lastly, knuckling is produced by disease of the suspensory ligament or of the flexor tendons, whereby they are shortened, and by disease of the fetlock joints.   (See p. 372.)

Treatment.—In young foals no treatment is necessary, unless there is some deformity present, since the legs straighten up without interference in the course of a few weeks. When knuckling has commenced, the indications are to relieve the tendons and ligaments by proper shoeing. The foot is to be prepared for the shoe by shortening the toe as much as possible, leaving the heels high; or if the foot is prepared in the usual way the shoe should be thin in front, with thick heels or high calks. For the hind feet a long-heeled shoe with calks seems to do best. Of course, when possible, the causes of knuckling are to be removed; since this can not always be done, however, the time may come when the patient can no longer perform any service, particularly in those cases in which both fore legs are affected, and it becomes necessary either to destroy the animal or obtain relief by surgical interference. In such cases the tendons between the fetlock and knee may be divided for the purpose of obtaining temporary relief. Firing and blistering the parts responsible for the knuckling may, in some instances, effect a cure; but a consideration of these measures belongs properly to the treatment of the disease in which knuckling appears simply as a sequel.

WINDGALL.

Joints and tendons are furnished with sacs containing a lubricating fluid called synovia. When these sacs are overdistended by reason of an excessive secretion of synovia, they are called windgalls. They form a soft, puffy tumor about the size of a hickory nut, and are most often found in the fore leg, at the upper part of the fetlock joint, between the tendon and the shin bone. When they develop in the hind leg it is not unusual to see them reach the size of a walnut. Occasionally they appear in front of the fetlock on the border of the tendon. The majority of horses are not subject to them after colthood has passed.   (See also p. 355.)

Causes.—Windgalls are often seen in young, overgrown horses, in which the body seems to have outgrown the ability of the joints to sustain the weight. In cart and other horses used to hard work, in trotters with excessive knee action, in hurdle racers and hunters, and in most cow ponies there is a predisposition to windgalls. Street-car horses and others used to start heavy loads on slippery streets are the ones most liable to develop windgalls in the hind legs.

Symptoms.—The tumor is more or less firm and tense when the foot is on the ground, but is soft and compressible when the foot is off the ground. In old horses windgalls generally develop slowly and cause no inconvenience. If they are caused by excessive tension of the joint the tumor develops rapidly, is tense, hot, and painful, and the animal is exceedingly lame. The patient stands with the joint flexed, and walks with short steps, the toe only being placed on the ground. When the tumor is large and situated upon the inside of the leg it may be injured by interfering, causing stumbling and inflammation of the sac. Rest generally causes the tumor to diminish in size, only to fill up again after renewed labor. In old cases the tumors are hardened, and may become converted into bone by a deposit of the lime salts.

Treatment.—The large, puffy joints of suckling colts, as a rule, require no treatment, for as the animal grows older the parts clean up and after a time the swelling entirely disappears.

When the trouble is from an injury, complete rest is to be obtained by the use of slings and a high-heeled shoe. Cold-water douches should be used once or twice a day, followed by cold-water bandages, until the fever has subsided and the soreness is largely removed, when a blister is to be applied.

In old windgalls, which cause more or less stiffness, some relief may be had by the use of cold-compress bandages, elastic boots, or the red iodid of mercury blisters. Opening the sacs, as recommended by some authors, is of doubtful utility, and should be adopted only by the surgeon capable of treating the wound he has made. Enforced rest until complete recovery is effected should always be insisted upon, since a too early return to work is sure to be followed by relapse.

SPRAIN OF THE FETLOCK.

Sprain of the fetlock joint is most common in the fore legs, and, as a rule, affects but one at a time. Horses doing fast work, as trotters, runners, steeplechasers, hunters, cow ponies, and those that interfere, are particularly liable to this injury.

Causes.—Horses knuckling at the fetlock, and all those with diseases which impair the powers of locomotion, such as navicular disease, contracted heels, sidebones, chronic laminitis, etc., are predisposed to sprains of the fetlock. It generally happens from a misstep, stumbling, or slipping, which results in the joint being extended or flexed to excess. The same result may happen where the foot is caught in a rut, a hole in a bridge, or in a car track, and the animal falls or struggles violently. Direct blows and punctured wounds may also set up inflammation of the joint.

Symptoms.—The symptoms of sprain of the fetlock vary with the severity of the injury. If slight, there may be no lameness, but simply a little soreness, especially when the foot strikes on uneven ground and the joint is twisted a little. In more severe cases the joint swells, is hot and puffy, and the lameness may be so intense as to compel the animal to hobble on three legs. While at rest the leg is flexed at the joint affected, and the toe rests on the ground.

Treatment.—If the injury is slight, cold-water bandages and a few days' rest are sufficient to effect recovery. When there is an intense lameness, swelling, etc., the leg should be placed under a constant stream of cold water, as described in the treatment for quittor. When the inflammation has subsided, a blister to the joint should be applied.

In some cases, especially in old horses long accustomed to fast work, the ligaments of the joints are ruptured, in whole or in part, and the lameness may last a long time. In these cases the joint should be kept completely at rest; this condition is best obtained by the application of plaster of Paris bandages, as in cases of fracture. As a rule, patients take kindly to this bandage, and, while wearing it, may be given the freedom of a roomy box or yard. If they are disposed to tear it off, or if sufficient rest can not otherwise be obtained, the patient must be kept in slings.

In the majority of instances the plaster bandage should remain on from two to four weeks. If the lameness returns when the bandage is removed, a new one should be put on. The swelling, which always remains after the other evidences of the disease have disappeared, may be largely dissipated and the joint strengthened by the use of the firing iron and blisters.

A joint once injured by a severe sprain never entirely regains its original strength, and is ever after particularly liable to a repetition of the injury.

RUPTURE OF THE SUSPENSORY LIGAMENT.

Sprain with or without rupture of the suspensory ligament may happen in either the fore or hind legs, and is occasionally seen in horses of all classes and at all ages. Old animals, however, and especially hunters, runners, and trotters, are the most subject to this injury, and with them the seat of the trouble is nearly always in one or both the fore legs. Horses used for heavy draft are more liable to have the ligament of the hind legs affected.

When the strain upon the suspensory ligament becomes too great, one or both of the branches may be torn from the sesamoid bones, one or both of the branches may be torn completely across, or the ligament may rupture above the point of division.

Symptoms.—The most common injury to the suspensory ligament is sprain of the internal branch in one of the fore legs. The trouble is indicated by lameness, heat, swelling, and tenderness of the affected branch, beginning just above the sesamoid bone and extending obliquely downward and forward to the front of the ankle. If the whole ligament is involved, the swelling comes on gradually, and is found above the fetlock and in front of the flexor tendons. The patient stands or walks upon the toe as much as possible, keeping the fetlock joint flexed so as to relieve the ligament of tension.

When both branches are torn from their attachments to the sesamoids, or both are torn across, the lameness comes on suddenly and is most intense; the fetlock descends, the toe turns up, and, as the animal attempts to walk, the leg has the appearance of being broken off at the fetlock. These symptoms, followed by heat, pain, and swelling of the parts at the point of injury, will enable anyone to make a diagnosis.

Treatment.—Sprain of the suspensory ligament, no matter how mild it may be, should always be treated by enforced rest of at least a month, and the application of cold douches and cold-water bandages, firmly applied until the fever has subsided, when a cantharides blister should be put on and repeated in two or three weeks if necessary. When rupture has taken place the patient should be put into slings and a constant stream of cold water allowed to trickle over the seat of injury until the fever is reduced. In the course of a week or ten days a plaster of Paris splint, such as is used in fractures, is to be applied and left on for a month or six weeks. When this is taken off, blisters may be used to remove the remaining soreness; but it is useless to expect a removal of all the thickening, for, in the process of repair, new tissue has been formed which will always remain.

In old cases of sprain the firing iron may often be used with good results. As a rule, severe injuries to the suspensory ligament incapacitate the subject for anything but slow, light work.

OVERREACH.

When the shoe of the hind foot strikes and injures the heel or quarter of the forefoot the horse is said to overreach. It rarely happens except when the animal is going fast; hence is most common in trotting and running horses. In trotters the accident generally happens when the animal breaks from a trot to a run. The outside heels and quarters are most liable to the injury.

Symptoms.—The coronet at the heel or quarter is bruised or cut, the injury in some instances involving the horn as well. When the hind foot strikes well back on the heel of the fore foot—an accident known among horsemen as "grabbing"—the shoe may be torn from the forefoot or the animal may fall to its knees. Horses accustomed to overreaching are often "bad breakers," for the reason that the pain of the injury so excites them that they can not readily be brought back to the trotting gait.

Treatment.—If the injury is but a slight bruise, cold-water bandages applied for a few days will remove all the soreness. If the parts are deeply cut, more or less suppuration will follow, and, as a rule, it is well to poultice the parts for a day or two, after which cold baths may be used, or the wounds dressed with tincture of aloes, oakum, and a roller bandage.

When an animal is known to be subject to overreaching, he should never be driven fast without quarter boots, which are specially made for the protection of the heels and quarters.

If there is a disposition to "grab" the forward shoes, the trouble may be remedied by having the heels of these shoes made as short as possible, while the toe of the hind foot should project well over the shoe. When circumstances permit of their use, the fore feet may be shod with the "tips" instead of the common shoe, as described in treatment for contracted heels.

CALK WOUNDS.

Horses wearing shoes with sharp calks are liable to wounds of the coronary region, either from trampling on themselves or on each other. These injuries are most common in heavy draft horses, especially on rough roads and slippery streets. The fore feet are more liable than the hind ones, and the seat of injury is commonly on the quarters. In the hind feet the wound often results from the animal resting with the heel of one foot set directly over the front of the other. In these cases the injury is generally close to the horn, and often involves the coronary band, the sensitive laminæ, the extensor tendon, and even the coffin bone.

Treatment.—Preventive measures include the use of boots to protect the coronet of the hind foot and of a blunt calk on the outside heel of the fore shoe, since this is generally the offending instrument when the fore feet are injured. If the wound is not deep and the soreness slight, cold-water bandages and a light protective dressing, such as carbolized cosmoline, will be all that is needed. When the injury is deep, followed by inflammation and suppuration of the coronary band, lateral cartilages, sensitive laminæ, etc., active measures must be resorted to. Cold, astringent baths, made by adding 2 ounces of sulphate of iron to 1 gallon of water, should be used, followed by poultices, if it is necessary to hasten the cleansing of the wound by stimulating the sloughing process. If the wound is deep between the horn and the skin, especially over the anterior tendon, the horn should be cut away so that the injured tissues may be exposed. The subsequent treatment in these cases should follow the directions given in the article on toe cracks.

FROSTBITES.

Excepting the ears, the feet and legs are about the only parts of the horse liable to become frostbitten. The cases most commonly seen are found in cities, especially among car horses, where salt is used for the purpose of melting the snow on curves and switches.

This mixture of snow and salt is splashed over the feet and legs, rapidly lowering the temperature of the parts to the freezing point. In mountainous districts, where the snowfall is heavy and the cold often intense, frostbites are not uncommon, even among animals running at large.

Symptoms.—When the frosting is slight the skin becomes pale and bloodless, followed soon after by intense redness, heat, pain, and swelling. In these cases the hair may fall out and the epidermis peel off, but the inflammation soon subsides, the swelling disappears, and only an increased sensitiveness to cold remains.

In more severe cases irregular patches of skin are destroyed and after a few days slough away, leaving slow-healing ulcers behind. If produced by low temperatures and deep snow, the coronary band is the part most often affected.

In many instances there is no destruction of the skin, but simply a temporary suspension of the horn-producing function of the coronary band. The fore feet are more often affected than the hind ones, and the heels and quarters are less often involved than the front part of the foot. The coronary band becomes hot, swollen, and painful, and after two or three days the horn separates from the band and slight suppuration follows. For a few days the animal is lame, but as the suppuration disappears the lameness subsides. New horn, often of an inferior quality, is produced by the coronary band, and in time the cleft is grown off and complete recovery is effected. The frog is occasionally frostbitten and may slough off, exposing the soft tissues beneath and causing severe lameness for a time.

Treatment.—Simple frostbites are best treated by cold fomentations followed by applications of a 5 per cent solution of carbolized oil. When portions of the skin are destroyed, their early separation should be hastened by warm fomentations and poultices. Ulcers are to be treated by the application of stimulating dressings, such as carbolized oil, a 1 per cent solution of nitrate of silver or of chlorid of zinc, with pads of oakum and flannel bandages. In many of these cases recovery is exceedingly slow. The new tissue by which the destroyed skin is replaced always shrinks in healing, and, as a consequence, unsightly scars are unavoidable. When the coronary band is involved it is generally advisable to blister the coronet over the seat of injury as soon as the suppuration ceases, for the purpose of stimulating the growth of new horn. Where a crevasse is formed between the old and the new horn no serious trouble is liable to be met with until the cleft is nearly grown out, when the soft tissues may be exposed by a breaking off of the partly detached horn. But even if this accident happens final recovery is effected by poulticing the foot until a sufficient growth of horn protects the parts from injury.

QUITTOR.

Quittor is a term applied to various affections of the foot wherein the tissues which are involved undergo a process of degeneration that results in the formation of a slough followed by the elimination of the diseased structures by means of a more or less extensive suppuration.

For convenience of consideration quittors may be divided into four classes, as suggested by Girard: (1) Cutaneous quittor, which is known also as simple quittor, skin quittor, and carbuncle of the coronet; (2) tendinous quittor; (3) subhorny quittor; and (4) cartilaginous quittor.

CUTANEOUS QUITTOR.

Simple quittor consists in a local inflammation of the skin and subcutaneous connective tissue on some part of the coronet, followed by a slough and the formation of an ulcer which heals by suppuration.

It is an extremely painful disease, owing to the dense character of the tissues involved; for in all dense structures the swelling which accompanies inflammation always produces intense pressure. This pressure not only adds to the patient's suffering but may at the same time endanger the life of the affected parts by strangulating the blood vessels. It is held by some writers that simple quittor is most often met with in the hind feet, but in my experience more than two-thirds of the cases have developed in the fore feet. While any part of the coronet may become the seat of attack, the heels and quarters are undoubtedly most liable.

Causes.—Bruises and other wounds of the coronet are often the cause of cutaneous quittor, yet there can be no question that in the great majority of cases the disease develops without any known cause. For some reason not yet satisfactorily explained most cases happen in the fall of the year. One explanation of this fact has been attempted in the statement that the disease is due to the injurious action of cold and mud. This claim, however, seems to lose force when it is remembered that in many parts of this country the most mud, accompanied with freezing and thawing weather, is seen in the early springtime without a corresponding increase of quittor. Furthermore, the serious outbreaks of this disease in the mountainous regions of Colorado, Wyoming, and Montana are seen in the fall and winter seasons, when the weather is the driest. It may be claimed, and perhaps with justice, that during these seasons, when the water is low, animals are compelled to wade through more mud to drink from lakes and pools than is necessary at other seasons of the year, when these lakes and pools are full. Add to these conditions the further fact that much of this mud is impregnated with alkaline salts which, like the mineral substances always found in the mud of cities, are more or less irritating, and it seems fair to conclude that under certain circumstances mud may become an important factor in the production of quittor.[1]

While this disease attacks any and all classes of horses, it is the large, common breeds, with thick skins, heavy coats, and coarse legs that are most often affected. Horses well groomed and cared for in stables seem to be less liable to the disease than those running at large or than those which are kept and worked under adverse circumstances.

Symptoms.—Lameness, lasting from one to three or four days, nearly always precedes the development of the strictly local evidences of quittor. The next sign is the appearance of a small, tense, hot, and painful tumor in the skin of the coronary region. If the skin of the affected foot is white, the inflamed portion will present a dark-red or even a purplish appearance near the center. Within a few hours the ankle, or even the whole leg as high as the knee or hock, becomes much swollen. The lameness is now so great that the patient refuses to use the foot at all, but carries it if compelled to move. As a consequence, the opposite leg is required to do the work of both, and if the animal persists in standing a greater part of the time it, too, becomes swollen. In many of these cases the suffering is so intense during the first few days as to cause general fever, dullness, loss of appetite, and increased thirst. Generally the tumor shows signs of suppuration within 48 to 72 hours after its first appearance; the summit softens, a fluctuating fluid is felt beneath the skin, which soon ulcerates completely through, causing the discharge of a thick, yellow, bloody pus, containing shreds of dead tissue which have sloughed away. The sore is now converted into an open ulcer, generally deep, nearly or quite circular in outline, and with hardened base and edges. In exceptional cases large patches of skin, varying from 1 to $2\frac{1}{2}$ inches in diameter, slough away at once, leaving an ugly superficial ulcer. These sores, especially when deep, suppurate freely, and if there are no complications they tend to heal rapidly as soon as the degenerated tissue has softened and is entirely removed. When suppuration is fully established, the lameness and general symptoms subside. When but a single tumor and abscess form, the disease progresses rapidly, and recovery, under proper treatment, may be ef-

---

[1] An outbreak of quittor near Cheyenne, Wyo., which came under the author's observation, was caused by the mud through which the horses had to wade to reach the watering troughs. These troughs were furnished with water by windmills, and the mudholes were caused by the waste water. More than 50 cases developed inside of two months, or during September and October. In these 50 cases all forms of the disease and all possible complications were presented. During the rainy season at Leadville, Colo., outbreaks of quittor are common, and the disease is so virulent that it has long been known as the "Leadville foot rot." The soil being rich in mineral matters is no doubt the cause of the outbreaks. In the city of Montreal quittor is said to be very common in the early springtime, when the streets are muddy from the melting snow and ice.

fected in from two to three weeks; but when two or more tumors are developed at once, or if the formation of one tumor is rapidly succeeded by another for an indefinite time, the sufferings of the patient are greatly increased, the case is more difficult to treat, and recovery is more slow and less certain.

This form of quittor is often complicated with the tendinous and subhorny quittors by an extension of the sloughing process.

Treatment.—The first step in the treatment of an outbreak of quittor should be the removal of all exciting causes. Crowding animals into small corrals and stables, where injuries to the coronet are likely to happen from trampling, especially among unbroken range horses, must be avoided as much as possible.

Watering places accessible without having to wade through mud should be provided. In towns, where the mud or dust is largely impregnated with mineral products, it is not possible to adopt complete preventive measures. Much can be done, however, by careful cleansing of the feet and legs as soon as the animal returns from work. Warm water should be used to remove the mud and dirt, after which the parts are to be thoroughly dried with soft cloths.

The means which are to be adopted for the cure of cutaneous quittor vary with the stage of the disease at the time the case is presented for treatment. If the case is seen early—that is, before any of the signs of suppuration have developed—the affected foot is to be placed under a constant stream of cold water, with the object of arresting a further extension of the inflammatory process. To accomplish this, put the patient in slings in a narrow stall having a slat or open floor. Bandage the foot and leg to the knee or hock, as the case may be, with flannel bandages loosely applied. Set a tub or barrel filled with cold water above the patient, and by the use of a small rubber hose of sufficient length make a siphon which will carry the water from the bottom of the tub to the leg at the top of the bandage. The stream of water should be quite small, and is to be continued until the inflammation has entirely subsided or until the presence of pus can be detected in the tumor. When suppuration has commenced, the process should be aided by the use of warm baths and poultices of lineseed meal or boiled turnips. If the tumor is of rapid growth, accompanied with intense pain, relief is obtained and sloughing largely limited by a free incision of the parts. The incision should be vertical and deep into the tumor, care being taken not to divide the coronary band entirely. If the tumor is large, more than one incision may be necessary.

The foot should now be placed in a warm bath for half an hour or longer and then poulticed. The hemorrhage produced by the cutting and encouraged by the warm bath is generally very copious and soon gives relief to the overtension of the parts

In other cases it will be found that suppuration is well under way, so that the center of the tumor is soft when the patient is first presented for treatment. It is always good surgery to relieve the tumor of pus whenever its presence can be detected; hence, in these cases a free incision must be made into the softened parts, the pus evacuated, and the foot poulticed.

By surgical interference the tumor is now converted into an open sore or ulcer, which, after it has been well cleaned by warm baths and poultices applied for two or three days, needs to be protected by proper dressings. The best of all protective dressings is made of small balls, or pledgets, of oakum, carefully packed into the wound and held in place by a roller bandage 4 yards long, from 3 to 4 inches wide, made of common bedticking and skillfully applied.

The remedies which may be used to stimulate the healing process are many, and, as a rule, they are applied in the form of solutions or tinctures.

In my own practice I prefer a solution of bichlorid of mercury 1 part, water 500 parts, with a few drops of muriatic acid or a few grains of muriate of ammonia added to dissolve the mercury. The balls of oakum are wet with this solution before they are applied to the wound.

Among the other remedies which may be used, and perhaps with equally as good results, will be noted the sulphate of copper, iron, and zinc, 5 grains of either to the ounce of water; chlorid of zinc, 5 grains to the ounce; carbolic acid, 20 drops dissolved in an equal quantity of glycerin and added to 1 ounce of water; and nitrate of silver, 10 grains to the ounce of water.

If the wound is slow to heal, it will be found of advantage to change the remedies every few days.

If the wound is pale in color, the granulations transparent and glistening, the tincture of aloes, tincture of gentian, or the spirits of camphor may do best.

When the sore is red in color and healing rapidly, an ointment made of 1 part of carbolic acid to 40 parts of cosmoline or vaseline is all that is needed.

If the granulations continue to grow until a tumor is formed which projects beyond the surrounding skin, it should be cut off with a sharp, clean knife, and the foot poulticed for twenty-four hours, after which the wound is to be well cauterized daily with lunar caustic and the bandages applied with great firmness.

The question as to how often the dressings should be renewed must be determined by the condition of the wound, etc. If the sore is suppurating freely, it will be necessary to renew the dressing every 24 or 48 hours; if the discharge is small in quantity and the patient comfortable, the dressing may be left on for several days; in fact, the less often the wound is disturbed, the better, so long as the healing process is healthy. When the sore commences to "skin over," the edges should be lightly touched with lunar caustic at each dressing. The patient may now be given a little exercise daily, but the bandages must be kept on until the wound is entirely healed.

TENDINOUS QUITTOR.

This form of quittor differs from the cutaneous in that it not only affects the skin and subcutaneous tissues, but involves also the tendons of the leg, the ligaments of the joints, and, in many cases, the bones of the foot as well.

Fortunately, this form of quittor is less common than the preceding, yet any case beginning as simple cutaneous quittor may at any time during its course become complicated by the death of some part of the tendons, by gangrene of the ligaments, sloughing of the coronary band, caries of the bones, or inflammation and suppuration of the synovial sacs and joints, thereby converting a simple quittor into one which will, in all probability, either destroy the patient's life or maim him for all time.

Causes.—Tendinous quittor is caused by the same injuries and influences that produce the simple form. Zundel believes it to be a not infrequent accompaniment of distemper. In my own experience I have seen nothing to verify this belief, but I am convinced that young animals are more liable to have tendinous quittor than older ones, and that they are much more likely to make a good recovery.

Symptoms.—When a case of simple quittor is transformed into the tendinous variety the change is announced by a sudden increase in the severity of all the symptoms. On the other hand, if the attack primarily is one of tendinous quittor, the earliest symptom seen is a well-marked lameness. In those cases due to causes other than injuries this lameness is at first very slight, and the animal limps no more in trotting than in walking; later on, generally during the next 48 hours, the lameness increases to such extent that the patient often refuses to use the leg at all. An examination made during the first two days rarely discloses any cause for this lameness; it may not be possible even to say with certainty that the foot is the seat of the trouble. On the third or fourth day, sometimes as late as the fifth, a doughy-feeling tumor will be found forming on the heel or quarter. This tumor grows rapidly, feels hot to the touch, and is extremely painful. As the tumor develops, all the other symptoms increase in intensity; the pulse is rapid and hard; the breathing quick; the temperature elevated 3° or 4°; the appetite is gone; thirst increased; and the lameness so great that the foot is carried if locomotion is attempted. At this stage of the disease the patient generally seeks relief by lying upon the broad side, with outstretched legs; the coat is bedewed with a clammy sweat, and every respiration is accompanied with a moan. The leg soon swells to the fetlock; later this swelling gradually extends to the knee or hock, and in some cases reaches the body. As a rule, several days elapse before the disease develops a well-defined abscess, for, owing to the dense structure of the bones, ligaments, and tendons, the suppurative process is a slow one, and the pus is prevented from readily collecting in a mass.

I made a post-mortem examination on a typical case of this disease, in which the animal had died on the fourth day after being found on the range slightly lame. The suffering had been intense, yet the only external evidences of the disease consisted in the shedding of the hoof from the right fore foot and a limited swelling of the leg to the knee. The sloughing of the hoof took place two or three hours before death, and was accompanied with but little suppuration and no hemorrhage. The skin from the knee to the foot was thickened from watery infiltration (edema), and on the inside quarter three holes, each about one-half inch in diameter, were found. All had ragged edges, while but one had gone deep enough to perforate the coronary band. The loose connective tissue beneath the skin was distended, with a gelatinous infiltration over the whole course of the flexor tendons and to the fetlock joint over the tendon in front. The soft tissues covering the coffin bone were loosened in patches by collections of pus which had formed beneath the sensitive laminæ. The coffin and pastern joints were inflamed, as were also the coffin, navicular, and coronet bones, while the outside toe of the coffin bone had become softened from suppuration until it readily crumbled between the fingers. The coronary band was largely destroyed and completely separated from the other tissues of the foot. The inner lateral cartilage was gangrenous, as was also a small spot on the extensor tendon near its point of attachment on the coffin bone. Several small collections of pus were found deep in the connective tissue of the coronary region; along the course of the sesamoid ligaments; in the sheath of the flexor tendons; under the tendon just below the fetlock joint in front; and in the coffin joint.

But all cases of tendinous quittor are by no means so complicated as this one was. In rare instances the swelling is slight, and after a few days the lameness and other symptoms subside, without any discharge of pus from an external opening. In most cases, however, from one to half a dozen or more soft points arise on the skin of the coronet, open, and discharge slowly a thick, yellow, fetid, and bloody matter. In other cases the suppurative process is largely confined to the sensitive laminæ and plantar cushion, when the suffering is intense until the pus finds an avenue of escape by separating the hoof from the coronary band, at or near the heels, without causing a loss of the whole horny box. When the flexor tendon is involved deep in the foot, the discharge of pus usually takes place from an opening in the follow of the heel; if the sesamoid ligament or the sheath of the flexors are affected, the opening is nearer the fetlock joint, although in most of these cases the suppuration spreads along the course of the tendons until the navicular joint is involved, and extensive sloughing of the deeper parts follows.

Treatment.—The treatment of tendinous quittor is to be directed toward the saving of the foot. First of all an effort must be made to prevent suppuration; if the patient is seen at the beginning, cold irrigation, recommended in the treatment for cutaneous quittor, is to be resorted to. Later, when the tumor is forming on the coronet, the knife must be used, and a free and deep incision made into the swelling. Whenever openings appear, from which pus escapes, they should be carefully probed; in all instances these fistulous tracts lead down to dead tissue which nature is trying to remove by the process of sloughing. If a counter opening can be made, which will enable a more ready escape of the pus, it should be done at once; for instance, if the probe shows that the discharge originates from the bottom of the foot, the sole must be pared through over the seat of trouble. Whenever suppuration has commenced the process is to be stimulated by the use of warm baths and poultices. The pus which accumulates in the deeper parts, especially along the tendons, around the joints, and in the hoof, is to be removed by pressure and injections made with a small syringe, repeated two or three times a day. As soon as the discharge assumes a healthy character and diminishes in quantity, stimulating solutions are to be injected into the open wounds. When the tendons, ligaments, and other deeper parts are affected, a strong solution of carbolic acid—1 to 4—should be used at first; or strong solutions of tincture of iodin, sulphate of iron, sulphate of copper, bichlorid of mercury, etc., may be used in place of the carbolic; after this the remedies and dressings directed for use in simple quittor are to be used. In those cases in which the fistulous tracts refuse to heal it is often necessary to burn them out with a saturated solution of caustic soda, equal parts of muriatic acid and water, or, better still, with a long, thin iron, heated white hot.

But no matter what treatment is adopted, a large percentage of the cases of tendinous quittor fail to make good recoveries. If the entire hoof sloughs away, the growth of a new, but soft and imperfect hoof may be obtained by carefully protecting the exposed tissues with proper bandages. When the joints are opened by deep sloughing, recovery may eventually take place, but the joint remains immovable ever after. If caries of a small part of the coffin bone takes place, it may be removed by an operation; but if much of the bone is affected, or if the navicular and coronet bones are involved in the carious process, the only hope for a cure is in the amputation of the foot. This operation is advisable only when the animal is valuable for breeding purposes. In all other cases in which there is no hope for recovery the patient's suffering should be relieved by death. In tendinous quittor much thickening of the coronary region, and sometimes of the ankle and fetlock, remains after suppuration has ceased and the fistulous tracts have healed. To stimulate the reabsorption of this new and unnecessary tissue, the parts should be fired with the hot iron, or, in its absence, repeated blistering with the biniodid of mercury ointment may largely accomplish the same results.

SUBHORNY QUITTOR.

This is the most common form of the disease. It is generally seen in but one foot at a time, and more often in the fore than in the hind feet. It nearly always attacks the inside quarter, but may affect the outside, the band in front, or the heel, where it is of but little consequence. It consists in the inflammation of a small part of the coronary band and adjacent skin, followed by sloughing and suppuration, which in most cases extends to the neighboring sensitive laminæ.

Causes.—Injuries to the coronet, such as bruises, overreaching, and calk wounds, are considered as the common causes of this disease. Still, cases occur in which there appears to be no existing cause, just as in the other forms of quittor, and it seems fair to conclude that subhorny quittor may also be produced by internal causes.

Symptoms.—At the outset the lameness is always severe, and the patient often refuses to use the affected foot. Swelling of the coronet close to the top of the hoof causes the quarter to protrude beyond the wall. This tumor is extremely sensitive, and the whole foot is hot and painful. After a few days a small spot in the skin, over the most elevated part of the tumor, softens and opens or the hoof separates from the coronary band at the quarter or well back toward the heel. From this opening, wherever it may be, a thin, watery, often dark, offensive discharge escapes, at times mixed with blood and always containing a considerable percentage of pus.

Probing will now disclose a fistulous tract leading to the bottom of the diseased tissues. If the opening is small, there is a tendency upon the part of the suppurative process to spread downward; the pus gradually separates the hoof from the sensitive laminæ until the sole is reached, and even a portion of this may be undermined.

As a rule, the slough in this form of quittor is not deep, and if the case receives early and proper treatment complications are generally avoided; but if the case is neglected, and, occasionally, even in spite of the best treatment, the disease spreads until the tendon in front, the lateral cartilage, or the coffin bone and joint as well are involved.

In all cases of subhorny quittor much relief is experienced when the slough comes away, and rapid recovery is made. If, however, after the lapse of a few days, the lameness remains and the wound continues to discharge a thin, unhealthy matter, the probabilities are that the disease is spreading, and pus collecting in the deeper parts of the foot. In Zundel's opinion, if the use of the probe now detects a pus cavity below the opening, a cartilaginous quittor is in the course of development.

Treatment.—Hot baths and poultices are to be used until the presence of pus can be determined, when the tumor is to be opened with a knife or sharp-pointed iron heated white hot. The hot baths and poultices are now continued for a few days or until the entire slough has come away and the discharge is diminished, when dressings recommended in the treatment for cutaneous quittor are to be used until recovery is completed. In cases in which the discharge comes from a cleft between the upper border of the hoof and the coronary band, always pare away the loosened horn, so that the soft tissues beneath are fully exposed, care being taken not to injure the healthy parts. This operation permits of a thorough inspection of the diseased parts, the easy removal of all gangrenous tissue, and a better application of the necessary remedies and dressings. The only objection to the operation is that the patient is prevented from being early returned to work.

When the probe shows that pus has collected under the coffin bone the sole must be pared through, and, if caries of the bone is present, the dead parts cut away. After either of these operations the wound is to be dressed with the oakum balls, saturated in the bichlorid of mercury solution, as previously directed, and the bandages tightly applied. Generally the discharge for the first two or three days is so great that the dressings need to be changed every 24 hours; but when the discharge diminishes, the dressing may be left on from one to two weeks. Before the patient is returned to work, a bar shoe should be applied, since the removed quarter or heel can only be made perfect again by a new growth from the coronary band.

Tendinous or cartilaginous complications are to be treated as directed under those headings.

CARTILAGINOUS QUITTOR.

This form of quittor may commence as a primary inflammation of the lateral cartilage, but in the great majority of cases it appears as a sequel to cutaneous or subhorny quittor. It may affect either the fore or hind feet, but is most commonly seen in the former. As a rule, it attacks but one foot at a time, and but one of the cartilages, generally the inner one. It is always a serious affection for the reason that, in many cases, it can only be cured by a surgical operation, requiring a thorough knowledge of the anatomy of the parts involved, and much surgical skill.

Causes.—Direct injuries to the coronet, such as trampling, pricks, burns, and the blow of some heavy falling object which may puncture, bruise, or crush the cartilage, are the common direct causes of cartilaginous quittor. Besides being a sequel to the other forms of quittor, it sometimes develops as a complication in suppurative corn, canker, grease, laminitis, and punctured wounds of the foot. Animals used for heavy draft, and those with flat feet and low heels, are more liable to the disease than others, for the reason that they are more exposed to injury. Rough roads also predispose to the disease by increasing liability to injury.

Symptoms.—When the disease commences as a primary inflammation of the cartilage, lameness develops with the formation of a swelling on the side of the coronet over the quarter. The severity of this lameness depends largely upon the part of the cartilage which is diseased, for if the disease is situated in that part of the cartilage nearest the heel, where the surrounding tissues are soft and spongy, the lameness may be very slight, especially if the patient is required to go no faster than a walk; but when the middle and anterior parts of the cartilage are diseased, the pain and consequent lameness are much greater, for the tissues are less elastic and the coffin joint is more liable to become affected.

Except in the cases to be noted hereafter, one or more fistulous openings finally appear in the tumor on the coronet. These openings are surrounded by a small mass of granulations which are elevated above the adjacent skin and bleed readily if handled. A probe shows these fistulous tracts to be more or less sinuous, but always leading to one point—the gangrenous cartilage. When cartilaginous quittor happens as a complication of suppurative corn, or from punctured wounds of the foot, the fistulous tract may open alone at the point of injury on the sole.

The discharge in this form of quittor is generally thin, watery, and contains pus enough to give it a pale-yellow color; it is offensive to the sense of smell, due to the detachment of small flakes of cartilage which have become gangrenous and are seen in the discharge as small, greenish-colored particles. In old cases it is not unusual to find some of the fistulous openings heal at the surface; this is followed by the gradual collection of pus in the deeper parts, forming an abscess, which in a short time opens at a new point. The wall of the hoof, over the affected quarter and heel, in very old cases becomes rough and wrinkled like the horn of a ram, and generally it is thicker than the corresponding quarter, owing to the stimulating effect which the disease has upon the coronary band.

Complications may arise by an extension of the disease to the lateral ligament of the coffin joint, to the joint itself, to the plantar cushion, and by caries of the coffin bone.

Treatment.—Before recovery can take place all the dead cartilage must be removed. In rare instances this is effected by nature without assistance. Usually, however, the disease does not tend to recovery, and active curative measures must be adopted. The best and simplest treatment, in a majority of cases, is the injection of strong caustic solutions, which destroy the diseased cartilage and cause its discharge, along with the other products of suppuration. In favorable cases these injections will secure a healing of the wound in from two to three weeks. While the saturated solution of sulphate of copper, or a solution of 10 parts of bichlorid of mercury to 100 parts of water, has given the best results in my hands, equally as favorable success has been secured by others from the use of caustic soda, nitrate of silver, sulphate of zinc, tincture of iodin, etc. No matter which one of these remedies may be selected, however, it must be used at least twice a day for a time. The solution is injected into the various openings with force enough to drive it to the bottom of the wound, after which the foot is to be dressed with a pad of oakum, held in place by a roller bandage tightly applied. While it is not always necessary, it is often of advantage to relieve the pressure on the parts by rasping away the hoof over the seat of the cartilage; the coronary band and laminæ should not be injured in the operation.

If the caustic injections prove successful, the discharge will become healthy and gradually diminish, so that by the end of the second week the fistulous tracts are closing up and the injections are made with much difficulty.

If, on the other hand, there is but little or no improvement after this treatment has been used for three weeks, it may reasonably be concluded that the operation for the removal of the lateral cartilage must be resorted to for the cure of the trouble. As this operation can be safely undertaken only by an expert surgeon, it will not be described in this connection.

THRUSH.

Thrush is characterized by an excessive secretion of unhealthy matter from the cleft of the frog. While all classes of horses are liable to this affection, it is more often seen in the common draft horse than in any other breed, owing to the conditions of servitude and not to the fault of the breed. Country horses are much less subject to the disease, except in wet, marshy districts, than are the horses used in cities and towns.

Causes.—The most common cause of thrush is the filthy condition of the stable in which the animal is kept. Mares are more liable to contract the disease in the hind feet when filth is the cause, while the gelding and stallion are more liable to develop it in the fore feet. Hard work on rough and stony roads may also induce the disease, as may a change from dryness to excessive moisture. The latter cause is often seen to operate in old track horses, whose feet are constantly soaked in the bathtub for the purpose of relieving soreness. Muddy streets and roads, especially where mineral substances are plentiful, excite this abnormal condition of the frog. Contracted heels, scratches, and navicular disease predispose to thrush, while by some a constitutional tendency is believed to exist among certain animals which otherwise present a perfect frog.

Symptoms.—At first there is simply an increased moisture in the cleft of the frog, accompanied with an offensive smell. After a time a considerable discharge takes place—thin, watery, and highly offensive, changing gradually to a thicker puriform matter, which rapidly destroys the horn of the frog. Only in old and severe cases is the patient lame and the foot feverish—cases in which the whole frog is involved in the diseased process.

Treatment.—Thrushes are to be treated by cleanliness, the removal of all exciting causes, and a return of the frog to its normal condition. As a rule, the diseased and ragged portions of horn are to be pared away and the foot poulticed for a day or two with boiled turnips, to which may be added a few drops of carbolic acid or a handful of powdered charcoal to destroy the offensive smell. The cleft of the frog and the grooves on its edges are then to be cleaned and well filled with dry calomel and the foot dressed with oakum and a roller bandage. If the discharge is profuse, the dressing should be changed daily; otherwise it may be left on two or three days. Where a constitutional taint is supposed to exist, with swelling of the legs, grease, etc., a purgative, followed by dram doses of sulphate of iron, repeated daily, may be prescribed. In cases where the growth of horn seems too slow a Spanish-fly blister applied to the heels is often followed by good results. Feet in which the disease is readily induced may be protected in the stable with a leather boot. If the thrush is but a sequel to other disease, a permanent cure may not be possible.

CANKER.

Canker of the foot is due to the rapid reproduction of a vegetable parasite. It not only destroys the sole and frog, but, by setting up a chronic inflammation in the deeper tissues, prevents the growth of a healthy horn by which the injury may be repaired. Heavy cart horses are more often affected than those of any other class.

Causes.—The essential element in the production of canker is the parasite; consequently the disease may be called contagious. As in all other diseases due to specific causes, however, the seeds of the disorder must find a suitable soil in which to grow before they are reproduced. It may be said, then, that the conditions which favor the preparation of the tissues for a reception of the seeds of this disease are simply predisposing causes.

The condition most favorable to the development of canker is dampness—in fact, dampness seems indispensable to the existence and growth of the parasite; the disease is rarely, if ever, seen in high, dry districts, and is much more common in rainy than in dry seasons. Filthy stables and muddy roads have been classed among the causes of canker; but it is very doubtful whether these conditions can do more than favor a preparation of the foot for the reception of the disease germ.

All injuries to the feet, by exposing the soft tissues, may render the animal susceptible to infection; but neither the injury nor the irritation and inflammation of the tissues which follow are sufficient to induce the disease.

For some unknown reason horses with lymphatic temperaments—thick skins, flat feet, fleshy frogs, heavy hair, and particularly with white feet and legs—are especially liable to canker.

Symptoms.—Usually, canker is confined to one foot; but it may attack two, three, or all of the feet at once; or, as is more commonly seen, the disease attacks first one then another, until all may have been successively affected. When the disease follows an injury which has exposed the soft tissues of the foot, the wound shows no tendency to heal, but instead there is secreted from the inflamed parts a profuse, thin, fetid, watery discharge, which gradually undermines and destroys the surrounding horn, until a large part of the sole and frog is diseased. The living tissues are swollen, dark colored, and covered at certain points with particles of new, soft, yellowish, thready horn, which are constantly undergoing maceration in the abundant liquid secretion by which they are immersed. As this secretion escapes to the surrounding parts, it dries and forms small, cheesy masses composed of partly dried horny matter, exceedingly offensive to the sense of smell. When the disease originates independently of an injury, the first evidences of the trouble are the offensive odor of the foot, the liquid secretion from the cleft and sides of the frog, and the rotting away of the horn of the frog and sole.

In the earlier stages there is no interference with locomotion, but later the foot becomes sensitive, particularly if the animal is used on rough roads, and, finally, when the sole and frog are largely destroyed the lameness is severe.

Treatment.—Since canker does not destroy the power of the tissues to produce horn, but rather excites them to an excessive production of an imperfect horn, the indications for treatment are to restore the parts to a normal condition, when healthy horn may again be secreted. In my experience, limited though it has been, the old practice of stripping off the entire sole and deep cauterization, with either the hot iron or strong acids, is not attended with uniformly good results.

I am of the opinion that recovery can generally be effected as surely and as speedily with measures which are less heroic and much less painful. True, the treatment of canker is likely to exhaust the patience, and sometimes the resources, of the attendant; but after all success depends more on the persistent application of simple remedies and great cleanliness than on the special virtues of any particular drug.

First, then, clean the foot with warm baths and apply a poultice containing powdered charcoal or carbolic acid. A handful of the charcoal or a tablespoonful of the acid mixed with the poultice serves to destroy much of the offensive odor. The diseased portions of horn are to be carefully removed with sharp instruments, until only healthy horn borders the affected parts. The edges of the sound horn are to be pared thin, so that the swollen soft tissues may not overlap their borders. With sharp scissors cut off all the prominent points on the soft tissues, shorten the walls of the foot, and nail on a broad, plain shoe. The foot is now ready for the dressings, and any of the many stimulating and drying remedies may be used; but it will be necessary to change frequently from one to another, until finally all may be tried.

The list from which a selection may be made comprises wood tar, gas tar, petroleum, creosote, phenic acid; sulphates of iron, copper, and zinc; chlorid of zinc, bichlorid of mercury, calomel, caustic soda, nitrate of silver, chlorid of lime; carbolic, nitric, and sulphuric acids.

In practice I prefer to give the newly shod foot a bath for an hour or two in a solution of the sulphate of iron made by adding 2 ounces of the powdered sulphate to a gallon of cold water. When the foot is removed from the bath it is dressed with oakum balls dipped in a mixture made of Barbados tar 1 part, oil of turpentine 8 parts, to which is slowly added 2 parts of sulphuric acid, and the mixture well stirred and cooled. The diseased parts being well covered with the balls, a pad of oakum sufficiently thick to cause considerable pressure is placed over them, and all are held in place by pieces of heavy tin fitted to slip under the shoe. The whole foot is now incased in a boot or folded gunny sack and the patient turned into a loose, dry box. The dressings are to be changed daily or even twice a day at first. When they are removed, all pieces of new horny matter which are now firmly adherent must be rubbed off with the finger or a tent of oakum. As the secretion diminishes, dry powders, such as calomel, sulphates of iron, copper, etc., may prove of most advantage. The sulphates should not be used pure, but are to be mixed with powdered animal charcoal in the proportion of one of the former to eight or ten of the latter. When the soft tissues are all horned over, the dressings should be continued for a time, weak solutions being used to prevent a recurrence of the disease. If the patient is run down in condition, bitter tonics, such as gentian, may be given in 2-dram doses twice a day and a liberal diet of grain allowed.

CORNS.

A corn is an injury to the living horn of the foot, involving the soft tissues beneath, whereby the capillary blood vessels are ruptured and a small quantity of blood escapes which, by permeating the horn in the immediate neighborhood, stains it a dark color. If the injury is continuously repeated, the horn becomes altered in character and the soft tissues may suppurate or a horny tumor develop. Corns always appear in the sole in the angle between the bar and the outside wall of the hoof. In many cases the laminæ of the bar, of the wall, or of both, are involved at the same time.

Three kinds of corns are commonly recognized—the dry, the moist, and the suppurative—a division based solely on the character of the conditions which follow the primary injury.

The fore feet are almost exclusively the subjects of the disease, for two reasons: First, because they support a greater part of the body; secondly, because the heel of the fore foot during progression is first placed upon the ground, whereby it receives much more concussion than the heel of the hind foot, in which the toe first strikes the ground.

Causes.—It may be said that all feet are exposed to corns, and that even the best feet may suffer from them when conditions necessary to the production of the peculiar injury are present. The heavier breeds of horses generally used for heavy work on rough roads and streets seem to be most liable to this trouble. Mules rarely have corns.

Among the causes and conditions which predispose to corns may be named high heels, which change the natural relative position of the bones of the foot and thereby increase the concussion to which these parts are subject; contracted heels, which in part destroy the elasticity of the foot, increase the pressure upon the soft tissues of the heel, and render lacerations more easy; long feet, which by removing the frog and heels too far from the ground deprive them of necessary moisture; this, in turn, reduces the elastic properties of the horn and diminishes the transverse diameter of the heels; weak feet, or those in which the horn of the wall is too thin to resist the tendency to spread, whereby the soft tissues are easily lacerated. Wide feet with low heels are always accompanied with a flat sole whose posterior wings either rest upon the ground or the shoe, and as a consequence are easily bruised; at the same time the arch of the sole is so broad and flat that it can not support the weight of the body, and in the displacement which happens when the foot is rested upon the ground the soft tissues are liable to become bruised or torn.

It is universally conceded that shoeing, either as a direct or predisposing cause, is most prolific in producing corns. One of the most serious as well as the most common of the errors in shoeing is to be found in the preparation of the foot. Instead of seeking to maintain the integrity of the arch, the first thing done is to weaken it by freely paring away the sole; nor does the mutilation end here, for the frog, which is nature's main support to the branches of the sole and the heels, is also largely cut away. This not only permits of an excessive downward movement of the contents of the horny box, but it at the same time removes the one great means by which concussion of the foot is destroyed. As adjuncts to the foregoing errors must be added the faults of construction in the shoe and in the way it is adjusted to the foot. An excess of concavity in the shoe, extending it too far back on the heels, high calks, thin heels which permit the shoe to spring, short heels with a calk set under the foot, and a shoe too light for the animal wearing it or for the work required of him, are all to be avoided as causes of corns. A shoe so set so as to press upon the sole or one that has been on so long that the hoof has overgrown it until the heels rest upon the sole and bars becomes a direct cause of corns. Indirectly the shoe becomes the cause of corns when small stones, hard, dry earth, or other objects collect between the sole and shoe. Lastly, a rapid gait and excessive knee action, especially on hard roads, predispose to this disease of the feet.

Symptoms.—Ordinarily a corn induces sufficient pain to cause lameness. It may be intense, as seen in suppurative corn, or it may be but a slight soreness, such as that which accompanies dry corn. It is by no means unusual in chronic corns to see old horses apparently so accustomed to the slight pain which they suffer as not to limp at all. But they are generally very restless. They paw their bedding behind them at night and often refuse to lie down for a long rest. The lameness of this disease, however, can hardly be said to be characteristic, for the reason that it varies so greatly in intensity; but the position of the leg while the patient is at rest is generally the same in all cases. The foot is so advanced that it is relieved of all weight, and the fetlock is flexed until all pressure by the contents of the hoof is removed from the heels. In suppurative corn the lameness subsides or entirely disappears as soon as the abscess opens. When the injured tissues are much inflamed, as may happen in severe and recent cases, the heel of the affected side, or even the whole foot, is hot and tender to pressure. In dry corn and in most chronic cases all evidences of local fever are often wanting. It is in these cases that the patient goes well when newly shod, for the smith cuts away the sole over the seat of injury until all pressure by the shoe is removed and lowers the heels so that concussion is reduced to a minimum.

If a corn is suspected, the foot should be examined for increased sensibility of the inside heel. Tapping the heel of the shoe with a hammer and grasping the wall and bar between the jaws of pincers with moderate pressure will cause more or less flinching if the disease is present. For further evidence the shoe is removed and the heel cut away with the drawing knife. As the horn is pared out, not only the sole in the angle is found discolored, but in many instances the insensible laminæ of the bar and wall adjacent are also stained with the escaped blood. In moist and suppurative corns this discoloration is less marked than in dry corn and even may be entirely wanting. In these cases the horn is soft, often white, and stringy or mealy, as seen in pumiced sole resulting from founder. When the whole thickness of the sole is discolored and the horn dry and brittle it is generally evidence that the corn is an old one and that the exciting cause has existed continuously. A moist corn differs from the dry one in that the injury is more severe. The parts affected are more or less inflamed, and the horn of the sole in the angle is undermined by a citron-colored fluid, which often permeates the injured sole and laminæ, causing the horn to become somewhat spongy.

A suppurative corn differs from others in that the inflammation ends in suppuration. The pus collects at the point of injury and finally escapes by working its way between the sensitive and insensible laminæ to the top of the hoof, where an opening is made between the wall and coronary band at or near the heels. This is the most serious form of corns, for the reason that it may induce gangrene of the plantar cushion, cartilaginous quittor, or caries of the coffin bone.

Treatment.—Since a diversity of opinion exists as to what measures must be adopted for the radical cure of corns, the author will advise the use of those which have proved most efficient in his hands.

As in all other troubles, the cause must be discovered, if possible, and removed. In the great majority of cases the shoeing is at fault. While sudden changes in the method of shoeing are not advisable, it may be said that all errors, either in the preparation of the foot, in the construction of the shoe, or in its application may very properly be corrected at any time. Circumstances may at times make it imperative that shoes be worn which are not free from objections;

as, for instance, the shoe with a high calk; but in such cases it is considered that the injuries liable to result from the use of calks are less serious than those which are sure to happen for the want of them.

For a sound foot perfectly formed, a flat shoe, with heels less thick than the toe, and which rests evenly on the wall proper, is the best. In flat feet it is often necessary to concave the shoe as much as possible on the upper surface, so that the sole may not be pressed upon. If the heels are very low the heels of the shoe may be made thicker. If the foot is very broad and the wall light toward the heels, a bar shoe resting upon the frog will aid to prevent excessive tension upon the soft tissues when the foot receives the weight of the body. A piece of leather placed between the foot and shoe serves largely to destroy concussion, and its use is absolutely necessary on some animals to enable them to work.

Last among the preventive measures may be mentioned those which serve to maintain the suppleness of the hoof. The dead horn upon the surface of the sole not only retains moisture for a long time, but protects the living horn beneath from the effects of evaporation; for this reason the sole should be pared as little as possible. Stuffing the feet with flaxseed meal, wet clay, or other like substances, or damp dirt floors or damp bedding of tanbark, greasy hoof ointments, etc., are all means which may be used to keep the feet from becoming too dry and hard.

As to the curative measures which are to be adopted much will depend upon the extent of the injury. If the case is one of chronic dry corn, with but slight lameness, the foot should be poulticed for a day or two and the discolored horn pared out, care being taken not to injure the soft tissues. The heel on the affected side is to be lowered until all pressure is removed and, if the patient's labor is required, the foot must be shod with a bar shoe or with one having stiff heels. Care must be taken to reset the shoe before the foot has grown too long, else the shoe will no longer rest on the wall, but on the sole and bar.

I believe in cutting moist corns out. If there is inflammation, cold baths and poultices should be used; when the horn is well softened and the fever allayed, pare out the diseased horn, lightly cauterize the soft tissues beneath, and poultice the foot for two or three days. When the granulations look red, dress the wound with oakum balls saturated in a weak solution of tincture of aloes or spirits of camphor and apply a roller bandage. Change the dressing every two or three days until a firm, healthy layer of new horn covers the wound, when the shoe may be put on, as in dry corn, and the patient returned to work.

In suppurative corns the loosened horn must be removed, so that the pus may freely escape. If the pus has worked a passage to the coronary band and escapes from an opening between the band and hoof, an opening must be made on the sole, and cold baths made astringent with a little sulphate of iron or copper are to be used for a day or two. When the discharge becomes healthy, the fistulous tracts may be injected daily with a weak solution of bichlorid of mercury, nitrate of silver, etc., and the foot dressed as after operation for moist corns. When complications arise, the treatment must be varied to meet the indications; if gangrene of the lateral cartilage takes place it must be treated as directed under the head of cartilaginous quittor; if the velvety tissue is gangrenous, it must be cut away; if the coffin bone is necrosed, it must be scraped, and the resulting wounds treated on general principles. After any of the operations for corns have been performed, in which the soft tissues have been laid bare, it is best to protect the foot by a sole of soft leather set beneath the shoe when the animal is returned to work. Only in rare instances are the complications of corns so serious as to destroy the life or usefulness of the patient. It is the wide, flat foot with low heels and thin wall which is most liable to resist all efforts toward effecting a complete cure.

BRUISE OF THE FROG.

When the frog is severely bruised the injury is followed by suppuration beneath the horn, and at times by partial gangrene of the plantar cushion.

Causes. A bruise of the frog generally happens from stepping on a rough stone or other hard object. It is more liable to take place when trotting, running, or jumping than when at a slower pace. A stone wedged in the shoe and pressing on the frog or between the sides of the frog and the shoe, if it remains for a time, produces the same results. A cut through the horny frog with some sharp instrument or a punctured wound by a blunt-pointed instrument may also cause suppuration and gangrene of the plantar cushion. Broad, flat feet with low heels and a fleshy frog are most liable to these injuries.

Symptoms.—Lameness, severe in proportion to the extent of the bruise and the consequent suppuration, is always an early symptom. When the animal moves, the toe only is placed to the ground or the foot is carried and the patient hobbles along on three legs. When he is at rest, the foot is set forward with the toe on the ground and the leg flexed at the fetlock joint. As soon as the pus finds its way to the surface the lameness improves. If the frog is examined early the injured spot may usually be found; later, if no opening exists, the pus may be discovered working its way toward the heels. The horn is loosened from the deeper tissues, and, if pared through, a thin, yellow, watery and offensive pus escapes. In other cases a ragged opening is found in the frog, leading down to a mass of dead, sloughing tissues, which are pale green in color if gangrene of the plantar cushion has set in. In rare cases the coffin bone may be involved in the injury and a small portion of it may become carious.

Treatment.—If the injury is seen at once, the foot should be placed in a bath of cold water to prevent suppuration. If suppuration has already set in, the horn of the frog, and of the bars and branches of the sole, if necessary, is to be pared thin so that all possible pressure may be removed, and the foot poulticed. When the pus has loosened the horn, all the detached portions are to be cut away. If the pus is discharging from an opening near the hair, the whole frog, or one-half of it, will generally be found separated from the plantar cushion, and is to be removed with the knife. After a few days the gangrenous portion of the cushion will slough off from the effects of the poultice; under rare circumstances only should the dead parts be removed by surgical interference. When the slough is all detached, the remaining wound is to be treated with simple stimulating dressings, such as tincture of aloes or turpentine; oakum balls, and bandages as directed in punctured wounds. When the lameness has subsided, and a thin layer of new horn has covered the exposed parts, the foot may be shod. Cover the frog with a thick pad of oakum, held in place by pieces of tin fitted to slide under the shoe, and return to slow work. Where caries of the coffin bone, etc., follow the injury the treatment recommended for these complications in punctured wounds of the foot must be resorted to.

PUNCTURED WOUNDS OF THE FOOT.

Of all the injuries to which the foot of the horse is liable, none are more common than punctured wounds, and none are more serious than these may be when involving the more important organs within the hoof. A nail is the most common instrument by which the injury is inflicted, yet wounds may happen from glass, wire, knives, sharp pieces of rock, etc.

A wound of the foot is more serious when made by a blunt-pointed instrument than when the point is sharp, and the nearer the injury is to the center of the foot the more liable are disastrous results to follow. Wounds in the heel and in the posterior parts of the frog are attended with but little danger, unless they are so deep as to injure the lateral cartilages, when quittor may follow. Punctured wounds of the anterior parts of the sole are more dangerous, for the reason that the coffin bone may be injured, and the suppuration, even when the wound is not deep, tends to spread and always gives rise to intense suffering. The most serious of the punctured wounds are those which happen to the center of the foot, and which, in proportion to their depth, involve the plantar cushion, the plantar aponeurosis, the sesamoid sheath, the navicular bone, or the coffin joint.

Punctured wounds are more liable to be deep in flat or convex feet than in well-made feet, and as a rule, recovery is neither so rapid nor so certain. These wounds are less serious in animals used for heavy draft than in those required to do faster work; for the former may be useful, even if complete recovery is not effected. Lastly, punctured wounds of the fore feet are more serious than of the hind feet, for the reason that in the former the instrument is liable to enter the foot in a nearly perpendicular line, and, consequently, is more liable to injure the deeper structures of the foot; in the hind foot, the injury is generally near the heels and the wound oblique and less deep.

Symptoms.—A nail or other sharp instrument may penetrate the frog and remain for several days without causing lameness; in fact, in many cases of punctured wound of the frog the first evidence of the injury is the finding of the nail or the appearance of an opening where the skin and frog unite, from which more or less pus escapes. Even when the sole is perforated, if the injury is not too deep, no lameness develops until suppuration is established. In all cases of foot lameness, especially if the cause is obscure, the foot should be examined for evidence of injury.

The lameness from punctured wounds, accompanied with suppuration, is generally severe, the patient often refusing to use the affected member at all. The pain being lancinating in character, he stands with the injured foot at rest or constantly moves it back and forth. In other cases the patient lies down most of the time with the feet outstretched; the breathing is rapid, the pulse fast, the temperature elevated, and the body covered with patches of sweat.

When the plantar aponeurosis is injured, the pus escapes with difficulty and the wound shows no signs of healing; the whole foot is hot and very painful. If the puncture involves the sesamoid sheath, the synovial fluid escapes. At first this fluid is pure, like joint water, but later becomes mixed with the products of suppuration and loses its clear, amber color. Suppuration generally extends up the course of the flexor tendon, an abscess forms in the hollow of the heel, and finally opens somewhere below the fetlock joint. The whole coronet is more or less swollen, the discharge is profuse and often mixed with blood, yet the suffering is greatly relieved from the moment the abscess opens.

If the puncture reaches the navicular bone the lameness is intense from the beginning; but the only certain way to determine the existence of this complication is by the use of the probe; and unless there is a free escape of synovia it must be used with the greatest of care, else the coffin joint may be opened.

If the coffin joint has been penetrated, either by the offending instrument or by the process of suppuration, acute inflammation of the joint follows, accompanied with high fever, loss of appetite, etc. The ankle and coronet are now greatly swollen, and dropsy of the leg to the knee or hock, or even to the body, often follows. If the process of suppuration continues, small abscesses appear at intervals on different parts of the coronet, the patient rapidly loses flesh, and may die from intense suffering and blood poisoning. In other cases the suppuration soon disappears, and recovery is effected by the joint becoming stiff (anchylosis).

When the wound is forward, near the toe, and deep enough to injure the coffin bone, caries always results. The presence of the dead pieces of bone can be determined by the use of the probe; the bone feels rough and gritty. Furthermore, there is no disposition upon the part of the wound to heal.

Besides the complications above mentioned, others equally as serious may be met with. The tendons may soften and rupture, the hoof may slough off, quittors develop, or sidebones and ringbones grow. Finally, laminatis of the opposite foot may happen if the patient persists in standing, or lockjaw may cause early death.

Treatment.—In all cases the horn around the seat of injury should be thinned down, a free opening made for the escape of the products of suppuration, and the foot placed in a poultice. If the injury is not serious, recovery takes place in a few days. When the wound is deeper it is better to put the foot into a cold bath or under a stream of cold water, as advised in the treatment for quittor.

If the bone is injured, cold baths, containing about 2 ounces each of sulphate of copper and sulphate of iron, may be used until the dead bone is well softened, when it should be removed by an operation. The animal must be cast for this operation. The sole is pared away until the diseased bone is exposed, when all the dead particles are to be removed with a drawing knife, and the wound dressed with 3 per cent compound cresol solution or a 5 per cent solution of carbolic acid, oakum balls, and a roller bandage.

Wounds of the bone which are made by a blunt-pointed instrument, like the square-pointed cut nail, in which a portion of the surface is driven into the deeper parts of the bone, always progress slowly, and should be operated upon as soon as the conditions are favorable. Even wounds of the navicular bone, accompanied with caries, may be operated on and the life of the patient saved; but the most skillful surgery is required and only the experienced operator should undertake their treatment.

If there is an escape of pure synovial fluid from a wound of the sole, without injury to the bone, a small pencil of corrosive sublimate should be introduced to the bottom of the wound and the foot dressed as directed above.

The other complications are to be treated as directed under their proper headings.

After healing of the wounds has been effected, lameness, with more or less swelling of the coronary region, may remain. In such cases the coronet should be blistered or even fired with the actual cautery, and the patient turned to pasture. If the lameness still persists, and is not due to a stiff joint, unnerving may be resorted to in many cases with very good results. If the joint is anchylosed, no treatment can relieve it, and the patient must either be put to very slow work or kept for breeding purposes only.

"*Prick in shoeing*" is an injury which should be considered under the head of punctured wounds of the foot. The nails by which the shoe is fastened to the hoof may produce an injury followed by inflammation and suppuration in two days, by penetrating the soft tissues directly or by being driven so deep that the inner layers of the horn of the wall are pressed against the soft tissues with such force as to crush them. In either case, unless the injury is at the toe, the animal generally goes lame soon after shoeing, when the first evidence of the trouble may be the discharge of pus at the coronet. If lameness follows close upon the setting of the shoes, without other appreciable cause, each nail should be lightly struck with a hammer, when the one at fault will be detected by the flinching of the animal.

Treatment consists in drawing the nail, and if the soft tissues have been penetrated or suppuration has commenced, the horn must be pared away until the diseased parts are exposed. The foot is now to be poulticed for a day or two, or until the lameness and suppuration have ceased. If the discharge of pus from the coronet is the first evidence of the disease, the offending nail must be found and removed, the horn pared out, and a weak solution of carbolic acid or compound cresol injected at the coronet until the fistulous tract has healed.

CONTRACTED HEELS, OR HOOFBOUND.

Contracted heels, or hoofbound, is a common disease among horses kept on hard floor in dry stables, and in such as are subject to much saddle work. It consists in an atrophy, or shrinking, of the tissues of the foot, whereby the lateral diameter of the heels is diminished. It affects the fore feet principally; but it is seen occasionally in the hind feet, where it is of less importance, for the reason that the hind foot first strikes the ground with the toe, and consequently less expansion of the heels is necessary than in the fore feet, where the weight is first received on the heels. Any interference with the expansibility of this part of the foot interferes with locomotion and ultimately gives rise to lameness. Usually but one foot is affected at a time, but when both are diseased the change is greater in one than in the other. Occasionally but one heel, and that the inner one, is contracted; in these cases there is less liable to be lameness and permanent impairment of the animal's usefulness. According to the opinion of some of the French veterinarians, hoofbound should be divided into two classes—total contraction, in which the whole foot is shrunken in size, and contraction of the heels, when the trouble extends only from the quarters backward. (Pl. XXXV, figs. 4 and 7.)

Causes.—Animals raised in wet or marshy districts, when taken to towns and kept on dry floors, are liable to have contracted heels, not alone because the horn becomes dry, but because fever of the feet and wasting away of the soft tissues result from the change. Another common cause of contracted heels is to be found in faulty shoeing, such as rasping the wall, cutting away the frog, heels, and bars; high calks and the use of nails too near the heels. Contracted heels may happen as one of the results of other diseases of the foot; for instance, it often accompanies thrush, sidebones, ringbones, canker, navicular disease, corns, sprains of the flexor tendons, of the sesamoid and suspensory ligaments, and from excessive knuckling of the fetlock joint.

Symptoms.—In contraction of the heels the foot has lost its circular shape, and the walls from the quarters backward approach to a straight line. The ground surface of the foot is now smaller than the coronary circumference; the frog is pinched between the inclosing heels, is much shrunken, and at times is affected with thrush. The sole is more concave than natural, the heels are higher, and the bars are long and nearly perpendicular. The whole hoof is dry and so hard that it can scarcely be cut; the parts toward the heels are scaly and often ridged like the horns of a ram, while fissures, more or less deep, may be seen at the quarters and heels following the direction of the horn fibers. (Plate XXXVI, fig. 10.) When the disease is well advanced lameness is present, while in the earlier stages there is only an uneasiness evinced by frequent shifting of the affected foot. Stumbling is common, especially on hard or rough roads. In most cases the animal comes out of the stable stiff and inclined to walk on the toe, but after exercise he may go free again. He wears his shoes off at the toe in a short time, no matter whether he works or remains in the stable. If the shoe is removed and the foot pared in old cases, a dry, mealy horn will be found where the sole and wall unite, extending upward in a narrow line toward the quarters.

Treatment.—First of all, the preventive measures must be considered. The feet are to be kept moist and the horn from drying out by the use of damp sawdust or other bedding; by occasional poultices of boiled turnips, linseed meal, etc., and greasy hoof ointments to the sole and walls of the feet. The wall of the foot should be spared from the abuse of the rasp; the frog, heels, and bars are not to be mutilated with the knife, nor should calks be used on the shoe except when absolutely necessary. The shoes should be reset at least once a month to prevent the feet from becoming too long, and daily exercise must be insisted on.

As to curative measures, a diversity of opinion exists. A number of kinds of special shoes have been invented, having for an object the spreading of the heels, and perhaps any of these, if properly used, would eventually effect the desired result. But a serious objection to most of these shoes is that they are expensive and often difficult to make and apply. The method of treatment which I have adopted is not only attended with good results, but is inexpensive, if the loss of the patient's services for a time is not considered a part of the question. It consists, first, in the use of poultices or baths of cold water until the horn is thoroughly softened. The foot is now prepared for the shoe in the usual way, except that the heels are lowered a little and the frog remains untouched. A shoe, called a "tip," is made by cutting off both branches at the center of the foot and drawing the ends down to an edge. The tapering of the branches should begin at the toe, and the shoe should be of the usual width, with both the upper and lower surfaces flat. This tip is to be fastened on with six or eight small nails, all set well forward, two being in the toe. With a common foot rasp begin at the heels, close to the coronet, and cut away the horn of the wall until only a thin layer covers the soft tissues beneath. Cut forward until the new surface meets the old $2\frac{1}{2}$ or 3 inches from the heel. The same sloping shape is to be observed in cutting downward toward the bottom of the foot, at which point the wall is to retain its normal thickness. The foot is now blistered all round the coronet with Spanish-fly ointment; when this is well set, the patient is to be turned to pasture in a damp field or meadow. The blister should be repeated in three or four weeks, and, as a rule, the patient can be returned to work in two or three months.

The object of the tip is to throw the weight on the frog and heels, which are readily spread after the horn has been cut away on the sides of the wall. The internal structures of the foot at the heels, being relieved of excessive pressure, regain their nomal condition if the disease is not of too long standing. The blister tends to relieve any inflammation which may be present, and stimulates a rapid growth of healthy horn, which, in most cases, ultimately forms a wide and normal heel. In old, chronic cases, with a shrunken frog and increased concavity of the sole, accompanied with excessive wasting of all the internal tissues of the foot, satisfactory results can not be expected and are rarely obtained. Still, much relief, if not an entire cure, may be effected by these measures.

When thrush is present as a complication, its cure must be sought by measures directed under that heading. If sidebones, ringbones, navicular disease, contracted tendons, or other diseases have been the cause of contracted heels, treatment will be useless until the cause is removed.

SAND CRACKS.

A sand crank is a fissure in the horn of the wall of the foot. These fissures are quite narrow, and, as a general rule, they follow the direction of the horny fibers. They may occur on any part of the wall, but ordinarily are only seen directly in front, when they are called toe cracks; or on the lateral parts of the walls, when they are known as quarter cracks. (Plate XXXVI.)

Toe cracks are most common in the hind feet, while quarter cracks nearly always affect the fore feet. The inside quarter is more liable to the injury than the outside, for the reason that this quarter is not only the thinner, but during locomotion receives a greater part of the weight of the body. A sand crack may be superficial, involving only the outer parts of the wall, or it may be deep, involving the whole thickness of the wall and the soft tissues beneath.

The toe crack is most likely to be complete—that is, extending from the coronary band to the sole—while the quarter crack is nearly always incomplete, at least when of comparatively recent origin. Sand cracks are most serious when they involve the coronary band in the injury. They may be complicated at any time by hemorrhage, inflammation of the laminæ, suppuration, gangrene of the lateral cartilage and of the extensor tendon, caries of the coffin bone, or the growth of a horny tumor known as a keraphyllocele.

Causes.—Relative dryness of the horn is the principal predisposing cause of sand cracks. Excessive dryness is perhaps not a more prolific cause of cracks in the horn than alternate changes from damp to dry. It is even claimed that these injuries are more common in animals working on wet roads than those working on roads that are rough and dry; at least these injuries are not common in mountainous countries. Animals used to running at pasture when transferred to stables with hard, dry floors are more liable to quarter cracks than those accustomed to stables. Small feet, with thick, hard hoofs, and feet which are excessively large, are more susceptible to sand cracks than those of better proportion. A predisposition to quarter cracks exists in contracted feet, and in those where the toe turns out or the inside quarter turns under.

Heavy shoes, large nails, and nails set too far back toward the heels, together with such diseases as canker, quittor, grease, and suppurative corns, must be included as occasional predisposing causes of sand cracks.

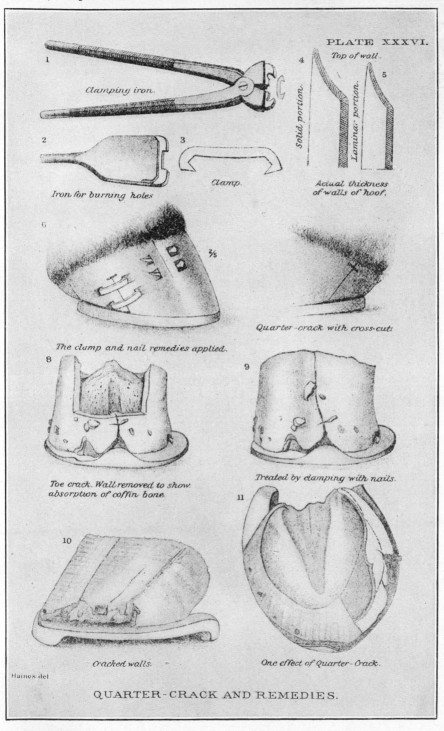

PLATE XXXVI.

1 Clamping iron.

2 Iron for burning holes

3 Clamp.

4 Top of wall. 5

Solid portion. Lamina portion.

Actual thickness of walls of hoof.

6 ⅜ The clamp and nail remedies applied.

Quarter-crack with cross-cut.

8 Toe crack. Wall removed to show absorption of coffin bone.

9 Treated by clamping with nails.

10 Cracked walls.

11 One effect of Quarter-Crack.

Haines del.

QUARTER-CRACK AND REMEDIES.

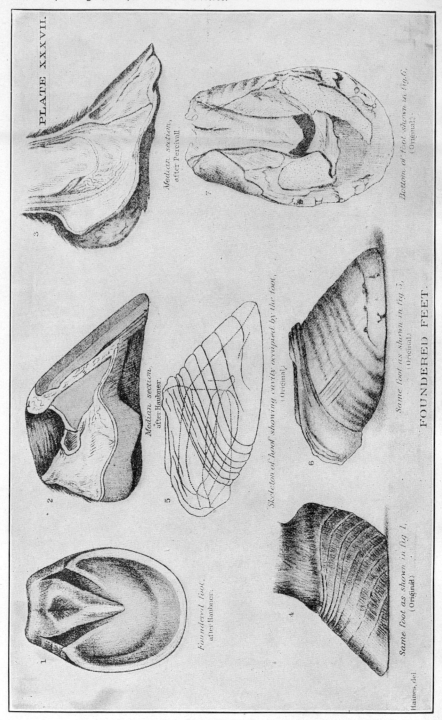

PLATE XXXVII.

3

Median section, after Percivall.

7

Bottom of foot shown in fig.6. (Original).

2

Median section, after Haubner.

5

Skeleton of hoof showing cavity occupied by the foot. (Original).

6

Same foot as shown in fig.3. (Original).

1

Foundered foot, after Haubner.

4

Same foot as shown in fig.1. (Original).

FOUNDERED FEET.

Haines, del.

Fast work on hard roads, jumping, and blows on the coronet, together with calk wounds of the feet, are accidental causes of quarter cracks in particular. Toe cracks are more likely to be caused by heavy pulling on slippery roads and pavements or on steep hills.

Symptoms.—The fissure in the horn is ofttimes the only evidence of the disease; even this may be accidentally or purposely hidden from casual view by mud, ointments, tar, wax, putty, gutta-percha, or by the long hairs of the coronet.

Sand cracks sometimes commence on the internal face of the wall, involving its whole thickness excepting a thin layer on the outer surface. In these cases the existence of the injury may be suspected from a slight depression, which begins near the coronary band and follows the direction of the horny fibers; but the trouble can only be positively diagnosed by paring away the outside layers of horn until the fissure is exposed. In toe cracks the walls of the fissure are in close apposition when the foot receives the weight of the body, but when the foot is raised from the ground the fissure opens. In quarter crack the opposition is true; the fissure closes when the weight is removed from the foot. As a rule, sand cracks begin at the coronary band, and as they become older they not only extend downward, but they also grow deeper. In old cases, particularly in toe cracks, the horn on the borders of the fissure loses its vitality and scales off, sometimes through the greater part of its thickness, leaving behind a rough and irregular channel extending from the coronet to the end of the toe.

In many cases of quarter crack, and in some cases of toe crack as well, if the edges remain close together, with but little motion, the fissure is dry; but in other cases a thin, offensive discharge issues from the crack and the ulcerated soft tissues, or a funguslike growth protrudes from the narrow opening.

When the cracks are deep and the motion of their edges considerable, so that the soft tissues are bruised and pinched with every movement, a constant inflammation of the parts is maintained and the lameness is severe.

Ordinarily the lameness of sand crack is slight when the patient walks, but it is greatly aggravated when he is made to trot, and the harder the road the worse he limps. Furthermore, the lameness is greater going downhill than up, for the reason that these conditions are favorable to an increased motion in the edges of the fissure. Lastly, more or less hemorrhage accompanies the inception of a sand crack when the whole thickness of the wall is involved. Subsequent hemorrhages may also take place from fast work, jumping, or a misstep.

Treatment.—So far as preventive measures are concerned, but little can be done. The suppleness of the horn is to be maintained by the use of ointments, damp floor, bedding, etc. The shoe is to be proportioned to the weight and work of the animal; the nails holding it in place are to be of proper size and not driven too near the heels; sufficient calks and toe pieces must be added to the shoes of horses working on slippery roads; also, the evils of jumping, fast driving, etc., are to be avoided.

When a fissure has made its appearance, means are to be adopted which will prevent it from growing longer or deeper; this can only be done by arresting all motion in the edges. The best and simplest artificial appliance for holding the borders of a toe crack together is the Vachette clasp. These clasps and the instruments necessary for their application can be had of any prominent maker of veterinary instruments. (Pl. XXXVI.) These instruments comprise a cautery iron, with which two notches are burned in the wall, one on each side of the crack, and forceps with which the clasps are closed into place in the bottom of the notches and the edges of the fissure brought close together. The clasps, being made of stiff steel wire, are strong enough to prevent all motion in the borders of the crack. Before these clasps are applied the fissure should be thoroughly cleansed and dried, and if the injury is of recent origin the crack may be filled with a putty made of 2 parts of gutta-percha and 1 part of gum ammoniac. The number of clasps to be used is to be determined by the length of the crack, the amount of motion to be arrested, etc. Generally the clasps are from one-half to three-quarters of an inch apart. The clasps answer equally as well in quarter crack if the wall is sufficiently thick and not too dry and brittle to withstand the strain.

In the absence of these instruments and clasps a hole may be drilled through the horn across the fissure and the crack closed with a thin nail made of tough iron, neatly clinched at both ends. A plate of steel or brass is sometimes fitted to the parts and fastened on with short screws; while this appliance may prevent much gaping of the fissure, it does not entirely arrest motion of the edges, for the reason that the plate and screw can not be rendered immobile.

If, for any reason, the measures above fail or can not be used, recourse must be had to an operation. The horn is softened by the use of warm baths and poultices, the patient cast, and the walls of the fissure entirely removed with the knife. The horn removed is in the shape of the letter V, with the base at the coronet. Care must be taken not to injure the coronary band and the laminæ. The wound is to be treated with mild stimulant dressings, such as compound cresol solution, a weak solution of carbolic acid, tincture of aloes, etc., oakum balls, and a roller bandage. After a few days the wound will be covered with a new, white horn, and only the oakum and bandages will be needed. As the new quarter grows out, the lameness disappears, and the patient may be shod with a bar shoe and returned to work.

In all cases of sand crack the growth of horn should be stimulated by cauterizing the coronary band or by the use of blisters. In simple quarter crack recovery will often take place if the coronet is blistered, the foot shod with a "tip," and the patient turned to pasture.

The shoe in toe crack should have a clip on each side of the fissure and should be thicker at the toe than at the heels. The foot should be lowered at the heels by paring, and spared at the toe, except directly under the fissure, where it is to be pared away until it sets free from the shoe.

When any of the complications referred to above arise, special measures must be resorted to. For the proper treatment of gangrene of the lateral cartilage and extensor tendon and caries of the coffin bone reference may be had to the articles on quittors. If the horny tumor, known as keraphyllocele, should develop, it is to be removed by the use of the knife. Since this tumor develops on the inside of the horny box and may involve other important organs of the foot in disease, its removal should only be undertaken by a skillful surgeon.

NAVICULAR DISEASE.

Navicular disease is an inflammation of the sesamoid sheath, induced by repeated bruising or laceration, and complicated in many cases by inflammation and caries of the navicular bone. In some instances the disease undoubtedly begins in the bone, and the sesamoid sheath becomes involved subsequently by an extension of the inflammatory process. (Plate XXXIV, fig. 5.)

The Thoroughbred horse is more commonly affected than any other, yet no class or breed of horses is entirely exempt. The mule, however, seems rarely, if ever, to suffer from it. For reasons which will appear when considering the causes of the disease, the hind feet are not liable to be affected. Usually but one fore foot suffers from the disease, but if both should be attacked the trouble has become chronic in the first before the second shows signs of the disease.

Causes.—To comprehend fully how navicular disease may be caused by conditions and usages common to nearly all animals, it is necessary to recall the peculiar anatomy of the parts involved in the process and the functions which they perform in locomotion.

It must be remembered that the fore legs largely support the weight of the body when the animal is at rest, and that the faster he moves the greater is the shock which the fore feet must receive as the body is thrown forward by the propelling force of the hind legs. This shock could not be withstood by the tissues of the fore feet and legs were it not that it is largely dissipated by the elastic muscles which bind the shoulder to the body, the ease with which the arm closes on the shoulder blade, and the spring of the fetlock joint. Even these means, however, are not sufficient within themselves to protect the foot from injury; so nature has further supplemented them by placing the coffin joint cn the hind part of the coffin bone instead of directly on top of it, whereby a large part of the shock of locomotion is dispersed before it can reach the vertical column represented by the cannon, knee, and arm bones. A still further provision is made by placing a soft, elastic pad—the frog and plantar cushion—at the heels to receive the sesamoid expansion of the flexor tendon as it is forced downward by the pressure of the coronet bone against the navicular. Extraordinary as these means may appear for the destruction of shock, and ample as they are when the animal is at a slow pace or unweighted by rider or load, they fail to relieve the parts completely from concussion and excessive pressure whenever the opposite conditions are present. The result, then, is that the coronet bone forces the navicular hard against the flexor tendon, which, in turn, presses firmly against the navicular as the force of the contracting muscles lifts the tendon into place. It is self-evident, then, that the more rapid the pace and the greater the load, the greater must these contending forces be, and the greater the liability to injury. For the same reason horses with excessive knee action are more liable to suffer from this disease than others, concussion of the foot and intense pressure on the tendon being common among such horses.

Besides the above-mentioned exciting causes must be considered those which predispose to the disease. Most prominent among these is heredity. It may be claimed, however, that an inherited predisposition to navicular disease consists not so much in a special susceptibility of the tissues which are involved in the process as in a vice of conformation which, as is well known, is liable to be transmitted from parent to offspring. The faults of conformation most likely to be followed by the development of navicular disease are an insufficient plantar cushion, a small frog, high heels, excessive knee action, and contracted heels. Finally, the environments of domestication and use, such as dry stables, heavy pulling, bad shoeing, punctured wounds, etc., all have their influence in developing this disease.

Symptoms.—In the early stages of navicular disease the symptoms are generally very obscure. When the disease begins in inflammation of the navicular bone, the animal while at rest points the affected foot a time before any lameness is seen. While at work he apparently travels as well as ever, but when placed in the stable one foot is set out in front of the other, resting on the toe, with fetlock and knee flexed. After a time, if the case is closely watched, the animal takes a few lame steps while at work, but the lameness disappears as suddenly as it came, and the driver doubts whether the animal was really lame at all. Later the patient has a lame spell which may last during a greater part of the day, but the next morning it is gone; he leaves the stable all right, but goes lame again during the day. In times he has a severe attack of lameness, which may last for a week or more, when a remission takes place and it may be weeks or months before another attack supervenes. Finally, he becomes constantly lame, and the more he is used the greater the lameness.

In the lameness from navicular disease the affected leg always takes a short step, and the toe of the foot first strikes the ground; so the shoe is most worn at this point. If the patient is made to move backward, the foot is set down with exceeding great care, and the weight rests upon the affected leg but a moment. When exercised he often stumbles, and if the road is rough he may fall on his knees. If he is lame in both feet the gait is stilty, the shoulders seem stiff, and, if made to work, he sweats profusely from intense pain. Early in the development of the disease a careful examination will reveal some increased heat in the heels and frog, particularly after work; as the disease progresses this becomes more marked, until the whole foot is hot to the touch. At the same time there is an increased sensibility of the foot, for the patient flinches from the percussion of a hammer lightly applied to the frog and heels or from the pressure of the smith's pincers. The frog is generally shrunken, often of a pale-red color, and at times is affected with thrush. If the heels are pared away so that all the weight is received on the frog, or if the same result is attained by the application of a bar shoe, the animal is excessively lame. The muscles of the leg and shoulder shrink away and often tremble as the animal stands at rest. After months of lameness the foot is found to be shrunken in its diameter and apparently lengthened; the horn is dry and brittle and has lost its natural gloss, while circular ridges, developed most toward the heels, cover the upper part of the hoof. When both feet are affected the animal points first one foot then the other, and stands with the hind feet well forward beneath the body, so as to relieve the fore feet as much as possible from bearing weight. In old cases the wasting of the muscles and the knuckling at the fetlock become so great that the leg can not be straightened and locomotion can scarcely be performed. The disease generally makes a steady progress without inclining to recovery—the remission of symptoms in the earlier stages should not be interpreted as evidence that the process has terminated. The complications usually seen are ringbones, sidebones, thrush, contracted heels, quartercracks, and fractures of the navicular, coronet, and pastern bones.

Treatment.—But few cases of navicular disease recover. In the early stages the wall of the heels should be rasped away, as directed in the treatment for contracted heels, until the horn is quite thin; the coronet should be well blistered with Spanish-fly ointment, and the patient turned to grass in a damp field or meadow. After three or four weeks the blister should be repeated. This treatment is to be continued for two or three months. Plane shoes are to be put on when the patient is returned to work. In chronic cases the animal should be put to slow, easy work. To relieve the pain, neurotomy may be performed—an operation in which the sense of feeling is destroyed in the foot by cutting out pieces of the nerve at the fetlock. This operation in nowise cures the disease, and, since it may be attended with serious results, can be advised only in certain favorable cases, to be determined by the veterinarian.

SIDEBONES.

A sidebone consists in a transformation of the lateral cartilages found on the wings of the coffin bone into bony matter by the deposition of lime salts. The disease is a common one, especially in heavy horses used for draft, in cavalry horses, cow ponies, and other saddle horses, and in runners and trotters.

Sidebones are peculiar to the fore feet, yet they occasionally develop in the hind feet, where they are of little importance since they cause no lameness. In many instances sidebones are of slow growth and, being unaccompanied with acute inflammation, they cause no lameness until such time as, by reason of their size, they interfere with the action of the joint. (Plate XXXIV, fig. 4.)

Causes.—Sidebones often grow in heavy horses without any apparent injury, and their development has been attributed to the over-expansion of the cartilages caused by the great weight of the animal. Blows and other injuries to the cartilages may set up an inflammatory process which ends in the formation of these bony growths. High-heeled shoes, high calks, and long feet are always classed among the conditions which may excite the growth of sidebones. They are often seen in connection with contracted heels, ringbones, navicular disease, punctured wounds of the foot, quarter cracks, and occasionally as a sequel to founder.

Symptoms.—In the earlier stages of the disease, if inflammation is present, the only evidence of the trouble to be detected is a little fever over the seat of the affected cartilage and a slight lameness. In the lameness of sidebones the toe of the foot first strikes the ground and the step is shorter than natural. The subject comes out of the stable stiff and sore, but the gait is more free after exercise.

Since the deposit of bony matter often begins in that part of the cartilage where it is attached to the coffin bone, the diseased process may exist for some time before the bony growth can be seen or felt. Later, however, the cartilage can be felt to have lost its elastic character, and by standing in front of the animal a prominence of the coronary region at the quarters can be seen. Occasionally these bones become so large as to bulge the hoof outward, and by pressing on the joint they so interfere with locomotion that the animal becomes entirely useless.

Treatment.—So soon as the disease can be diagnosed active treatment should be adopted. Cold-water bandages are to be used for a few days to relieve the fever and soreness.

The improvement consequent on the use of these simple measures often leads to the belief that the disease has recovered; but with a return to work the lameness, fever, etc., reappears. For this reason the use of blisters, or, better still, the firing iron, should follow on the discontinuance of the cold bandages.

But in many instances no treatment will arrest the growth of these bony tumors, and as a palliative measure neurotomy must be resorted to. Generally this operation will so relieve the pain of locomotion that the patient may be used for slow work; but in animals used for fast driving or for saddle purposes, the operation is practically useless. Some years ago at Fort Leavenworth I unnerved a number of cavalry horses that were suffering from sidebones, and the records show that in less than seven months all were more lame than ever. Since a predisposition to develop sidebones may be inherited, animals suffering from this disease should not be used for breeding purposes unless the trouble is known to have originated from an accident.

RINGBONE.

A ringbone is the growth of a bony tumor on the ankle. This tumor is, in fact, not the disease, but simply the result of an inflammatory action set up in the periosteum and bone tissue proper of the pastern bones. (Plate XXXIV, fig. 1.) (See also p. 313.)

Causes.—Injuries, such as blows, sprains, overwork in young, undeveloped animals, fast work on hard roads, jumping, etc., are among the principal exciting causes of ringbone. Horses most disposed to this disease are those with short, upright pasterns, for the reason that the shock of locomotion is but imperfectly dissipated in the fore legs of these animals. Improper shoeing, such as the use of high calks, a too great shortening of the toe and correspondingly high heels, predispose to this disease by increasing the concussion to the feet.

Symptoms.—The first symptom of an actively developed ringbone is the appearance of a lameness more or less acute. If the bony tumor forms on the side or upper parts of the large pastern, its growth is generally unattended with acute inflammatory action, and consequently produces no lameness or evident fever. These are called "false" ringbones. But when the tumors form on the whole circumference of the ankle, or simply in front under the extensor tendon, or behind under the flexor tendons, or if they involve the joints between the two pastern bones, or between the small pastern and the coffin bone, the lameness is always severe. These constitute the true ringbone. Besides lameness, the ankle of the affected limb presents more or less heat, and in many instances a rather firm, though limited, swelling of the deeper tissues over the seat of the inflammatory process. The lameness of ringbone is characteristic in that the heel is first placed on the ground when the disease is in a fore leg, and the ankle is kept as rigid as possible. In the hind leg, however, the toe strikes the ground first, when the ringbone is high on the ankle, just as in health, but the ankle is maintained in a rigid position. If the bony growth is under the front tendon of the hind leg, or if it involves the coffin joint, the heel is brought to the ground first. In the early stages of the disease it is not always easy to diagnose ringbone, but when the deposits have reached some size they can be felt and seen as well.

The importance of a ringbone depends on its seat and often on its size. If it interferes with the joints or with the tendons it may cause an incurable lameness, even though small. If it is on the sides of the large pastern, the lameness generally disappears as soon as the tumor has reached its growth and the inflammation subsides. Even when the pastern joint is involved, if complete anchylosis results, the patient may recover from the lameness with simply an imperfect action of the foot remaining, due to the stiff joint.

Treatment.—Before the bony growth has commenced the inflammatory process may be cut short by the use of cold baths and wet bandages, followed by one or more blisters. If the bony deposits have begun, the firing iron should always be used. Even when the tumors are large and the pastern joint involved, firing often hastens the process of anchylosis and should always be tried.

When the lower joint is involved, or if the tumor interferes with the action of the tendons, recovery is not to be expected. In many of these latter cases, however, the animal may be made serviceable by proper shoeing. If the patient walks with the toe on the ground, the foot should be shod with a high-heeled shoe and a short toe. On the other hand, if he walks on the heel, a thick-toed and thin-heeled shoe must be worn.

Since ringbone is considered to be one of the hereditary diseases, no animal suffering from this trouble should ever be used for breeding purposes.

LAMINITIS, OR FOUNDER.

Laminitis is a simple inflammation of the sensitive laminæ of the feet, characterized by the general phenomena attending inflammation of the skin and mucous membranes, producing no constitutional disturbances except those dependent upon the local disease, and having a strong tendency, in severe cases, to destructive disorganization of the tissues affected.

Causes.—The causes of laminitis are as wide and variable as in any of the local inflammations, and may be divided into two classes—the predisposing and the exciting.

Predisposing causes.—From personal observation I do not know that any particular construction of foot or any special breed of horses is predisposed to this disease, neither can I find anything to warrant the assumption that it is in any way hereditary; so that while we may easily cultivate a predisposition to the disease, it does not originate without an exciting cause. Like most other tissues, a predisposition to inflammation may be induced in the sensitive laminæ by any cause which lessens their power of withstanding the work imposed on them. It exists to an extent in those animals unaccustomed to work, particularly if they are plethoric, and in all that have been previous subjects of the disease, for the same rule holds good here that we find in so many diseases—i. e., that one attack impairs the functional activity of the affected tissues and renders them more easy of a subsequent inflammation. Unusual excitement by determining an excessive blood supply, bad shoeing, careless paring of the feet by removing the sole support, and high calkings without corresponding toe pieces must be included under this head.

Exciting causes.—The exciting causes of laminitis are many and varied. The most common are concussion, overexertion, exhaustion, rapid changes of temperature, ingestion of certain feeds, purgatives, and the oft-mentioned metastasis.

(1) Concussion produces this disease by local overstimulation. The excessive excitement is followed by an almost complete exhaustion of the functional activity of the laminated tissues, the exhaustion by congestion, and eventually by inflammation. But congestion here, as in all other tissues, is not necessarily followed by inflammation; for, although the principal symptoms belonging to true laminitis are present, the congestion may be relieved before the processes of inflammation are fully established. This is the condition in the many so-called cases of laminitis which recover in from 24 to 48 hours. They should be called congestion of the laminæ.

Laminitis from concussion is common in trotting horses that are raced when not in condition, especially if they carry the obnoxious toe weights, and in green horses put to work on city pavements to which they are unaccustomed. Concussion from long drives on dirt roads is at times productive of the same results, notably when the weather is extremely warm, or at least when the relative change of temperature is great. But the exhaustion of these circumstances must prove an exciting cause as well as the long-continued concussion. This combination of causes must also determine the disease at times in hunters, for the weight of the rider increases the demands made upon the function of these tissues, and their powers are the sooner exhausted.

(2) Overexertion, as heavy pulling or rapid work, even when there is no immoderate concussion, occasionally results in this disease. Here also exhaustion is a conjunctive cause, for overexertion can not be long continued without exhaustion.

(3) Exhaustion is nearly as prolific a source of laminitis as is concussion, for when the physical strength is impaired, even though temporarily, some part of the economy is rendered more vulnerable to disease than others. To this cause we must ascribe those cases which follow a hard day's work, in which at no time has there been overexertion or immoderate concussion.

The tendency to laminitis in horses on sea voyages results from the continual constrained position the animal maintains on account of the rocking motion of the vessel.

If one foot has been blistered, or if one limb is incapacitated from any cause, the opposite member, doing double duty, soon becomes exhausted, and congestion, followed by inflammation, results. When one foot only becomes laminitic, it is customary to find the corresponding member participating at a later date; not always because of sympathy, but because one foot had to do the work of two.

(4) Rapid changes of temperature act as an exciting cause of laminitis by impairing the normal blood supply.

This change of temperature may be induced by drinking large quantities of cold water while in an overheated condition. Here the internal heat is rapidly reduced, the neighboring tissues and blood vessels constrained, and the blood supply to these organs greatly diminished, while the quantity sent to the surface is correspondingly increased. True, in many cases there has not been sufficient labor performed to impair the powers of the laminæ, and laminitis is more readily induced than congestion or inflammation of the skin or other surface organs, because the laminæ can not relieve themselves of threatened congestion by the general safety valve of perspiration. A cold wind or relatively cold air allowed to play upon the body when heated and wet with sweat has virtually the same result, for it arrests evaporation and rapidly cools the external surface, thereby determining an excess of blood to such organs and tissues as are protected from this outside influence. In many instances this happens to be some of the internal organs, as the lungs, if the previous work has been rapid and their functional activity impaired; but in numerous other instances the determination is toward the feet, and that it is so depends upon two very palpable facts: First, that these tissues have been greatly excited and are already receiving as much blood as they can accommodate consistently with health; second, even though these tissues are classed with those of the surface, their protection from atmospheric influences by means of the thick box of horn incasing them renders them in this respect equivalent to internal organs.

A more limited local action of cold may excite this disease, by driving through water or washing the feet and legs while the animal is warm or just in from work. Here a very marked reaction takes place in the surface tissues of the limbs, and passive congestion of the foot results from an interference with the return flow of blood which is being sent to these organs in excess. These are more liable to be simple cases of congestion, soon to recover, yet they may become true cases of laminitis.

(5) Why it is that certain kinds of grain will cause laminitis does not seem to be clearly understood. Certainly they possess no specific action upon the laminæ, for all animals are not alike affected; neither do they always produce these results in the same animal. Some of these feeds cause a strong tendency to indigestion, and the consequent irritation of the alimentary canal may be so great as to warrant the belief that the laminæ are affected through sympathy. In other instances there is no apparent interference with digestion nor evidence of any irritation of the mucous membranes, yet the disease is in some manner dependent upon the feed for its inception. Barley, wheat, and sometimes corn are the grains most liable to cause this disease. With some horses there appears to be a particular susceptibility to this influence of corn, and the use of this grain is followed by inflammation of the feet, lasting from a few days to two weeks. In these animals, to all appearances healthy, the corn neither induces colic, indigestion, nor purging, and apparently no irritation whatever of the alimentary canal.

(6) Fortunately purgative medicines rarely cause inflammation of the laminæ. That it is, then, the result of sympathetic action is no doubt more than hypothetical, for when there is no derangement of the alimentary canal a dose of cathartic medicine will at times bring on severe laminitis.

(7) Almost all the older authorities were agreed that metastatic laminitis is a reality. In my opinion metastatic laminitis is nothing more nor less than concurrent laminitis, and presents little in any

way peculiar outside the imperfectly understood exciting cause. The practitioner who allows the acute symptoms of the laminitis to mislead him, simply because their severity has overshadowed those of the primary disease, may lose his case through unguarded subsequent treatment. This form of laminitis is by no means commonly met with. It may be found in conjunction with pneumonia, according to Youatt with inflammation of the bowels and eyes, and according to Law and Williams sometimes with bronchitis.

Symptoms.—Laminitis is characterized by a congregation of symptoms so well marked as scarcely to be misinterpreted by the most casual observer. They are nearly constant in their manifestations, modified by the number of feet affected, the cause which has induced the disease, the previous condition of the patient, and the various other influences which to some extent operate in all diseases. They may be divided into general symptoms, which are concomitants of all cases of the disease, subject to variations in degree only, and special symptoms, or those which serve to determine the feet affected and the complications which may arise.

General symptoms.—Usually, the first symptom is the interference with lomomotion. Occasionally the other symptoms are presented first. As the lameness develops the pulse becomes accelerated, full, hard, and strikes the finger strongly; the temperature soon rises several degrees above the normal, reaching sometimes 106° F.; it generally ranges between 102.5° and 105° F. The respirations are rapid and panting in character, the nostrils widely dilated, and the mucous membranes highly injected. The facial expression is anxious and indicative of the most acute suffering, while the body is more or less bedewed with sweat. At first there may be a tendency to diarrhea, or it may appear later as the result of the medicines used. The urine is high colored, scant in quantity, and of increased specific gravity, owing to the water being eliminated by the skin instead of the kidneys. The appetite is impaired, sometimes entirely lost, but thirst is greatly increased. The affected feet are hot and dry, and as much as possible are relieved from bearing weight. Rapping them with a hammer, or compelling the animal to stand upon one affected member, causes intense pain. The artery at the fetlock throbs beneath the finger.

Special symptoms.—Liability to affection varies in the different feet according to the exciting cause. Any one or more of the feet may become the subject of this disease, although it appears more often in the fore feet than in the hind ones. This is due to the difference of the function, i. e., that the fore feet are the bases of the columns of support, receiving nearly all the body weight during progression and consequently most of the concussion, while the hind feet become simply the fulcra of the levers of progression, and are almost exempt from concussion.

One foot.—Injuries and excessive functional performance are the causes of the disease in only one foot. The general symptoms, as a rule, are not severe, there being often no loss of appetite and no unusual thirst, while the pulse, temperature, and respiration remain about normal. The weight of the body is early thrown upon the opposite foot, and the affected one is extended, repeatedly raised from the floor, and then carefully replaced. When made to move forward the lame foot is either carried in the air while progression is accomplished by hopping with the healthy one, or else the heel of the first is placed upon the ground and receives little weight while the sound limb is quickly advanced. Progression in a straight line is more easy than turning toward the lame side.

Both fore feet.—When both fore feet are affected the symptoms are well marked. The lameness is excessive and the animal almost immovable. When standing the head hangs low down, or rests upon the manger as a means of support and to relieve the feet; the fore feet are well extended so that the weight is thrown upon the heels, where the tissues are least sensitive, least inflamed, and most capable of relief by free effusion. The hind feet are brought forward beneath the body to receive as much weight as possible, thereby relieving the diseased ones. If progression is attempted, which rarely happens voluntarily during the first three or four days, it is accomplished with very great pain and lameness at the starting, which usually subsides to an extent after a few minutes' exercise. During this exercise, if the animal happens to step upon a small stone or other hard substance, he stumbles painfully and is excessively lame in the offended member for a number of steps, owing to the acute pain which pressure upon the sole causes in the tissues beneath. The manner of the progression is pathognomonic of the complaint. Sometimes the affected feet are simultaneously raised from the ground (the hind ones sustaining the weight), then advanced a short distance and carefully replaced; at almost the same moment the hind ones are quickly shuffled forward near to the center of gravitation.

In other instances one foot at a time is advanced and placed with the heel upon the ground in the same careful manner, all causes of concussion being carefully avoided. In attempting to back the animal he is found to be almost stationary, simply swaying the body backward on the haunches and elevating the toes of the diseased feet as they rest upon their heels. In attempting to turn either to the right or left he allows his head to be drawn to the one side to its full extent before moving, then makes his hind feet the axis around which the forward ones describe a shuffling circle.

In most of cases of laminitis in the fore feet the animal persists in standing until he is nearly recovered. In other cases he as persistently lies, standing only when necessity seems to compel it, and then for as short a time as possible. If the recumbent position is once assumed, the relief experienced tempts the patient to seek it again; so we often find him down a greater part of the time. But this is not true of all cases; sometimes he will make the experiment, then cautiously guard against a repetition. Even in cases of enforced recumbency, he ofttimes takes advantage of the first opportunity and gets upon his feet, doggedly remaining there until again laid upon his side. How to explain this diversity of action I do not know; theoretically the recumbent position is the only appropriate one, except when complications exist, and the one which should give the most comfort, yet it is rejected by very many patients and, no doubt, for some good reason. It has been suggested as an explanation that when the animal gets upon his feet after lying for a time the suffering is so greatly augmented that the memory of this experience deters him from an attempted repetition. If this were true, the horse with the first attack must necessarily make the experiment before knowing the after effects of lying down, yet many remain standing without even an attempt at gaining this experimental knowledge.

The most-favored position of the animal when down is on the broadside, with the feet and legs extended. While in this position the general symptoms greatly subside; the respirations and pulse become almost normal; the temperature falls and the perspiration dries. It is with difficulty that he is made to rise. When he attempts it he gets up rapidly and "all of a heap," as it were, shifting quickly from one to the other foot until they become accustomed to the weight thrown upon them. Occasionally a patient will get up like a cow, rising upon the hind feet first. Although enforced exercise relieves the soreness to some extent, it is but temporary, for after a few minutes' rest it returns with all its former severity.

Both hind feet.—When only both hind feet are affected, they are, while standing, maintained in the same position as when only the fore ones are the subjects of the disease, but with an entirely different object in view. Instead of being there to receive weight, they are so advanced that the heels only may receive what little weight is necessarily imposed on them; the fore feet at the same time are placed well back beneath the body, where they become the main supports; the animal standing, as Williams describes it, "all of a heap."

Progression is even more difficult now than when the disease is confined to the anterior extremities. The fore feet are dubiously advanced a short distance and the hind ones brought forward with a sort of kangaroo hop that results in an apparent loss of equilibrium which the animal is a few moments in regaining. The general symptoms, or, in other words, the degree of suffering, seem more severe than when the disease affects the fore feet alone. The standing position is not often maintained, the patient seeking relief in recumbency. This fact is easily understood when we consider how cramped and unnatural is the position he assumes while standing and, if it were maintained for any considerable length of time, would, no doubt, excite the disease in the fore feet, as explained by D'Arboval.

All four feet.—Laminitis of all four feet is but uncommonly met with. The author has seen but three such cases. In all these the position assumed was nearly normal. All the feet were slightly advanced, and first one, then another, momentarily raised from the ground and carefully replaced, this action being kept up almost continually during the time the animal remained standing. The suffering is most acute, the appetite lost, and, although the patient lies most of the time, the temperature remains too high. The pulse and respirations are greatly accelerated, the body covered with sweat, and bed sores are unpleasant accompaniments.

Course.—The course which laminitis takes varies greatly in different cases, being influenced more or less by the exciting cause, the animal's previous condition, the acuteness of the attack, and the subsequent treatment. The first symptoms rarely exhibit themselves while the animal is at his work, although we occasionally see the gait impaired by stumbling, the body covered with a profuse sweat, and the respirations become blowing in character as premonitions of the oncoming disease; but, as a rule, nothing amiss with the animal is noted until he has stood for some time after coming in from work, when, in attempting to move him, he is found very stiff. Like all congestions, the early symptoms usually develop rapidly; yet this is not always the case, for often there appears to be no well-defined period of congestion, the disease seemingly commencing at a point and gradually spreading until a large territory is involved in the morbid process.

Simple congestion.—Those cases of simple congestion of the laminæ, which we erroneously call laminitis, are rapidly developed, the symptoms are but moderately severe, and but one to three days are required for recovery. There are no structural changes and but a moderate exudate. This is rapidly reabsorbed, leaving the parts in the same condition as they were previous to the attack. If the congestion has been excessive, a rupture of some of the capillaries will be found, a condition more liable to exist if the animal is made to continue work after a development of symptoms has begun.

True, the majority of these last-described cases prove to be the laminitis in fact, yet the congestion may pass away and the extravasated blood be absorbed without inflammation sufficient to warrant calling it laminitis. The seat of greatest congestion will always be found in the neighborhood of the toe, because of the increased vascularity of that part, and, although at times it is limited to the podophyllous tissue alone, any or all parts of the keratogenous membrane may be affected by the congestion and followed finally by inflammation.

Acute.—In the acute form of laminitis the symptoms may all develop rapidly, or it may commence by the appearance of a little soreness of the feet which in 24 or 48 hours develops into a well-marked case. This peculiarity of development is due to one of two causes. Either the congestion is general, but takes place slowly, or it begins in one or more points and gradually spreads throughout the laminæ. These acute cases generally run their course in from one to two weeks. Usually a culmination of the symptoms is reached, if the patient is properly treated, in from three to five days; then evidences of recovery are discernible in favorable cases. The lameness improves, the other symptoms gradually subside, and eventually health is regained. It is in these cases that a strong tendency to disorganization of a destructive character exists; hence it is we see so many recover imperfectly, with marked structural changes permanently remaining.

Subacute.—Subacute laminitis is most often seen as a termination of the acute form, although it may exist independent of or precede an acute attack. It is characterized by the mildness of its symptoms, slow course, and moderate tissue changes. It may be present a long time before any pathological lesions result other than those found in the acute form, and when these changes do take place they should be viewed rather as complications.

Chronic.—Chronic laminitis is a term used by many to designate any of the sequelæ of the acute and subacute forms of this disease. Pure, chronic inflammation of the laminæ is not very commonly met with, but is most frequent in horses that have long done fast track work. They have " fever in the feet " at all times and are continually sore, both conditions being aggravated by work. Like chronic inflammation of other parts, there is a strong tendency to the development of new connective tissue which, by its pressure upon the blood vessels, interferes with nutrition. Wasting of the coffin bone and inflammation of its covering with caries is not unusual. The continued fever and impaired function of secretion result in the production of a horn deficient in elasticity, somewhat spongy in character, and inclined to crumble. In some cases of " soreness " in horses used to hard or fast work there is evident weakness of the coats of the vessels, brought on by repeated functional exhaustion. Here slight work brings on congestion, which results in serous effusion and temporary symptoms similar to those of chronic laminitis.

Complications.—Complications concurrent with or supervening upon laminitis are frequent and varied, and are often dependent upon causes not fully understood.

Excessive purgation is one of the simplest of these, and not usually attended with dangerous consequences. It rarely occurs unless induced by a purgative, and the excessive action of the medicine is probably to be explained upon the theory that the mucous membrane sympathizes with the diseased laminæ, is irritable, and readily becomes overexcited. The discharges are thin and watery, sometimes offensively odorous, and occasionally persist in spite of treatment. It may prove disastrous to the welfare of the patient by the rapid exhaustion which it causes, preventing resolution of the laminitis, and may even cause death.

Septicemia and pyemia.—Septicemia and pyemia are unusual complications and are seen only in the most severe cases in which bed sores are present or suppuration of the laminæ results. They die, as a rule, within three days after showing signs of the complication.

Pneumonia—the so-called metastatic—needs no special consideration, for in its lesions and symptoms it does not differ from ordinary pneumonia, although it may be overlooked entirely by the practitioner. Examinations of the chest should be made every day, so as to detect the disease at its onset and render proper aid.

Sidebones.—A rapid development of sidebones is one of the complications, or, perhaps better, a sequel of laminitis not often met with in practice. Here the inflammatory process extends to the lateral cartilages, with a strong tendency to calcification. The deposition of the lime salts is sometimes most rapid, so that the " bones " are developed in a few weeks; in other instances they are deposited slowly and their growth is not noted until long after the subsidence of the laminitis, so that the exciting cause is not suspected. This change in the cartilages may commence as early as the first of the laminitis; and although the trouble in the laminæ is removed in the course of a fortnight the symptoms do not entirely subside, the animal retains the shuffling gait, the sidebones continue to grow, and the patient usually remains quite lame. This alteration of the cartilages generally prevents the patient from recovering his natural gait, and the practitioner receives unjust censure for a condition of affairs he could neither foresee nor prevent.

The laminitic process occasionally extends to the covering of the coronet bone, or at least concurrent with and subsequent to laminitis the development of "low ringbone" is seen, and it is apparently dependent upon the disease of the laminæ for its exciting cause. The impairment of function and consequent symptoms are much less marked here than in sidebones. The coronet remains hot and sensitive and somewhat thickened after the laminitis subsides, and a little lameness is present. This lameness persists, and the deposits of new bone may readily be detected.

Suppuration of the sensitive membrane is a somewhat common complication, and even when present in its most limited form is always a serious matter; but when it becomes extensive, and especially when the suppurative process extends to the periosteum, the results are liable to be fatal. When suppuration occurs the exudation does not appear to be excessive. It is rich in leucocytes and seems to have caused detachment of the sensitive tissues from the horn prior to the formation of pus in some instances; in others the tissues are still attached to the horn, and the suppuration takes place in the deeper tissues.

Limited suppuration may take place in any part of the sensitive tissues of the foot during laminitis, and may ultimately be reabsorbed instead of being discharged upon the surface, but generally the process begins in the neighborhood of the toe and spreads backward and upward toward the coronet, finally separating the horn from the coronary band at the quarters. At the same time it spreads over the sole and eventually the entire hoof is loosened and sloughs away, leaving the tissues beneath entirely unprotected. In other instances— and these are generally the cases not considered unusually severe—the suppuration begins at the coronary band. It extends but a short distance into the tissues, yet destroys the patient by separating the hoof from the coronary band, upon which it depends for support and growth. This form of the suppurative process usually begins in front. It is this part of the coronary band that is always most actively affected with inflammation, and consequently it is here that impairments first occur.

Suppuration of the sensitive sole is more common than of the sensitive laminæ and coronary band. It is present in the majority of cases in which there is a dropping of the coffin bone, and in other instances when the effusion at this point is so great as to arrest the production of horn and uncover the sensitive tissues. Except when the result of injury it begins at the toe and spreads backward, and, if not relieved by opening the sole, escapes at the heel. Suppuration of the sole is much less serious than in other parts of the foot.

If the acute constitutional symptoms developed from sloughing of the foot do not result in death, a new hoof of very imperfect horn may be developed after a time; but unless the animal is to be kept for breeding purposes alone the foot will ever be useless for work and death should relieve the suffering. When only the sole sloughs, recovery takes place with proper treatment.

Peditis.—This is the term that Williams applies to that serious complication of laminitis in which not only the laminæ, but the periosteum membrane covering the bone and coffin bone also are subjects of the inflammatory process. Neither is this all; in some of these cases of peditis acute inflammation of the coffin joint is present, and occasionally suppuration of the joint. A mild form of periostitis, in which the exudation is in the outer layer of the periosteum only, is a more common condition than is recognized generally by practitioners. Intimate contiguity of structures is the predisposing cause, for the disease either spreads from the original seat or the complication occurs as one of the primary results of the exciting cause. In the severer cases in which the exudate separates the periosteum from the bone, suppuration, gangrene, and superficial caries are common results. If infiltration of the bone tissues is rapid the blood supply is cut off by pressure upon the vessels and death of the coffin bone follows. Grave constitutional symptoms mark these changes, which soon prove fatal.

In the mild cases of periostitis it is by no means easy positively to determine its presence, for there are no special symptoms by which it may be distinguished from pure laminitis. In a majority of acute cases, though, which show no signs of improvement by the fifth to seventh day, it is safe to suspect periostitis, particularly if the coronets are very hot, the pulse full and hard, and the lameness acute. In the fortunately rare cases in which the bone is affected with inflammation and suppuration the agony of the patient is intense; he occupies the recumbent position almost continually, never standing for more than a few minutes at a time; suffers from the most careful handling of the affected feet; maintains a rapid pulse and respiration, high temperature, loss of appetite, and great thirst. It is in these cases that the patient continually grows worse, and the appearance of suppuration at the top of the hoof in about two weeks after the inception of the disease proves the inefficiency of any treatment which may have been used and the hopelessness of the case. These patients die usually between the tenth and twentieth days either from exhaustion or pyemic infection.

Gangrene occurs in the periosteum as the result of excessive detachment from the bone and compression due to excessive exudation. Other parts of the sensitive tissues are subject occasionally to the same fate, and at times large areas will be found dead.

Pumiced sole is that condition in which the horny sole in the neighborhood of the toe readily crumbles away and leaves the sensitive tissues more or less exposed. It is not a complication of laminitis only, for it is seen under other conditions. Williams has described the horny tissue of pumiced sole as "weak, cheesy, or spongy, like macerated horn, or even grumous (thick, clotted)." Crumbling horn, when critically examined, shows almost an entire absence of the cohesive matter which unites the healthy fibers, while the fibers themselves are irregular and granular in appearance. Pumiced sole depends upon an impairment of the horn-secreting powers of the sensitive sole or upon a separation of the horny from the soft tissues which maintain its vitality.

Punctured wounds of the foot, accompanied with any considerable destruction of the soft tissues, present the same peculiarities of horn in the immediate neighborhood of the injury. Bruises of the sole are followed by this change when the exudation has been excessive and has separated the horn from the living tissues. True, in these cases we rarely see the soft tissues laid bare, for the reason that new horn is constantly secreted and replaces that undergoing disintegration.

Laminitis presents three conditions under which pumiced sole may appear: First, when free exudation separates the horn from the other tissues, or when the process of inflammation arrests the production of horn by impairing or destroying the horn-secreting membrane; second, when depression of the coffin bone causes pressure upon and arrests the formation of horn; and, third, when the elevation of the sole compresses the soft tissues against the pedal bone and induces the same condition.

Pumiced sole, from simple exudation and separation of tissues, is of little importance for the reason given above in connection with bruises; but when suppuration occurs in restricted portions of the foot in conjunction with laminitis, it always lays bare the tissues beneath and temporarily impairs the animal's value. Recovery takes place after a few weeks by the tissues "horning over," as in injuries attended by the same process. Depression of the coffin bone is not sufficient within itself to cause pumiced sole; for, if the relative change in the bone takes place slowly, or if the horn is thin, the sole becomes convex from gradual pressure and the soft tissues adapt themselves to the change without having their function materially impaired. But when the dropping is sudden and the soft tissues are destroyed, the horn rapidly crumbles away and the toe of the bone comes through. In many of these cases the soft tissues remain uncovered for months. When they are eventually covered it is with a thin, slightly adherent horn that stands but little or no wear. The sole being now convex, the diseased tissues bear unusual weight by coming in contact with the ground, and hence it is that these animals are generally incurable cripples.

In most cases in which the sole is raised to meet the pedal bone and pumiced sole occurs it is due not to pressure of the bone from within (for the tissues are capable of adapting themselves to the gradual change) but to impaired vitality of the sensitive tissues from the inflammation and to the constant concussion and pressure applied from without during progression. To this is to be added the paring away of the horn when applying the shoe, thereby keeping the sole at this point too thin.

Turning up of the toe.—In many cases of laminitis which have become chronic it is found that the toe of the foot turns up; that the heels are longer than natural; while the hoof near the coronary band is circled with ridges like the horn of a ram. Even in cases in which recovery has taken place, and in other diseases than laminitis, these ridges may be found in the wall of the foot. In such cases, however, the ridges are equally distant from one another all around the foot, while in turning up of the toe the ridges are wide apart at the heels and close together in front, as seen in the figure. (Plate XXXVII, fig. 4.) These ridges are produced by periods of interference with the growth of horn alternating with periods during which a normal or nearly normal growth takes place. When the toe turns up it is because the coronary band in front produces horn very slowly, while at the heels it grows much faster, causing marked deformity.

Animals so affected always place the abnormally long heel first upon the ground, not alone because the heel is too long, nor as in acute or subacute laminitis to relieve the pain, but for the reason that the toe is too short and lifted away from its natural position. To bring the toe to the ground the leg knuckles at the fetlock joint.

The pain and impairment of function in these cases always result in marked atrophy of the muscles of the forearm and shoulder, and to some extent of the pectorals, while the position of the fore legs advances the shoulder joints so far forward as to cause a sunken appearance of the breast, which the laity recognize as "chest founder."

The lesions of turning up of the toe are permanent, and are the most interesting pathologically of all the complications of laminitis.

Treatment.—The treatment of laminitis is probably more varied than of any other disease, and yet a large number of cases recover for even the poorest practitioner.

Prevention.—To guard against and prevent disease, or to render an unpreventable attack less serious than it otherwise would be, is the highest practice of the healing art. In a disease so prone to result from the simplest causes, especially when the soundest judgment may not be able to determine the extent of the disease-resisting powers of the tissues which are liable to be affected, or of what shall in every instance constitute an overexcitement, it is not strange that horse owners find themselves in trouble from untintentional transgression. If the disease were dependent upon specific causes, or if the stability of the tissues were of a fixed or more nearly determinate quality, some measures might be instituted that would prove generally preventive; but the predisposing causes are common conditions and often can not be remedied. That which is gentle work in one instance may incite disease in another. That which is feed to-day may to-morrow prove disastrous to health. Finally, necessary medical interference, no matter how judicious, may cause a more serious complaint than that which was being treated. Notwithstanding these difficulties there are some general rules to be observed that will in part serve to prevent the development of an unusual number of cases. First of all the predisposing causes must be removed when possible; when impossible, unusual care must be taken not to bring an exciting cause into operation. Under no circumstances should fat animals have hard work. If the weather is warm or the variation of temperature great, all horses should have but slow, gentle labor until they become inured to it, the tissues hardened, and their excitability reduced to a minimum. Green horses should have moderate work, particularly when taken from the farm and dirt roads to city pavements; for under these circumstances increased concussion, changed hygienic conditions, and artificial living readily become active causes of the disease. Army horses just out of winter quarters, track horses with insufficient preparation, and farmers' horses put to work in the spring are among the most susceptible classes, and must be protected by work that is easy and gradual. If long marches or drives are imperative, the incumbrances must be as light as possible and the journey interspersed with frequent rests, for this allows the laminæ to regain their impaired functional activity and to withstand much more work without danger. Furthermore, it permits early detection of an attack, and prevents working after the disease begins, which renders subsequent medication more effective by cutting the process short at the stage of congestion.

All animals when resting immediately after work should be protected from cold air or drafts. If placed in a stable that is warm and without draft, no covering is necessary; under opposite conditions blankets should be used until the excitement and exhaustion of labor have entirely passed away. It is still better that all animals coming in warm from work be "cooled out" by slow walking until the perspiration has dried and the circulation and respiration are again normal. Animals stopped on the road even for a few moments should always be protected from rapid change of temperature by appropriate clothing. If it can be avoided, horses that are working should never be driven or ridden through water. If unavoidable, they should be cooled off before passing through, and then kept moving until completely dried. The same care is to be practiced with washing the legs in cold water when just in from work, for occasionally it proves to be the cause of a most acute attack of this disease.

Unusual changes in the manner of applying the shoes should not be hastily made. If a plane shoe has been worn, high heels or toes must not be substituted at once; but the change, if necessary, should gradually be made, so that the different tissues may adapt themselves to the altered conditions. If radical changes are imperative, as is sometimes the case, the work must be so reduced in quantity and quality that it can not excite the disease.

Laminitis from the effects of purgatives can scarcely be guarded against. I can not determine from the cases in which I have seen this result that there are any conditions present that would warn us of danger. The trouble does not seem to depend upon the size of the purgative, the length of time before purgation begins, or the activity and severity with which the remedy acts. Medicines known to have unusually irritating effects on the alimentary canal should be used only when necessity demands it, and then in moderate doses.

Experience alone will determine what animals are liable to suffer from this diesease through the use of feeds. When an attack can be ascribed to any particular feed it should be withheld, unless in small quantities. Horses that have never been fed upon Indian corn should receive but a little of it at a time, mixed with bran, oats, or other feed, until it has been determined that no danger exists. Corn is less safe in warm than in cold weather, and for this reason it should always be fed with caution during spring and summer months.

When an animal is excessively lame in one foot the shoe of the opposite member should be removed, and cold water frequently applied to the well foot. At the same time, if the subject remains standing, the slings should be used. Horses should under no circumstances be overworked; to guard against this, previous work, nature of roads, state of weather, and various other influences must be carefully considered. Watering while warm is a pernicious habit, and, unless the animal is accustomed to it, is liable to result in some disorder, ofttimes in laminitis.

Curative measures.—In cases of simple congestion of the laminæ the body should be warmly clothed and warm drinks administered. The feet should be placed in a warm bath to increase the return flow of blood. In course of an hour the feet may be changed to cold water and kept there until recovery is completed. If the constitutional symptoms demand it, diuretics should be given. Half-ounce doses of saltpeter three times a day in the water answer the purpose. In cases of active congestion the warm footbaths should be omitted and cold ones used from the commencement. Subacute laminitis demands the same treatment, with laxatives if there is constipation, and the addition of low-heeled shoes. The diuretics may need to be continued for some time and their frequency increased. Regarding acute laminitis, what has been called the "American treatment" is simple and efficient. It consists solely in the administration of large doses of nitrate of potash and the continued application to the feet and ankles of cold water.

Three to four ounces of saltpeter in a pint of water, repeated every six hours, is a proper dose. The laminitis frequently subsides within a week. These large doses may be continued for a week without danger. Under no circumstances have I seen the kidneys irritated to excess or other unfavorable effects produced.

The feet should be kept in a tub of water at a temperature of 45° to 50° F., unless the animal is lying down, when swabs are to be used and wet every half hour with the cold water. The water keeps the horn soft and moist and acts directly upon the inflamed tissues by reducing the temperature. Cold maintains the vitality and disease-resisting qualities of the soft tissues, tones up the coats of the blood vessels, diminishes the supply of blood, and limits the exudation. Furthermore, it has an anesthetic effect upon the diseased tissues and relieves the pain.

Aconite may be given in conjunction with the niter when the heart is greatly excited and beats strongly. Ten-drop doses, repeated every 2 hours for 24 hours, are sufficient. The use of cathartics is dangerous, for they may excite superpurgation. Usually the niter will relieve the constipation; yet if it should prove obstinate, laxatives may be carefully given. Bleeding, both general and local, should be guarded against. The shoes must be early removed and the soles left unpared.

Paring of the soles presents two objections: First, while it may temporarily relieve the pain by relieving pressure, it favors greater exudation, which may more than counterbalance the good effects. Secondly, it makes the feet tender and subject to bruises when the animal again goes to work. The shoes should be replaced when convalescence sets in and the animal is ready to take exercise. Exercise should never be enforced until the inflammation has subsided; for although it temporarily relieves the pain and soreness it maintains the irritation, increases the exudation, and postpones recovery.

If at the end of the fifth or sixth day prominent symptoms of recovery are not apparent, apply a stiff blister of cantharides around the coronet and omit the niter for about 48 hours. When the blister is well set, the feet may again receive wet swabs. If one blister does not remove the soreness it may be repeated, or the actual cautery applied. The same treatment should be adopted where sidebones form or inflammation of the coronet bone follows. When the sole breaks through, exposing the soft tissues, the feet must be carefully shod with thin heels and thick toes if there is a tendency to walk on the heels, and the sole must be well protected with appropriate dressings and pressure over the exposed parts. When there is turning up of the toe, blistering of the coronet, *in front only*, sometimes stimulates the growth of horn, but as a rule judicious shoeing is the only treatment that will enable the animal to do light, slow work.

When suppuration of the laminæ is profuse, it is better to destroy your patient at once and relieve his suffering; but if the suppuration is limited to a small extent of tissue, especially of the sole, treatment, as in acute cases, may induce recovery and should always be tried. If from bed sores or other causes septicemia or pyemia is feared, the bisulphite of soda, in half-ounce doses, may be given in conjunction with tonics and such other treatment as is indicated in these diseases.

As to enforced recumbency I doubt the propriety of insisting on it in the majority of cases, for I think the patient usually assumes whatever position gives most comfort. No doubt recumbency diminishes the amount of blood sent to the feet, and may greatly relieve the pain, so that forcing the patient to lie down may be tried, yet should not be renewed if he thereafter persists in standing.

When the animal persistently stands, or constant lying indicates it (to prevent extensive sores), the patient should be placed in slings. When all four feet are affected it may be impossible to use slings, for the reason that the patient refuses to support any of his weight and simply hangs in them. Lastly, convalescent cases must not be returned to work too early, else permanent recovery may never be effected.

DISEASES OF THE SKIN.

By JAMES LAW, F. R. C. V. S.,

Formerly Professor of Veterinary Science, etc., Cornell University.

As we find them described in systematic works, the diseases of the skin are very numerous and complex, which may be largely accounted for by the fact that the cutaneous covering is exposed to view at all points, so that shades of difference in inflammatory and other diseased processes are easily seen and distinguished from one another. In the horse the hairy covering serves to some extent to mask the symptoms, and hence the nonprofessional man is tempted to apply the term "mange" to all alike, and it is only a step further to apply the same treatment to all these widely different disorders. Yet even in the hairy quadruped the distinction can be made in a way which can not be done in disorders of that counterpart and prolongation of the skin—the mucous membrane, which lines the air passages, the digestive organs, the urinary and generative apparatus. Diseased processes, therefore, which in these organs it might be difficult or impossible to distinguish from one another, can usually be separated and recognized when appearing in the skin.

Nor is this differentiation unimportant. The cutaneous covering presents such an extensive surface for the secretion of cuticular scales, hairs, horn, sebaceous matter, sweat, and other excretory matters, that any extensive disorder in its functions may lead to serious internal disease and death. Again, the intimate nervous sympathy of different points of the skin with particular internal organs renders certain skin disorders causative of internal disease and certain internal diseases causative of affections of the skin. The mere painting of the skin with an impermeable coating of glue is speedily fatal; a cold draft striking on the chest causes inflammation of the lungs or pleura; a skin eruption speedily follows certain disorders of the stomach, the liver, the kidneys, or even the lungs; simple burns of the skin cause inflammations of internal organs, and inflammation of such organs cause in their turn eruptions on the skin. The relations—nervous, secretory, and absorptive—between the skin and internal organs are most extensive and varied, and therefore a visible disorder in the skin may point at once and specifically to a particular fault in diet, to an injudicious use of cold water when the system is heated, to a fault in drainage, ventilation, or lighting of the stables, to indigestion, to liver disease, to urinary disorder, etc.

458

PLATE XXXVIII.

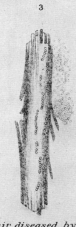

Vertical section through skin.
after Chauveau.

Hair diseased by
Trichophyton Tonsurans
after Mégnin.

E. *Epidermis* D. *Derma.* 1 *Horny layer of the epidermis.*
2. *Stratum mucosum.* 3 *Papillary layer of the derma.*
4. *Excretory duct of a sudoriparous gland.*
5. *Glomerule of a sudoriparous gland.* 6 *Hair follicle.*
7. *Sebaceous gland.* 8. *Internal sheath of the hair follicle.*
9. *Bulb of the hair.* 10. *Mass of adipose tissue.*

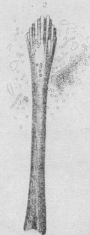

Microsporon Adouinii from
Parasitic Pityriasis in the horse
after Mégnin

Hair diseased by
Achorion Schonleini
after Mégnin.

THE SKIN AND ITS DISEASES.

STRUCTURE OF THE SKIN.

The skin consists primarily of two parts: (1) The superficial non-vascular (without blood vessels) layer, the cuticle, or epidermis; and (2) the deep vascular (with blood vessels) layer, the corium, dermis, or true skin. (See Pl. XXXVIII, fig. 1.)

The cuticle is made up of cells placed side by side and more or less modified in shape by their mutual compression and by surface evaporation and drying. The superficial stratum consists of the cells dried in the form of scales, which fall off continually and form dandruff. The deep stratum (the mucous layer) is formed of somewhat rounded cells with large central nuclei, and in colored skin containing numerous pigment granules. These cells have prolongations, or branches, by which they communicate with one another and with the superficial layer of cells in the true skin beneath. Through these prolongations they receive nutrient liquids for their growth and increase, and pass on liquids absorbed by the skin into the vessels of the true skin beneath. The living matter in the cells exercises an equally selective power on what they shall take up for their own nourishment and on what they shall admit into the circulation from without. Thus, certain agents, like iodin and belladonna, are readily admitted, whereas others, like arsenic, are excluded by the sound, unbroken epidermis. Between the deep and superficial layers of the epidermis there is a thin, translucent layer (septum lucidum) consisting of a double stratum of cells, and forming a medium of transition from the deep spheroidal to the superficial scaly cuticle.

The true skin, or dermis, has a framework of interlacing bundles of white and yellow fibers, large and coarse in the deeper layers, and fine in the superficial, where they approach the cuticle. Between the fibrous bundles are left interspaces which, like the bundles, become finer as they approach the surface, and inclose cells, vessels, nerves, glands, gland ducts, hairs, and in the deeper layers fat.

The superficial layer of the dermis is formed into a series of minute, conical elevations, or papillæ, projecting into the deep portion of the cuticle, from which they are separated by a very fine transparent membrane. This papillary layer is very richly supplied with capillary blood vessels and nerves, and is at once the seat of acute sensation and the point from which the nutrient liquid is supplied to the cells of the cuticle above. It is also at this point that the active changes of inflammation are especially concentrated; it is the immediately superposed cell layers (mucous) that become morbidly increased in the earlier stages of inflammation; it is on the surface of the papillary layer that the liquid is thrown out which raises the cuticle in the form of a blister, and it is at this point mainly that pus forms in the ordinary pustule.

The fibrous bundles of the true skin contain plain, muscular fibers, which are not controlled by the will, but contract under the influence of cold and under certain nervous influences, as in some skin diseases and in the chill of a fever, and lead to contraction, tightening, or corrugation of the skin, contributing to produce the " hidebound " of the horseman. Other minute, muscular filaments are extended from the surface of the dermis to the hair follicle on the side to which the hair is inclined, and under the same stimulating influences produce that erection of the hair which is familiarly known as " staring coat." Besides these, the horse's skin is furnished with an expansion of red, voluntary muscle, firmly attached to the fibrous bundles, and by which the animal can not only dislodge insects and other irritants, but even shake off the harness. This fleshy envelope covers the sides of the trunk and the lower portions of the neck and head, the parts unprotected by the mane and tail, and serves to throw the skin of these parts into puckers, or ridges, in certain irritating skin diseases.

The hairs are cuticular products growing from an enlarged papilla lodged in the depth of a follicle or sac, hollowed out in the skin and extending to its deepest layers. The hair follicle is lined by cells of epidermis, which at the bottom are reflected on the papilla and become the root of the hair. The hair itself is formed of the same kind of cells firmly adherent to one another by a tough, intercellular substance, and overlapping each other, like slates on a roof, in a direction toward the free end.

The sebaceous glands are branching tubes ending in follicles or sacs and opening into the hair follicles, lined by a very vascular fibrous network representing the dermis, and an internal layer of cells representing the mucous layer of the cuticle. The oily secretion gives gloss to the hair and prevents its becoming dry and brittle, and keeps the skin soft and supple, protecting it at once against undue exhalation of water and undue absorption when immersed in that medium. Besides those connected with the hair follicles there are numerous, isolated, sebaceous glands, opening directly on the surface of the skin, producing a somewhat thicker and more odorous secretion. They are found in large numbers in the folds of the skin, where chafing would be liable if the surface were dry, as on the sheath, scrotum, mammary glands, and inner side of the thigh, around the anus and vulva, in the hollow of the heel, beneath the fine horn of the frog, on the inner side of the elbow, on the lips, nostrils, and eyelids. When closed by dried secretion or otherwise these glands may become distended so as to form various-sized swellings on the skin, and when inflamed they may throw out offensive, liquid discharges, as in " grease," or produce red, tender, fungous growths (" grapes.")

The sweat glands of the horse, like those of man, are composed of simple tubes, which extend down through the cuticle and dermis in a spiral manner, and are coiled into balls in the deeper layer of the true skin. In addition to their importance in throwing offensive waste products out of the system, these glands tend to cool the skin and the entire economy of the animal through the evaporation of their watery secretion. Their activity is therefore a matter of no small moment, as besides regulating the animal heat and excreting impurities, they influence largely the internal organs through the intimate sympathy maintained between them and the skin.

Diseases of the skin may be conveniently divided, according to their most marked features, into—

(1) Those in which congestion and inflammation are the most marked features, varying according to the grade or form into (*a*) congestion with simple redness, dryness, and heat, but no eruption (erythema); (*b*) inflammation with red-pointed elevations, but no blisters (papules); (*c*) inflammation with fine, conical elevations, each surmounted by a minute blister (vesicle); (*d*) inflammation with a similar eruption but with larger blisters, like half a pea and upwards (bullæ); (*e*) inflammation with a similar eruption, but with a small sac of white, creamy pus on the summit of each elevation (pustules); (*f*) the formation of pustules implicating the superficial layer of the true skin, a small portion of which dies and is thrown off as a slough, or "core" (boils); (*g*) the formation of round, nodular, transient swellings in the true skin (tubercles); and (*h*) the excessive production of scales, or dandruff (scaly or squamous affections).

(2) Diseases in which there are only deranged sensations of itching, heat, tenderness, etc. (neurosis).

(3) Diseased growths, such as warts, callosities, horny growths, cancer, etc.

(4) Diseases from parasites, animal and vegetable.

(5) Diseases connected with a specific poison, such as horsepox, erysipelas, anthrax, farcy, or cutaneous glanders, etc.

(6) Physical injuries, like wounds, burns, scalds, etc.

CONGESTION (RED EFFLORESCENCE, OR ERYTHEMA).

This is a congested or slightly inflamed condition of the skin, unattended with any eruption. The part is slightly swollen, hot, tender, or itchy, and dry, and if the skin is white there is redness. The redness is effaced by pressure, but reappears instantly when it is removed. Except in transient cases the hairs are liable to be shed. It may be looked on as the first stage of inflammation, and therefore when it becomes aggravated it may merge in part or in whole into a papular, vesicular, or pustular eruption.

Erythema may arise from a variety of causes, and is often named in accordance with its most prominent cause. Thus the chilling, or partial freezing, of a part will give rise to a severe reaction and congestion. When snowy or icy streets have been salted this may extend to severe inflammation, with vesicles, pustules, or even sloughs of circumscribed portions of the skin of the pastern (chilblain, frostbite). Heat and burning have a similar effect, and this often comes from exposure to the direct rays of the sun. The skin that does not perspire is the most subject, and hence the white face or white limb of a horse becoming dried by the intensity of the sun's rays often suffers to the exclusion of the rest of the body (white face and foot disease). The febrile state of the general system is also a potent cause; hence the white-skinned horse is rendered the more liable if kept on a heating ration of buckwheat, or even of wheat or maize. Contact of the skin with oil of turpentine or other essential oils, with irritant liquids, vegetable or mineral, with rancid fats, with the acrid secretions of certain animals, like the irritating toad, with pus, sweat, tears, urine, or liquid feces, will produce congestion or even inflammation. Chafing is a common cause, and is especially liable to affect the fat horse between the thighs, by the side of the sheath or scrotum, on the inner side of the elbow, or where the harness chafes on the poll, shoulder, back, breastbone, and under the tail. The accumulation of sweat and dust between the folds of the skin and on the surface of the harness, and the specially acrid character of the sweat in certain horses, contribute to chafing or " intertrigo." The heels often become congested owing to the irritation caused by the short, bristly hairs in clipped heels. Again, congestion may occur from friction by halter, harness, or other foreign body under the pastern, or inside the thigh or arm, or by reason of blows from another foot (cutting, interfering, overreach). Finally, erythema is especially liable to occur in spring, when the coat is being shed, and the hair follicles and general surface are exposed and irritable in connection with the dropping of the hairs.

If due only to a local irritant, congestion will usually disappear when the cause has been removed, but when the feeding or system is at fault these conditions must be first corrected. While the coat is being shed the susceptibility will continue, and the aim should be to prevent the disease from developing and advancing so as to weaken the skin, render the susceptibility permanent, and lay the foundation of persistent or frequently recurring skin disease. Therefore at such times the diet should be nonstimulating, any excess of grain, and above all of buckwheat, Indian corn, or wheat, being avoided. A large grain ration should not be given at once on return from hard work, when the general system and stomach are unable to cope with it; the animal should not be given more than a swallow or two of cold water when perspiring and fatigued, nor should he be allowed a full supply of water just after his grain ration; he should not be over-heated or exhausted by work, nor should dried sweat and dust be allowed to accumulate on the skin or on the harness pressing on it. The exposure of the affected heels to damp, mud, and snow, and, above all, to melting snow, should be guarded against; light, smooth, well-fitting harness must be obtained, and where the saddle or collar irritates an incision should be made in them above and below the part that chafes, and, the padding between having been removed, the lining should be beaten so as to make a hollow. A zinc shield in the upper angle of the collar will often prevent chafing in front of the withers.

Treatment.—Wash the chafed skin and apply salt water (one-half ounce to the quart), extract of witch-hazel, a weak solution of oak bark, or camphorated spirit. If the surface is raw use bland powders, such as oxid of zinc, lycopodium, starch, or smear the surface with vaseline, or with 1 ounce of vaseline intimately mixed with one-half dram each of opium and sugar of lead. In cases of chafing rest must be strictly enjoined. If there is constitutional disorder or acrid sweat, 1 ounce cream of tartar or a teaspoonful of bicarbonate of soda may be given twice daily.

CONGESTION, WITH SMALL PIMPLES, OR PAPULES.

In this affection there is the general blush, heat, etc., of erythema, together with a crop of elevations from the size of a poppy seed to a coffee bean, visible when the hair is reversed or to be felt with the finger where the hair is scanty. In white skins they vary from the palest to the darkest red. All do not retain the papular type, but some go on to form blisters (eczema, bullæ) or pustules, or dry up into scales, or break out into open sores, or extend into larger swellings (tubercles). The majority, however, remaining as pimples, characterize the disease. When very itchy the rubbing breaks them open, and the resulting sores and scales hide the true nature of the eruption.

The general and local causes may be the same as for erythema, and in the same subject one portion of the skin may have simple congestion and another adjacent papules. As the inflammatory action is more pronounced, so the irritation and itching are usually greater, the animal rubbing and biting himself severely. This itching is espe-cially severe in the forms which attack the roots of the mane and tail, and there the disease is often so persistent and troublesome that the horse is rendered virtually useless.

The bites of insects often produce a papular eruption, but in many such cases the swelling extends wider into a buttonlike elevation, one-half to an inch in diameter. The same remarks apply to the effects of the poison ivy and poison sumac.

Treatment.—In papular eruption first remove the cause, then apply the same general remedies as for simple congestion. In the more inveterate cases use a lotion of one-half ounce sulphid of potassium in 2 quarts of water, to which a little Castile soap has been added, or use a wash with one-half ounce oil of tar, 2 ounces Castile soap, and 20 ounces water.

INFLAMMATION WITH BLISTERS, OR ECZEMA.

In this the skin is congested, thickened, warm (white skins are reddened), and shows a thick crop of little blisters formed by effusions of a straw-colored fluid between the true skin and the cuticle. The blisters may be of any size from a millet seed to a pea, and often crack open and allow the escape of the fluid, which concretes as a slightly yellowish scab or crust around the roots of the hairs. This exudation and the incrustation are especially common where the hairs are long, thick, and numerous, as in the region of the pastern of heavy draft horses. The term eczema is now applied very generally to eruptions of all kinds that depend on internal disorders or constitutional conditions and that tend to recurrences and inveteracy. Eczema may appear on any part of the body, but in horses it is especially common on the heels and the lower parts of the limbs, and less frequently on the neck, shoulder, and abdomen. The limbs appear to be especially liable because of their dependent position, all blood having to return from them against the action of gravity and congestions and swellings being common, because of the abundance of blood vessels in this part of the skin and because of the frequent contact with the irritant dung and urine and their ammoniacal emanations. The legs further suffer from contact with wet and mud when at work, from snow and ice, from drafts of cold air on the wet limbs, from washing with caustic soaps, or from the relaxing effects of a too deep and abundant litter. Among other causes may be named indigestion and the presence of irritant matters in the blood and sweat, the result of patent medicated feeds and condition powders (aromatics, stimulants), green food, new hay, new oats, buckwheat, wheat, maize, diseased potatoes, smut, or ergot in grains, decomposing green feed, brewers' grains, or kitchen garbage. The excitement in the skin, caused by shedding the coat, lack of grooming, hot weather, hot, boiled, or steamed feed conduces to the eruption. Lastly, any sudden change of feed may induce it.

The blisters may in part go on to suppuration so that vesicles and pustules often appear on the same patch, and, when raw from rubbing, the true nature of the eruption may be completely masked. In well-fed horses, kept in close stables with little work, eczema of the limbs may last for months and years. It is a very troublesome affection in draft stallions.

Treatment.—This disease is so often the result of indigestion that a laxative of 1 pound Glauber's salt in 3 or 4 quarts water or 1½ pints olive oil is often demanded to clear away irritants from the alimentary canal. Following this, in recent and acute cases, give 2 drams of acetate or bicarbonate of potash twice a day in the drinking water. If the bowels still become costive, give daily 1 ounce sulphate of soda and 20 grains of powdered nux vomica. In debilitated horses combine the nux vomica with one-half ounce powdered gentian root. As a wash for the skin use 1 dram bicarbonate of soda and 1 dram carbolic acid in a quart of water, after having cleansed the surface with tepid water. Employ the same precautions as regards feeding, stabling, and care of harness as in simple congestion of the skin.

In the more inveterate forms of eczema more active treatment is required. Soak the scabs in fresh sweet oil, and in a few hours remove these with tepid water and Castile soap; then apply an ointment of sulphur or iodid of sulphur day by day. If this seems to be losing its effect after a week, change for mercurial ointment or a solution of sulphid of potassium, or of hyposulphite of soda, 3 drams to the quart of water. In these cases the animal may take a course of sulphur (1 ounce daily), bisulphite of soda (one-half ounce daily), or of arsenic (5 grains daily) mixed with 1 dram bicarbonate of soda.

INFLAMMATION WITH PUSTULES.

In this affection the individual elevations on the inflamed skin show in the center a small sac of white, creamy pus, in place of the clear liquid of a blister. They vary in size from a millet seed to a hazelnut. The pustules of glanders (farcy buds) are to be distinguished by the watery contents and the cordlike swelling, extending from the pustules along the line of the veins, and those of boils by the inflammation and sloughing out of a core of the true skin. The hair on the pustule stands erect, and is often shed with the scab which results. When itching is severe the parts become excoriated by rubbing, and, as in the other forms of skin disease, the character of the eruption may become indistinct. Old horses suffer mainly at the root of the mane and tail and about the heels, and suckling foals around the mouth, on the face, inside the thighs, and under the tail.

Pustules, like eczema, are especially liable to result from unwholesome feed and indigestion, from a sudden change of feed—above all, from dry to green. In foals it may result from overheating of the mare and allowing the first milk after she returns, or by milk rendered unwholesome by faulty feeding of the dam. If a foal is brought up by hand the souring and other decompositions in the milk derange the digestion and cause such eruption. Vetches and other plants affected with honeydew and buckwheat have been the cause of these eruptions on white portions of the skin. Disorders of the kidneys or liver are common causes of this affection.

Treatment.—Apply soothing ointments, such as benzoinated oxid of zinc, or vaseline with 1 dram oxid of zinc in each ounce. Or a wash of 1 dram sugar of lead or 2 drams hyposulphite of soda in a quart of water may be freely applied. If the skin is already abraded and scabby, smear thickly with vaseline for some hours, then wash with soapsuds and apply the above dressings. When the excoriations are indolent they may be painted with a solution of lunar caustic 2 grains to 1 ounce of distilled water. Internally counteract costiveness and remove intestinal irritants by the same means as in eczema, and follow this with one-half ounce doses daily of hyposulphite of soda, and one-half ounce doses of gentian. Inveterate cases may often be benefited by a course of sulphur, bisulphite of soda, or arsenic. In all, the greatest care must be taken with regard to feed, feeding, watering, cleanliness, and work. In wet and cold seasons predisposed animals should, so far as possible, be protected from wet, mud, snow, and melted snow—above all, from that which has been melted by salt.

BOILS, OR FURUNCLES.

These may appear on any part of the skin, but are especially common on the lower parts of the limbs, and on the shoulders and back where the skin is irritated by accumulated secretion and chafing with the harness. In other cases the cause is constitutional, or attended with unwholesome diet and overwork with loss of general health and condition. They also follow on weakening diseases, notably strangles, in which irritants are retained in the system from overproduction of poisons and effete matter during fever, and imperfect elimination. There is also the presence of a pyogenic bacterium, by which the disease may be maintained and propagated.

While boils are pus producing, they differ from simple pustule in affecting the deepest layers of the true skin, and even the superficial layers of the connective tissues beneath, and in the death and sloughing out of the central part of the inflamed mass (core). The depth of the hard, indurated, painful swelling, and the formation of this central mass or core, which is bathed in pus and slowly separated from surrounding parts, serve to distinguish the boil alike from the pustule, from the farcy bud, and from a superficial abscess.

Treatment.—To treat very painful boils a free incision with a lancet in two directions, followed by a dressing with one-half an ounce carbolic acid in a pint of water, bound on with cotton wool or lint, may cut them short. The more common course is to apply a warm poultice of linseed meal or wheat bran, and renew daily until the center of the boil softens, when it should be lanced and the core pressed out.

If the boil is smeared with a blistering ointment of Spanish flies and a poultice put over it, the formation of matter and separation of the core is often hastened. A mixture of sugar and soap laid on the boil is equally good. Cleanliness of the skin and the avoidance of all causes of irritation are important items, and a teaspoonful of bicarbonate of soda once or twice a day will sometimes assist in warding off a new crop.

NETTLERASH (SURFEIT, OR URTICARIA).

This is an eruption in the form of cutaneous nodules, in size from a hazelnut to a hickory nut, transient, with little disposition to the formation of either blister or pustule, and usually connected with shedding of the coat, sudden changes of weather, and unwholesomeness or sudden change in the feed. It is most frequent in the spring and in young and vigorous animals (good feeders). The swelling embraces the entire thickness of the skin and terminates by an abrupt margin in place of shading off into surrounding parts. When the individual swellings run together there are formed extensive patches of thickened integument. These may appear on any part of the body, and may be general; the eyelids may be closed, the lips rendered immovable, or the nostrils so thickened that breathing becomes difficult and snuffling. It may be attended with constipation or diarrhea or by colicky pains. The eruption is sudden, the whole skin being sometimes covered in a few hours, and it may disappear with equal rapidity or persist for six or eight days.

Treatment.—This consists in clearing out the bowels by 5 drams Barbados aloes, or 1 pound Glauber's salt, and follow the operation of these by daily doses of one-half ounce powdered gentian and 1 ounce Glauber's salt. A weak solution of alum may be applied to the swellings.

PITYRIASIS, OR SCALY SKIN DISEASE.

This affection is characterized by an excessive production and detachment of dry scales from the surface of the skin (dandruff). It is usually dependent on some fault in digestion and an imperfect secretion from the sebaceous glands and is most common in old horses with spare habit of body. Williams attributes it to feed rich in saccharine matter (carrots, turnips) and to the excretion of oxalic acid by the skin. He has found it in horses irregularly worked and well fed and advises the administration of pitch for a length of time and the avoidance of saccharine feed. Otherwise the horse may take a laxative followed by dram doses of carbonate of potash, and the affected parts may be bathed with soft, tepid water and smeared with an ointment made with vaseline and sulphur. In obstinate cases sulphur may be given daily in the feed.

PRURITUS, OR NERVOUS IRRITATION OF THE SKIN.

This is seen in horses fed to excess on grain and hay, kept in close stables, and worked irregularly. Though most common in summer, it is often severe in hot, close stables in winter. Pimples, vesicles, and abrasions may result, but as the itching is quite as severe on other parts of the skin, these may be the result of scratching merely. It is especially common and inveterate about the roots of the mane and tail.

Treatment consists in a purgative (Glauber's salt, 1 pound), restricted, laxative diet, and a wash of water slightly soured with oil of vitriol and rendered sweet by carbolic acid. If obstinate, give daily 1 ounce of sulphur and 20 grains nux vomica. If the acid lotion fails, 2 drams carbonate of potash and 2 grains of cyanid of potassium in a quart of water will sometimes benefit. If from pinworms in the rectum, the itching of the tail may be remedied by an occasional injection of a quart of water in which chips of quassia wood have been steeped for 12 hours.

HERPES.

This name has been applied to a disease in which there is an eruption of minute vesicles in circular groups or clusters, with little tendency to burst, but rather to dry up into fine scabs. If the vesicles break, they exude a slight, gummy discharge which concretes into a small, hard scab. It is apparently noncontagious and not appreciably connected with any disorder of internal organs. It sometimes accompanies or follows specific fevers, and is, on the whole, most frequent at the seasons of changing the coat—spring and autumn. It is seen on the lips and pastern, but may appear on any part of the body. The duration of the eruption is two weeks or even more, the tendency being to spontaneous recovery. The affected part is very irritable, causing a sensitiveness and a disposition to rub out of proportion to the extent of the eruption.

Treatment.—It may be treated by oxid of zinc ointment, and to relieve the irritation a solution of opium or belladonna in water, or of sugar of lead or oil of peppermint. A course of bitters (one-half an ounce of Peruvian bark daily for a week) may be serviceable in bracing the system and producing an indisposition to the eruption.

BLEEDING SKIN ERUPTIONS, OR DERMATORRHAGIA PARASITICA.

In China, Hungary, Spain, and other countries, horses frequently suffer from the presence of a threadworm (*Setaria hæmorrhagica* (Railliet) = *Filaria multipapillosa* Condamine and Drouilly) in the subcutaneous, intermuscular, and interfascicular connective tissues, causing effusions of blood under the scurf skin and incrustations of dried blood on the surface. The eruptions, which appear mainly on the sides of the trunk, but may cover any part of the body, are rounded elevations about the size of a small pea, or larger, containing blood which bursts through the scurf skin and dries like a reddish scab around the erect, rigid hairs. These swellings appear in groups, which remain out for several days, gradually diminishing in size; new groups appear after an interval of three or four weeks, the manifestation being confined to three or four months of spring and disappearing in winter. A horse will suffer for several years in succession and then permanently recover, although fatal cases sometimes occur. It is reported that when cases of the disease are imported into France the disease appears in attenuated form the second year and then disappears without treatment. To find the worm the hair is shaved from the part where the elevations are felt, and as soon as a bleeding point is shown the superficial layer is laid open with the knife, when the parasite will be seen drawing itself back into the parts beneath. The worm is about 1 inch to almost 3 inches long and like a stout thread, thicker toward the head than toward the tail, and with numerous little papilliform elevations around the head. The adult female worm produces numerous eggs which contain embryos when deposited. Apparently the eggs hatch in the blood. In all probability the worm has an intermediate host, perhaps an insect, which transmits it from one horse to another.

Treatment is not satisfactory, but the affected surface should be kept clean by sponging, and the pressure of harness on any affected part must be avoided. The part may be frequently washed with a strong solution of potassium sulphid. Rest may be essential to recovery.

SUMMER SORES.

The summer sores of horses (dermatitis granulosa, boils) have been traced to the presence in the skin of a roundworm 3 millimeters in length and very slender. These worms were long known as *Filaria irritans*, but have been found to be the larvæ of the stomach worms, *Habronema* spp., of the horse. The sores may be as small as a millet seed, but more frequently the size of a pea, and may become an inch in diameter. They may appear on any point, but are especially obnoxious where the harness presses, or on the lower parts of the limbs. They cause intense and insupportable itching, and the victim rubs and bites the part until extensive raw surfaces are produced. Aside from the effects of such friction, the sore is covered by a brownish-red, soft, pulpy material with cracks or furrows filled with serous pus. In the midst of the softened mass are small, firm, rounded granulations, fibrinous, and even caseated, and when the soft, pultaceous material has been scraped off, the surface bears a resemblance to the fine, yellow points of miliary tuberculosis in the lung. The worm or its débris is found in the center of such masses. These sores are very obstinate, resisting treatment for months in summer, and even after apparent recovery during the cold season they may appear anew the following summer. In bad cases the rubbing and biting may cause exposure of synovial sacs and tendons, and cause irremediable injury. Even in winter, however, when the diseased process seems arrested, there remain the hard, firm, resistant patches of the skin with points in which the diseased product has become softened like cheese.

The apparent subsidence of the disease in winter is attributed to the coldness and comparative bloodlessness of the skin, whereas in summer, with high temperature, active circulation, and rapid cell growth, inflammation is increased, itching follows, and from the animal rubbing the part the irritation is persistently increased. The hotter the climate the more troublesome the disease.[1]

Treatment consists, first, in placing the animal in a cool place and showering the surface with cold water. The parasite may be destroyed by rubbing the surface of the wound with iodoform and covering it with a layer of collodion, and repeating the applications every 24 hours for 15 days, or until the sores heal up. Ether or chloroform, poured on cotton wool and applied to the sore for two minutes before painting it with collodion, may be used in place of iodoform.[2]

CRACKED HEELS (SCRATCHES, OR CHAPS ON KNEE AND HOCK).

This usually sets in with swelling, heat, and tenderness of the hollow of the heel, with erections of the hairs and redness (in white

[1] Descazeaux and others have shown that the worms found in these summer sores are larval forms of the stomach worms of the horse, especially *Habronema megastoma* and *H. muscæ*. Ransom and others have shown that the larvæ of these worms develop in the common house fly and other flies, the fly becoming infested as a maggot in horse manure. *H. microstoma*, however, usually develops in stable flies and rarely in house flies. Infestation with the adult worms in the stomach of the horse (Pl. V, fig. 4) may take place through the ingestion of such infested flies, or by the escape of larvæ from the proboscis of the fly as it feeds on the moist lips of the horse. In view of this it may be surmised that summer sores may arise as the result of flies so infested feeding on the moisture on the skin of the horse, and this theory has the support of some experimental and clinical evidence.

Preventive measures consist in the removal of the adult worms from the stomach of the horse by the use of anthelmintics, the destruction of the embryos in the manure, fly-control measures, and the use of clean bedding. The protection of all wounds and skin abrasions from flies by means of bandages, fly repellents, etc., is also of importance in regions where summer sores occur. Such anthelmintics as carbon bisulphid and carbon tetrachlorid will probably kill the stomach worms of horses whenever the worms are exposed to the action of the drugs, but the worms which are embedded in the mucosa or in nodules are probably not accessible to any drugs used at present.—M. C. HALL.

[2] Descazeaux recommends the application and injection of 2 to 3 per cent trypan blue, though he states that the only truly efficacious treatment is the early and complete ablation of the invaded tissue.—M. C. HALL.

skins), with stiffness and lameness, which may be extreme in irritable horses. Soon slight cracks appear transversely, and may gain in depth and width, and may even suppurate. More frequently they become covered at the edges or throughout by firm incrustations resulting from the drying of the liquids thrown out, and the skin becomes increasingly thick and rigid. A similar condition occurs behind the knee and in front of the hock (malanders and salanders), and may extend from these points to the hoof, virtually incasing that side of the limb in a permanent incrusting sheath.

Causes.—Besides a heavy lymphatic constitution, which predisposes to this affection, the causes are overfeeding on grain, unwholesome fodder, close, hot, dirty stables, constant contact with dung and urine and their emanations, working in deep, irritant mud; above all, in limestone districts, irritation by dry limestones or sandy dust in dry weather on dirt roads; also cold drafts, snow, and freezing mud, washing the legs with caustic soap, wrapping the wet legs in thick woolen bandages which soak the skin and render it sensitive when exposed next day, clipping the heels, weak heart and circulation, natural or supervening on overwork, imperfect nourishment, impure air, lack of sunshine, chronic exhausting, or debilitating diseases, or functional or structural diseases of the heart, liver, or kidneys. These last induce dropsical swelling of the limbs (stocking), weaken the parts, and induce cracking. Finally the cicatrix of a preexisting crack, weak, rigid, and unyielding, is liable to reopen under any severe exertion; hence rapid paces and heavy draft are active causes.

Treatment.—In treatment the first step is to ascertain and remove the cause whenever possible. If there is much local heat and inflammation, a laxative (5 drams aloes or 1 pound Glauber's salt) may be given, and for the pampered animal the grair should be reduced or replaced altogether by bran mashes, flaxseed, and other laxative, non-stimulating feed. In the debilitated, on the other hand, nutritious food and bitter tonics may be given, and even a course of arsenic (5 grains arsenic with 1 dram bicarbonate of soda daily). When the legs swell, exercise on dry roads, hand rubbing, and evenly applied bandages are good, and mild astringents, like extract of witch-hazel, may be applied and the part subsequently rubbed dry and bandaged. If there is much heat but unbroken skin, a lotion of 2 drams sugar of lead to 1 quart of water may be applied on a thin bandage, covered in cold weather with a dry one. The same may be used after the cracks appear, or a solution of sulphurous acid 1 part, glycerin 1 part, and water 1 part, applied on cotton and well covered by a bandage. In case these should prove unsuitable to the particular case, the part may be smeared with vaseline 1 ounce, sugar of lead 1 dram, and carbolic acid 10 drops.

INFLAMMATION OF THE HEELS WITH SEBACEOUS SECRETION (GREASE, OR CANKER).

This is a specific affection of the heels of horses usually associated with the growth of a parasitic fungus, an offensive discharge from the numerous sebaceous glands, and, in bad cases, the formation of red, raw excrescences (grapes) from the surface. It is to be distinguished (1) from simple inflammation in which the special fetid discharge and the tendency to the formation of " grapes " are absent; (2) from horsepox, in which the abundant exudate forms a firm, yellow incrustation around the roots of the hair, and is embedded at intervals in the pits formed by the individual pocks, and in which there is no vascular excrescence; (3) from foot scabies (mange), in which the presence of an acarus is distinctive; (4) from lymphangitis, in which the swelling appears suddenly, extending around the entire limb as high as the hock, and on the inner side of the thigh along the line of the vein to the groin, and in which there is active fever, and (5) from erysipelas, in which there is active fever (wanting in grease), the implication of the deeper layers of the skin and of the parts beneath giving a boggy feeling to the parts, the absence of the fetid, greasy discharge, and finally a tendency to form pus loosely in the tissues without any limiting membrane, as in abscess. Another distinctive feature of grease is its tendency to implicate the skin which secretes the bulbs or heels of the horny frog and in the cleft of the frog, constituting the disease known as canker.

Causes.—The predisposing causes of grease are essentially the same as those of simple inflammation of the heel, so that the reader may consult the preceding section. Though a specific fungus and bacteria of different kinds are present, they tend mainly to aggravation of the disease, and are not proved to be essential factors in causation.

Symptoms.—The symptoms vary according to whether the disease comes on suddenly or more tardily. In the first case there is a sudden swelling of the skin in the heel, with heat, tenderness, itching, and stiffness, which is lessened during exercise. In the slower forms there is seen only a slight swelling after rest, and with little heat or inflammation for a week or more. Even at this early stage, a slight, serous oozing may be detected. As the swelling increases, extending up toward the hock or knees, the hairs stand erect, and are bedewed by moisture no longer clear and odorless, but grayish, milky, and fetid. The fetor of the discharge draws attention to the part whenever one enters the stable, and the swollen pastern and wet, matted hairs on the heel draw attention to the seat of the malady. If actively treated, the disease may not advance further, but if neglected the tense, tender skin cracks open, leaving open sores from which vascular bleeding growths grow up, constituting the " grapes." The hair is shed, and the heel may appear but as one mass of rounded, red, angry excrescences which bleed on handling and are covered with the now repulsively fetid, decomposing discharge. During this time there is little or no fever, the animal feeds well, and but for its local trouble it might continue at work. When the malady extends to the frog, there is a fetid discharge from its cleft or from the depressions at its sides, and this gradually extends to its whole surface and upon the adjacent parts of the sole. The horn meanwhile becomes soft, whitish, and fleshy in aspect, its constituent tubes being greatly enlarged and losing their natural cohesion; it grows rapidly above the level of the surrounding horn, and when pared is found to be penetrated to an unusual depth by the secreting papillæ, and that at intervals these have bulged out into a vascular fungous mass comparable to the " grapes."

Treatment.—In treatment hygienic measures occupy a front rank, but are in themselves insufficient to establish a cure. All local and general conditions which favor the production and persistence of the disease must be guarded against. Above all, cleanliness and purity of the stable and air must be obtained; also nourishing diet, regular exercise, and the avoidance of local irritants—septic, muddy, chilling, etc. At the outset benzoated oxid of zinc ointment may be used with advantage. A still better dressing is made with 1 ounce vaseline, 2 drams oxid of zinc, and 20 drops iodized phenol. If the surface is much swollen and tender, a flaxseed poultice may be applied, over the surface of which has been poured some of the following lotion: Sugar of lead, one-half ounce; carbolic acid, 1 dram; water, 1 quart. All the astringents of the pharmacopœia have been employed with more or less advantage, and some particular one seems to suit particular cases or patients. To destroy the grapes, they may be rubbed daily with strong caustics (copperas, bluestone, lunar caustic), or each may be tied round its neck with a stout, waxed thread, or, finally and more speedily, they may be cut off by a blacksmith's shovel heated to redness and applied with its sharp edge toward the neck of the excrescence, over a cold shovel held between it and the skin to protect the skin from the heat. The cold shovel must be kept cool by frequent dipping in water. After the removal of the grapes the astringent dressing must be persistently applied to the surface. When the frog is affected, it must be pared to the quick and dressed with dry caustic powders (quicklime, copperas, bluestone) or carbolic acid and subjected to pressure, the dressing being renewed every day at least.

ERYSIPELAS.

This is a specific contagious disease, characterized by spreading, dropsical inflammation of the skin and subcutaneous tissues, attended with general fever. It differs from most specific diseases in the absence of a definite period of incubation, a regular course and duration, and a conferring of immunity on the subject after recovery. On the contrary, one attack of erysipelas predisposes to another, partly, doubtless, by the loss of tone and vitality in the affected tissues, but also, perhaps, because of the survival of the infecting germ.

Cause.—It is no longer to be doubted that the microbes found in the inflammatory product are the true cause of erysipelas, as by their means the disease can be successfully transferred from man to animals and from one animal to another. This transition may be direct or through the medium of infected buildings or other articles. Yet from the varying severity of erysipelas in different outbreaks and localities it has been surmised that various different microbes are operative in this disease, and a perfect knowledge of them might perhaps enable us to divide erysipelas into two or more distinct affections. At present we must recognize it as a specific inflammation due to a bacterial poison and closely allied to septicemia. Erysipelas was formerly known as surgical when it spread from a wound (through which the germ had gained access) and medical, or idiopathic, when it started independently of any recognizable lesion. Depending as it does, however, upon a germ distinct from the body, the disease must be looked upon as such, no matter by what channel the germ found an entrance. Erysipelas which follows a wound is usually much more violent than the other form, the difference being doubtless partly due to the lowered vitality of the wounded tissues and to the oxidation and septic changes which are invited on the raw, exposed surface. As apparently idiopathic cases may be due to infection through bites of insects, the small amount of poison inserted may serve to moderate the violence.

This affection may attack a wound on any part of the horse's body, while, apart from wounds, it is most frequent about the head and the hind limbs. It is to be distinguished from ordinary inflammations by its gradual extension from the point first attacked, by the abundant liquid exudation into the affected part, by the tension of the skin over the affected part, by its soft, boggy feeling, allowing it to be deeply indented by the finger, by the abrupt line of limitation between the diseased and the healthy skin, the former descending suddenly to the healthy level instead of shading off slowly toward it, by the tendency of the inflammation to extend deeply into the subjacent tissues and into the muscles and other structures, by the great tendency to death and sloughing of portions of skin and of the structures beneath, by the formation of pus at various different points throughout the diseased parts without any surrounding sac to protect the surrounding structures from its destructive action, and without the usual disposition of pus to advance harmlessly toward the surface and escape; and, finally, by a low, prostrating type of fever, with elevated temperature of the body, coated tongue, excited breathing, and loss of appetite. The pus when escaping through a lancet wound is grayish, brownish, or reddish, with a heavy or fetid odor, and intermixed with shreds of broken-down tissues. The most destructive form, however, is that in which pus is deficient and gangrene and sloughing more speedy and extensive.

Treatment resolves itself mainly into the elimination from the system of the poisonous products of the bacteria by laxatives and diuretics, the sustaining of the failing vitality by tonics and stimulants, above all those of the nature of antiferments, and the local application of astringent and antiseptic agents. Internal treatment may consist in 4 drams tincture of muriate of iron and one-half dram muriate of ammonia or chlorate of potash, given in a pint of water every two hours. Locally a strong solution of iron, alum, or of sulphate of iron and laudanum may be used; or the affected part may be painted with tincture of muriate of iron or with iodized phenol. In mild cases a lotion of 4 drams sugar of lead and 2 ounces laudanum in a quart of water may be applied. It is desirable to avoid the formation of wounds and the consequent septic action, yet when pus has formed and is felt by fluctuation under the finger to be approaching the surface it should be freely opened with a clean, sharp lancet, and the wound thereafter disinfected daily with carbolic acid 1 part to water 10 parts, with a saturated solution of hyposulphite of soda, or with powders of iodoform or salol.

HORSEPOX, ANTHRAX, AND CUTANEOUS GLANDERS (FARCY).

These subjects are discussed under the head of contagious diseases.

CALLOSITIES.

These are simple thickening and induration of the cuticle by reason of continued pressure, notably in lying down on a hard surface. Being devoid of hair, they cause blemishes; hence, smooth floors and good bedding should be provided as preventives.

HORNY SLOUGHS (SITFASTS), OR SLOUGHING CALLOSITIES.

These are circumscribed sloughs of limited portions of the skin, the result of pressure by badly fitting harness or by irritating masses of dirt, sweat, and hairs under the harness. They are most common under the saddle, but may be found under collar or breeching as well.

The sitfast is a piece of dead tissue which would be thrown off but that it has formed firm connections with the fibrous skin beneath, or even deeper with the fibrous layers (fascia) of the muscles, or with the bones, and is thus bound in its place as a persistent source of irritation. The hornlike slough may thus involve the superficial part of the skin only, or the whole thickness of the skin, and even of some of the structures beneath. The first object is to remove the dead irritant by dissecting it off with a sharp knife, after which the sore may be treated with simple wet cloths or a weak carbolic-acid lotion, like a common wound. If the outline of the dead mass is too indefinite, a linseed-meal poultice will make its outline more evident to the operator. If the fascia or bone has become gangrenous, the dead portion must be removed with the hornlike skin. During and after treatment the horse must be kept at rest or the harness must be so adjusted that no pressure can come near the affected parts. (See also page 496.)

WARTS.

These are essentially a morbid overgrowth of the superficial papillary layer of the skin and of the investing cuticular layer. They are mostly seen in young horses, about the lips, eyelids, cheeks, ears, beneath the belly, and on the sheath, but may develop anywhere. The smaller ones may be clipped off with scissors and the raw surface cauterized with bluestone. The larger may be sliced off with a sharp knife, or if with a narrow neck they may be twisted off and then cauterized. If very vascular they may be strangled by a wax thread or cord tied around their necks, at least three turns being made around and the ends being fixed by passing them beneath the last preceding turn of the cord, so that they can be tightened day by day as they slacken by shrinkage of the tissues. If the neck is too broad it may be transfixed several times with a double-threaded needle and then be tied in sections. Very broad warts that can not be treated in this way may be burned down with a soldering bolt at a red heat to beneath the surface of the skin, and any subsequent tendency to overgrowth kept down by bluestone.

BLACK PIGMENT TUMORS, OR MELANOSIS.

These are common in gray and in white horses on the naturally black parts of the skin at the roots of the tail, around the anus, vulva, udder, sheath, eyelids, and lips. They are readily recognized by their inky-black color, which extends throughout the whole mass. They may appear as simple, pealike masses, or as multiple tumors aggregating many pounds, especially around the tail. In the horse these are usually simple tumors, and may be removed with the knife. In exceptional cases they prove cancerous, as they usually are in man.

EPITHELIAL CANCER, OR EPITHELIOMA.

This sometimes occurs on the lips at the angle of the mouth and elsewhere in the horse. It begins as a small, wartlike tumor, which grows slowly at first, but finally bursts open, ulcerates, and extends laterally and deeply in the skin and other tissues, destroying them as it advances (rodent ulcer). It is made up of a fibrous framework and numerous round, ovoid, or cylindrical cavities, lined with masses of epithelial cells, which may be squeezed out as a fetid, caseous material. Early and thorough removal with the knife is the most successful treatment.

VEGETABLE PARASITES OF THE SKIN.

(Pl. XXXVIII, figs. 2, 3, 4.)

PARASITE: *Trichophyton tonsurans.* MALADY: *Tinea tonsurans, or circinate ringworm.*—This is especially common in young horses coming into training and work, in low-conditioned colts in winter and spring after confinement indoors, during molting, in lymphatic rather than nervous subjects, and at the same time in several animals that have herded together. The disease is common to man, and among the domestic animals to horse, ox, goat, dog, cat, and in rare instances to sheep and swine. Hence it is common to find animals of different species and their attendants suffering at once, the diseases having been propagated from one to the other.

Symptoms.—In the horse the symptoms are the formation of a circular, scurfy patch where the fungus has established itself, the hairs of the affected spot being erect, bristly, twisted, broken, or split up and dropping off. Later the spot first affected has become entirely bald, and a circular row of hairs around this are erect, bristly, broken, and split. These in turn are shed and a new row outside passes through the same process, so that the extension is made in more or less circular outline. The central bald spot, covered with a grayish scurf and surrounded by a circle of broken and split hairs, is characteristic. If the scurf and diseased hairs are treated with caustic-potash solution and put under the microscope, the natural cells of the cuticle and hair will be seen to have become transparent, while the groups of spherical cells and branching filaments of the fungus stand out prominently in the substance of both, dark and unchanged. The eruption usually appears on the back, loins, croup, chest, and head. It tends to spontaneous recovery in a month or two, leaving for a time a dappled coat from the spots of short, light-colored hair of the new growth.

The most effective way of reaching the parasite in the hair follicles is to extract the hairs individually, but in the horse the mere shaving of the affected part is usually enough. It may then be painted with tincture of iodin twice a day for two weeks. Germs about the stable may be covered up or destroyed by a whitewash of freshly burned quicklime, the harness, brushes, etc., may be washed with caustic soda, and then smeared with a solution of corrosive sublimate one-half dram and water 1 pint. The clothing may be boiled and dried.

PARASITE: *Achorion schönleini.* MALADY: *Favus, or honeycomb ringworm.*—Mégnin and Goyau, who describe this in the horse, say that it loses its characteristic honeycomb or cup-shaped appearance, and forms only a series of closely aggregated, dry, yellowish crusts the size of hemp seed on the trunk, shoulders, flanks, or thighs. They are accompanied by severe itching, especially at night. The cryptogam, formed of spherical cells with a few filaments only, grows in the hair follicles and on the cuticle, and thus a crust often forms around the root of a hair. Like the other cryptogams, their color, as seen under the microscope, is unaffected by acetic acid, alcohol, ether, or oil of turpentine, while the cells are turned bluish by iodin. For treatment, remove the hair and apply tincture of iodin or corrosive sublimate lotion, as advised under the last paragraph.

PARASITE: *Microsporon furfur.* MALADY: *Parasitic pityriasis.*— This attacks the horse's head where the harness presses, and leads to dropping of the hair, leaving bald patches covered with a branlike scurf, without any eruption, heat, tenderness, swelling, or rigidity of the skin. A lotion of carbolic acid 1 dram and water $2\frac{1}{2}$ ounces is usually applied to effect a cure.

ANIMAL PARASITES OF THE SKIN.[1]

ACARIASIS, OR MANGE.

This affection is due to the irritation of the skin caused by the presence of nearly microscopic acari, or mites. The disease varies, however, according to the species of mite which infests the skin, so that we must treat of several different kinds of mange.

PARASITE: *Sarcoptes scabiei equi.* MALADY: *Sarcoptic acariasis.*— This is the special *Sarcoptes* of the horse, but under favorable conditions it can be transmitted to ass and mule, and even to man, and may live for some time on the human skin. The mite (Pl. XXXIX, fig. 1) is nearly microscopical, but may be detected with a magnifying lens among moving scurf taken from the infected skin. Like all *Sarcoptes*, it burrows little galleries in and beneath the scurf skin, where it hides and lays its eggs and where its young are hatched. It is therefore often difficult to find the parasite on the surface, unless the skin has been heated by a temporary exposure to the sun or in a warm room. The mite may be detected more readily by placing scrapings on black cardboard and warming, or better by macerating

---

[1] Revised by M. C. Hall.

scabs or scrapings in a solution of caustic soda or potash and then examining them microscopically. Like other mites, this mite is wonderfully prolific, a new generation of fifteen individuals being possible every fifteen days, so that in three months the offspring of a single pair may produce generations aggregating 1,500,000 young. The *Sarcoptes* have less vitality than the nonburrowing mites, as they die in an hour when kept apart from the skin in dry air at a heat of 145° F. They live 12 to 14 days apart from the skin in the damp air of a stable. On a piece of damp hide they lived till the twenty-fourth day, when they began to die, and all were dead on the twenty-eighth in an experimental test.

Symptoms.—The symptoms are an incessant, intolerable, and increasing itching of some part of the skin (head, mane, tail, back, etc.), the horse inclining himself toward the hand that scratches him, and moving his lips as if himself scratching. The hairs may be broken and rubbed off, but the part is never entirely bald, as in ringworm, and there may be papules or any kind of eruption or open sores from the energy of the scratching. Scabs of varying thickness may form, but the special features are the intense itching and the presence of the mite.

Treatment consists in the removal of the scabs by soapsuds, and, if necessary, a brush and the thorough application of tobacco 1½ ounces and water 2 pints, prepared by boiling. This may be applied more than once, and should always be repeated in 10 to 14 days, to destroy the new brood that may have been hatched in the interval. All harness and stable utensils should be similarly treated; blankets and rubbers may be boiled, and the stalls should be covered with a whitewash of quicklime, containing one-fourth pound of chlorid of lime to the gallon.

When there are too many animals to treat by means of hand dressings, the lime-and-sulphur dip or the tobacco dip may be used and are very effective, though the cresol dips are fairly effective. These dips may be puchased and made up in the dilution called for on the container. The affected animals may be dipped when the number warrants it and facilities are available; otherwise the dips may be applied with a swab or a spray pump. Directions for constructing a dipping vat may be obtained from the United States Department of Agriculture on application. Any treatment used should be repeated in the course of 10 to 14 days. If the stables are not disinfected, animals should be removed after treatment and put in clean stables or on clean pasture for at least a month to allow the mites in the infested stables to die. Otherwise the disease may recur.

PARASITE: *Psoroptes equi* (*Dermatocoptes equi, Dermatodectes equi*). MALADY: *Psoroptic acariasis.*—Psoroptic mange is less common than sarcoptic mange in horses, and as the parasite (Pl. XXXIX, fig. 3) only bites the surface and lives among the crusts under the shelter of the hair, it is very easily discovered. It reproduces rapidly and causes symptoms similar to those produced by the *Sarcoptes*. The same treatment will suffice and is more promptly effectual. The disinfection of the stable must be thorough, as the *Psoroptes* will survive twenty to thirty days in the moist atmosphere of a stable, and may even revive after six or eight weeks when subjected to moist warmth. Infested pastures will therefore prove dangerous to horses for that length of time, and such pastures, with infected rubbing posts, etc., should not be used for over two months.

PARASITE: *Chorioptes equi* (*Symbiotes equi*, *Dermatophagus equi*, *Chorioptes spathiferus*). MALADY: *Foot mange.*—The mite (Pl. XXXIX, fig. 2) attacks the heels and lower parts of the legs, especially the hind ones, and may be present for years without extending upon the body. Like the *Psoroptes*, it lives on the surface, on the hairs, and among the scabs. It gives rise to great itching, stamping, rubbing of the one leg with the other, and the formation of papules, wounds, ulcerous sores, and scabs. The intense itching will always suggest this parasite, and the discovery of the mite will identify the disease. The treatment is the same as for the *Sarcoptes*, but may be confined to the legs and the parts with which they come in contact.

PARASITE: *Dermanyssus gallinæ, or chicken acari.* MALADY: *Poultry acariasis.*—This is a large-sized mite, though usually miscalled "hen louse," and the disease "poultry lousiness." The mite (Pl. XXXIX, fig. 4) lives in droppings and in crevices of chicken houses, but temporarily passes on to the skin of man and of the horse and other quadrupeds, when occasion serves. It causes much irritation, with the eruption of papules or vesicles and the formation of sores and scabs. The examination of the skin is usually fruitless, as the attacks are mostly made at night and the effects only may be seen during the day. The proximity of hen manure swarming with the mites explains the trouble, and the removal of this and a white-washing with quicklime, with or without chlorid of lime, will prevent future attacks. The skin may still require bland ointments or lotions, as for congestion.

PARASITE: *Larva of a Trombicula, Leptus americanus, or harvest mite, commonly called chigger.* MALADY: *Autumn mange.*—This parasite is a brick-red acarus, visible to the naked eye on a dark ground, and living on green vegetation in many localities. It attacks man, and the horse, ox, dog, etc., attaching to the skin and giving rise to small papules and intolerable irritation. This continues for two or three days only from a single invasion, but will last until cold weather sets in if there is a fresh invasion daily. Horses at pasture suffer mainly on the lower part of the face. If they are kept indoors the disease will disappear, or if left at pasture a weak tar water or solution of tobacco may be applied to the face. The application of sulphur ointment is very beneficial, and of flowers of sulphur is protective.

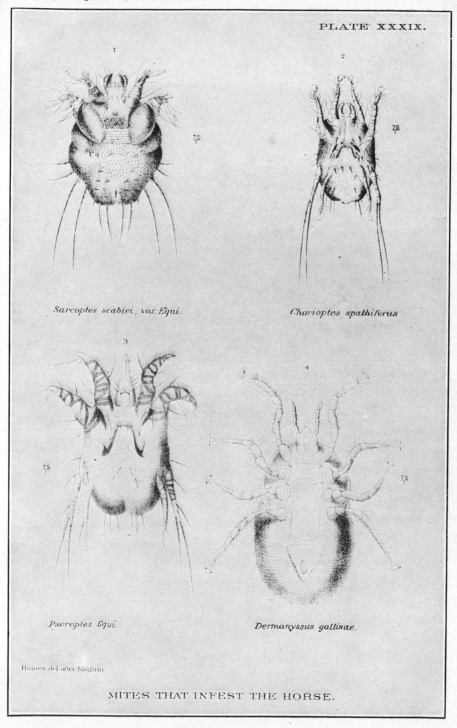

PLATE XXXIX.

1

7.5

Sarcoptes scabiei, var. Equi.

2

7.5

Chorioptes spathiferus

3

7.5

Psoroptes Equi.

4

7.5

Dermanyssus gallinae.

Haines del after Mégnin

MITES THAT INFEST THE HORSE.

TICKS.

The wood ticks are familiar to inhabitants of uncultivated lands and prove troublesome parasites to man and beast alike. The tick lives on bushes, and attaches itself to the mammal to feed. When it is gorged it drops off to molt, and finally the female drops to lay eggs on the soil. The tick produces great irritation by boring into the skin with its armed proboscis. If pulled out, the head and thorax are often left in the skin. The ticks may be covered with oil to shut out the air from their breathing pores, or by touching them with a hot penknife they will be impelled to let go their hold. The application of crude oil or the arsenical dips used for cattle is fatal to ticks on horses.

GRUBS IN SKIN.

PARASITE: *Hypoderma lineatum.* MALADY: *Larvæ (grubs) under the skin.*—The larvæ of a fly (usually *Hypoderma lineatum*), commonly in the skin of cattle and known as "warbles," are occasionally found in little sacs beneath the skin of horses. The mature larva escapes in early summer and develops into a fly. In districts where they exist the grubs should be pressed out of the skin in the course of the winter and destroyed.

LARVÆ (GRUBS) ON THE SKIN, OR FLYBLOW.

The following flies, among others, deposit their eggs on open sores or on wet, filthy parts of the skin, where their larvæ or grubs give rise to serious trouble: *Lucilia cæsar* (bluebottle), *Chrysomyia macellaria* (screw-worm fly), *Musca vomitoria* (meat fly), and *Sarcophaga carnaria* (flesh fly). To prevent their attacks, wet, filthy hair should be removed and wounds kept clean and rendered antiseptic by a lotion of carbolic acid 1 part, water 50 parts, or by a mixture of 1 ounce oil of tar in 20 ounces sweet oil, or by some other antiseptic. If the grubs are already present they should be picked off and one of these dressings freely applied. For deep wounds a mixture of chloroform, 1 part, and a bland oil, 7 parts, is recommended.

FLIES.

A number of flies attack horses and suck their blood, producing great annoyance and in some instances death. These insects not only suck the blood, but also often instill an acid poison into the skin, and in exceptional cases transfer infectious diseases from animal to animal by inoculation.

Various devices are resorted to to prevent the attacks, as to sponge the skin with a decoction of walnut or elder leaves, of tobacco, to dust with Persian insect powder, to keep a light blanket or fly net on the horse, to close doors and windows with fine screens and destroy by pyrethrum any flies that have gained admission, to remove all manure heaps that would prove breeding places for flies, to keep the stalls clean, deodorize by gypsum, and to spread in them trays of dry chlorid of lime. For the poisoned bites apply ammonia, or a solution of 1 part of carbolic acid in 20 parts of sweet oil or glycerin, or one-fourth ounce bicarbonate of soda and 1 dram of carbolic acid in a quart of water may be used.

A large number of fly repellents have been recommended, but most of them must be applied daily in order to maintain the protective effect. Among the things used are carbolic solutions, pine tar, oil of tar, fish oil, laurel oil, oil of citronella, oil of sassafras, oil of camphor, and cod-liver oil. Some of these things must be used judiciously or they will result in poisoning or removal of the hair from the animal in some instances. Ten per cent oil of tar in Beaumont oil or in cottonseed oil was found to be safe and efficacious by Graybill.

The use of the fly-maggot trap noted under stomach worms of the horse, and of the various forms of the Hodge flytrap, is recommended.

FLEAS.

The flea of man and those of poultry, when numerous, will bite the horse and give rise to rounded swellings on the skin. To dispose of them it is needful to clear the surroundings of the grublike larvæ as well as to treat the victim. The soil may be sprinkled with quicklime, carbolic acid, coal tar, or petroleum; the stalls may be deluged with boiling water and afterwards painted with oil of turpentine and littered with fresh pine sawdust, and all blankets should be boiled. The skin may be sponged with a solution of 1 part carbolic acid in 50 parts of water. Other animals should be kept free from fleas or kept away from the vicinity of the stable.

The chigoe (*Pulex penetrans*) of the Gulf coast is still more injurious, because it burrows under the surface and develops to the size of a small pea. The tumor formed by it should be laid open and the parasite extracted. This can be done more easily a day or two after its entrance into the skin than on the first day. It is best enucleated by means of a blunt pin or some similar instrument.

LICE, OR PEDICULI.

Two kinds of lice attack the horse, one of them having a narrow head and a proboscis for perforating the skin and sucking the blood, and the other—the broad-headed kind—having strong mandibles with which it bites the skin. Poor condition, itching, and loss of hair should lead to the suspicion that lice are present, and a close examination will usually disclose the lice. They may be destroyed by rubbing the horse's skin with sulphur ointment, or with sulphuret of potassium, 4 ounces in water, 1 gallon, or with coal-tar-creosote preparations, or the skin may be sponged with benzine. The application should be repeated 10 to 12 days later to destroy all lice hatched from the nits in the interval. Where only biting lice are present, one treatment with a mixture of commercial sodium fluorid, 1 part, and flour, 5 parts, thoroughly dusted into the skin, will destroy all the biting lice present. The sodium fluorid may be used without the flour, or may be used in solution, as a spray, at the rate of 1 ounce to 1 gallon of water. Sodium fluorid should not be applied to, or in the vicinity of, the mucous surfaces, such as the mouth, vulva, anus, etc., as it may cause considerable irritation. Properly used, it is a valuable substance for controlling biting lice in winter, the time when they are most prevalent and annoying. It is advisable to dip twice for lice in the fall, in order to avoid having to apply treatments under the unfavorable conditions prevailing in winter.

STINGS OF BEES, WASPS, AND HORNETS.

These are much more irritating than the bites of flies, partly because the barbed sting is left in the wound and partly because of the quantity and quality of the venom. When a swarm attacks an animal the result may prove fatal.

Treatment consists in the application of wet clay, or of a lotion of soda or ammonia, or of carbolic acid, or permanganate of potash, 2 grains to the ounce; or of sugar of lead 2 drams, laudanum 1 ounce, and water 1 pint. The embedded stings should be extracted with fine forceps or even with the finger nails.

TARANTULA AND SCORPION.

The bite of the first and the sting of the second are poisonous, and may be treated like other insect venom, by carbolated glycerin, or a strong solution of ammonia, or permanganate of potash.

SNAKE BITES.

These are marked by the double incision caused by the two fangs, by the excessive doughy (dark red) swelling around the wounds, and in bad cases by the general symptoms of giddiness, weakness, and prostration. They are best treated by aqua ammonia very largely diluted in water, the object being to sustain life until the poison shall have spent its power. As local treatment, if the wound is in a limb, the latter may have a handkerchief or cord tied around it above the injury and drawn tight by a stick twisted into it. In this way absorption may be checked until the poison can be destroyed by the application of a hot iron or a piece of nitrate of silver or other caustic. A poultice of tobacco leaves is a favorite remedy, and may be used to soothe the sore after cauterization.

A treatment which has been highly recommended consists in prompt and vigorous scarification at the site of puncture and rubbing crystals of potassium permanganate into the wound.

BURNS AND SCALDS.

These subjects are discussed in the following chapter.

WOUNDS OF THE SKIN.

Wounds of the skin are fully discussed in the next chapter.

WOUNDS AND THEIR TREATMENT.

By Ch. B. Michener, V. S.

[Revised by John R. Mohler, V. M. D., A. M.]

DESCRIPTION OF WOUNDS.

A wound is an injury to any part of the body involving a solution of continuity or disruption of the affected parts and is caused by violence, with or without laceration of the skin. In accordance with this definition we have the following varieties of wounds: Incised, punctured, contused, lacerated, gunshot, and poisoned. They may further be classified as superficial, deep, or penetrating, and also as unclean, if hair, dirt, or splinters of wood are present; as infected when contaminated with germs, and as aseptic if the wound does not contain germs.

An incised wound is a simple cut made with a sharp body, like a knife, producing merely a division of the tissues. The duller the body the more force is required, the more tissues destroyed, and a greater time will be required for healing. In a cut wound the edges are even and definite, while those of a lacerated wound are irregular and torn. Three conditions are present as a result of an incised wound: (1) Pain, (2) hemorrhage, (3) gaping of the wound. The first pain is due to the crushing and tearing of the nerve fibers. In using a sharp knife and by cutting quickly, the animal suffers less pain and healing occurs more rapidly. The secondary pain is usually due to the action of the air and inflammatory processes. When air is kept from the wound pain ceases soon after the lesion is produced. Hemorrhage is absent only in wounds of nonvascular tissues, as the cornea of the eye, the cartilage of joints, and other similar structures. Bleeding may be from the arteries, veins, or capillaries. In the last form of bleeding the blood oozes from the part in drops. Hemorrhage from the veins is dark red and issues in a steady stream without spurting. In arterial bleeding the blood is bright red and spurts with each heart beat. This latter variety of hemorrhage is the most dangerous, and should be stopped at once before attempting any further treatment. Bleeding from small veins and capillaries ceases in a short time spontaneously, while larger vessels, especially arteries, require some form of treatment to cause complete stoppage of the hemorrhage.

HEMOSTASIA.

By this term is meant the checking of the flow of blood. It may be accomplished by several methods, such as compress bandages, torsion, hot iron, and ligatures. The heat from a hot iron will cause the immediate clotting of the blood in the vessels, and this clot is further supported by the production of a scab, or crust, over the portion seared. The iron should be at a red heat. If at a white heat, the tissue is charred, which makes it brittle and the bleeding is liable to be renewed. If the iron is at a black heat, the tissue will stick to the iron and will pull away from the surface of the wound. Cold water and ice bags quickly stop capillary bleeding, while hot water is preferable in more excessive hemorrhages. Some drugs, called styptics, possess the power of contracting the walls of blood vessels and also of clotting the blood. A solution of the chlorid of iron placed on a wound alone or by means of cotton drenched in the liquid produces a rapid and hard clot. Tannic acid, alum, acetic acid, alcohol, and oil of turpentine are all more or less active in this respect. To check bleeding from large vessels compression may be adopted. When it is rapid and dangerous and from an artery, the fingers may be used for pressing between the wound and the heart (digital compression), but if from a vein, the pressure should be exerted on the other side of the wound. Tourniquet may also be used by passing a strap around the part and tightening after placing a pad over the hemorrhage. The rubber ligature has now replaced the tourniquet and is bound tightly around the limb to arrest the bleeding. Tampons, such as cotton, tow, or oakum, may be packed tightly in the wound and then sewed up. After remaining there for twenty-four or forty-eight hours they are removed. Bleeding may sometimes be easily checked by passing a pin under the vessel and by taking a horsehair and forming a figure 8 by running it above and below the pin, thus causing pressure on the vessel. Torsion is the twisting of the blood vessel until the walls come together and form a barrier to the flow of blood. It may be accomplished by the fingers, forceps, or by running a pin through the vessel, turning it several times, and then running the point into the tissue to keep it in a fixed position.

Ligation is the third method for stopping a hemorrhage. The blood vessel should be seized with the artery forceps, a clean thread of silk passed around it, and tied about one-half inch from its end. The silk should be sterilized by placing it in an antiseptic solution so as not to impede the healing process or cause blood poisoning or lockjaw, which often follows the ligation of a vein with unsterilized material. Sometimes it will be impossible to reach the bleeding vessel, so it is necessary to pass the ligature around a mass of tissue which includes the blood vessel. Ligation is the most useful method of arresting hemorrhage, since it disturbs healing least and gives the greatest security against secondary hemorrhage.

SUTURES.

After the bleeding has been controlled and all foreign bodies removed from the wound, the gaping of the wound is noticeable. It is caused by the contraction of the muscles and elastic fibers, and its degree depends on the extent, direction, and nature of the cut. This gaping will hinder the healing process so that it must be overcome by bringing the edges together by some sort of sutures or pins or by a bandage applied from below upward. As suture material, ordinary cotton thread is good, if well sterilized, as are also horsehair, catgut, silk, and various kinds of wire. If the suture is made too tight the subsequent swelling may cause the stitch to tear out. In order to make a firm suture the depth of the stitch should be the same as the distance the stitch is from the edge of the wound. The deeper the suture the more tissue is embraced and the fewer the number of stitches required. In tying a suture the square or reef knot should be used. Closure of wounds by means of adhesive plaster, collodion, and metal clamps is not practiced to any great extent in veterinary practice.

PROCESS OF HEALING.

In those cases where perfect stoppage of bleeding, perfect coaptation of the edges of the wound, and perfect cleanliness are obtained, healing occurs within three days, without the formation of graulations, pus, or proud flesh, by what is termed first intention. If wounds do not heal in this manner they will gap somewhat and become warm and painful. Healing then occurs by granulation or suppuration, which is termed healing by second intention. The sides of the wound become covered with granulation tissue which may fill the wound and sometimes overlap the lips, forming a fungoid growth called proud flesh. Under favorable conditions the edges of the wound appear to grow together by the end of the first week, and the whole surface gradually becomes dry, and finally covered with pigmented skin, when the wound is healed. The cause of pus formation in wounds is usually the presence of germs. For this reason the utmost care should be adopted to keep clean wounds aseptic, or free from germs, and to make unclean wounds antiseptic by using antiseptic fluids to kill the microbes present in the wound. The less the injurious action of this fluid on the wound and the greater its power to kill germs, the more valuable it becomes. All antiseptics are not equally destructive, and some germs are more susceptible to one antiseptic than to another. The most important are (1) bichlorid of mercury, which is to be preferred on horses. It becomes weakened in its action if placed in a wooden pail or on an oily or greasy surface. It is used in the strength of 1 part of bichlorid to 1,000 to 5,000 parts of water, according to the delicacy of the tissue to which it is applied. (2) Carbolic acid in from 2 to 5 per cent solution is used on infected wounds and for cleaning instruments, dressings, and sponges. It unites well with oil and is preferred to the bichlorid on a greasy surface. A 5 per cent solution in oil is often used under the name of carbolized oil. (3) Aluminum acetate is an efficient and cheap antiseptic, and is composed of 1 part alum and 5 parts acetate of lead, mixed in 20 parts of water. (4) Boric acid is good, in a 2 to 4 per cent solution, to cleanse wounds and wash eyes. Compound cresol may be used in a 1 to 3 per cent solution in water. Iodoform is one of the most used of the antiseptics, and it also acts as an anodyne, stimulates granulation, and checks wound secretion. A very efficacious and inexpensive powder is made by taking 5 parts of iodoform and 95 parts of sugar, making what is called iodoform sugar. Tannic acid is a useful drug in the treatment of wounds, as it arrests hemorrhage, checks secretion, and favors the formation of a scab. A mixture of 1 part tannic acid and 3 parts iodoform is good in suppurating wounds. Iodol, white sugar, ground and roasted coffee, and powdered charcoal are all used as protectives and absorbents on suppurating surfaces. More depends on the care and the method of application of the drug than on the drug itself. On aseptic wounds use only those antiseptics that do not irritate the tissue. If care is used in the application of the antiseptic, corrosive sublimate or carbolic acid is to be recommended. In order to keep air from the wound and to absorb all wound secretions rapidly, a dressing should be applied. If the wound is aseptic, the dressing should be likewise, such as cotton gauze, sterile cotton, oakum, or tow. This dressing should be applied with uniform pressure at all times and secured by a bandage. Allow it to remain for a week or ten days if the wound is aseptic or if the dressing does not become loose or misplaced or become drenched with secretions from the wound, or if pain, fever, or loss of appetitie does not develop. The dressing should then be removed, the wound treated antiseptically, and a sterilized dressing applied.

HEALING UNDER A SCAB.

This often occurs in small superficial wounds that have been kept aseptic. In order that a scab may form, the wound must not gap, secrete freely, or become infected with germs. The formation of scab is favored by astringents and styptics, such as tannic acid, iodoform, and 5 per cent solution of zinc chlorid. In case of fistulous withers, open joints, or other large, hollow wounds that can not be dressed, antisepsis may be obtained by warm-water irrigation with or without an antiseptic fluid. It should continue day and night, and never be interrupted for more than eight hours, for germs will then have gained headway and will be difficult to remove. Four or five days of irrigation will be sufficient, for granulations will then have formed and pus will remain on the outside if it forms. For permanent irrigation the stream should be very small, or drop by drop, but should play over the entire surface of the wound. It is always better to heal an infected wound under a scab, or treat it as an open wound, than it is to suture it, thus favoring the growth of the inclosed germs and retarding ultimate healing. In the latter case pus may develop in the wound, form pockets by sinking into the tissues, and cause various complications. The pockets should be well drained, either through incisions at the bottom or by drainage tubes or setons. They should then be frequently syringed out or continuously irrigated. In case proud flesh appears it should be kept down either by pressure or by caustics, as powdered bluestone, silver nitrate, chlorid of antimony, or by astringents, such as burnt alum. If they prove resistant to this treatment they may be removed by scissors, the knife, or by searing with the hot iron. The following rules for the treatment of wounds should be followed: (1) See that the wound is clean, removing all foreign bodies. (2) For this purpose use a clean finger rather than a probe. (3) All hemorrhage should be arrested before closing the wound. (4) Antiseptics should only be used if you suspect the wound to be infected. (5) When pus is present treat without closing the wound. (6) This may be accomplished by drainage tubes, absorbent dressings, setons, or continuous irrigations. (7) Protect the wound against infection while healing.

LACERATED AND CONTUSED WOUNDS.

Lacerated and contused wounds may be described together although there is, of course, this difference, that in contused wounds there is no break or laceration of the skin. Lacerated wounds, however, are, as a rule, also contused—the surrounding tissues are bruised to a greater or lesser extent. While at first sight such wounds may not appear to be as serious as incised wounds, they are commonly very much more so. Lacerations and contusions, when extensive, are always to be regarded as dangerous. Many horses die from septic infection or mortification as a result of these injuries. We find in severe contusions an infiltration of blood into the surrounding tissues; disorganization and mortification follow, and involve often the deeper seated structures. Abscesses, single or multiple, may also result and call for special treatment.

In wounds that are lacerated the amount of hemorrhage is mostly inconsiderable; even very large blood vessels may be torn apart without inducing a fatal result. The edges of the wound are ragged and uneven. These wounds are produced by barbed wire or some blunt object, as when a horse runs against fences, board piles, the corners of buildings, or when he is struck by the pole or shafts of another team, falling on rough, irregular stones, etc.

Contused wounds are caused by blunt instruments moving with sufficient velocity to bruise and crush the tissues, as kicks, running against objects, or falling on large, hard masses.

Treatment.—In lacerated wounds great care must at first be exercised in examining or probing to the very bottom of the rent or tear, to see whether any foreign body is present. Very often splinters of wood or bits of stone or dirt are thus lodged, and unless removed prevent the wound from healing; or if it should heal, the wound soon opens again, discharging a thin, gluey matter that is characteristic of the presence of some object in the part. After a thorough exploration these wounds are to be carefully and patiently fomented with warm water, to which has been added carbolic acid in the proportion of 1 part to 100 of water. Rarely, if ever, are stitches to be inserted in lacerated wounds. The surrounding tissues and skin are so weakened in vitality and structure by the contusions that stitches will not hold; they only irritate the parts. It is better to endeavor to obtain coaptation by means of bandages, plasters, or collodion. One essential in the treatment of lacerated wounds is to provide a free exit for the pus. If the orifice of the wound is too high, or if pus is found to be burrowing in the tissues beneath the opening, we must then make a counter opening as low as possible. This will admit of the wound being thoroughly washed out, at first with warm water, and afterwards injected with some mild astringent and antiseptic wash, as chlorid of zinc, 1 dram to a pint of water. A dependent opening must be maintained until the wound ceases to discharge. Repeated hot fomentations over the region of lacerated wounds afford much relief and should be persisted in.

BRUISES.

Bruises are nothing but contused wounds where the skin has not been ruptured. There is often considerable solution of continuity of the parts under the skin, subcutaneous hemorrhage, etc., which may result in local death (mortification) and slough of the bruised parts. If the bruise or contusion is not so severe, many cases are quickly cured by constant fomentation with hot water for from two to four hours. The water should be allowed about this time to become cool gradually and then cold. Cold fomentation must then be kept up for another hour or two. The parts should be thoroughly and quickly dried and bathed freely with camphor 1 ounce, sweet oil 8 ounces, or with equal parts of lead water and laudanum. A dry, light bandage should then be applied, the horse allowed to rest, and if necessary the treatment may be repeated each day for two or three days. If, however, the wound is so severe that sloughing must ensue, we should encourage it by poultices made of linseed meal, wheat bran, turnips, onions, bread and milk, or hops. Charcoal is to be sprinkled over the surface of the poultice when the wound is bad smelling. After the slough has fallen off the wound is to be dressed with warm washes of carbolic acid, chlorid of zinc, permanganate of potash, or other antiseptic. If granulating (filling up) too fast, use burnt alum or air-slaked lime. Besides this local treatment, we find that the constitutional symptoms of fever and inflammation call for measures to prevent or control them. This is best done by placing the injured animal on soft or green feed. A physic of Barbados aloes, 1 ounce, should be given as soon as possible after the accident. Sedatives, such as tincture of aconite root, 15 drops, three times a day, or ounce doses of saltpeter every four hours, may also be administered. When the symptoms of fever are abated, and if the discharges from the wound are abundant, the strength of the patient must be supported by good feed and tonics. One of the best tonics is as follows: Powdered sulphate of iron, powdered gentian, and powdered ginger, of each 4 ounces. Mix thoroughly and give a heaping tablespoonful twice a day, on the feed or as a drench.

PUNCTURED WOUNDS.

Punctured wounds are produced by the penetration of a sharp or blunt-pointed substance, such as a thorn, fork, nail, etc., and the orifice of these wounds is always small in proportion to their depth. In veterinary practice punctured wounds are much more common than the others. They involve the feet most frequently, next the legs, and often the head and face from nails protruding through the stalls and trough. They are not only the most frequent, but they are also the most serious, owing to the difficulty of obtaining thorough disinfection. Another circumstance rendering them so is the lack of attention that they at first receive. The external wound is so small that but little or no importance is attached to it, yet in a short time swelling, pain, and acute inflammation, often of a serious character, are manifested.

Considering the most common of the punctured wounds, we must give precedence to those of the feet. Horses worked in cities, about iron works, around building places, etc., are most likely to receive "nails in the feet." The animal treads upon nails, pieces of iron or screws, forcing them into the soles of the feet. If the nail, or whatever it is that has punctured the foot, is fast in some large or heavy body, and is withdrawn as the horse lifts his foot, lameness may last for only a few steps; but unless properly attended to at once he will be found in a day or two to be very lame in the injured member. If the foreign body remains in the foot, he gradually grows worse from the time of puncture until the cause is discovered and removed. If, when shoeing, a nail is driven into the " quick " (sensitive laminæ) and allowed to remain, the horse gradually evinces more pain from day to day; but if the nail has at once been removed by the smith, lameness does not, as a rule, show itself for some days; or, if the nail is simply driven " too close," not actually pricking the horse, he may not show any lameness for a week or even much longer. At this point it is due to the blacksmith to say that, considering how thin the walls of some feet are, the uneasiness of many horses while shoeing, the ease with which a nail is diverted from its course by striking an old piece of nail left in the wall, or from the nail itself splitting, the wonder is not that so many horses are pricked or nails driven " too close," but rather that many more are not so injured. It is not, by any means, always carelessness or ignorance on the part of the smith that is to account for this accident. Bad and careless shoers we do meet with, but let us be honest and say that the rarity of these accidents points rather to the general care and attention given by these much-abused mechanics.

From the construction of the horse's foot (being incased in an impermeable, horny box), and from the elasticity of the horn closing the orifice, punctured wounds of the feet are almost always productive of lameness. Inflammation results, and as there is no relief afforded by swelling and no escape for the product of inflammation, this matter must and does burrow between the sole or wall and the sensitive parts within it until it generally opens " between hair and hoof." We can thus see why pain is so much more severe, why tetanus (lockjaw) more frequently follows wounds of the feet, and why, from the extensive, or at times complete, separation and " casting" of the hoof, these wounds must always be regarded with grave apprehension.

Symptoms and treatment.—A practice which, if never deviated from—that of picking up each foot, cleaning the sole, and thoroughly examining the foot each and every time the horse comes into the stable—will enable us to reduce to the minimum the serious consequences of punctured wounds of the feet. If the wound has resulted from pricking, lameness follows soon after shoeing; if from the nails being driven too close, it usually appears from four to five days or a week afterwards. We should always inquire as to the time of shoeing, examine the shoe carefully, and see whether it has been partially pulled and the horse has stepped back upon some of the nails or the clip. The pain from these wounds is lancinating; the horse is seen to raise and lower the limb or hold it from the ground altogether; often he points the foot, flexes the leg, and knuckles at the fetlock. Swelling of the fetlock and back tendons is also frequently seen and is liable to mislead us. The foot must be carefully examined, and this can not be properly done without removing the shoe. The nails should be drawn separately and carefully examined. If there is no escape of pus from the nail holes, or if the nails themselves are not moist, we must continue our examination of the foot by carefully pinching or tapping it at all parts. With a little practice we can detect the spot where pain is the greatest or discover the delicate line or scar left at the point of entrance of the foreign body. The entire sole is then to be thinned, after which we are carefully to cut down upon the point where pain is greatest upon pressure, and, finally, through the sole at this spot. When the matter has escaped, the sole, so far as it was undermined by pus, is to to be removed. The foot must now be poulticed for one or two days and afterwards dressed with a compress of oakum saturated with carbolic-acid solution or other antiseptic dressing.

If we discover a nail or other object in the foot, the principal direction, after having removed the offending body, is to cut away the sole, in a funnel shape, down to the sensitive parts beneath. This is imperative, and if a good free opening has been made and is maintained for a few days, and hot fomentations and antiseptic dressings applied, the cure is mostly easy, simple, quick, and permanent. The horse should be shod with a leather sole under the shoe, first of all applying tar and oakum to prevent any dirt from entering the wound. In some instances nails may puncture the flexor tendons, the coffin bone, or enter the coffin joint. Such injuries are always serious, their recovery slow and tedious, and the treatment so varied and difficult that the services of a veterinarian will be necessary.

PUNCTURED WOUNDS OF JOINTS, OR OPEN JOINTS.

These wounds are more or less frequent. They are always serious, and often result in anchylosis (stiffening) of the joint or the death of the animal. The joints mostly punctured are the hock, fetlock, or knee, though other joints may, of course, suffer this injury. As the symptoms and treatment are much the same for all, only the accident as it occurs in the hock joint will be described. Probably the most common mode of injury is from the stab of a fork, but it may result from the kick of another horse that is newly shod, or in many other ways. At first the horse evinces but slight pain or lameness. The owner discovers a small wound scarcely larger than a pea, and pays but little attention to it. In a few days, however, the pain and lameness become excessive; the horse can no longer bear any weight upon the injured leg; the joint is very much swollen and painful upon pressure; there are well-marked symptoms of constitutional disturbance—quick pulse, hurried breathing, high temperature, 103°

to 106° F., the appetite is lost, thirst is present, the horse reeks with sweat, and his anxious countenance shows the pain he suffers. He may lie down, though mostly he persists in standing, and the opposite limb becomes greatly swollen from bearing the entire weight and strain for so long a time. The wound, which at first appeared so insignificant, is now constantly discharging a thin, whitish or yellowish fluid—joint oil or water, which becomes coagulated about the mouth of the wound and adheres to the part in clots like jelly, or resembling somewhat the white of an egg. Not infrequently the joint opens at different places, discharging at first a thin, bloody fluid that soon assumes the character above described.

Treatment of these wounds is most difficult and unsatisfactory. We can do much to prevent this array of symptoms if the case is seen early—within the first 24 or 48 hours after the injury; but when inflammation of the joint is once fairly established the case becomes one of grave tendencies. Whenever a punctured wound of a joint is noticed, even though apparently of but small moment, we should apply without the least delay a strong cantharides blister over the entire joint, being even careful to fill the orifice of the wound with the blistering ointment. This treatment is almost always effectual. It operates to perform a cure in two ways—first, the swelling of the skin and tissues underneath it completely closes the wound and prevents the ingress of air; second, by the superficial inflammation established it acts to check and abate all deep-seated inflammation. In the great majority of instances, if pursued soon after the accident, this treatment performs a cure in about one week; but should the changes described as occurring later in the joint have already taken place, we must then treat by cooling lotions and the application to the wound of chlorid of zinc, 10 grains to the ounce of water, or a paste made of flour and alum. A bandage is to hold these applications in place, which is only to be removed when swelling of the leg or increasing febrile symptoms demand it. In the treatment of open joints our chief aim must be to close the orifice as soon as possible. For this reason repeated probing or even injections are contraindicated. The only probing of an open joint that is to be sanctioned is on our first visit, when we should carefully examine the wound for foreign bodies or dirt, and after removing them the probe must not again be used. The medicines used to coagulate the synovial discharge are best simply applied to the surface of the wound, on pledgets of tow, and held in place by bandages. Internal treatment is also indicated in those cases of open joints in which the suffering is great. At first we should administer a light physic and follow this up with sedatives and anodynes, as directed for contused wounds. Later, however, we should give quinin or salicylic acid in 1-dram doses two or three times a day.

WOUNDS OF THE TENDON SHEATHS.

Wounds of tendon sheaths are similar to open joints in that there is an escape of synovial fluid, "sinew water." Where the tendons are simply punctured by a thorn, nail, or fork, we must, after a thorough exploration of the wound for any remaining foreign substance, treat with the flour-and-alum paste, bandages, etc., as for open joint. Should the skin and tendons be divided the case is even more serious and is often incurable. There is always a large bed of granulations (proud flesh) at the seat of injury, and a thickening more or less pronounced remains. When the back tendons of the leg are severed we should apply at once a high-heel shoe (which is to be gradually lowered as healing advances) and bandage firmly with a compress moistened with a 10-grain chlorid of zinc solution. When proud flesh appears it is best kept under control by repeated applications of a red-hot iron. Mares that are valuable as brood animals and stock horses should always be treated for this injury, as, even though blemished, their value is not seriously impaired. If the subject is old and comparatively valueless, the length of time required and the expense of treatment will cause us to hesitate in attempting a cure.

GUNSHOT WOUNDS.

These wounds vary in size and character, depending on the size and quality of the projectile and also the tissue injured. They are so seldom met with in our animals that an extended reference to them seems unnecessary. If a wound has been made by a bullet a careful examination should be made to ascertain whether the ball has passed through or out of the body. If it has not we must then probe for it, and if it can be located it is to be cut out when practicable to do so. Oftentimes a ball may be so lodged that it can not be removed, and it then may become encysted and remain for years without giving rise to any inconvenience. It is often difficult to locate a bullet, as it is very readily deflected by resistances met with after entering the body.

The entering wound is the size of the projectile, the edges are inverted and often scorched. The wound produced in case of the bullet's exit is larger than the projectile, the edges are turned out and ragged. A bullet heated by the friction of the barrel or air often softens and becomes flattened on striking a bone or other tissue. Modern bullets that have an outer steel layer may pass through bone without splintering it. Lead bullets may split, producing two exit wounds. Spent bullets may only produce a bruise. Should bones be struck by a ball they are sometimes shattered and splintered to such an extent as to warrant us in having the animal destroyed. A gunshot wound, when irreparable injury has not been done, is to be treated the same as punctured wounds, i. e., stop the hemorrhage, remove the foreign body if possible, and apply hot fomentations or poultices to the wound until suppuration is fairly established. Antiseptic and disinfectant injections may then be used. Should pus accumulate in the tissues, openings must be made at the most depending parts for its escape. Wounds from shotguns fired close to the animals are serious. They are virtually lacerated and contused wounds. Remove all the shot possible from the wound and treat as directed for contusions. When small shot strike the horse from a distance they stick in the skin or only go through it. The shot grains must be picked out, but as a rule this "peppering" of the skin amounts to but little.

POISONED WOUNDS.

These injuries are the result of bites of snakes, rabid dogs, stings of bees, wasps, etc. A single sting is not dangerous, but an animal is often stung by a swarm of insects, when the chief danger occurs from the swelling produced. If stung about the head, the nostrils may be closed as a result of the swelling, causing labored breathing and possibly asphyxiation. Intoxication may be produced by the absorption of this poison and is manifested by staggering gait, spreading of the legs, paralysis of the muscles, difficult respiration, and a rise of temperature. Death may follow in five to ten hours.

Treatment.—Douse animal with cold water and apply any alkaline liquid, such as soapsuds, bicarbonate of soda, or weak solution of ammonia. Internally give alcohol, ether, or camphor to strengthen the heart. In case of bites by rattlesnakes, moccasin, or other poisonous snakes, a painful swelling occurs about the bitten part, which is followed by labored breathing, weakness, retching, fever, and death from collapse. The animal usually recovers if it can be kept alive over the third day. In treating the animal, a tight ligature should be passed about the part above the wound to keep the poison from entering the general circulation. Wash out the wound thoroughly with antiseptics and then apply a caustic, such as silver nitrate, or burn with a hot instrument. A subcutaneous injection of one-fourth dram of 1 per cent solution of chromic acid above the wound is also beneficial. Cold water may be applied to the wound to combat the inflammation. Bites of rabid dogs produce an infected wound, and the virus of rabies introduced in this manner should be removed or destroyed in the wound. Therefore produce considerable bleeding by incising the wound, wash out thoroughly with 10 per cent solution of zinc chlorid, and then apply caustics or the actual cautery.

HARNESS GALLS (SITFASTS).

Wounds or abrasions of the skin are frequently caused by ill-fitting harness or saddles. When a horse has been resting from steady work for some time, particularly after being idle in a stable on a scanty allowance of grain, as in winter, he is soft and tender and sweats easily when put to work again. In this condition he is liable to sweat and chafe under the harness, especially if it is hard and poorly fitted. This chafing is likely to cause abrasions of the skin, and thus pave the way for an abscess or for a chronic blemish, unless attended to very promptly. Besides causing the animal considerable pain, chafing, if long continued, leads to the formation of a callosity. This may be superficial, involving only the skin, or it may be deep-seated, involving the subcutaneous fibrous tissue and sometimes the muscle and even the bone. This causes a dry slough to form, which is both inconvenient and unsightly. Sloughs of this kind are commonly called "sitfasts" and, while they occur in other places, are most frequently found under the saddle. (See also p. 475.)

Treatment.—Abrasions are best prevented by bringing the animal gradually into working shape after it has had a prolonged rest, in order that the muscles may be hard and the skin tough. The harness should be well fitted, neither too large nor too small, and it should be cleaned and oiled to remove all dirt and to make it soft and pliable. Saddles should be properly fitted so as to prevent direct pressure on the spine, and the saddle blankets should be clean and dry. Parts of the horse where chafing is likely to occur, as on the back under the saddle, should be cleaned and brushed free of dirt.

The remedies for simple harness galls are numerous. Among them may be mentioned alcohol, 1 pint, in which are well shaken the whites of two eggs; a solution of nitrate of silver, 10 grains to the ounce of water; sugar of lead or sulphate of zinc, 20 grains to an ounce of water; carbolic acid, 1 part in 15 parts of glycerin, and so on almost without end. Any simple astringent wash or powder will effect a cure, provided the sores are not irritated by friction.

If a sitfast has developed, the dead hornlike slough must be carefully dissected out and the wound treated carefully with antiseptics. During treatment it is always best to allow the animal to rest, but if this is inconvenient care should be taken to prevent injury to the abraded or wounded surface by padding the harness so that chafing can not occur.

BURNS AND SCALDS.

These wounds of domestic animals are fortunately of rare occurrence; however, when they do occur, if at all extensive, they prove to be quite troublesome and in many cases are fatal. According to the severity of the burn we distinguish three degrees: First degree, where there is a simple reddening of the skin; second degree, where there is a formation of vesicles, or blisters; third degree, where there is a complete destruction of vitality of the tissues, such as would occur is charring from direct contact with flames or from escaping steam. Besides the burns caused by flames and steam, there are other causative agents, such as chemicals (caustic alkalies and acids), lightning stroke, and occasionally the broken trolley wires of electric railways. When a large surface of the skin is burned or scalded, the animal (if it does not die at once from shock) will soon show signs of fever—shivering, coldness of the extremities, weakness, restlessness, quick and feeble pulse, and labored breathing. No matter which agent is a factor in the production of burns, the lesions are practically of the same nature. The extent and site of the burn should lead one in the determination and course of treatment. Burns of the shoulder and those about the region of the elbow or other parts where there is much movement of the tissues are grave, and, if at all extensive, treatment should not be attempted, but the immediate destruction of the animal is advised. A burn of the third degree, where there is a destruction of the vitality of large areas of tissue, even on parts not subject to much motion, is extremely tedious to treat; in fact, it is questionable whether the treatment and keep of the animal will ever be compensated for, even though recovery does take place; this, in any event, will require at least six or eight weeks. Burns caused by lightning stroke and trolley wires are liable to occur in irregular lines, and, unless death occurs at once, they generally are not serious.

Treatment.—Treatment should be prompt and effective. If the burns are extensive, the constitutional symptoms should be combated with ammonia carbonate, strychnin, caffein, or other stimulant to prevent shock. In the local treatment, to alleviate the pain, the application of cold water in some form and the hypodermic injection of morphin are to be recommended. In burns of the first degree, where there is only a superficial inflammation, lead carbonate (white lead) ointment is very good. Carron oil (limewater and linseed oil, equal parts) is a standard remedy, but a modification of it known as Stahl's liniment is perhaps better. This is composed of linseed oil and limewater each 200 parts, bicarbonate of soda 100 parts, and thymol 1 part. The scorched surface should be covered with this liniment and then with a layer of borated gauze or absorbent cotton, to protect from the air. The application should be frequently renewed. Carbolated vaseline may be used in place of the above. In case the burn is more extensive, the following solution may be used: Picric acid 2 parts, alcohol 40 parts, water 400 parts. The lesion should be thoroughly cleansed with this solution used on absorbent cotton. The vesicles, if any appear, should be opened with a clean needle, allowing the skin to remain. Strips of gauze or absorbent cotton saturated with the solution should now be applied and renewed only occasionally. In burns of the second and third degrees more satisfactory results may be obtained with nonpoisonous, dry dressing powder, such as is used in ordinary open wounds, as tannic acid 8 parts and iodoform 1 part, or a salve made of this powder and a sufficient quantity of vaseline. When sloughing of the tissues takes place the wounds should be cleansed with a warm 3 per cent solution of carbolic acid, all loose fragments of tissue removed, and either a dry, antiseptic dressing powder or carbolated vaseline ointment applied to exclude the air. Granulation tissue (proud flesh) should be controlled by the application of silver nitrate in the form of a caustic pencil.

Burns due to mineral acids may be first treated by flushing the parts with a copious quantity of cold water or by the application of whiting or chalk. Either use a large quantity of water at the start or use the chalk first, then wash with water. If the irritant has been a caustic alkali, such as potash, lye, ammonia, or soda, then vinegar should be the first application. Stahl's liniment is probably the best general application for all burns for the first week; then this should be followed by the ordinary antiseptic wound dressings.

GANGRENE.

Gangrene, or mortification, denotes the death of the affected part, and is mostly found attacking soft tissue near the surface of the body. Gangrenous areas may occur as a result of shutting off their blood supply. Constitutional diseases, such as ergotism, anthrax, and septicemia, predispose to gangrene. As external causes we have acids and alkalies, freezing and burning, contusions and continuous pressure that interrupt the circulation. There are two forms of gangrene—dry and moist. Dry gangrene is most often seen in horses from continuous lying down (decubitus) or from uneven pressure of some portion of the harness.

Symptoms.—There is a lack of sensation due to the death of nerves. In dry gangrene the skin is leathery and harsh, while in moist gangrene the tissues are soft, wrinkled, and friable; the hair is disturbed, and the skin is usually moist and soapy and sometimes covered with blebs. The tissue surrounding the moist gangrenous patch is usually inflamed, swollen, and hot, but this is less noticeable in the case of dry gangrene. Moist gangrene often spreads and involves deeper tissue, sheaths of tendons and joints producing septic synovitis or septic arthritis leading to pyemia and death. Dry gangrene is seldom dangerous, but the rapidity of its spread will indicate its virulence.

Treatment.—The preventive treatment consists in avoiding all the influences that tend to disturb the nutrition of the tissues, such as excessive cold or heat or continuous pressure. Gangrene following decubitus may be prevented by using soft bedding and frequently turning the animal from one side to the other. In dry gangrene moist heat in the form of poultices or anointing the tissue with oils and fats will be found beneficial in hastening the dead tissue to slough off. When the outer skin begins to suppurate, it should be removed with a pair of pincers, and the patch treated as an open wound. In moist gangrene the tissue should be thoroughly disinfected with a 3 per cent solution of compound cresol, or particularly an alcoholic tincture of camphor. Continuous irritation with antiseptic fluids prevents the accumulation and absorption of poisonous liquids. Incisions into the dead tissue may be made, and when sloughing commences the tissue should be removed with forceps and the resulting wound treated as in dry gangrene.

ULCERATION.

An ulcer is a circumscribed area of necrosis occurring on the skin or mucous membrane and covered with granulation tissue. It is a process of destruction, and when this process is going on faster than regeneration can take place, we have a gnawing, or eating, ulcer. When such an ulcer increases rapidly in size it is termed a phagedenic ulcer. A fungoid ulcer is one in which the bottom of the ulcer projects beyond the edge of the skin. These ulcers secrete milky or bloody-white liquid called ichor. When the ulcer is of an ashen or leaden color, with the bottom and sides formed of dense, hard connective tissue, which gives but little discharge and is not sensitive, it is termed callous, torpid, or indolent ulcer.

Causes.—As in the case of gangrene, disturbances of circulation are among the most frequent causes. A wound to a tissue with slight recuperative power may be followed by ulceration, as in tumors. Certain germs may produce ulcers, as the glanders bacilli, which cause the ulcerations on the nasal septum in glanders.

Treatment.—This consists in removing the exciting cause at once. The secretions of the ulcer should be washed off with antiseptic solutions and the formation of granulation tissues stimulated by antiseptic salves, such as carbolated vaseline, lead ointment, or by dressings of camphor. Air should be kept from the ulcer by occlusive dressings. Where the ulcers are inflamed, warm lead water or lead water and laudanum will be found efficacious. Callous ulcers are best removed by a curette, knife, or hot iron and then treated like a common wound. Mechanical irritation should be avoided.

ABSCESSES.

These consist of accumulations of pus within circumscribed walls, at different parts of the body, and may be classed as acute and cold or chronic abscesses.

When an abscess occurs about a hair follicle it is called a boil or furuncle; when several hair follicles are involved, resulting in the formation of more than one exit for the inflammatory products, it is called a carbuncle.

ACUTE ABSCESSES.

Acute abscesses follow as the result of local inflammation in glands, muscular tissue, or even bones. They are very common in the two former. The abscesses most commonly met with in the horse (and the ones which will be here described) are those of the salivary glands, occurring during the existence of " strangles," or " colt distemper." The glands behind or under the jaw are seen to increase slowly in size, becoming firm, hard, hot, and painful. At first the swelling is uniformly hard and resisting over its entire surface, but in a little while becomes soft (fluctuating) at some portion, mostly in the center. From this time on the abscess is said to be " pointing," or " coming to a head," which is shown by a small elevated or projecting prominence, which at first is dry, but soon becomes moist with transuded serum. The hairs over this part loosen and fall off, and in a short time the abscess opens, the contents escape, and the cavity gradually fills up—heals by granulations.

Abscesses in muscular tissue are usually the result of bruises or injuries. In all cases in which abscesses are forming we should hurry the ripening process by frequent hot fomentations and poultices. When they are very tardy in their development a blister over their surface is advisable. It is a common rule with surgeons to open an abscess as soon as pus can be plainly felt, but this practice can scarcely be recommended indiscriminately to owners of stock, since this little operation frequently requires an exact knowledge of anatomy. It will usually be found the better plan to encourage the full ripening of an abscess and allow it to open of itself. This is imperative if the abscess is in the region of joints, etc. When open, we must not squeeze the walls of the abscess to any extent. They may be very gently pressed with the fingers at first to remove the clots—inspissated pus—but after this the orifice is simply to be kept open by the introduction of a clean probe, should it be disposed to heal too soon. If the opening is at too high a level another should be made into the lowest portion of the abscess so as to permit the most complete drainage. Hot fomentations or poultices are sometimes required for a day or two after an abscess has opened, and are particularly indicated when the base of the abscess is hard and indurated.

The cavity should be thoroughly washed with stimulating antiseptic solutions, such as 3 per cent solution of carbolic acid, 3 per cent solution of compound cresol, 1 to 1,000 bichlorid of mercury, or 1 per cent permanganate of potash solution. If the abscesses are foul and bad smelling, their cavities should first be syringed with 1 part of hydrogen peroxid to 2 parts of water and then followed by the injection of any of the above-mentioned antiseptics.

COLD ABSCESSES.

Cold abscess is the term applied to those large, indolent swellings that are the result of a low or chronic form of inflammation, in the center of which there is a small collection of pus. They are often seen near the point of the shoulder, forming the so-called breast boil. The swelling is diffuse and of enormous extent, but slightly hotter than surrounding parts, and not very painful upon pressure. A pronounced stiffness, rather than pain, is evinced upon moving the animal. Such abscesses have the appearance of a hard tumor, surrounded by a softer edematous swelling, involving the tissues to the extent of a foot or more in all directions from the tumor. This diffused swelling gradually subsides and leaves the large, hardened mass somewhat well defined. One of the characteristics of cold abscesses is their tendency to remain in the same condition for a great length of time. There is neither heat nor soreness; no increase nor lessening in the size of the tumor; it remains in statu quo. If, however, the animal should be put to work for a short time the irritation of the collar causes the surrounding tissues to assume again an edematous condition, which after a few days' rest disappears, leaving the tumor as before or but slightly larger. Upon careful manipulation we may discover what appears to be a fluid deep seated in the center of the mass. The quantity of matter so contained is very small—often not more than a tablespoonful—and for this reason it can not, in all cases, be detected.

Cold abscesses are mostly, if not always, caused by the long-continued irritation of a loose and badly fitting collar. There is a slow inflammatory action going on, which results in the formation of a small quantity of matter inclosed in very thick and but partially organized walls that are not so well defined as is the circumference of fibrous tumors, which they most resemble.

Treatment.—The means recommended to bring the acute abscess " to a head " are but rarely effectual with this variety; or, if successful, too much time has been occupied in the cure. We must look for other and more rapid methods of treatment. These consist, first of all, in carefully exploring the tumor for the presence of pus. The incisions must be made over the softest part and carried deep into the tumor—to its very bottom, if necessary—and the matter allowed to escape. After this, and whether we have found matter or not, we must induce an active inflammation of the tumor, in order to promote solution of the thick walls of the abscess. This may be done by inserting well into the incision a piece of oakum or cotton saturated with turpentine, carbolic acid, tincture of iodin, etc., or we may pack the incision with powdered sulphate of zinc and keep the orifice plugged for 24 hours. These agents set up a destructive inflammation of the walls. Suppuration follows, and this should now be encouraged by hot fomentations and poultices. The orifice must be kept open, and should it be disposed to heal we must again introduce some of the agents above described. A favored treatment with many, and it is probably the best, is to plunge a red-hot iron to the bottom of the incision and thoroughly sear all parts of the walls of the abscess. This is to be repeated after the first slough has taken place if the walls remain thickened and indurated.

It is useless to waste time with fomentations, poultices, or blisters in the treatment of cold abscesses, since though apparently removed by such methods, they almost invariably return when the horse is put to work. Extirpation by the knife is not practicable, as the walls of the tumor are not sufficiently defined. If treated as above directed, and properly fitted with a good collar after healing, there will not remain any track or trace of the large, unsightly mass.

FISTULAS.

Definition.—The word fistula is applied to any ulcerous lesion upon the external surface of the body which is connected by ducts, or passages, with some internal cavity. Because of this particular formation the term fistulous tract is often used synonymously with the word fistula. Fistulas may exist in any part of the body, but the name has come to be commonly accepted as applicable only to such lesions when found upon the withers. Poll evil is a fistula upon the poll, and in no sense differs from fistulous withers except in location. The description of fistula will apply, then, in the main, to poll evil equally well. Quittor presents the characteristic tubular passages of a fistula and may, therefore, be considered and treated as fistula of the foot. Fistulous passages may also be developed upon the sides of the face, through which saliva is discharged instead of flowing into the mouth, and are called salivary fistulas. A dental fistula may arise from the necrosis of the root of a tooth. Again, a fistula is sometimes noted at the umbilicus associated with hernia, and rectovaginal fistulas have been developed in mares, following difficult parturition. Fistulas may arise from wounds of glandular organs or their ducts, and thus we have the so-called mammary or lacrimal fistulas.

Fistulous tracts are lined with a false, or adventitious, membrane and show no disposition to heal. They constantly afford means of exit to the pus or ichorous material discharged by the unhealthy parts below. They are particularly liable to develop at the withers or poll because of the exposed positions which these parts occupy, and, having once become located there, they usually assert a tendency to further extension, because the vertical and laminated formation of the muscles and tendons of these parts allows the forces of gravitation to assist the pus in gaining the deeper-lying structures and also favors its retention among them.

Causes.—Fistulas follow as a result of abscesses, bruises, wounds, or long-continued irritation by the harness. Among the more common causes of fistula of the poll (poll evil) are chafing by the halter or heavy bridle; blows from the butt end of the whip; the horse striking his head against the hayrack, beams of the ceiling, low doors, etc. Fistulous withers are seen mostly in those horses that have thick necks as well as those that are very high in the withers; or, among saddle horses, those that are very low in the withers, the saddle here riding forward and bruising the parts. In either of these locations ulcers of the skin, or simple abscesses, if not properly and punctually treated, may become fistulas. They are often caused by bad-fitting collars or saddles, by direct injuries from blows, and from the horse rolling upon rough or sharp stones. The pus burrows and finds lodgment deep down between the muscles, and escapes only when the sinus becomes surcharged or when, during motion of the parts, the matter is forced to the surface.

Symptoms.—These, of course, will vary according to the progress made by the fistula. Following an injury we may often notice soreness or stiffness of the front legs, and upon careful examination of the withers we see small tortuous lines running from the point of irritation downward and backward over the region of the shoulder. These are superficial lymphatics, and are swollen and painful to the touch. In a day or two a swelling is noticed on one or both sides of the dorsal vertebræ, which is hot, painful, and rapidly enlarging. The stiffness of the limbs may disappear at this time, and the heat and soreness of the parts may become less noticeable, but the swelling remains and continues to enlarge.

A fistulous ulcer of the poll may be first indicated by the opposition which the animal offers to the application of stable brush or bridle. At this time the parts are so sore and sensitive that there is some danger that unless handled with the greatest care the patient will acquire disagreeable stable habits. The disease in its early stages may be recognized as a soft, fluctuating tumor surrounded by inflammatory swelling, with the presence of enlarged lymphatic vessels and stiffness of the neck. Later the inflammation of the surrounding tissues may disappear, leaving a prominent tumor. The swelling, whether situated upon the head or the withers, may open and form a running ulcer, or its contents may dry up and leave a tumor which gradually develops the common characteristics of a fibrous tumor. When the enlargement has opened we should carefully examine its cavity, as upon its condition will wholly depend our treatment.

Treatment.—In the earliest stage, when there is soreness, enlarged lymphatics, but no well-marked swelling, the trouble may frequently be aborted. To do this requires both general and local treatment. A physic should be given, and the horse receive 1 ounce of powdered saltpeter three times a day in his water or feed. If the fever runs high, 20-drop doses of tincture of aconite root every two hours may be administered. The local application of cold water to the inflamed spot for an hour at a time three or four times a day has often proved very beneficial, and has afforded great relief.

Cooling lotions, muriate of ammonia, or saltpeter and water; sedative washes, such as tincture of opium and aconite, chloroform liniment, or camphorated oil, are also to be frequently applied. Should this treatment fail to check the progress of the trouble, the formation of pus should be hastened as rapidly as possible. Hot fomentations and poultices are to be constantly used, and as soon as the presence of pus can be detected, the abscess wall is to be opened at its lowest point. In this procedure lies our hope of a speedy cure. As with any simple abscess, if drainage can be so provided that the pus will run off as fast as formed without remaining within the interstices of the tissues, the healing will be rapid and satisfactory.

Attention is again called to the directions given above as to the necessity of probing the cavity when opened. If upon a careful examination with the probe we find that there are no pockets, no sinuses, but a simple, regular abscess wall, the indication for treatment is to make an opening from below so that all the matter must escape. Rarely is anything more needed than to keep the orifice open and to bathe or inject the parts with some simple antiseptic wash that is not irritant or caustic. A low opening and cleanliness constitute the essential and rational treatment.

If the abscess has already opened, giving vent to a quantity of purulent matter, and the pipes and tubes leading from the opening are found to be extensive and surrounded with thick fungoid membranes, there is considerable danger that the internal ligaments or even some of the bones have become affected, in which case the condition has assumed a serious aspect. Or, on the other hand, if the abscess has existed for some time without a rupture, its contents will frequently be found to consist of dried purulent matter, firm and dense, and the walls surrounding the mass will be found greatly thickened. In such a case we must generally have recourse to the application of caustics which will cause a sloughing of all of the unhealthy tissue, and will also stimulate a rapid increase of healthy organized material to replace that destroyed in the course of the development and treatment of the disease. Threads or cords soaked in gum-arabic solution and rolled in powdered corrosive sublimate may be introduced into the canal and allowed to remain. The skin on all parts of the shoulder and leg beneath the fistula should be carefully greased with lard or oil, as this will prevent the discharge that comes from the opening after the caustic is introduced from irritating or blistering the skin over which it flows. In obstinate cases a piece of caustic potash (fused) 1 to 2 inches in length may be introduced into the opening and should be covered with oakum or cotton. The horse should then be secured so that he can not reach the part with his teeth. After the caustic plug has been in place for 24 hours, it may be removed and hot fomentations applied. As soon as the discharge has become again established the abscess should be opened from its lowest extremity, and the passage thus formed may be kept open by the introduction of a seton. If the pipes become established in the deep tissues beneath the shoulder blade or among the spines of the vertebral column, it will often be found impossible to provide proper drainage for the abscess from below, and treatment must consist of caustic solutions carefully injected into all parts of the suppurating sinuses. A very effective remedy for this purpose consists of 1 ounce of chlorid of zinc in half a pint of water, injected three times during a week, after which a weak solution of the same may be occasionally injected. Injections of Villate's solution or alcoholic solution of corrosive sublimate, strong carbolic acid, or possibly oil of turpentine will also prove beneficial. Pressure should be applied from below, and endeavors made to heal the various pipes from the bottom.

Should the swelling become general, without forming a well-defined tumor, the placing of 20 to 30 grains of arsenious acid, wrapped in a single layer of tissue paper, in a shallow incision beneath the skin, will often produce a sloughing of the affected parts in a week or 10 days, after which the formation of healthy tissue follows. The surrounding parts of the skin should be protected from any damage from escaping caustics by the application of lard or oil, as previously suggested.

Although the successful treatment of fistulas requires time and patience, the majority of cases are curable. The sinuses must be opened at their lowest extremity and kept open. Caustic applications must be thoroughly used once or twice, after which mild astringent antiseptic washes should be persistently used until a cure is reached.

It sometimes happens that the erosions have burrowed so deeply or in such a direction that the opening of a drainage passage becomes impracticable. In other cases the bones may be attacked in some inaccessible location, or the joints may be affected, and in these cases it is often best to destroy the horse at once.

The reappearance of the fistula after it has apparently healed is not uncommon. The secondary attack in these cases is seldom serious. The lesion should be carefully cleaned and afterwards injected with a solution of zinc sulphate, 20 grains to the ounce of water, every second or third day until a cure is effected.

In fistula of the foot we see the same tendency toward the burrowing of pus downward to lower structures, or in some cases upward toward the coronet. Prior to the development of a quittor there is always swelling at the coronet, accompanied with heat and pain. Every effort should now be made to prevent the formation of an abscess at the point of injury. Wounds caused by nails, gravel, or any other foreign body which may have lodged in the sole of the foot should be opened at once from below, so as to allow free exit to all purulent discharges. Should the injury have occurred directly to the coronet the application of cold fomentations may prove efficient in preventing the formation of an abscess.

When a quittor becomes fully established it should be treated precisely as a fistula situated in any other part of the body; that is, the sinuses should all be opened from their lowest extremities, so as to afford constant drainage. All fragments of diseased tissue should be trimmed away, antiseptic solutions injected, and, after covering the wound with a pad of oakum saturated with some good antiseptic wash, the whole foot may be carefully covered with clean bandages, which will afford valuable assistance to the healing process by excluding all dirt from the affected part.

Another form of treatment for this class of infections consists in the use of bacterial vaccines. Such treatment appears to be well adapted for the purpose, and according to current veterinary literature has met with success. These vaccines are composed of several strains of the organisms usually found in these pustular infections of the horse. Two kinds of vaccines are used: First, autogenic vaccines, which consist of heated (killed) cultures of the organism or organisms which are causing the trouble and which have been isolated from the lesions; second, stock vaccines, consisting of dead organisms of certain species generally found in these lesions and which are used in diseased conditions caused by one or the other of these germs. The vaccine is administered subcutaneously by means of a syringe, but the quantity of the vaccine to be injected and the number of doses to be used should be left to the judgment of a competent veterinarian.

INFECTIOUS DISEASES.

By Rush Shippen Huidekoper, M. D., Vet.

[Revised by A. Eichhorn, D. V. S.]

GENERAL DISCUSSION.

An infectious disease may be defined as any malady caused by the introduction into the body of minute organisms of the vegetable or animal kingdom which have the power to multiply indefinitely and set free certain peculiar poisons which are chiefly responsible for morbid changes. Nearly all diseases of animals for which a definite cause may be attributed are caused by bacteria; such are tuberculosis, anthrax, blackleg, lockjaw, and others. There are some diseases, as, for instance, Texas fever and rabies, which are caused by a minute animal parasite known as protozoa, while others again, like lumpy jaw and aspergillosis, are caused by fungi. Besides there are infectious diseases in which the causative agents have never been successfully isolated, as they are so small that they can not be detected by the aid of the most powerful microscope, and accordingly they are termed as ultravisible viruses. Hog cholera, foot-and-mouth disease, smallpox, and others belong to this group.

Bacteria may be defined as very minute unicellular organisms of plantlike character. They multiply either by simple division or by spore formation, the latter usually taking place when the conditions pertaining to the growth of the bacteria become unfavorable. The spores are much more resistant to destruction than the bacteria which produce them.

Another group of parasites producing disease is known as protozoa. These are more complex than bacteria, and their artificial cultivation is also much more difficult than is the case with the bacterial parasites. Of the representatives of this group, causing disease in animals, are the trypanosomes, which are the causative factors of dourine and surra, and the piroplasma, which induce Texas fever in cattle and malaria or biliary fever of horses. There are also disease-producing fungi which are responsible for certain affections in horses; among these the most important are mycotic lymphangitis, or sporotrichosis, and streptotrichosis.

The introduction of the infection may take place in various ways. The most frequent method is by ingestion. Further, the entrance of the germs may occur by inhalation, skin abrasions, wounds of any kind, through the genital organs, and at times also through the milk ducts of the teats. As a general rule infectious diseases have a period of incubation which comprises the time elapsing between the exposure to the infection and the actual appearance of the disease. This period varies in the different diseases.

The treatment of infectious diseases is, as a rule, unsatisfactory. When the symptoms have once appeared a disease is liable to run its course in spite of treatment, and if it is one from which animals usually recover, all that can be done is to put them into the most favorable surroundings. Many infectious diseases lead sooner or later to death; treatment is useless so far as the sick animals are concerned, and it may be worse than useless for those not yet affected. All animals suffering with infectious diseases are more or less directly a menace to all others. They represent for the time being manufactories of disease germs, and they are giving them off more or less abundantly during the period of disease. They may infect others directly or they may scatter the virus about and the surroundings may become the future source of infection.

Therefore, in the control of infectious diseases prevention is the most important procedure. The isolation or segregation of healthy animals from infected ones should be primarily considered, and if at any time an animal manifests the symptoms of an infectious disease it is essential to protect the others from such a source of danger. In some of the infectious diseases it may become advisable to kill the infected animals in order to avoid the spread of the disease. This is especially important in diseases which are slow in their course, such as tuberculosis. At times when diseases appear in a country where they have not been prevalent it becomes advisable and necessary to protect the healthy herds by the slaughter of all the infected animals. Pursuance of this policy has resulted in control of the foot-and-mouth disease, and has proved to be a very satisfactory method of eradication.

DISINFECTION.

Disinfection is a very important phase in the control of infectious disease. This consists in the use of certain substances which possess the power to destroy bacteria or their spores, or both. The cheapest and most available for animal diseases are ordinary freshly slaked lime, or unslaked lime in powder form, chlorid of lime, crude carbolic acid, corrosive sublimate, formalin, formaldehyde gas, cresol, etc.

In the disinfection of stables and premises it is essential to execute the work in a most thorough manner. This may be satisfactorily accomplished by carrying out the following directions:

1. Sweep ceilings, side walls, stall partitions, floors, and other surfaces until free from cobwebs and dust.

2. Scrape away all accumulation of filth, and if woodwork has become decayed, porous, or absorbent, it should be removed, burned, and replaced with new material.

3. If floor is of earth, remove 4 inches from the surface, and in places stained with urine a sufficient depth should be replaced to expose fresh earth. All earth removed should be replaced with earth from an uncontaminated source; it would be better still to lay a new floor of concrete, which is very durable and easily cleaned.

4. All refuse and material from stable and barnyard should be removed to a place not accessible to cattle or hogs. The manure should be spread on fields and turned under, while the wood should be burned.

5. The entire interior of the stable, especially the feeding troughs and drains, should be saturated with a disinfectant, as liquor cresolis compositus (U. S. P.), or carbolic acid, 6 ounces to every gallon of water, to which 4 ounces of chlorid of lime should be added. The best method of applying the disinfectant and the lime wash is by means of a strong spray pump, such as those used by orchardists. This method is efficient in disinfection against most of the contagious and infectious diseases of animals, and should be applied immediately following any outbreak, and, as a matter of precaution, it may be used once or twice yearly.

6. It is important that arrangements be made to admit a plentiful supply of sunlight and fresh air by providing an ample number of windows, thereby eliminating dampness, bad odor, and other insanitary conditions. Good drainage is also very necessary.

If the use of liquor cresolis compositus, carbolic acid, or other coal-tar products is inadmissible because of the readiness with which their odor is imparted to milk and other dairy products, bichlorid of mercury may be used in proportion of 1 to 800, or 1 pound of bichlorid to 100 gallons of water. All portions of the stable soiled with manure, however, should first be thoroughly scraped and cleaned, as the albumin contained in manure would otherwise greatly diminish the disinfecting power of the bichlorid. Disinfection with this material should be supervised by a veterinarian or other person trained in the handling of poisonous drugs and chemicals, as the bichlorid is a powerful, corrosive poison. The mangers and the feed boxes, after drying, following spraying with this material, should be washed out with hot water, as cattle are especially susceptible to mercurial poisoning. The bichlorid solution should be applied by means of a spray pump, as recommended for the liquor cresolis compositus.

VACCINATION.

In recent years vaccination for the prevention of certain infectious diseases has been successfully developed, and without a doubt the future has a great deal in store for this phase of prevention. At the present time vaccination has been found effective against blackleg, hog cholera, anthrax, lockjaw, strangles, rabies, white scours, etc. It is always essential, of course, that the products used for the vaccination be pure and potent; also they should be employed only with the advice of competent authorities and with proper care. The biological products prepared for the cure and prevention of infections are prepared by manufacturers who, in order to conduct an interstate business, are required to obtain a license from the United States Department of Agriculture for the manufacture of such preparations.

Since July 1, 1913, the Department of Agriculture, by an act of Congress of March 4, 1913, has had control of the manufacture of biological products for the treatment of domestic animals. The numerous complaints which were received from time to time relative to the impotency of some of the preparations, and also the fact that in some instances the use of the products were directly responsible in causing outbreaks of disease, made the necessity for such control obvious. This supervision is no doubt of far-reaching importance, as it assures the users that the preparations are reliable.

INFLUENZA.

Synonyms.—Pinkeye, typhoid fever, epizooty, epihippic fever, hepatic fever, bilious fever, etc.; fièvre typhoïde, grippe (French); Pferdestaupe (German); gastro-enteritis of Vatel and d'Arboval; febris erysipelatodes, Zundel; typhus of Delafond.

Definition.—The term influenza is applied to a febrile, contagious, infectious disease of horses, which is characterized by a blood infection, with inflammation of the mucous membranes, which frequently involves the lungs. Inflammatory complications also occur in the form of swellings of the subcutis, tendons, and tendinous sheaths and laminæ of the feet. One attack usually protects the animal from future ones of the same disease, but not always. An apparently complete recovery is sometimes followed by serious sequelæ of the nervous and blood-vessel systems. Under certain conditions of the atmosphere or from unknown causes, the disease is very liable to assume an epizootic form, with tendency to complications of especial organs, as, at one period, the lungs, at another the intestines, etc.

The first description of influenza is given by Laurentius Rusius in 1301, when it spread over a considerable portion of Italy, causing great loss among the war horses of Rome and the surrounding district. Later, in 1648, an epizootic of this disease visited Germany and spread to other parts of Europe. In 1711, under the name of "epidemica equorum," it followed the tracks of the great armies all over Europe, causing immense losses among the horses, while rinderpest was scourging the cattle of the same regions. The two diseases were confounded with each other, and were, by the scientists of the day, supposed to be allied to the typhus, which was a plague to the human race at the same time. We find the first advent of this disease to the British Islands in an epizootic among the horses of London and the southern counties of England in 1732, which is described by Gibson. In 1758 Robert Whytt recounts the devastation of the horses of the north of Scotland from the same trouble. Throughout the eighteenth century a number of epizootics occurred in Hanover and other portions of Germany and in France, which were renewed early in the present century, with complications of the intestinal tract, which obtained for it its name of gastroenteritis. In 1766 it first attacked the horses in North America, but is not described as again occurring in a severe form until 1870–1872, when it spread over the entire country, from Canada south to Ohio, and then eastward to the Atlantic and westward to California. It is now a permanent disease in our large cities, selecting for the continuance of its virulence young or especially susceptible horses which pass through the large and ill-ventilated and uncleaned stables of dealers, and assumes from time to time an enzootic form, when from some reason its virulence increases. It assumes this form also when, from reasons of rural economy and commerce, large numbers of young and more susceptible animals are exposed to its contagion.

Etiology.—The experiments of Dieckerhoff many years ago proved that the disease may be transmitted to healthy animals by intravenous injection of warm blood from affected horses.

Further investigations revealed the fact that blood from affected horses, even when passed through porcelain filters, may transmit the disease, thereby proving that the causative agent belongs to the so-called filterable viruses. This has been further substantiated by Gaffky, who showed in his recent experiments that the disease may be transmitted with defibrinated as well as with filtered blood, in which cases the typical form of influenza developed in inoculated animals in from five to six days. These findings were also substantiated by Basset. Further observations have also proved that apparently recovered animals may harbor the infection for a long time and still be capable of transmitting the disease. Such virus carriers are no doubt responsible for numerous outbreaks of this disease when, in a locality free from the disease, it certainly appears after the introduction of an apparently healthy animal.

As one attack is usually self-protective, numbers of old horses, having had an earlier attack, are not capable of contracting it again; but, aside from this, young horses, especially those about four or five years of age, are much more predisposed to be attacked, while the older ones, even if they have not had the disease, are less liable to it. Again, the former age is that in which the horse is brought from the farm, where it has been free from the risk of exposure, and is sold to pass through the stables of the country taverns, the dirty, infected railway cars, and the foul stockyards and damp stables of dealers in our large cities. Overfed, fat, young horses which have just come through the sales stables are much more susceptible to contagion than the same horses are after a few months of steady work.

Pilger, in 1805, was the first to recognize infection as the direct cause of the disease. Roll and others studied the contagiousness of influenza, and, finding it so much more virulent and permanent in old stables than elsewhere, classed it as a " stall miasm." The contagion will remain in the straw bedding and droppings of the animal and in the feed in an infected stable for a considerable time and if these are removed to other localities it may be carried in them. It may be carried in the clothing of those who have been in attendance on horses suffering from the disease. The drinking water in troughs and even running water may hold the virus and be a means of its communication to other animals, even at a distance.

The studies of Dieckerhoff, in 1881, in regard to the contagion of influenza were especially interesting. He found that during a local enzootic, produced by the introduction of infected horses into an extensive stable otherwise perfectly healthy, the infection took place in what at first seemed to be a most irregular manner, but which was shown later to be dependent on the ventilation and currents of air through the various buildings. His experiments showed that the virus of influenza is excessively diffusible, and that it will spread rapidly to the roof of a building and pass by the apertures of ventilation to others in the neighborhood. The writer has seen cases that have appeared to spread through a brick wall and attack animals on the opposite side before others even in the same stable were affected. Brick walls, old woodwork, and the dirt which is too frequently left about the feed boxes of a horse stall will hold the contagion for several days, if not weeks, and communicate it to susceptible animals when placed in the same locality. On two successive mornings a 4-year-old colt belonging to the writer stood for about 10 minutes at the open door, fully 40 feet from the stalls, of a stable in which two cases of influenza had broken out the day before; in six days the colt developed the disease. On the morning when the trouble in the colt was recognized it stood in an infirmary with a dozen horses that were being treated for various diseases, but was immediately isolated; within one week two-thirds of the other horses had contracted the disease.

Symptoms.—After the exposure of a susceptible horse to infection a period of incubation of from four to seven days elapses, during which the animal seems in perfect health, before any symptom is visible. When the symptoms of influenza develop they may be intense, or so moderate as to occasion but little alarm, but the latter condition frequently exposes the animal to use and to the danger of the exciting causes of complications which would not have happened had it been left quietly in its stall in place of being worked or driven out to show to prospective purchasers. The disease may run a simple course as a specific fever, with alterations only of the blood, or at any period it may become complicated by local inflammatory troubles, the gravity of which is augmented by developing in an animal with an impoverished blood, an already irritated, rapid circulation, and defective nutritive and reparative functions.

The first symptoms are those of a rapidly developing fever, which becomes intense within a very short period. The animal becomes dejected and inattentive to surrounding objects; stands with its head down, and not back on the halter as in serious lung diseases. In the flanks, the muscles of the croup and of the shoulders, or of the entire body it has chills lasting from 15 to 30 minutes, and frequently a grinding of the teeth which warns one that a severe attack may be expected. The hairs become dry and rough and stand on end. The body temperature increases to 104°, 104.5°, and 105° F., or even in severe cases to 107° F., within the first twelve or eighteen hours. The horse becomes stupid, stands immobile with its head hanging, the ears listless, and it pays but little attention to the surrounding attendants or the crack of a whip. The stupor becomes rapidly more marked, the eyes become puffy and swollen with excessive lacrimation, so that the tears run from the internal canthus of the eye over the cheeks and may blister the skin in their course. The respiration becomes accelerated to 25 or 30 in a minute, and the pulse is quickened to 70, 80, or even 100, moderate in volume and in force. There is great depression of muscular force; the animal stands limp, as if excessively fatigued. There is diminution, or in some cases total loss, of sensibility of the skin, so that it may be pricked or handled without attracting the attention of the animal. On movement, the horse staggers and shows a want of coordination of all the muscles of its limbs. The senses of hearing, sight, and taste are diminished, if not entirely destroyed. The visible mucous membranes (as the conjunctiva), from which it received the name pinkeye, and the mouth, and the natural openings become of a deep saffron, ocher, or violet-red color. This latter is especially noticeable on the rim of the gums and is a condition not found in any other disease, so that it is an almost diagnostic symptom. In some outbreaks there is much more swelling of the lids and weeping from the eyes than in others. If the animal is bled at this period the blood is found more coagulable than normal, but at a later period it becomes of a dark color and less coagulable. There is great diminution or total loss of appetite, with an excessive thirst, but in many cases cold-blooded horses may retain a certain amount of appetite, eating slowly at hay, oats, or other feed. There is some irritation of the mucous membrane of the respiratory tract, as shown by discharge of mucus from the nose, and by cough. Pregnant mares are liable to abort.

We have, following the fever, a tumefaction, or edema, of the subcutaneous tissues at the fetlocks, of the under surface of the belly, and of the sheath of the penis, which may be excessive. The infiltration is noninflammatory in character and produces an insensibility of the skin like the excessive stocking which we see in debilitated animals after exposure to cold. In ordinary cases the temperature has reached its maximum of 105° or 106° F. in from 24 to 48 hours from the origin of the fever. It remains stationary for a period of from 3 to 4 days without so much variation between morning and evening temperature as we have in pneumonia or other serious diseases of the lungs. At the termination of the specific course of the disease, which is generally from 6 to 10 days, the fever abates, the swelling of the legs and under surface of belly diminishes, the appetite returns, the strength is rapidly regained, the mucous membranes lose their yellowish color, which they attain so rapidly at the commencement of the disease, and the animal convalesces promptly to its ordinary good condition and health, and rapidly regains the large amount of weight which it lost in the early part of the disease, a loss which frequently reaches 30, 50, or even 75 pounds each 24 hours. For the first three days of the high temperature there is a great tendency to constipation, which should be avoided if possible by the use of the means recommended below, for, if it has been marked, it may be followed by a troublesome diarrhea.

Terminations.—The terminations of simple influenza may be death by extreme fever, with failure of the heart's action; from excessive coma, due generally to a rapid congestion of the brain; to the poisonous effects of the débris of the disintegrated blood corpuscles and the toxin of the disease; to an asphyxia, following congestion of the lungs; or the disease terminates by subsidence of the fever, return of the appetite and nutritive functions of the organs, and rapid convalescence; or, in an unfortunately large number of cases, the course of the disease is complicated by local inflammatory troubles, whose gravity is greater in influenza than it is when they occur as sporadic diseases.

Complications.—The complications are congestions, followed by inflammatory phenomena in the various organs of the body, but they are most commonly located in the intestines, lungs, brain, or vascular laminæ of the feet. Atmospheric influence or other surrounding influences of unknown quality seem to be an important factor in the determination of the local lesions. At certain seasons of the year, and in certain epizootics, we find 40 and 50 per cent or even a greater percentage of the cases rendered more serious by complication of the intestines; at other seasons of the year, or in other epizootics, we find the same percentage of cases complicated by inflammation of the lungs, while at the same time a small percentage of them are complicated by troubles of the other organs; inflammatory changes of the brain, of the laminæ, more rarely commence in epizootic form, but are to be found in a certain small percentage of cases in all epizootics.

Exciting causes are important factors in complicating individual cases of influenza, or in localizing special lesions, during either enzootics or epizootics. These exciting or determining causes act much as they would in sporadic inflammatory diseases, but in this case we find the animal much more susceptible and predisposed to be acted upon than ordinary healthy animals. With a temperature already elevated, with the heart's action driving the blood in increased quantity into the distended blood vessels, which become dilated and lose their contractility, with a congestion of all the vascular organs already established, it takes but little additional irritation to carry the congestion one step further and produce inflammation.

Complication of the intestines.—When any cause acts as an irritant to the intestinal tract during the course of this specific fever it may produce inflammation of the organs belonging to it. This cause may be constipation, which can find relief only in a congestion which offers to increase the function of the glands and relieve the inertia caused by a temporary cessation of activity; or irritant medicines, especially any increased use of antimony, turpentine, or the more active remedies; the taking of indigestible feed, or of feed in too great quantities, or that has been altered in any way by fungus or other injurious alterations; the swallowing of too cold water; or any other irritant may cause congestion. This complication is ushered in by colics. The animal paws with the fore feet and evinces a great sensibility of the belly; it looks with the head from side to side, and may lie down and get up, not with violence, but with care for itself, perfectly protecting the surface of the belly from any violence. At first we find a decided constipation; the droppings if passed are small and hard, coated with a viscous varnish or even with false membranes. In from 36 to 40 hours the constipation is followed by diarrhea. The alimentary discharge becomes mixed with a sero-mucous exudation, which is followed by a certain amount of suppurative matter. The animal becomes rapidly exhausted and unstable, staggers on movement, losing the little appetite which may have remained, and has exacerbations of fever. The pulse becomes softer and weaker, the respiration becomes gradually more rapid, the temperature is about 1° to 1.5° F. higher. If a fatal result is not produced by the extensive diarrhea the discharge is arrested in from 5 to 10 days and a rapid recovery takes place.

Complication of the lungs.—If at any time during the course of the fever the animal is exposed to cold or drafts of air, or in any other way to the causes of repercussion, the lungs may become affected. In the majority of cases, however, after three, four, or five days of the fever, congestion of the lungs commences without any exposure or apparent exciting cause. Unless this congestion of the lungs is soon relieved it is followed by an inflammation constituting pneumonia. This pneumonia, while it is in its essence the same, differs from an ordinary pneumonia at the commencement by an insidious course. The animal commences to breathe heavily, which is distinctly visible in the heaving of the flanks, the dilatation of the nostrils, and frequently in the swaying movement of the unsteady body. The respirations increase in number, what little appetite remained is lost, the temperature increases from 1° to 2°, the pulse becomes more rapid, and at times, for a short period, more tense and full, but the previous poisoning of the specific disease has so weakened the tissues that it never becomes the characteristic full, tense pulse of a simple pneumonia.

On percussion of the chest dullness is found over the inflamed areas; on auscultation at the base of the neck over the trachea a tubular murmur is heard. The crepitant râles and tubular murmurs of pneumonia are heard on the sides of the chest if the pneumonia is peripheral, but in pneumonia complicating influenza the inflamed portions are frequently disseminated in islands of variable size and are sometimes deep-seated, in which case the characteristic auscultory symptoms are sometimes wanting. From this time on the symptoms of the animal are those of an ordinary grave pneumonia, rendered more severe by occurring in a debilitated animal. The cough is at first hacky and aborted; later, more full and moist. There is discharge from the nostrils, which may be mucopurulent, purulent, or hemorrhagic. As in simple pneumonia, in the outset this discharge may be "rusty," owing to capillary hemorrhages. We find that the blood is thoroughly mixed with the matter, staining it evenly, instead of being mixed with it in the form of clots. At the commencement of the complication the animal may be subject to chills, which may again occur in the course of the disease, in which case, if severe, an unfavorable termination by gangrene may be looked for. If gangrene occurs it is shown by preliminary chills, a rapid elevation of temperature, a tumultuous heart, a flaky discharge from the nostrils, and a fetid breath; the symptoms are identical with those which occur in gangrene complicating other diseases.

Complication of the brain.—At any time during the course of the disease congestion of the brain may occur; at an early period if the fever has been intense from the outset, but in ordinary cases more frequently after three or four days. The animal, which has been stupid and immobile, becomes suddenly restless, walks forward in the stall until it fastens its head in the corner. If in a box stall and it becomes displaced from its position, it follows the wall with the nose and eyes, rubbing it along until it reaches the corner and again fastens itself. It may become more violent and rear and plunge. If disturbed by the entrance of the attendant or any loud noise or bright light, it will stamp with its fore feet and strike with its hind feet, but is not definite in fixing the object which it is resisting, which is a diagnostic point between meningitis and rabies and which renders the animal with the former disease less dangerous to handle. If fastened by a rope to a stake or post, the animal will wander in a circle at the end of the rope. It wanders almost invariably in one direction. The pupils may be dilated or contracted, or we may find one condition in one eye and the opposite in the other.

The period of excitement is followed by one of profound coma, in which the animal is immobile, the head hanging and placed against the corner of the stall, the body limp, and the motion, if demanded of the animal, unsteady. Little or no attention is paid to the surrounding noises, the crack of a whip, or even a blow on the surface of the body. The respiration becomes slower, the pulsations are diminished, the coma lasts for variable time, to be followed by excesses of violence, after which the two alternate, but if severe the period of coma becomes longer and longer until the animal dies of spasms of the lungs or of heart failure. It may die from injuries which occur in the ungovernable attacks of violence.

Complication of the feet.—The feet are the organs which are next in frequency predisposed to congestion. This congestion takes place in the laminæ (podophyllous structures) of the feet. The stupefied animal is roused from its condition by excessive pain in the feet and assumes the position of a foundered horse; that is, if the fore feet alone are affected, they are carried forward until they rest on the heels; and if the hind feet are affected, all the feet are carried forward, resting on their heels, the hind ones as near the center of gravity as possible. In some cases the stupor of the animal is so great that the pain is not felt, and little or no change of the position of the animal is noticeable. The foot is found hot to the touch, and after a given time the depressed convex sole of typical founder is recognized.

Pleurisy.—This is a rare complication, but when it does occur it is ushered in by the usual symptoms of depression, rapid pulse, small respiration, elevation of the temperature, subcutaneous edema of the legs and under surface of the belly, and we find a line of dullness on either side of the chest and an absence of respiratory murmur at the lower part. If it is severe, there may be an effusion filling one-fourth to one-third of the thoracic cavity in from 36 to 48 hours.

Pericarditis is an occasional complication of influenza. It is ushered in by chills, elevation of the temperature; the pulse becomes rapid, thready, and imperceptible. The heart murmurs become indistinct or can not be heard. A venous pulse is seen on the line of the jugular veins along the neck. Respiration becomes more difficult and rapid. If the animal is moved the symptoms become more marked or it may drop dead from heart failure.

Peritonitis, or inflammation of the membranes lining the belly and covering the organs contained in it, sometimes takes place. The general symptoms are similar to those of a commencing pericarditis. The local symptoms are those of pain, especially to pressure on side of the flanks and belly, distention of the latter, and sometimes the formation of flatus, or gas, and constipation.

Other occasional complications are nephritis, hepatitis, inflammation of the flexor tendons and rupture of them, and abscesses.

Diagnosis.—The diagnosis of influenza is based upon continued fever, with great depression and symptoms of stupor and coma; the rapidly developing, dark-saffron, ocher, yellowish discoloration of the mucous membranes, swelling of the legs and soft tissues of the genitals. When these symptoms have become manifested the diagnosis of a local complication is based upon the same symptoms that are produced in the local diseases from other causes, but in influenza the local symptoms are frequently masked or even entirely hidden by the intense stupor of the animal, which renders it insensible to pain. The evidence of colic and congestion, which is followed by diarrhea, indicates enteritis. The rapid breathing or difficulty of respiration points to a complication of the lungs, but, as we have seen in the study of the symptoms, the local evidences of lung lesions are frequently hidden. Again, we have seen that inflammation of the feet, or founder, complicating influenza is frequently not shown on account of the insensibility to pain on the part of the animal, which indicates the importance of running the hand daily over the hoofs to detect any sudden elevation of temperature on their surface.

The diagnosis of brain trouble is based upon the excessive violence which occurs in the course of the disease, for during the intervening period or coma there is no means of determining that it is due to this complication. Severe cases of influenza may simulate anthrax in the horse. In both we have stupor, the intense coloration of the mucous membranes of the eyes, and a certain amount of swelling of the legs and under surface of the belly. The diagnosis here can be made only by microscopic examination of the blood. In strangles, equine variola, and scalma we have an intensely red, rosy coloration of the mucous membranes, full, tense pulse, and although in these diseases we may have depression, we do not have the stupor and coma except in severe cases which have lasted for several days. In influenza we have no evidence of the formation of pus on the mucous membranes as in the other diseases, except sometimes in the conjunctivæ.

In severe pneumonia (lung fever) we may find profound coma, dark-yellowish coloration of the mucous membranes, and swelling of the under surface of the belly and legs; but in pneumonia we have the history of the difficulty of breathing and an acute fever of a strong type from the outset, and the other symptoms do not occur for several days, while in influenza we have the history of characteristic symptoms for several days before the rapid breathing and difficulty of respiration indicate the appearance of the complication. Without the history it is frequently difficult to diagnose a case of influenza of several days' standing, complicated by pneumonia, from a case of severe pneumonia of five or six days' standing, but from a prognostic point of view it is immaterial, as the treatment of both are identical. The fact that other horses in the same stable or neighborhood have influenza may aid in the diagnosis.

Prognosis.—Influenza is a serious disease chiefly on account of its numerous complications. Uncomplicated influenza is a comparatively simple malady, and is fatal in but 1 to 5 per cent of all cases. In some outbreaks, however, complications of one kind or another preponderate; in such instances the rate of mortality is much increased.

Alterations.—The chief alteration of influenza occurs in the digestive tract, and consists of hyperemia, infiltration, and swelling of the mucous membrane, and especially of the Peyer's patches near the ileocecal valve. The tissues throughout the body are found stained, and of a more or less yellowish hue. There is always found a congested condition of all the organs, muscles, and interstitial tissues of the body. The coverings of the brain and spinal cord partake in the congested and discolored condition of the rest of the tissues.

Other alterations are dependent entirely upon the complications. If the lungs have been affected, we find effusions identical in their intimate nature with those of simple pneumonia, but they differ somewhat in their general appearance in not being so circumscribed in their area of invasion. The alterations of meningitis and laminitis are identical with those of sporadic cases of founder and inflammation of the brain.

Treatment.—While the appetite remains the patient should have a moderate quantity of sound hay, good oats, and bran; or even a little fresh clover, if obtainable, can be given in small quantities. It is not so important that a special diet shall be observed as that the horse shall eat a moderate quantity of nourishing feed, and he may be tempted with any feed of good quality that he relishes. He should be placed in a well-ventilated box stall away from other horses. Grass, roots, apples, and milk may be offered and, if relished, allowed freely. To reduce the temperature the safest simple plan is to inject large quantities of cold water into the rectum. Antipyrene may be used with strychnia. Derivatives in the form of essential oils and mustard poultices, baths of turpentine and hot water, after which the animal must be immediately dried and blanketed, serve to waken the animal from the stupor and relieve the congestion of the internal organs. This treatment is especially indicated when complication by congestion of the lungs, intestines, or of the brain is threatened. Quinin and salicylic acid in 1-dram doses will lower the temperature, but too continuous use of the former in some cases increases the depression. Iodid of potash reduces the excessive nutrition of the congested organs and thereby reduces the temperature; again, this drug in moderate quantities is a stimulant to the digestive tract and acts as a diuretic, causing the elimination of waste matter by the kidneys. Small doses of Glauber's salt and bicarbonate of soda, used from the outset, stimulate the digestive tract and prevent constipation and its evil results.

In cases of severe depression and weakness of the heart digitalis can be used with advantage.

In complications of the intestines camphor and asafetida are most frequently used to relieve the pain causing the colics; diarrhea is also relieved by the use of bicarbonate of soda, nitrate of potash, and drinks made from boiled rice or starch, to which may be added small doses of laudanum.

In complication of the lungs iodid of potash and digitalis are most frequently indicated, in addition to the remedies used for the disease itself.

Founder occurring as a complication of influenza is difficult to treat. It is, unfortunately, frequently not recognized until inflammatory changes have gone on for several days. If recognized at once, local bleeding and the use of hot or cold water, as the condition of the animal may permit, are most useful, but in the majority of cases the stupefied animal is unable to be moved satisfactorily or to have one foot lifted for local treatment; the only treatment consists in local bleeding above the coronary bands and the application of poultices.

During convalescence small doses of alkalines may be kept up for a short time, but the greatest care must be used, while furnishing the animal with plenty of nutritious, easily digestible feed, not to overload the intestinal tract, causing constipation and consequent diarrhea. Special care must be taken for several weeks not to expose the animal to cold.

Prevention.—In order to prevent the introduction of the disease it is advisable to isolate newly purchased animals for at least a week. Further, the stabling of healthy horses in sales and feed stables should also be guarded against. At the beginning of an outbreak the disease may be checked by immediate isolation of the affected horses, by taking the temperatures of the healthy animals, and by the segregation of those showing a marked elevation.

Bacterial vaccines are now being prepared for the prevention of this disease and also for its cure, but to date the results are not convincing as to the beneficial action of these products. Since the cause of the disease has not yet been satisfactorily determined it is difficult to conceive how immunity could be produced with the aid of the germs which enter into the preparation of these products. The reports would indicate, however, that vaccines exert a favorable influence upon the course of the disease, probably preventing severe complications which under ordinary conditions are the principal factors in determining the severity of the outbreak.

CONTAGIOUS PNEUMONIA.

Synonyms.—Edematous pneumonia; stable pneumonia; equine pleuropneumonia; influenza pectoralis equorum; pleuropneumonia; influenzal pneumonia; Brustseuche (German).

Contagious pleuropnuemonia is an acute contagious disease of horses manifesting itself either as a croupous pneumonia or a pleuropneumonia with complications in the form of serous infiltrations of the subcutaneous tissues and tendons.

Etiology.—Investigators of this disease incriminated various kinds of microorganisms as the cause of this affection. Transmission experiments were usually negative with these organisms. This was also the case in attempts to transmit the disease by feeding with affected parts of the lungs, intestinal contents, and nasal discharge; likewise by intravenous or subcutaneous injections of blood and of emulsions made from nasal discharge, urine, the lung, and other organs.

The most recent experimental results of Gaffky and Lüher proved that at least at the beginning of the disease the bronchial secretion contains the infection. Upon killing horses affected with the typical forms of the disease on the third or fourth day of the affection the air passages are usually found to be filled with a yellowish, tenacious, germ-free secretion with which they succeeded in infecting healthy colts The virus has not been isolated. The possibility of its being a protozoan is suggested by the above-named investigators through their observations of round or rod-shaped bodies in the round cells of the secretions.

Two organisms were formerly especially considered to play an important part in the cause of the disease, the *Streptococcus pyogenes equi*, which has been isolated from most cases of the disease, and the *Bacillus equisepticus*, which by some investigators was considered to be the cause of contagious pleuropenumonia. Although there is no doubt as to the presence of these microorganisms in most of the cases, their association with the cause of this disease, however, is now doubted, especially since attempts to transmit the disease with pure cultures of these germs failed to reproduce the typical form of the disease. They, however, are of great significance in connection with the pathological changes occurring in connection with the infection and probably are the determining factor in the course of the disease. They exert their action after the animal has already been attacked by the true virus, and then produce the inflammatory changes attributed to these secondary invaders.

This disease is the adynamic pneumonia of the older veterinarians, who did not recognize any essential difference in its nature from an ordinary inflammation of the lungs, except in the profound sedation of the force of the animal affected with it, which is a prominent symptom from the outset of the disease. Again, this same prostration of the vital force of the animal, combined with the staggering movement and want of coordination of the muscles, caused it for a long time to be confounded with influenza, with which at certain periods it certainly has a strong analogy of symptoms, but from which, as from sporadic pneumonia, it can be separated very readily if the case can be followed throughout its whole course.

Infectious pneumonia is a specific inflammation of the lungs, accompanied with interstitial edema and inflammation of the tissues of these organs and a constitutional disturbance and fever. It causes a profound sedation of the nervous system, which may be so great as to cause death. It is sometimes attended with pleurisy, inflammation of the heart or septic complications, which also prove fatal.

Old, cold, damp, foul, unclean, and badly drained and ventilated stables allow rapid dissemination of the disease to other horses in the same stable and act as rich reservoirs for preserving the contagion, which may be retained for over a year.

The virus is but moderately volatile, and in a stable seems rather to follow the lines of the walls and irregular courses than the direct currents of air and the tracts of ventilation. Prof. Dieckerhoff found that the contagion of influenza was readily diffusible throughout an entire stable and through any opening to other buildings, but he also found that the contagion of infectious pneumonia is not transmissible at any great distance, nor is it very diffusible in the atmosphere. A brick wall 8 feet in height served, in one instance, to prevent the infection of other animals placed on the opposite side from a horse ill with the disease, while others placed on the same side and separated from the focus of contagion only by open bars in the stall were infected and developed the disease in its typical form.

Symptoms.—The symptoms differ slightly from those of a frank, fibrinous pneumonia, but not so much by the introduction of new symptoms as by the want of or absence of the distinct evidences of local lesions which are found in the latter disease. All the pneumonias throughout the whole course of the trouble are less marked and less clearly defined.

The symptoms may develop slowly or rapidly. If slowly, there is fever and the animal gives a rare cough which resembles that of a heavy horse affected with a slight chronic bronchitis; it becomes somewhat dejected and dull, at times somnolent, and has a diminished appetite. This condition lasts for several days, or the disease may begin with high fever, and the symptoms described below are severe and delevop in rapid sequence. The respiration increases to 24, 30, or 36 to the minute, and a small, running, soft pulse attains a rhythm of 50, 70, or even more beats in the sixty seconds. The heart, however, contrary to the debilitated condition of the pulse, is found beating violently and tumultuously, as it does in anthrax and septic intoxication. The mucous membranes of the eyes and mouth and of the genital organs are found somewhat edematous, and they rapidly assume a dirty, saffron color, at times approaching an ocher, but distinguishable from the similar coloration in influenza by the want of the luster belonging to the latter and by the muddy, dull tint, which is characteristic throughout the disease.

Suddenly, without the preliminary râles which precede grave lesions of the lungs in other diseases, the blowing murmur of pneumonia is heard over a variable area of the chest, usually, however, much more distinctly over the trachea at the base of the neck and directly behind the shoulder on each side of the chest. In some cases the evidence of lung lesion can be detected only over the trachea.

The lesions of the lungs may be scattered throughout both lungs, involving numerous small areas, or they may be confined to and more or less fully occupy one or two lobes. Occasionally there is a general involvement of both lungs. The body temperature has now reached 104° or 105° F., or in extreme cases even a degree higher. The debility of the animal is great without the stupefaction or evidence of cerebral trouble, which is constant with such grave constitutional phenomena in influenza or severe pneumonia. The animal is subject to occasional chills, and staggers in its gait. The yellow coloration of the visible mucous membrane is rendered pale by infiltration of the liquid of the blood into the tissues; the pulse may become so soft as to be almost imperceptible, the heart movement and sounds being at the same time exaggerated. The animal loses flesh rapidly, and dropsies of the extremities, of the under surface of the belly, or of the internal organs may show themselves.

Terminations.—These symptoms may gradually subside after five to eight days, with an improved appetite the inanition may cease and the animal commence to nourish its impoverished blood and tissues; the pulse becomes stronger and the heart more regular and less tumultuous; the mucous membranes assume a brighter and more distinct color; the difficulty of respiration is removed, and the animal may make a recovery. When death occurs it is usually directly due to heart failure; in some cases it is caused by asphyxia, owing to the great amount of exudation into the lung tissue, rendering its further function impossible.

Complications.—The pulmonary complications of infectious pneumonia are secondary inflammatory or necrotic changes in the lungs themselves. Suppuration at times takes place in the bronchi and may extend to the lung tissue. In this case mucous râles develop which are most distinctly heard over the trachea and on the sides of the chest directly behind the shoulders. With the development of the mucous râles, to be heard on auscultation, we have a more purulent discharge from the nostrils, similar to that of a chronic or subacute bronchitis. If the inflammation has been of some standing, cavernous râles may be heard, indicating the destruction of a considerable portion of lung tissue and the formation of a cavity. The effects of this more acute inflammatory process are not appreciable in the general condition of the animal, except to weaken it still further and add to its debilitated and emaciated cachexia. Gangrene sometimes occurs. A sudden rise of the body temperature of 1° or 2°, with a more enfeebled pulse and a still more tumultous heart, develop simultaneously with the appearance of a discharge from the nostrils. This discharge is gray in color, serous or watery in consistency, mixed with the detritus of broken-down lung tissue, and sometimes contains clots of blood, or in more serious cases may be marked by a quantity of fluid blood from a hemorrhage, which proves fatal. The discharge is fetid to the smell. The animal emaciates rapidly. On examination of the lungs mucous râles are heard in the larger bronchi, cavities may be found at any part of these organs, and points of lobular pneumonia may be detected.

A very serious complication is an inflammation of the heart muscle. This is shown by a very weak and rapid pulse, great prostration, some filling of the lungs. This complication nearly always terminates in death. Other complications which may be mentioned are inflammation of the kidneys, blood poisoning, congestion of the brain, and inflammation of the tendinous sheaths and the tendons of the legs.

Diagnosis.—As fever is the first symptom of infectious pneumonia, it is useful during an outbreak of this disease to make daily temperature measurements of the exposed horses, so that the first indication of disease may be discovered and the horse removed from contact with those that are sound.

Prognosis.—The mortality in this disease may be as high as 25 per cent, but it is usually not more than 10 per cent. If there is a special tendency to complications of some sort, the mortality is increased.

Alterations.—At the time of death from infectious pneumonia we frequently find septic changes and the evidences of putrefaction. The solidification of the lung tissue is found irregular in shape and high around the root of the lungs and the large bronchi, and is generally covered by sound lung tissue. The anterior lobes of the lungs are usually entirely affected. The diseased portion appears of a gray-yellowish color, somewhat watery, and tears readily. Matter is found in the air tubes which form gutters through the jellylike mass of the diseased lung. Abscesses from the size of a nut to larger masses may be found throughout the lungs. The blood is dark in color, fluid, or only clotted into soft, jellylike masses. Masses of gangrenous or dead-black tissue may be present.

Treatment.—Bleeding is not to be used, because it would only still further weaken an already enfeebled animal; antimony or the alterants would increase the depression of a too-depraved constitution. There is in this disease no acute congestion of a particular organ to draw off by depletive measures, nor any violent blood current to be retarded, for fear of hypernutrition of any special part.

Revulsives do good, as they excite the nervous system and awaken the torpor of the weakened blood vessels, which aid in the reestablishment of the functions. As in other diseases, mustard poultices may be applied over the belly and sides of the chest, but caution must be used in the employment of blisters, as ugly ulcers may result from their action on a tissue of weakened vitality. Setons are dangerous from the great tendency in this disease to septic complications. Repeated friction of the legs by hand-rubbing and warmth by bandaging and by rubbing the surface of the body with turpentine and alcohol, which is immediately to be dried by rough towels, will excite the circulation and stimulate the emunctories of the skin.

Stimulants are given internally from the outset of the disease. Turpentine in 1-dram doses regulates the heart and excites the kidneys to carry off waste matter, but if repeated too frequently may disturb the already delicate digestive system. The aromatics and bitter tonics are useful; gentian and tea in warm decoction form a useful menstruum for other remedies. Digitalis is a useful remedy. Strychnin and quinin may be given throughout almost the whole course of the disease. The various preparations of iron are astringents and excitants to the digestive system. Creosote is an antiputrid which is of marked benefit in edematous pneumonia; it may be given in doses of 15 to 30 minims in a pint of milk.

Salicylic acid may be given in 1 or 2 dram doses every few hours. It is much used for troubles of the serous membranes, lowers the temperature, and is of value in this disease in preventing the exudation into the tissue of the lungs. The alkalines, as the sulphate and bicarbonate of soda, the nitrate of potash, and very small doses of the iodid of potash, should be employed to regulate the digestive tract, the kidneys, and the other excreting glands, and to stimulate absorption of the waste matter.

The biological products enumerated under the treatment of the catarrhal form of influenza are also recommended for this disease. The bacterial vaccines in particular are being employed to a great extent, but the results are not uniformly satisfactory, especially with regard to prevention. They might, however, exert a beneficial influence against an attack of the secondary invaders and complications. A serum is also being prepared especially for the treatment of this disease, and since this is obtained from animals which have been highly immunized against the various organisms found in association with influenza it no doubt is beneficial, especially when the life of the animal is threatened. Such serum, however, should be used in sufficiently large doses, as repeated experience has proved that small doses have no beneficial action on the disease.

More recently salvarsan is being highly recommended for the treatment of the pneumonic form of influenza, and by many investigators it is considered as a specific for this affection. A single injection of this preparation is supposed to result in a rapid clearing of the lungs and the recovery of the animal is hastened. The cost of this product, however, at the present time, is exorbitant, and it should be considered only in the treatment of very valuable animals.

The same procedure as given for influenza should be carried out in the prevention of this affection.

The diet demands the strictest attention from the outset. In many of the fevers the feed has to be diminished in quantity and regulated in the quality of its heat-producing components during the acute part of the disease, so as to lessen the material for combustion in the inflamed organs. In edematous pneumonia, on the contrary, all the feed that can possibly be digested and assimilated must be given. Choice must be made of the richest material which can be handled by the weakened stomach and intestines without fatiguing them. Good, sound hay should be chopped short and dampened or partly boiled; in the latter case the hay tea can be reserved to use as a drink. Oats may be preferred dry or in other cases are taken better scalded; in most cases, however, it is better to give slops of oatmeal, to which may be added a little bran, barley flour, or boiled milk and wheat flour. Pure cow's milk, not too rich in fatty matter, may be given alone or with beaten eggs; frequently the horse has to be coaxed with the milk diluted with several parts of water at first, but will soon learn to drink the pure milk. Apples and carrots cut up raw or boiled are useful, and fresh clover in small quantities will frequently stimulate the appetite. In other words, various feeds and combinations should be given to the horse. Throughout the course of the disease and during convalescence the greatest attention must be taken to cleaning the coat thoroughly so as to keep the glands of the skin in working order, and light, warm covering must be used to protect the animal from cold or drafts of air.

STRANGLES.

Synonyms.—Distemper; colt-ill; catarrhal fever; one form of shipping fever; febris pyogenica.

Definition.—Strangles is an infectious disease of the horse, mule, and ass, seen most frequently in young animals, and usually leaving them immune from future trouble of the same kind.

It appears as a fever lasting for a few days, and is usually associated with an abscess formation of lymph glands, especially those under the jaw, which have a tendency to break on the outside. It usually leaves the animal after convalescence perfectly healthy and as good as it was before, but sometimes leaves it a roarer or is followed by the development of deep-seated abscesses which may prove fatal.

Causes.—The cause of strangles is infection by direct contact with an animal suffering from the disease, or indirectly through contact with the discharges from an infected animal, or by means of the atmosphere in which an infected animal has been. There are many predisposing causes which render some animals much more subject to contract the disease than others. Early age, which has given it the popular name of colt-ill, offers many more subjects than the later periods of life do, for the animal can contract the disease but once, and the large majority of adult and old animals have derived an immunity from previous attacks. At 3, 4, or 5 years of age the colt, which has been at home, safe on a meadow or in a cozy barnyard, far from all intercourse with other animals or sources of contagion, is first put to work and driven to the market town or county fairs to be exposed to an atmosphere or to stables contaminated by other horses suffering from disease and serving as infecting agents. If it fails to contract it there, it is sold and shipped in foul, undisinfected railway cars to dealers' stables, equally unclean, where it meets many opportunities of infection. If it escapes so far, it reaches the time for heavier work and daily contact on the streets of towns or large cities, with numerous other horses and mules, some of which are sure to be the bearers of the germs of this or some other infectious disease, and at last it succumbs.

The period of the eruption of the last permanent teeth, or the end of the period of development from the colt to an adult horse, at which time the animals usually have a tendency to fatten and be excessively full-blooded, also seems to be a predisposing period for the contraction of this as well as of the other infectious diseases. Thoroughbred colts are very susceptible, and frequently contract strangles at a somewhat earlier age than those of more humble origin. Mules and asses are much less susceptible and are but rarely affected. Other animals are not subject to this disease, but there is a certain analogy between it and distemper in dogs. After exposure to infection there is a period of incubation of the disease, lasting from two to four days, during which the animal enjoys its ordinary health.

Symptoms.—The horse at first is a little sluggish if used, or when placed in its stable is somewhat dejected, paying but moderate attention to the various disturbing surroundings. Its appetite is somewhat diminished in many cases, while in some cases the animal eats well throughout. Thirst is increased, but not a great deal of water is taken at one time. If a bucket of water is placed in the manger the patient will dip its nose into it and swallow a few mouthfuls, allowing some of it to drip back and then stop, to return to it in a short time. The coat becomes dry and the hairs stand on end. At times the horse will have chills of one or the other leg, the fore quarters, or hind quarters, or in severe cases of the whole body, with trembling of the muscles and dryness of the skin.

If the eyes and mouth are examined the membranes are found reddened to a bright rosy color. The pulse is quickened and the breathing may be slightly accelerated. At the end of two days a cough is heard and a discharge begins to come from the nostrils. This discharge is at first watery; it then becomes thicker, somewhat bluish in color, and sticky, and finally it assumes the yellowish color of matter and increases greatly in quantity.

At the outset the colt may sneeze occasionally and a cough is heard. The cough is at first repeated and harsh, but soon becomes softer and moist as the discharge increases. Again, the cough varies according to the source of the discharge, for in light cases this may be only a catarrh of the nasal canals, or it may be from the throat, the windpipe, or the air tubes of the lungs, or even from the lungs themselves. According to the organ affected the symptoms and character of cough are similar to those of a laryngitis, bronchitis, or lung fever caused by ordinary cold.

Shortly after the discharge is seen a swelling takes place under the jaw, or in the intermaxillary space. This is at first puffy, somewhat hot and tender, and finally becomes distinctly so, and an abscess is felt, or having broken itself the discharge is seen dripping from a small opening. When the discharge from the nostrils has fully developed the fever usually disappears and the animal regains its appetite, unless the swelling is sufficient to interfere with the function of the throat, causing pain on any attempt to swallow. At the end of four or six days the discharge lessens, the soreness around the throat diminishes, the horse regains its appetite, and in two weeks has regained its usual condition. Old and strong horses may have the disease in so light a form that the fever is not noticeable; they may continue to eat and perform their ordinary work as usual and no symptom may be seen beyond a slight discharge from the nose and a rare cough, which is not sufficient to worry any but the most particular owner. But, on the other hand, the disease may assume a malignant form or become complicated so as to become a most serious disease, and even prove fatal in many cases. Inflammation of the larynx and bronchi, if excessive, produce violent, harsh coughing, which may almost asphyxiate the animal. The large amount of discharge may be mixed with air by the difficult breathing, and the nostrils, the front of the animal, manger, and surrounding objects become covered with a white foam. The inflammation may be in the lung itself (lobular pneumonia) and cause the animal to breathe heavily, heave at the flanks, and show great distress. In this condition marked symptoms of fever are seen, the appetite is lost, the coat

54763°—23——34

is dry, the horse stands back in its stall at the end of the halter strap with its neck extended and its legs propped apart to favor breathing. This condition may end by resolution, leaving the horse for some time with a severe cough, or the animal may die from choking up of the lungs (asphyxia).

The swelling under the jaw may be excessive, and if the abscess is not opened it burrows toward the throat or to the side and causes inflammation of the parotid glands and breaks in annoying fistulas at the sides of the throat and even up as high as the ears. Roaring may occur either during a moderately severe attack from inflammation of the throat (larynx), or at a later period as the result of continued lung trouble. Abscesses may develop in other parts of the body, in the poll, in the withers, or in the spaces of loose tissue under the arms, in the fold of the thigh, and, in entire horses, in the testicles.

During the course of the disease, or later, when the animal seems to be on the road to perfect recovery, abscesses may form in the internal organs and produce symptoms characteristic of disease of those parts.

Roaring, plunging, wandering in a circle, or standing with the head wedged in a corner of the stall indicate the collection of matter in the brain. Sudden and severe lung symptoms, without previous discharge, point to an abscess between the lungs, in the mediastinum; colic, which is often continuous for days, is the result of the formation of an abscess in some part of the abdominal cavity, usually in the mesentery.

Pathology.—The lesions of strangles are found on the surface of the mucous membranes, essentially of the respiratory system, and in the loose connective tissue fibers of the internal organs and glands, and consist of acute inflammatory changes, tending to the formation of matter. The blood is unaltered, though it is rich in fibrin, and if the animal has died of asphyxia it is found dark colored and uncoagulated when the body is first opened. If the animal has died while suffering from high fever the ordinary alterations throughout the body, which are produced by any fever not attended by alteration of blood, are found.

Prevention.—Healthy horses should be separated from the infected animals, and the stables in which the disease has occurred should be thoroughly disinfected. Since the disease frequently occurs annually on infected premises, systematic disinfection should be practiced after an outbreak. The stables, as well as all utensils which might have come in contact with the infection, should be thoroughly disinfected. By such practices recurrences of the disease may be prevented.

Treatment.—Ordinary light cases require but little treatment beyond diet, warm washes, moistened hay, warm coverings, and protection from exposure to cold. The latter is urgently called for, as lung complications, severe bronchitis, and laryngitis are often the results of neglect of this precaution. If the fever is excessive, the horse may receive small quantities of Glauber's salt (handful three times a day) as a laxative, bicarbonate of soda or niter in one-dram doses every few hours, and small doses of antimony, iodid of potash, aconite, or quinin. Steaming the head with the vapor of warm water poured over a bucket of bran and hay, in which belladonna leaves or tar have been placed, will allay the inflammation of the mucous membranes and greatly ease the cough.

The swelling of the glands should be promptly treated by flaxseed poultices and bathing with warm water, and as soon as there is any evidence of the formation of matter it should be opened. Prompt action in this will often save serious complications. Blisters and irritating liniments should *not* be applied to the throat. When lung complications show themselves the horse should have mustard applied to the belly and to the sides of the chest. When convalescence begins great care must be taken not to expose the animal to cold, which may bring on relapses, and while exercise is of great advantage it must not be turned into work until the animal has entirely regained its strength.

Bacterial vaccines are now being extensively used for the prevention and treatment of this disease. They are prepared from the specific germ of the disease and frequently exert a very beneficial influence. A serum is also being prepared from horses, which is injected with gradually increasing doses of this germ. This serum possesses considerable curative value and may prove especially valuable in cases in which the animals have failed to respond to other forms of treatment, or when valuable animals are affected with the disease.

PURPURA HEMORRHAGICA.

Synonyms.—Anasarca; petechial fever; morbus maculosus.

Definition.—This disease is a septic bacterial intoxication, acute and infectious in character, and is manifested by edematous swellings of the subcutaneous connective tissue, and hemorrhages on the mucous membrane and in the internal organs.

A previous attack of influenza is a common predisposing cause of this disease, which appears most frequently a few weeks after convalescence is established. It occurs more frequently in those animals which have made a rapid convalescence and are apparently perfectly well than it does in those which have made a slower recovery.

Anasarca commences by symptoms which are excessively variable. The local lesions may be confined to a small portion of the animal's body and the constitutional phenomena be nil. The appearance and gravity of the local lesions may be so unlike, from difference of location, that they seem to belong to a separate disease, and complications may completely mask the original trouble.

In the simplest form the first symptom noticed is a swelling, or several swellings, occurring on the surface of the body—on the forearm, the leg, the under surface of the belly, or the side of the head. The tumefaction is at first the size of a hen's egg; not hot, little sensitive, and distinctly circumscribed by a marked line from the surrounding healthy tissue. These tumors gradually extend until they coalesce, and in a few hours we have swelling of the legs, legs and belly, or the head, to an enormous size; they have always the characteristic constricted border, which looks as if it had been tied with a cord. In the nostrils are found small reddish spots, or petechiæ, which gradually assume a brownish and freqently a black color. Examination of the mouth will frequently reveal similar lesions on the surface of the tongue, along the lingual gutter, and on the frænum. If the external swelling has been on the head, the petechiæ of the mucous membranes are liable to be more numerous and to coalesce into patches of larger size than when the dropsy is confined to the legs. The animal may be rendered stiff by the swelling of the legs, or be annoyed by an awkward swollen head, which at times may be so enormous as to resemble that of a hippopotamus rather than that of a horse. During this period the temperature remains normal; the pulse, if altered at all, is only a little weaker; the respiration is only hurried if the swelling of the head infringes on the caliber of the nostrils. The appetite remains normal. The animal is attentive to all that is going on, and, except for the swelling, apparently in perfect health.

In from two to four days, in severe cases, the tissues can no longer resist the pressure of the exuded fluid. Over the surface of the skin which covers the dropsy we find a slight serous sweating, which loosens the epidermis and dries so as to simulate the eruption of some cutaneous disease. If this is excessive we may see irritated spots which are suppurating. In the nasal fossæ the hemorrhagic spots have acted as irritants, and, inviting an increased amount of blood to the Schneiderian membrane, produce a coryza or even a catarrh. We may now find some enlargement and peripheral edema of the lymphatic glands, which are fed from the affected part. The thermometer indicates a slight rise in the body temperature, while the pulse and respiration are somewhat accelerated. The appetite usually remains good. In the course of a few days the temperature may have reached 102°, 103°, or 104° F.

Fever is established, not an essential or specific fever in any way, but a simple secondary fever produced by the dead material from the surface or superficial suppuration, and by the oxidization and absorption of the colloid mass contained in the tissues. The skin may suppurate or slough more or less over the areas of greatest tension or where it is irritated by blows or pressure. The great swelling about the head may by closure of the nostrils interfere seriously with breathing. Internal edema may occur in the throat, lungs, or intestines. Septicemia, or blood poisoning, may result from anasarca.

Terminations.—The simple form of the disease most frequently terminates favorably on the eighth or tenth day by resolution or absorption of the effusion, with usually a profuse diuresis, and with or without diarrhea. The appetite remains good or is at times capricious.

Death may occur from mechanical asphyxia, produced by closure of the nostrils or closure of the glottis. Metastasis to the lungs is almost invariably fatal, causing death by asphyxia. Metastasis to the intestines may cause death from pain, enteritis, or hemorrhage.

Excessive suppuration, lymphangitis, and gangrene are causes of a fatal termination by exhaustion. Mortal exhaustion is again produced by inability to swallow in cases of excessive swelling of the head.

Peritonitis may arise secondary to the enteric edema, or by perforation of the stomach or intestines by a gangrenous spot. Septicemia terminates fatally with its usual train of symptoms.

Alterations.—The essential alterations of anasarca are exceedingly simple; the capillaries are dilated, the lymphatic spaces between the fibers of the connective tissue are filled with serum, and the coagulable portion of the blood presents a yellowish or citrine mass, jellylike in consistency, which has stretched out the tissue like the meshes of a sponge. Where the effusion has occurred between the muscles, as in the head, these are found dissected and separated from each other like those of a hog's head by the masses of fat. The surface of the skin is desquamated and frequently denuded of the hair. Frequently there are traces of suppuration and of ulceration. The mucous membrane of the nose is found studded with small, hemorrhagic spots, sometimes red, more frequently brown or black, often coalesced with each other in irregular-sized patches and surrounded by a reddish zone, the product of irritation. If edema of the intestines has occurred, the membrane is found four or five times its normal thickness, reddish in color, with hemorrhages on the free surface. Edema of the lungs leaves these organs distended. The secondary alterations vary according to the complications. There are frequently the lesions of asphyxia; externally we find ulcers, abscesses, and gangrenous spots and the deep ulcers resulting from the latter. The lymphatic cords and glands are found with all the lesions of lymphangitis. Again are found the traces of excessive emaciation, or the lesions of septicemia. Except from the complications the blood is not altered in anasarca.

Diagnosis.—The diagnosis of anasarca must principally be made from farcy or glanders. In anasarca the swelling is nonsensitive, while sensitive in the acute swelling of farcy. The nodes of farcy are distinct and hard and never circumscribed, as in the other disease. The eruption of glanders on the mucous membranes is nodular, hard, and pelletlike. The redness disappears on pressure. In case of excessive swelling of the head in anasarca, there may occur an extensive serofibrinous exudation from the mucous membranes of the nose, poured out as a semifluid mass or as a cast of the nasal fossæ, never having the appearance or typical oily character which it has in glanders. The inflammation of the lymphatic cords and glands in anasarca does not produce the indurated character which is found in farcy.

Prognosis.—While anasarca is not an excessively fatal disease, the prognosis must always be guarded. The majority of cases run a simple course and terminate favorably at the end of 8 or 10 days, or possibly, after one to two relapses, requiring several weeks for complete recovery. Effusion into the head renders the prognosis much more grave from the possible danger of mechanical asphyxia. Threatened mechanical asphyxia is especially dangerous on account of the risk of blood poisoning after an operation of tracheotomy. Edema of the viscera is a most serious complication. The prognosis is based on the complications, their extent, and their individual gravity, existing, as they do here, in an already debilitated subject.

Treatment.—The treatment of anasarca may be as variable as are the lesions. The indications are at once shown by the alterations and mechanism of the disease, which we have just studied.

Hygiene comes into play as the most important factor. Oats, oat-and-hay tea, milk, eggs—anything which the stomach or rectum can be coaxed to take care of—must be employed to give the nutriment, which is the only thing that will permanently strengthen the tissues; they must be strengthened in order to keep the capillaries at their proper caliber.

Laxatives, diaphoretics, and diuretics must be used to stimulate the emunctories so that they may carry off the large amount of the products of decomposition which result from the stagnated effusions of anasarca. Of these the sulphate of soda in small, repeated doses, the nitrate of potash and bicarbonate of soda in small quantity, or the chlorate of potash in single large doses will be found useful. Williams cites the chlorate of potash as an antiputrid. Stimulants and astringents are directly indicated. Spirits of turpentine serves the double purpose of a cardiac stimulant and a powerful, warm diuretic, for the kidneys in this disease will stand a wonderful amount of work. Camphor can be used with advantage. Coffee and tea are two of the diffusible stimulants which are too much neglected in veterinary medicine; both are valuable adjuncts in treatment of anasarca, as they are during convalescence at the end of any grave disease which has tended to render the patient anemic. Dilute sulphuric and hydrochloric acids are, perhaps, the best examples of a combination of stimulant, astringent, and tonic which can be employed. The simple astringents of mineral origin, sulphates of iron, copper, etc., are useful as digestive tonics; I doubt whether they have any constitutional effect. The vegetable astringents, tannic acid, etc., have not proved efficacious in my hands. Iodid of potash in small doses serves the triple purpose of digestive tonic, denutritive for inflammantion, and diuretic. Among the newer forms of treatment are diluted Lugol's solution injected into the trachea, antistreptococcus serum and colloidal silver solution injected into the circulation. No one but a qualified veterinarian would be competent to apply these remedies.

Externally.—Sponging the swollen parts, especially the head, when the swelling occurs there, is most useful. The bath should be at an extreme of temperature—either ice cold to constrict the tissues or hot water to act as an emolient and to favor circulation. Vinegar may be added as an astringent. When we have excessively denuded surfaces, suppuration, or open wounds, disinfectants should be added to the wash.

In cases of excessive swelling, especially of the head, mechanical relief may be required. Even in country practice, punctures of the part should be made with the hot iron, as no other disease so predisposes to septic contamination. When mechanical asphyxia is threatened tracheotomy may be demanded. With the first evidence of dyspnea, not due to closing of the nostrils or glottis, or with the first pawing which gives rise to a suspicion of colic, a mustard plaster should be applied over the whole belly and chest. The sinapism will draw the current of the circulation to the exterior, the metastasis to the lungs or intestines is prevented, and the enfeebled nervous system is stimulated to renewed vigor by the peripheral irritation. The organs are encouraged by it to renewed functional activity; the local inflammation produced by it favors absorption of the exudation. The objection to the use of blisters is their more severe action and the danger of mortification. Septicemia, when occurring as a complication, requires the ordinary treatment for the putrid diseases, with little hope of a good result.

After recovery the animal regains its ordinary health, and there is no predisposition to a return of the disease.

HORSEPOX, OR EQUINE VARIOLA.

Synonyms.—Variola equina; pustular grease; phlyctenoid herpes.

Definition.—Horsepox is a specific, infectious fever of the horse, attended by an eruption of pustules, or pocks, over any part of the skin or on the mucous membranes lining the various cavities in the body, but chiefly, and often exclusively, upon the pasterns and fetlocks. The eruption may commence upon the lips, or about the nostrils or eyes.

This disease was described by the early Roman agricultural writers and by the veterinarians of the eighteenth century. It received its first important notice from the great Jenner, who confounded it with grease in horses, since animals with this disease are very liable to have the eruption of variola appear on the fetlocks. He saw these cases transmit the disease to cattle in the byres and to the stablemen and milkmaids who attended them, and furnish the latter with immunity from smallpox, which led to the discovery of vaccination. Horsepox is also frequently mistaken for the exanthemata attending some forms of venereal disease in horses.

Variola in the horse, while it is identical in principle, general course, complications, and lesions with variola in other animals, is a disease of the horse itself, and is not transmissible in the form of variola to any other animal; nor is the variola of any other animal transmissible to the horse. Cattle and men, if inoculated from a case of horsepox, develop vaccinia, but vaccinia from the latter animals is not so readily reinoculated into the horse with success. If it does develop, it produces the original disease.

Causes.—The direct cause of horsepox is infection. A large number of predisposing causes favor the development of the disease, as in the case of strangles, and this trouble, like almost all contagious diseases, renders the animal which has had one attack immune. The chief predisposing cause is youthfulness. Old horses which have not been affected are less liable to become infected when exposed than younger ones. The exposure incident to shipment, through public stables, cars, etc., acts as a predisposing cause, as in the other infectious diseases. The period of final dentition is a time which renders it peculiarly susceptible.

Dupaul states that the infection is transmissible through the atmosphere for several hundred yards. The more common means of contagion is by direct contact or by means of fomites. Feed boxes and bridles previously used by horses affected with variola are probably the most frequent carriers of the virus, and we find the lesions in the majority of cases developed in the neighborhood of the lips and nostrils. Coition is a frequent cause. A stallion suffering from this disease may be the cause of a considerable epizootic, as he transmits it to a number of brood mares and they in turn return to the farms where they are surrounded by young animals to which they convey the contagion. The saddle and croup straps are frequent agents of infection. The presence of a wound greatly favors the inoculation of the disease, which is also sometimes carried by surgical instruments or sponges. Trasbot recites a case in which a set of hobbles, which had been used on an animal suffering from variola, were used on a horse for a quittor operation and transmitted the disease, which developed on the edges of the wound.

Symptoms.—There is a period of incubation, after an animal has been exposed, of from five to eight days, during which there is no appreciable alteration in the health. This period is shorter in summer than in winter. At the end of this time small nodes develop at the point of inoculation and the animal becomes feverish. The horse is dull and dejected, loses its appetite, and has a rough, dry coat with the hairs on end. There is moderate thirst. The respirations are somewhat quickened and the pulse becomes rapid and full. The body temperature is elevated, frequently reaching 104° or 105° F. within 36 or 48 hours from the appearance of the first symptoms.

The visible mucous membranes, especially the conjunctivæ, are of a bright rosy red. In the lymphatic, cold-blooded, and more common horses these symptoms of fever are less marked; even with a comparatively high temperature the animal may retain its appetite and work comparatively well, but these cases, if worked and overheated, are liable to develop serious complications.

At the end of from three and a half to four days the eruption breaks out, the fever abates, and the general symptoms improve. The eruption in severe cases may be generalized; it may be confined to the softer skin of the nose and lips, the genital organs, and the inside of the thighs, or it may be localized in the neighborhood of a wound or in the irritated skin of a pair of greasy heels. It consists of a varying number of little nodes which, on a mucous membrane, as in the nostrils or vagina, or on soft, unpigmented skin, appear red and feel at first like shot under the epidermis. These nodes soften and show a yellowish spot in the center when they become pustules. The epidermis is dissolved and the matter escapes as a viscid fluid at first citrine and later cloudy and purulent, which dries rapidly, forming scabs; if these fall off or are removed they leave a little shallow, concave ulcer which heals in the course of five or six days. In the softer skin if pigmented the cicatrices are white and frequently remain so for about a year, when the pigment returns. The lips or genital organs of a colored horse, if covered with a number of small white spots about the size of a pea, will usually indicate that the animal has been affected with the horsepox.

At times the pustules may become confluent and produce large, superficial, serpentine ulcers on the membrane of the nostrils, around the lips or eyelids, or on the borders of wounds and in greasy heels; in this case the part becomes swollen, hot, painful, and is covered with a profuse discharge of matter. In this form there is frequently a secondary fever lasting for a day or two.

In severe cases there may be a suppurative adenitis, or inflammation of the lymphatic glands which are fed from the affected part. If the eruption is around the nostrils and lips, the glands between the jaws (submaxillary) form abscesses as in a case of strangles; if the eruption is in a pair of greasy heels abscesses may form in the fold of the groin (inguinal). There may be so much tumefaction of the nostrils as to produce difficulty in breathing.

Complications.—A case of horsepox may be attended with various complications of varying degrees of importance. Adenitis, or suppuration of the glands, has just been mentioned. Confluent eruptions irritate the part and induce the animal to rub the inflamed part against the manger or scratch it in other ways and thus produce troublesome ulcers, which may leave ugly scars. Irritation of the mucous membrane of the nose causes severe coryza with purulent discharge.

The eruption may occur in the throat or in the air tubes to the lungs, developing an acute laryngitis or bronchitis. If the animal is exposed to cold, or worked so as to engorge the lungs with blood at the termination of the specific fever, just when the eruption is about to localize, it may be determined to the lungs. In this case we have a short, dry cough, labored breathing, the development of a secondary fever of some gravity, and all the external symptoms of a pneumonia. This pneumonia differs, however, from an ordinary pneumonia in the symptoms furnished by the examination of the lungs themselves. In place of a large mass of the lung tissue being affected the inflammation is disseminated in smaller spots over the entire lung.

Diagnosis.—The diagnosis of horsepox is to be based on the presence of a continuous fever, with rosy mucous membranes, for several days and the appearance of the characteristic eruption. If the eruption is in the nasal cavities, marked by a considerable discharge and attended with submaxillary abscesses, it may be confounded with strangles. If the throat is affected, it may be confounded with an angina (laryngitis or pharyngitis), but in the latter the local trouble precedes or is concomitant with the fever, while in the former the fever precedes the local trouble by several days. Variola may be confounded with bronchitis or pneumonia if complicated with these troubles and the eruption is absent from the exterior, but it is of little moment, as the treatment for both is much the same. When the eruption is in the neighborhood of the genital organs the disease has been mistaken for dourine. In variola the eruption is a temporary one; the nodes and pustules are followed by shallow ulcers and rapid cicatrization unless continued in the vagina or on the penis by the rubbing of the walls and filth which accumulates; there are apt to be pustules at other parts of the body. In the venereal disease the local trouble commences as a papule and breaks into an ulcer without having formed a pustule. The ulcer has not the convex rosy appearance of that of the less serious discharge; the symptoms last for a longer period, by which time others aid in differentiating the two. In glanders the tubercle is hard and, after breaking into an ulcer, the indurated bottom remains, grayish or dirty white in color, ragged, and exuding a viscous, oily discharge. There is no disposition to suppuration of the neighboring glands. In variola the rosy shallow ulcer and healthy pus, with the acutely tumefied glands, should not be mistaken, at least after a day. I have seen in mules acute glanders which required a day's delay to differentiate from strangles; at that time the farcy buds appeared.

Prognosis.—The average case of horsepox runs a course of dejection, loss of appetite, and more or less fever for about four days, followed by a rapid convalescence, and leaves the animal as well and as sound as before. If the eruption has been excessive or confluent, the ulcerations may act as irritants and render the animal unfit for use for several weeks. Laryngitis, pharyngitis, bronchitis, and pneumonia in this disease are not of greater gravity than they are when occurring from other causes. The spots denuded of pigment left by the pustules on the lips and genitals may temporarily depreciate the value of the animal to a slight degree.

Treatment.—As this is a disease unattended by alterations of the blood itself, although a specific fever, and is of a sthenic type, active remedies are admissible and indicated. The horse should be placed on a low diet (little or no oats)—bran mashes, a moderate quantity of good, sound hay, a few carrots or apples, which will act as laxatives; also slop feed. Barley flour is more cooling for mashes than bran or oatmeal. Water may be given as the animal desires it, but it should not be cold; if a half bucketful of water is kept in the manger, the horse will take but a few swallows at a time. One-dram doses of nitrate of potash or 1-ounce doses of sweet spirits of niter are useful in the drinking water. If the fever is high, the antipyretics are indicated: Sulphate of quinin in 1-dram doses; iodid of potash in 1-dram doses; infusion of pine tops, of juniper leaves, of the aromatic herbs, or of English breakfast tea are useful in the later stages. If complications of the air passages or lungs are threatened, a large mustard poultice should be applied to the belly and sides of the chest. Oxid of zinc ointment should be used on confluent eruptions, and if the ulceration is excessive it may have to be touched with caustic.

Great care must be taken to keep the animal protected from cold drafts of air or other exposure. Blankets or sheets should be used on the body and bandages on the legs. After convalescence is established, nutritious feed of easy digestion and walking exercise are all that is needed, except perhaps a little Glauber's salt to prevent constipation.

Prophylactic treatment.—When horsepox breaks out among a large number of horses, especially on a farm where there are a number of colts, it may be assumed that the greater majority will contract the disease, and it is more economical that they should have it and be through with it at once. If the weather is moderate, all the animals which have not been affected can be inoculated, which will produce the disease in a mild form, with the eruption at a point of election, and render the danger of complication a minimum one. For inoculation the discharge from the pustules of a mild case should be selected and inoculated by scarification on the belly or the under surface of the neck.

ANTHRAX.

Synonyms: Carbuncle, splenic fever, splenic apoplexy, etc.; charbon, sang de rate (French); Miltzbrand (German).

Definition.—Anthrax is a severe and usually fatal contagious disease, characterized by chills, great depression and stupor of the animal, and a profound alteration of the blood. It is caused by the entrance into the animal's body of a bacterium, known as the *Bacillus anthracis*, or its spores.

Practically all animals are susceptible to anthrax. The herbivora are especially susceptible, in the following order: The sheep, the ox, and the horse. The guinea pig, the hog, the rabbit, mice, and other animals die quickly from its effects. Man, the dog, and other omnivora and carnivora may be attacked by it in a constitutional form as fatal as in the herbivora, but fortunately in many cases develop from it only local trouble, followed by recovery.

Anthrax has been a scourge of the animals of the civilized world since the first written history we have of any of their diseases. In 1709–1712 extensive outbreaks of anthrax occurred in Germany, Hungary, and Poland. In the first half of the nineteenth century it had become an extensively spread disease in Russia, Holland, and England, and for the last century has been gradually spreading in the Americas, more so in South America than here. In 1864, in the five governments of Petersburg, Novgorod, Olonetz, Twer, and Jaroslaw, in Russia, more than 10,000 horses and nearly 1,000 persons perished from the disease.

Causes.—The causes of anthrax were for a long time attributed entirely to climatic influence, soil, and atmospheric temperature, and they are still recognized as predisposing factors in the development of the disease, for it is usually found, especially when outbreaks in a great number of animals occur, in low, damp, marshy countries during the warm seasons. It is more frequent in districts where marshy lands dry out during the heat of summer and are then covered with light rains. Decaying vegetable matter seems most favorable for nourishing and preserving the virus.

The direct cause of anthrax is always infection of a previously sound animal, either directly from a diseased animal or through various media which contain excretions or the débris from the body of one previously infected.

The specific virus of anthrax was first discovered by Davaine in 1851. He recognized microscopic bodies in the form of little rods in the blood of animals suffering from anthrax. It was not, however, till a quarter of a century later that Pasteur defined the exact nature of the bacillus, the mode of its propagation, and its exact relationship to anthrax as the sole cause of the disease. In the animal body the bacilli have a tendency to accumulate in the spleen, liver, and elsewhere, so that these organs are much more virulent than the muscles or less vascular tissues. When eliminated from the animal in the excretions, or when exposed to outside influences by the death of the animal and the disintegration of the tissues, the body of the rod is destroyed and the spores only remain. These spores, which may be called the seeds of the bacilli, retain their vitality for a long period; they resist ordinary putrefaction; they are unchanged by moisture; and they are not affected by moderate heat. If scattered with the débris of a dead animal on the surface of the ground, they may remain around the roots of the grass in a pasture or may be washed to the nearest low-lying ground or marsh. If buried in the body of an animal dead from anthrax, they may be washed deep into the ground, and in later years (in one proved case 17 years) be brought to the surface and infect other animals. They are frequently brought to the surface of the earth, having been swallowed by earthworms, in the bodies of which they have been found.

This accounts for the outbreaks at the time of the first rains after a dry season. During the latter the earthworm goes deep in the ground in search of moisture; it finds the spore which has been washed there in past years, swallows it, and afterwards brings it to the surface. The virus is carried with the wool from infected sheep and remains in it through the process of manufacture into cloth. The spores remain in the hides of animals which have died of anthrax and retain their vitality throughout months of soaking in the tanners' pits, the working of the harness maker or the cobbler, and after the oiling of the completed leather. The dried spores in the dust from any of these products may be carried by the atmosphere.

Infection of an animal takes place through inoculation or contact of the bacillus or its spores with an abraded surface or mucous membrane, on a sound animal. In an infected district horses may eat with impunity the rich pasturage of spring and early summer, but when grass gets low they crop it close to the ground, pull up the roots around which the virus may be lodged, and under these conditions the animals are more apt to have abrasions of the lips or tongue by contact with dried stubble and the dirt on the roots; this favors the introduction of the germs into the system. The virus may be introduced with feed and enter the blood-vessel system from the stomach and intestines. If in the dust, dried hay, or on the parched pasture of late summer, the virus may be inhaled and be absorbed from the lining of the lungs. If in harness leather; it needs but an abrasion of the skin, as the harness rubs it, to transfer the spore from the leather to the circulation of the animal.

The writer saw a case of anthrax occur in a groom from the use of a new horse brush. The strap which passes over the back of the hand inoculated an abrasion on the knuckle of the first finger, and in 12 hours a "pustule" had formed and the arm had become infected.

Symptoms.—The symptoms of anthrax usually develop with extreme rapidity. The horse is dejected and falls into a state of profound stupor, attended with great muscular weakness. The feeble, indolent animal, if forced to move, drags its legs. There are severe chills, agitation of the muscles, symptoms of vertigo, and at times colicky pains. The mucous membranes turn a deep ocher or bluish-red color. The body temperature is rapidly elevated to 104° or 105° F. The breathing is increased to 30 or 40 respirations in the minute and the pulse is greatly accelerated, but while the arteries are soft and almost imperceptible, the heart beats can be felt and heard, violent and tumultuous. In some cases, when inoculation is through the skin, large subcutaneous swellings appear; these may involve a leg, a shoulder, one side of the body, or the neck or head. The swelling is at first hot and painful, but afterwards it becomes necrotic and sensation is lost. The symptoms last but two, three, or four days at most, when the case usually terminates fatally. An examination of the blood shows a dark fluid which will not clot, and which remains black after exposure to the air. After death the bodies putrefy rapidly and bloat up; the tissues are filled with gases, and a bloody foam exudes from the mouth, nostrils, and anus, and frequently the mucous membrane of the rectum protrudes from the latter. The hairs detach from the skin. Congestion of all the organs and tissues is found, with interstitial hemorrhages. The muscles are friable and are covered with ecchymotic spots. This is especially marked in the heart.

The black, uncoagulated, and incoagulable blood shows an iridescent scum on its surface, which is due to the fat of the animal dissolved by the ammonia produced by the decomposed tissues. The serum oozes out of every tissue and contains broken-down blood, which, when examined microscopically, is found to have the red globules crenated and the leucocytes granular. A high power of the microscope also reveals the bacteria in the shape of little .rodlike bodies of homogeneous texture with their brilliant spores.

The lymphatic ganglia are increased four, five, six, or ten times their natural size, enlarged by the engorgement of blood. The spleen shows nodulated black spots containing a muddy blood, which is found teeming with the virus. This organ is much enlarged and is quite friable. The mucous membranes of the intestines are congested and reddish brown; the surface of the intestines is in many places denuded of its lining membrane, showing fissures and hemorrhagic spots. The liver has a cooked appearance; the kidneys are congested and friable; the urine is red; the pleura, lungs, and the meninges are congested, and the bronchi of the lungs contain a bloody foam.

Treatment.—Treatment of anthrax in animals by medicinal means has not proved satisfactory. In cases of local anthrax an incision of the swelling followed by the application of disinfectants sometimes causes good results. In such cases, however, the danger of disseminating the infection from the wounds tends to make this procedure inadvisable unless great care is taken.

Good results are obtained from the use of serum in the treatment of the disease. For this purpose 30 to 100 cubic centimeters should be administered subcutaneously or intravenously. If no improvement is noticed within 24 hours the injection should be repeated. In a number of instances afforded to test the curative value of the serum in cases of anthrax in man and animals splendid results were obtained.

The prophylactic treatment formerly consisted in the avoidance of certain fields and marshes which were recognized as contaminated. It underwent, however, a revolution after the discovery by Pasteur of the possibility of a prophylactic inoculation or vaccination which granted immunity from future attacks of the disease similar to that granted by the recovery of an animal from an ordinary attack of the disease.

This treatment consists in the use of a vaccine which is made by the artificial cultivation of the virus of anthrax in broth and its continued exposure to a high temperature for a certain time, which weakens the virus to such extent that it is capable of producing only a very mild and not dangerous attack of anthrax in the animal in which it is inoculated, and thus protects the animal from inoculation of a stronger virus. The production of this virus, which is carried on in some countries at the expense of the governments and is furnished at a small cost to the farmers in regions where the disease prevails, in this country is made in private laboratories only.

At the present time very good results are being obtained with vaccination consisting of an injection of highly potent anthrax serum on one side of the animal and a vaccine on the other side. This method of treatment requires only a single handling of the animals and further possesses advantages over the Pasteur treatment in that it immediately makes animals immune. In the numerous applications of this form of treatment very good results have been obtained and the immunity produced thereby usually lasts at least one year. The vaccinated animals should be kept for a period of ten days to two weeks from exposure, since during that period they are at times even more susceptible to the disease, and therefore care should be taken not to reduce their vitality.

Prevention.—In attempts to control the disease it is essential, aside from protective vaccination, to prevent the reinfection of localities. For this purpose it is essential, if possible, to drain thoroughly and keep under cultivation the infected areas before animals are permitted to pasture on them. The complete destruction of all anthrax carcasses is also very important. This is best accomplished by burning, but as this method of disposal is impracticable in many localities, deep burial may be found to be better. Covering the carcasses within their graves with quicklime adds another valuable precaution against further dissemination of the infection. No animal dying from anthrax should ever be skinned or cut open, as the blood from these sources is one of the most dangerous means of spreading the infection, being charged, while in the animal, with great numbers of bacilli, which quickly turn into spores as soon as spread about upon the face of the ground. All discharges from the body openings should also be burned or buried deeply, as they are frequently of a virulent character.

GLANDERS AND FARCY.

(Pls. XL–XLII.)

Definition.—Let it be understood at the outset that glanders and farcy are one and the same disease, differing only in that the first term is applied to the disease when the local lesions predominate in the internal organs, especially in the nostrils, lungs, and air tubes, and that the second term is applied to it when the principal manifestation is an outbreak of the lesions on the exterior or skin of the animal. The term glanders applies to the disease in both forms, while the term farcy is limited to the visible appearance of external trouble only; but in the latter case internal lesions always exist, although they may not be evident.

Glanders is a contagious constitutional disease of the genus *Equus* (the horse, ass, and mule), readily communicable to man, the dog, the cat, the rabbit, and the guinea pig. It is transmitted with diffi-

PLATE XL.

ZEESE-WILKINSON CO., INC., N.Y.

GLANDERS.

Nasal septum of horse, right side, showing acute lesions.

Haines.

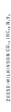

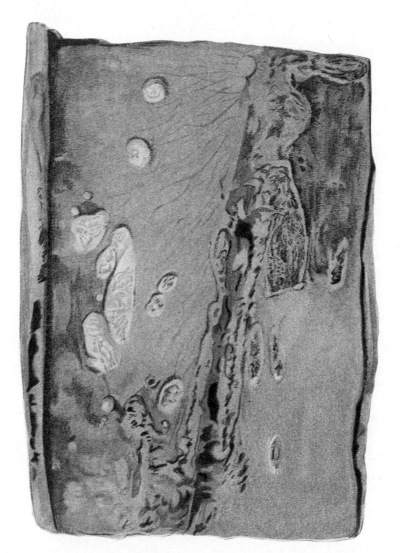

ZEESE-WILKINSON CO., INC., N.Y.

GLANDERS.

Middle region of nasal septum, left side, showing ulcers.

Haines.

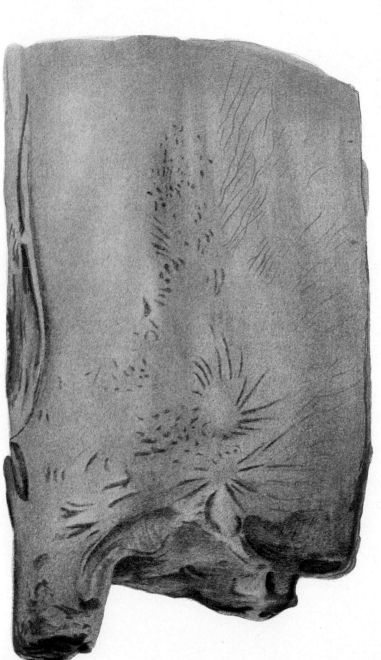

GLANDERS.

Posterior half of nasal septum, right side, showing cicatrices.

Haines.

culty to sheep and goats, and cattle seem to be entirely immune. It runs a variable course and usually produces the death of the animal affected with it. It is characterized by the formation of neoplasms, or nodules, of connective tissue, which degenerate into ulcers, from which exude a peculiar discharge. It is accompanied with a variable degree of fever, according to the rapidity of its course. It is subject to various complications of the lymphatic glands, of the lungs, of the testicles, of the internal organs, and of the subcutaneous connective tissue.

History.—Glanders is one of the oldest diseases of which we have definite knowledge in the history of medicine. Absyrtus, the Greek veterinarian in the army of Constantine the Great, described it with considerable accuracy and recognized the contagiousness of its character. Another Greek veterinarian, Vegetius Renatus, who lived in the time of Theodosius (381 A. D.), described, under the name of "malleus humidus," a disease of the horse characterized by a nasal discharge and accompanied by superficial ulcers. He recognized the contagious properties of the discharge of the external ulcers, and recommended that all animals sick with the disease be separated at once with the greatest care from the others and should be pastured in separate fields, for fear the other animals should become affected.

In 1682 Sollysel, the stable master of Louis XIV, published an account of glanders and farcy, which he considered closely related to each other, although he did not recognize them as identical. He admitted the existence of a virus which communicated the disease from an infected animal to a sound one. He called special attention to the feed troughs and water buckets as being the media of contagion. He divided glanders into two forms—one malignant and contagious and the other benign—and he stated that there was always danger of infection.

Garsault in 1746 said that "as this disease is communicated very easily and can infect in a very short time a prodigious number of horses by means of the discharges which may be licked up, animals infected with glanders should be destroyed."

Bourgelat, the founder of veterinary schools, in his "Elements of Hippiatry," published in 1755, establishes glanders as a virulent disease.

Extensive outbreaks of glanders are described as prevailing in the great armies of continental Europe and England from time to time during the periods of all the wars of the last few centuries.

Glanders was imported into America at the close of the eighteenth century, and before the end of the first half of the last century had spread to a considerable degree among the horses of the Middle and immediately adjoining Southern States. This disease was unknown in Mexico until carried there during the Mexican War by the badly diseased horses of the United States Army. During the first half of the last century a large body of veterinarians and medical men protested against the contagious character of the disease, and by their opinion prevailed to such an extent against the common opinion that several of the Governments of Europe undertook a series of experiments to determine the right between the contesting parties.

At the veterinary school at Alfort and at the farm of Lamirault in France several hundred horses which had passed examination as sound had placed among them glandered horses under various conditions. The results of these experiments proved conclusively the contagious character of the disease.

In 1881 Bouchard, of the faculty of medicine in Paris, assisted by Capitan and Charrin, undertook a series of experiments with matter taken from the farcy ulcer of a human being. They afterwards continued their experiments with matter taken from horses, and in 1883 succeeded in showing that glanders is caused by a bacterium which is capable of propagation and reproduction of others of its own kind if placed in the proper media. In 1882 the specific germ of glanders was first discovered and described by Loeffler and Schuetz in Germany.

When we come to study the etiology of glanders, the difference of susceptibility on the part of different species of animals, or even on the part of individuals of the same species, and when we come to find proof of the slow incubation and latent character of the disease as it exists in certain individuals, we understand how in a section of country containing a number of glandered animals others can *seem* to contract and develop the disease without having apparently been exposed to contagion.

Causes.—The contagious nature of glanders, in no matter what form it appears, being to-day definitely demonstrated, we can recognize but one cause for all cases, and that is contagion by means of the specific virus of the disease. The causative organism is known as the *Bacillus mallei*.

In studying the writings of the older authors on glanders, and the works of those authors who contested the contagious nature of the disease, we find a large number of predisposing causes assigned as factors in the development of the malady.

While a virus from a case of glanders if inoculated into an animal of the genus *Equus* will inevitably produce the disease, we find a vast difference in the contagious activity of different cases of glanders. We find a great variation in the manner and rapidity of the development of the disease in different individuals and that the contagion is much more liable to be carried to sound animals under certain circumstances than it is under others. Only certain species of animals are susceptible of contracting the disease, and while some of these contract it as a general constitutional malady, in others it develops as only a local sore.

In acute glanders the contagion is found in its most virulent form, as is shown by the inevitable infection of susceptible animals inoculated with the disease, while the discharge from chronic semilatent glanders and farcy may at times be inoculated with a negative result; again, in acute glanders, as we have a free discharge, a much greater quantity of virus-containing matter is scattered in the neighborhood of an infected horse to serve as a contagion to others than is found in the small amount of discharge of the chronic cases.

The chances of contagion are much greater when sound horses, asses, or mules are placed in the immediate neighborhood of glandered horses, drink from the same bucket, stand in the next stall, or work in the same wagon, or are fed from feed boxes or mangers which have been impregnated by the saliva and soiled by the discharge of sick animals. Transmission occurs by direct contact of the discharges of a glandered animal with the tissues of a sound one, either on the exterior, when swallowed mixed with feed into the digestive tract, or when dried and inhaled as dust.

The stable attendants serve as one of the most common carriers of the virus. Dried or fresh discharges are collected from the infected animals in cleaning, harnessing, feeding, and by means of the hands, clothing, the teeth of the currycomb, the sponge, the bridle, and the halter, and are thus carried to other animals.

An animal affected with chronic glanders in a latent form is moved from one part of the stable to another, or works hitched with one horse and then with another, and may be an active agent in the spreading of the disease without the cause being recognized.

Glanders is found frequently in the most insidious forms, and we recognize that it can exist without being apparent; that is, it may affect a horse for a long period without showing any symptoms that will allow even the most experienced veterinarian to make a diagnosis. An old gray mare belonging to a tavern keeper was reserved for family use with good care and light work for a period of eight years, during which time other horses in the tavern stable were from time to time affected with glanders without an apparent cause. The mare, whose only trouble was an apparent attack of heaves, was sold to a huckster who placed her at hard work. Want of feed and overwork and exposure rapidly developed a case of acute glanders, from which the animal died, and at the autopsy were found the lesions of an acute pneumonia of glanders grafted on chronic lesions, consisting of old nodules which had undoubtedly existed for years.

In a case that once came under the care of the writer, a coach horse was examined for soundness and passed as sound by a prominent veterinarian, who a few months afterwards treated the horse for a skin eruption from which it recovered. Twelve months afterwards it came into the hands of the writer, hidebound, with a slight cough and a slight eruption of the skin, which was attributed to clipping and the rubbing of the harness, but which had nothing suspicious in its character. The horse was placed on tonics and put to regular light driving. In six weeks it developed a bronchitis without having been specially exposed, and in two days this trouble was followed by a lobular pneumonia and the breaking of an abscess in the right lung. Farcy buds developed on the surface of the body and the animal died. The autopsy showed the existence of a number of old glanderous nodules in the lungs which must have existed previous to purchase, more than a year before.

Public watering troughs and the feed boxes of boarding stables and the tavern stables of market towns are among the most common recipients for the virus of glanders, which is most dangerous in its fresh state, but cases have been known to be caused by feeding animals in the box or stall in which glandered animals had stood several months before. While the discharge from a case of chronic glanders is much less liable to contain many active bacilli than that from a case of acute glanders, the former, if it infects an animal, will produce the same disease as the latter. It may assume from the outset an acute or chronic form, according to the susceptibility of the animal infected, and this does not depend upon the character of the disease from which the virus was derived.

The animals of the genus *Equus*—the horse, the ass, and the mule—are those which are the most susceptible to contract glanders, but in these we find a much greater receptivity in the ass and mule than we do in the horse. In the ass and mule in almost all cases the period of incubation is short and the disease develops in an acute form. We find that the kind of horse infected has an influence on the character of the disease; in full-blooded, fat horses of a sanguinary temperament, the disease usually develops in an acute form, while in the lymphatic, cold-blooded, more common race of horses the disease usually assumes a chronic form. If the disease develops first in the chronic form in a horse in fair condition, starvation and overwork are liable to bring on an acute attack, but when the disease is inoculated into a debiliated and impoverished animal it is apt to start in the latent form. Inoculation on the lips or the exterior of the animal is frequently followed by an acute attack, while infection by ingestion of the virus and inoculation by means of the digestive tract is often followed by the trouble in the chronic latent form.

In the dog the inoculation of glanders may develop a constitutional disease with all the symptoms which are found in the horse, but more frequently the virus pullulates only at the point of inoculation, remaining for some time as a local sore, which may then heal, leaving a perfectly sound animal; but while the local sore is continuing to ulcerate, and specific virus exists in it, it may be the carrier of contagion to other animals. In man we find a greater receptivity to glanders than in the dog, and in many unfortunate cases the virus spreads from the point of inoculation to the entire system and destroys the wretched mortal by extensive ulcers of the face and hemorrhage or by destruction of the lung tissue; in other cases, however, glanders may develop, as in the dog, in local form only, not infecting the constitution and terminating in recovery, while the specific ulcer by proper treatment is turned into a simple one. In the feline species glanders is more destructive than in the dog. The point of inoculation ulcerates rapidly and the entire system becomes infected.

While a student the writer saw a lion in the service of Prof. Trasbot, at Alfort, which had contracted the disease by eating glandered meat and died with the lung riddled with nodules. A litter of kittens lapped the blood from the lungs of a glandered horse on which an autopsy was being made, and in four days almost their entire faces, including the nasal bones, were eaten away by rapid ulceration. Nodules were found in the lungs. A pack of wolves in the Philadelphia Zoological Garden died in 10 days after being fed with the meat of a glandered horse. The rabbit, guinea pig, and mice are especially susceptible to the inoculation of glanders, and these animals are convenient witnesses and proofs of the existence of suspected cases of the glanders in other animals by the results of successful inoculations.

The primary lesion in any form is a local point in which occurs a rapid proliferation of the cell elements which make up the animal tissue with formation of new connective tissue, with a crowding together of the elements until their own pressure on one another cuts off the circulation and nutrition, and death takes place in them in the form of ulceration or grangrene. Following this primary lesion we have an extension of infection by means of the spread of the bacilli into those tissues immediately surrounding the first infected spot, which are most suitable for the development of simple inflammatory phenomena or the specific virus. The primary symptoms are the result of specific reaction at the point of inoculation, but at a later time the virus is carried by means of the blood vessels and lymphatic vessels to other parts of the body and becomes lodged at different places and develops in them; again, when the disease has existed in the latent form in the lungs of the animal and the virus is wakened into action from any cause, we have it carried to various parts of the body and developing in the most susceptible regions or organs. The points of development are most frequently determined by the activity of the circulation and the effects of exterior irritants. For example, if a horse which has been so slightly affected with the virus of glanders that no symptoms are visible is exposed to cold, rain, or sleet, or by the rubbing of the harness on the body and the irritation of mud on the legs, the disease is liable to develop on the exterior in the form of farcy, while a full-blooded horse which is employed at speed and has its lungs and respiratory tract gorged with blood from the extreme use of these organs will develop glanders as the local manifestation of the disease in the respiratory tract.

The previous reference to the existence of glanders under the two forms more commonly differentiated as glanders and as farcy, and our reference to the various conditions in which it may exist as acute, chronic, and latent, show that the disease may assume several different phases. Without for a moment losing sight of the fact that all these varied conditions are identical in their origin and in their essence, for convenience of study we may divide glanders into three classes—chronic farcy, chronic glanders, and acute glanders with or without farcy.

CHRONIC FARCY.

Symptoms.—In farcy the symptoms commence by formation of little nodes on the under surface of the skin, which rapidly infringe on the tissues of the skin itself. These nodes, which are known as farcy "buds" and farcy "buttons," are from the size of a bullet to the size of a walnut. They are hot, sensitive to the touch, at first elastic and afterwards become soft; the tissue is destroyed, and infringing on the substance of the skin the disease produces an ulcer, which is known as a chancre. This ulcer is irregular in shape, with ragged edges which overhang the sore; it has a gray, dirty bottom and the discharge is sometimes thin and sometimes purulent; in either case it is mixed with a viscous, sticky, yellowish material like the white of an egg in consistency and like olive oil in appearance. The discharge is almost diagnostic; it resembles somewhat the discharge which we have in greasy heels and in certain attacks of lymphangitis, but to the expert the specific discharge is characteristic. The discharge accumulates on the hair surrounding the ulcer and over its surface and dries, forming scabs which become thicker by successive deposits on the under surface until they fall off, to be replaced by others of the same kind; and the excess of discharge may drop on the hairs below and form similar brownish yellow crusts. The farcy ulcers may retain their specific form for a considerable time—days or even weeks—but eventually the discharge becomes purulent in character and assumes the appearance of healthy matter. The surface of the gangrenous bottom of the ulcer is replaced by rosy granulations, the ragged edges are beveled off, and the chancre is turned into a simple ulcer which rapidly heals.

The farcy buttons occur most frequently on the sides of the lips, the sides of the neck, the lower part of the shoulders, the inside of the thighs, or the outside of the legs, but may occur on any part of the body.

We have next an irritation of the lymphatic vessels in the neighborhood of the chancres. Those become swollen and then indurated and appear like great ridges underneath the skin; they are hot to the touch and sensitive. The cords may remain for a considerable time and then gradually disappear, or they may ulcerate like a farcy bud itself, forming elongated, irregular, serpentine ulcers with a characteristic, dirty, gray bottom and ragged edges, and pour out a viscous, oily discharge like the chancres themselves.

The essential symptoms of farcy are, as above described, the button, the chancre, the cord, and the discharge. We have in addition to these symptoms a certain number of accessory symptoms, which, while not diagnostic in themselves, are of great service in aiding the diagnosis in cases where the eruption takes place in small quantities, and when the ulcers are not characteristic.

Epistaxis, or bleeding from the nose without previous work or other apparent cause, is one of the frequent concomitant symptoms in glanders, and such hemorrhage from the nostrils should always be regarded with suspicion. The animal with farcy frequently develops a cough, resembling much that which we find in heaves—a short, dry, aborted, hacking cough, with little or no discharge from the nostrils. With this we find an irregular movement of the flanks, and on auscultation of the lungs we find sibilant or at times a few mucous râles. Another common symptom is a sudden swelling of one of the hind legs; it is found suddenly swollen in the region of the cannon, the enlargement extending below to the pastern and above as high as the stifle. This swelling is hot and painful to the touch, and renders the animal stiff and lame. On pressure with the finger the swelling can be indented, but the pits so formed soon fill again on removal of the pressure. In severe cases we may have ulceration of the skin, and serum pours out from the surface, resembling the oozing which we have after a blister or in a case of grease. This swelling is not to be confounded with the stocking in lymphatic horses or the edema which we have in chronic heart or in kidney trouble, as in the last the swelling is cool, not painful, and the pitting on pressure remains for some time after the latter is withdrawn. It is not to be confounded with greasy heels. In these the disease commences in the neighborhood of the pastern and gradually extends up the leg, rarely passing beyond the neighborhood of the hock. The swollen leg in glanders almost invariably swells for the entire length in a single night or within a very short period. When greasy heels are complicated by lymphangitis we have a condition very much resembling that of farcy. The swelled leg in farcy is frequently followed by an outbreak of farcy buttons and ulcers over its surface. In the entire horse the testicles are frequently swollen and hot and sensitive to the touch, but they have no tendency to suppuration. The acute inflammation is rapidly followed by the specific induration, which corresponds to the local lesions in other parts of the body.

Chronic farcy in the ass and mule is an excessively rare condition, but sometimes occurs.

CHRONIC GLANDERS.

Symptoms.—In chronic glanders we find the same train of inflammatory phenomena, varying in appearance from those of chronic farcy only by the difference of the tissues in which they are situated. In chronic glanders there is first the nodule, from the size of a shot to that of a small pea, which forms in the mucous membranes of the respiratory tract. This may be just inside the wings of the nostrils or on the septum which divides the one nasal cavity from the other, and may be easily detected, or it may be higher in the nasal cavities on the turbinated bones, or it may form in the larnyx itself or on the surface of the trachea or deep in the lungs.

The nodules, which are first red and hard and consist of new connective tissue, soon soften and become yellow; the yellow spots break and we have a small ulcer the size of the preceding nodule, which has a gray, dirty bottom and ragged edges and is known as a chancre. This ulcer pours from its surface a viscous, oily discharge similar to that which we have seen in the farcy ulcer. The irritation of the discharge may ulcerate the lining mucous membrane of the nose, causing serpentine gutters with bottoms resembling those of the chancres themselves. If the nodules have formed in large numbers, we may have them causing an acute inflammation of the Schneiderian membrane, with a catarrhal discharge which may mark the specific discharge, or that which comes from the ulcers and resembles the discharge of strangles or simple inflammatory diseases.

The eruption of the ulcers and discharge soon cause an irritation of the neighboring lymphatics; and in the intermaxillary space, deep inside of the jaws, we find an enlargement of the glands, which for the first few days may seem soft and edematous, but which rapidly becomes confined to the glands, these being from the size of an almond to that of a small bunch of berries, exceedingly hard and nodulated. This enlargement of the glands is found high on the inside of the jaws, firmly adherent to the base of the tongue. It is not to be confounded with the puffy, edematous swelling, which is not separated from the skin and subcutaneous connective tissues found in strangles, in laryngitis, and in other simple inflammatory troubles.

These glands bear a great resemblance to the indurated glands which we find in connection with the collection of pus in the sinuses; but in the latter disease the glands have not the extreme nodulated feel which they have in glanders. With the glands we find indurated cords, feeling like balls of tangled wire or twine, fastening the glands together.

The essential symptoms of glanders are the nodule, the chancre, the glands, and the discharge. With the development of the nodules in the respiratory tract, according to their number and the amount of eruption which they cause, we may find a cough which resembles that of a coryza, a laryngitis, a bronchitis, or a broncho-pneumonia, according to the location of the lesions. In chronic glanders we find the same accessory symptoms that occur in chronic farcy, the hemorrhage of the nose, the swelling of the legs, the chronic cough, and, in the entire horse, the swelling of the testicles.

On healing, the chancres on the mucous membranes leave small, whitish, star-shaped scars, hard and indurated to the touch, and which remain for almost an indefinite time. The chancres heal and the other local symptoms disappear, with the exception of the enlargement of the glands, and we find these so diminished in size that they are scarcely perceptible on examination. During the subacute attacks, with a minimum quantity of local troubles, in chronic glanders and in chronic farcy the animal rarely shows any degree of fever, but does have a generally depraved appearance; it loses flesh and becomes hidebound; the skin becomes dry and the hairs stand on end. There is a cachexia, however, which resembles greatly that of any chronic, organic trouble, but is not diagnostic, although it has in it certain appearances and conditions which often render the animal suspicious to the eye of the expert veterinarian, while without the presence of local lesions he would be unable to state on what he has based his opinion.

ACUTE GLANDERS.

Symptoms.—In the acute form of glanders we find the symptoms which we have just studied in chronic farcy and in chronic glanders in a more acute and aggravated form. There is a rapid outbreak of nodules in the respiratory tract which rapidly degenerate into chancres and pour out a considerable discharge from the nostrils. There is a cough of more or less severity according to the amount and site of the local eruption. Over the surface of the body swellings occur which are rapidly followed by farcy buttons, which break into ulcers; we find the indurated cords and enlargement of the lymphatics.

Bleeding from the nose, sudden swelling of one of the hind legs, and the swelling of the testicles are liable to precede an acute eruption of glanders. As the symptoms become more marked the animal has difficulty of respiration, the flanks heave, the respiration becomes rapid, the pulse becomes quickened, and the temperature becomes elevated to 103°, 104°, or 105° F.

With the other symptoms of an acute fever the general appearance and station of the animal is that of one suffering from an acute pneumonia, but upon examination, while we may find sibilant and mucous râles over the side of the chest, and may possibly hear tubular murmurs at the base of the neck over the trachea, we fail to find the tubular murmur or the large area of dullness on percussion over the sides of the chest which belongs to simple pneumonia.

Diagnosis.—When there is doubt as to the diagnosis, the mallein test, the inoculation test, or the complement-fixation test may be employed. The mallein test is made by injecting mallein (a sterilized extract from a culture of glanders bacilli) beneath the skin. If the horse has glanders there results a febrile reaction and a swelling at the point of injection. If the horse does not have glanders the mallein has no effect or, at most, it produces a slight swelling only at the point of injection. The inoculation test consists in the inoculation of a susceptible animal (usually a guinea pig) with some of the suspected discharge from the nose or a farcy ulcer. If the material is properly used, and if it contains bacilli of glanders, the experimental animal will develop the disease.

The eye test is now universally accepted as a very satisfactory means of diagnosing glanders. This consists in dropping into an eye of a suspected animal a specially prepared solution of mallein, as a result of which in an infected animal the inflammation develops in the eye, resulting in a discharge which varies in intensity from a mucopurulent character to a thick, sticky pus. The eyelids may also swell and many times become glued together. The reaction usually appears in from 8 to 20 hours after the introduction of the mallein.

Neither of these tests should be put into use except by a competent veterinarian. The complement-fixation test is a highly specialized laboratory test and can be carried out only by one versed in laboratory technique. (See Bureau of Animal Industry Bulletin 136.)

The post-mortem examination of the lungs shows that the pneumonia of glanders is a lobular, V-shaped pneumonia scattered throughout the lungs and caused by the specific inflammatory process taking place at the divergence of the smaller air tubes of the lungs. In some cases of acute glanders the formation of nodules may so irritate the mucous membrane of the respiratory tract and cause such a profuse discharge of mucopurulent or purulent matter that the specific character of the original discharge is entirely masked. In this case, too, for a few days the submaxillary space may so swell as to resemble the edematous, inflamed glands of strangles, equine variola, or laryngitis. This condition is especially liable to be marked in an acute outbreak of glanders in a drove of mules.

Cases of chronic farcy and glanders, if not destroyed, may live in a depraved condition until the animal dies from general emaciation and anemia, but in the majority of cases, from some sudden exposure to cold, it develops an acute pneumonia or other simple inflammatory trouble which starts the latent disease and the animal has acute glanders.

In the ass, mule, and plethoric horses acute glanders usually terminates by lobular pneumonia. In other cases the general symptoms may subside. The symptoms of pneumonia gradually disappear, the temperature lowers, the pulse becomes slower, the ulcers heal, leaving small, indurated cicatrices, and the animal may return to apparent health, or may at least be able to do a small amount of work with but a few symptoms of the disease remaining in a chronic form. During the attack of acute glanders the inflammation of the nasal cavities frequently spreads into the sinuses or air cells, which are found in the forehead and in front of the eyes on either side of the face, and causes abscesses of these cavities, which may remain as the only visible symptom of the disease. An animal which has recovered from a case of acute glanders, like the animals which are affected by chronic glanders and chronic farcy, is liable to be affected with emphysema of the lungs (heaves), and to have a chronic cough. In this condition it may continue for a long period, serving as a dangerous source of contagion, the more so because the slight quantity of discharge does not serve as a warning to the owner or driver as profuse discharge does in the more acute cases.

At the post-mortem examination of an animal which has been destroyed or has died of glanders we find evidences of the various lesions which we have studied in the symptoms. In addition to this, we find nodules similar to those which we have seen on the exterior throughout the various organs of the body. Nodules may be found in the liver, in the spleen, and in the kidneys. We may find inflammation of the periosteum of the bones, and we have excessive alterations in the marrow in the interior of the bones themselves. Both these conditions during the life of the animal may have been the cause of the lamenesses which were difficult to diagnose.

In one case which came under the observation of the writer, a lame horse was destroyed and found to have a large abscess of the bone of the arm, with old nodules of the lungs. When an animal has died immediately after an attack of a primary, acute case of glanders, we find small V-shaped spots of acute pneumonia in the lungs. If the animal has made an apparent recovery from acute glanders, and in cases of chronic farcy and chronic glanders, no matter how few the external and visible symptoms may have been, there is a deposit of nodules—small, hard, indurated nodes—of new connective tissue to be found in the lungs. When these have existed for some time we may find a deposit of lime salts in them. These indurated nodules retain the virus and their power to give out contagion for almost an indefinite time, and predispose to the causes which we have studied as the common factors in developing a chronic case into an acute case; that is, an inflammatory process wakens their vitality and produces a reinfection of the entire animal. The blood of an animal suffering from chronic glanders and farcy is not virulent and is unaltered, but during the attack of acute glanders, while the animal has fever, the blood becomes virulent and remains so for a few days.

Treatment.—Almost the entire list of drugs in the pharmacopœia has been tested in the treatment of glanders. Good hygienic surroundings, good feed, with alteratives and tonics, frequently ameliorate the symptoms, and often do so to such an extent that the animal would pass the examination of any expert as a perfectly sound animal. While in this case the number of nodules of the lungs, which are invariably there, may be so few as not to cause sufficient disturbance in the respiration as to attract the attention of the examiner, yet they exist, and will remain there almost indefinitely, with the constant possibility of a return of acute symptoms.

It is probable that some horses may recover from glanders if the infection is slight, but it will not do to depend upon this except under the most stringent veterinary supervision. With good care, good feed, good surroundings and little work, an animal affected with glanders may live for months or even years in a state of apparently perfect health, but with the first deprivation of feed, with a few days of severe hard work, with exposure to cold or with the attack of a simple fever or inflammatory trouble from other causes, the latent seeds of the disease break out and develop the trouble again in an acute form.

In several celebrated cases horses which have been affected with glanders have been known to work for years and die from other causes without ever having had the return of symptoms; but allowing that these cases may occur, they are so few and far between, and the danger of infection of glanders to other horses and to the stable attendants is so great, that no animal which has once been affected with the disease should be allowed to live unless repeated mallein tests have shown him to have become free from taint of glanders.

In all civilized countries, with the exception of some of the States in the United States, the laws are most stringent regarding the prompt declaration on the part of the owner and attending veterinarian at the first suspicion of a case of glanders, and they allow indemnity for the animal. When this is done, in all cases the animal is destroyed and the articles with which it has been in contact are thoroughly disinfected. When the attendants have attempted to hide the presence of the disease in a community, punishment is meted out to the owner, attending veterinarian, or other responsible parties. Several States have passed excellent laws in regard to glanders, but these laws are not always carried out with the rigidity with which they should be.

SPOROTRICHOSIS (MYCOTIC LYMPHANGITIS).

By JOHN R. MOHLER, V. M. D., *Chief, Bureau of Animal Industry.*

This disease has previously been known in this country as epizootic lymphangitis, or pseudo-farcy. It is a chronic, contagious disease, particularly of equines, caused by a specific organism, the *Sporotrichum schenckii*, and characterized by a suppurative inflammation of the subcutaneous lymph vessels and the neighboring lymph glands. Owing to the fact that this affection does not spread as an epizootic and that its causal factor is a fungus, the name sporotrichosis has been suggested.

The disease in man was first described by Schenck and by Beurmann and Gougerot. Carougeau observed its occurrence among horses and mules in Madagascar, while in the United States it was first observed by Pearson in Pennsylvania in 1907, although it is probable that it had existed for many years in various parts of this country. Page and Frothingham were first to recognize its mycotic nature in the United States. More recently Meyer has also made valuable contributions with regard to the existence of this affection. Its presence has been definitely established in Ohio, Iowa, California, and North Dakota, and there is a probability of its existence in Indiana and several Western States.

Bacteriology.—The sporotrichum is 2 microns thick, cylindrical and segmented, having more or less branching threads, which bear spores at the end. In the pus they occur as slightly ovoid bodies 3 to 5 microns long, which are somewhat pointed toward the poles, have a sharp double contour, and only on artificial cultivation at a temperature of over 18° do they develop into the characteristic spore-carrying threads.

The period of incubation varies greatly, extending from three days to four months, or even longer. In artificial inoculations with pus through wounds in the skin, inflammation and swelling of the lymph vessels may be noticed in ten to sixty days; these vessels show in their course a development of hard nodules, from which abscesses form.

The natural infection without doubt is caused through superficial wounds, such as galls, barbed-wire cuts, or through various stable utensils, harness, bandages, insects, etc. Solipeds are mostly susceptible, but cattle may also be infected.

Symptoms.—The inflammation of the lymph vessels is usually first observed on the extremities, especially on one or both hind legs; it may also appear on the forelegs, shoulder, or neck, and more rarely on the rump, udder, and scrotum. The lesions, as a rule, develop in the tissue adjacent to the place of inoculation. In the early stages of the disease the lymph vessels appear very hard and thickened, and along their course hard nodules develop, ranging in size from a pea to a hen's egg. Later these nodules soften, burst spontaneously, and discharge a thick, yellowish pus. The surface of the resulting ulcers or abscess cavities soon fills up with exuberant granulations which protrude beyond the surface of the skin, giving it a fungoid appearance. The affected extremities are considerably enlarged, similar to cases of simple lymphangitis. In rare cases the mucous membrane of the nostrils may also become affected, showing yellowish flat elevations and ulcerations, and these may extend by metastasis to internal organs. In cases in which the mucous membrane is affected, the submaxillary lymph gland may also become enlarged and suppurate.

The constitutional symptoms accompanying this disease are not very marked and may be altogether absent. There is usually only a very slight fever, which seldom runs over 102° F. The appetite is not impaired except in the advanced cases.

Lesions.—The anatomical changes are most marked in the skin and the subcutaneous tissues. They may become 2 to 3 inches thick and indurated as the result of fibrous-tissue formation, owing to the inflammation present. On the baconlike cut surface suppurative areas and granulating sores may be noticed of various sizes, also enlarged lymph vessels filled with clotted lymph mixed with pus. The neighboring lymph glands are usually enlarged and frequently contain suppurating foci. Rarely the internal organs may show metastatic abscesses.

Diagnosis.—The diagnosis is based on the characteristic appearance of the ulcerations, which show exuberant granulation of a bright red color, inverted edges, and a thick, creamy, glutinous discharge. These manifestations differentiate the disease from glanders, in which the ulcers are craterlike, do contain exuberant granulations, and the discharge is of a viscous, oily character. The submaxillary and other nodes as well as the corded lymphatics in glanders are more firmly attached to the adjacent tissues, and are therefore less movable. In some chronic cases of sporotrichosis, however, the lesions may closely resemble those of farcy, and in these cases the microscopical examination of the pus will disclose the nature of the affection. In the pus the causative organism can be easily seen in the unstained specimen, and is recognized by its size, shape, and highly refractory double outline. Furthermore, the injection of mallein in cases of sporotrichosis will be attended with negative results.

Treatment.—At the onset of the disease treatment consists in entire extirpation of the nodules, in case the lesions are localized. In cases in which the nodules have formed abscesses, their opening is recommended, followed by the application of the actual cautery or a 1 to 250 solution of bichlorid of mercury. It must be borne in mind that the organism is quite resistant to antiseptics, and the best results will be obtained from the application of a solution of a strong antiseptic following the opening of the lesions. Internally, potassium iodid is recommended in 2-dram doses, dissolved in drinking water, twice a day.

In the most favorable cases recovery results in from five to seven weeks; as a rule, however, it requires several months.

In order to prevent the spreading of the disease the affected animals should be isolated, the products of the disease should be destroyed, and the stable should be disinfected with very strong liquid disinfectants in consideration of the resistance of the causative organism.

RABIES, HYDROPHOBIA, OR MADNESS.

Rabies is a contagious disease, which is usually transmitted by a bite and by the introduction of a virus contained in the saliva of an affected animal. It may, however, be transmitted in other ways. It is characterized by symptoms of aberration of the nervous system and invariably terminates fatally. It is accompanied with lesions, inflammation, and degeneration in the central nervous system. It is a disease that is most common in the dog, but is transmitted to the horse, either from dogs or from any other animal affected with it. (See also remarks on page 244.) As a disease of the horse it is invariably the result of the bite of a rabid animal, usually a dog.

Perhaps no disease in medicine has been the object of more controversy than rabies. Certain medical men of prominence have even doubted its existence, and many others have claimed for it a spontaneous origin. The experience of ages, however, has shown that contagion can be proved in the great majority of cases, and, by analogy with other contagious diseases, we may only believe that the development of one case requires the preexistence of a case from which the virus has been transmitted. Pasteur has further added to our knowledge of the disease by showing that a virus capable of cultivation exists in the nervous system, especially in the lower part of the brain (medulla oblongata) and in the anterior part of the spinal column. He has further shown that that portion of the nervous system which contains the virus, the exact nature of which has not yet been demonstrated, will retain it for a very long time if kept at a very low temperature or if left surrounded by carbolic acid; but if the nerve matter, which is virulent at first, is exposed to the air and is kept from putrefaction by substances which will absorb the surrounding moisture, it will gradually lose its virulence and become inoffensive in about fifteen days. He has also further shown that the action of a weak virus on an animal will prevent the development of a stronger virus, and from this he has formulated his method of prophylactic treatment. This treatment consists in the successive inoculation of portions of the nerve matter containing the virus from a rabid animal which has been exposed to the atmosphere for thirteen days, ten days, seven days, and four days, until the virulent matter which will produce rabies in any unprotected animal can be inoculated with impunity. A curious result of the experiments of Pasteur is that an animal which has first been inoculated with a virus of full strength can be protected by subsequent inoculations of attenuated virus repeated in doses of increasing strength.

Innumerable attempts have been made to discover the causative agent, and investigators have announced the finding of many of the lower forms of animal and vegetable life as the pathogenic factor. Among the recently described causes, certain protozoanlike bodies found in the ganglionic cells in 1903 by Negri, and termed Negri bodies, are of a very suggestive nature. Negri claims that these bodies are not only specific for rabies, but that they are protozoa and the cause of the disease. His work has been corroborated by investigators in all parts of the scientific world. An examination of the vitality of these bodies will show a striking resemblance to the vitality of an emulsion of the virulent tissue. Thus, they have been found to be quite resistant to external agencies, such as putrefaction, drying, etc., and are about the last portion of the nerve cell to survive the advance of decomposition. They are also found in more than 96 per cent of the cases of rabies examined, but have not been proved to exist in other diseases.

Valenti states, as his strongest evidence of the protozoan nature of the bodies, that the virus of rabies is neutralized in test tubes by quinin, while no other alkaloid has this property. As a result of the work performed in the New York City Board of Health laboratory, Park claims that Negri bodies are found in animals before the beginning of visible symptoms, and evidence is given that they may be found early enough to account for the infectiousness of the central nervous system. These bodies are now almost universally considered as diagnostic of rabies, and in the pathological laboratory of the Bureau of Animal Industry their detection in the nerve cells of the brain suffices for a diagnosis of rabies without animal inoculations. In case these granular bodies are not found in a suspected animal, the plexiform ganglion is next examined, and should negative results still be obtained, the inoculation of rabbits is then made as a last resort. It is indeed rare that positive results are obtained from the latter method after the first two methods have been negative, but it has occurred occasionally in cases in which the animal had been killed in the early stages of the disease.

Symptoms.—From the moment of inoculation by the bite of a rabid dog or other rabid animal or by other means, a variable time elapses before the development of any symptoms. This time may be eight days or it may be several months; it is usually about four weeks. The first symptom is an irritation of the original wound. This wound, which may have healed completely, commences to itch until the horse rubs or bites it into a new sore. The horse then becomes irritable and vicious, and it is especially susceptible to moving objects, excessive light, noises, the entrance of an attendant, or any other disturbance will cause the patient to be on the defensive. It apparently sees imaginary objects; the slightest noise is exaggerated into threatening violence; the approach of an attendant or another animal, especially a dog, is interpreted as an assault and the horse will strike and bite. The violence on the part of the rabid horse is not for a moment to be confounded with the fury of the same animal suffering from meningitis or any other trouble of the brain. But in rabies there is a volition, a premeditated method, in the attacks which the animal will make, which is not found in the other diseases. Between the attacks of fury the animal may become calm for a variable period. The writer attended a case in which, after a violent attack of an hour, the horse was sufficiently calm to be walked 10 miles and only developed violence again an hour after being placed in the new stable. In the period of fury the horse will bite at the reopened original wound; it will rear and attempt to break its halter and fastenings; it will bite at the woodwork and surrounding objects in the stable. If the animal lives long enough it shows paralytic symptoms and falls to the ground, unable to use two or more of its extremities, but in the majority of cases in its excesses of violence it does physical injury to itself. It breaks its jaws in biting at the manger or fractures other bones in throwing itself on the ground and dies of hemorrhage or internal injuries. At times throughout the course of the disease there is an excessive sensibility of the skin which, if irritated by the touch, will bring on attacks of violence. Throughout the course of the disease the animal may have appetite and desire water, but on attempting to swallow has a spasm of the throat which renders the act impossible. This latter condition, which is common in all rabid animals, has given the disease the name of hydrophobia (fear of water).

54763°—23——36

In a case under the care of the writer a horse, four weeks after being bitten on the forearm by a rabid dog, developed local irritation in the healed wound and tore it with its teeth into a large ulcer. This was healed by local treatment in 10 days, and the horse was kept under surveillance for more than a month. On the advice of another practitioner the horse was taken home and put to work; within 3 days it developed violent symptoms and had to be destroyed.

Diagnosis.—The diagnosis of rabies in the horse is to be made from the various brain troubles to which the animal is subject; first by the history of a previous bite of a rabid animal or inoculation by other means; second, by the evident volition and consciousness on the part of the animal in its attacks, offensive and defensive, on persons, animals, or other disturbing surroundings. The irritation and reopening of the original wound or point of inoculation is a valuable factor in diagnosis. Diagnosis after death may be made by microscopic examination for Negri bodies or by the inoculation of rabbits, as already mentioned.

Recovery from rabies may be considered as a question of the correctness of the original diagnosis. Rabies is always fatal.

Treatment.—No remedial treatment has ever been successful. All the anodynes and anesthetics, opium, belladonna, bromid of potash, ether, chloroform, etc., have been used without avail. The prophylactic treatment of successive inoculations is being used on human beings, and has experimentally proved efficacious in dogs, but would be impracticable in the horse unless the conditions were quite exceptional.

DOURINE.

By JOHN R. MOHLER, V. M. D., *Chief, Bureau of Animal Industry.*

Dourine (also known as maladie du coït, equine syphilis, covering disease, breeding paralysis) is a specific infectious disease affecting under normal conditions only the horse and ass, transmitted from animal to animal by the act of copulation, and due to an animal parasite, the *Trypanosoma equiperdum.*

History.—It is described as having existed as early as 1796 in the Eastern Hemisphere, and was more or less prevalent in several of the European countries, including France, Germany, Austria, and Switzerland, during the first half of the nineteenth century. Its presence was recognized for the first time in the United States in 1886, when an outbreak occurred in Illinois. Since then the existence of the disease has been observed at irregular intervals in numerous other States, including Nebraska, Iowa, Montana, Wyoming, New Mexico, North Dakota, and South Dakota.

Symptoms.—There are many variations in the symptoms of dourine, and this is particularly true of the disease as it occurs in this country. Two distinct stages may be noted which vary somewhat from those described in textbooks, but probably no more than could be expected when differences of climatic conditions and methods of handling are taken into consideration.

The first stage chiefly concerns the sexual organs and therefore differs somewhat in the male and female. In the second stage the symptoms indicating an affection of the nervous system are more prominent and are not dependent upon the sex of the animal.

Following a variable period of incubation of from 8 days to 2 months, there is seen in the stallion an irritation and swelling about the penis and sheath. In a few days small vesicles or blisters may appear on the penis, which later break, discharging a yellowish, serous fluid and having irregular, raw ulcers. The ulcers show a tendency to heal rapidly, leaving scars which are permanent. There may be more or less continuous dripping from the uretha of a yellowish, serouslike fluid. Stallions may show great excitement when brought in the vicinity of mares, but service is often impossible because of the fact that a complete erection of the penis does not occur.

In the mare the first symptoms may be so slight as to be overlooked. The disease, being the result of copulation, usually begins with inflammation of the vulva and vagina. There may be a muco-purulent discharge, which may be slight or profuse in quantity, agglutinating the hairs of the tail. The mare may appear uneasy and urinate frequently. Vesicles may appear on the external vulva and mucous membrane of the vulva and vagina which later rupture and form ulcers. On the dark skin of the external vulva the scars resulting from healing of the ulcers are white, more or less circular in outline, from one-eighth to half an inch in diameter, and pitlike. This depigmentation of the skin about the external genitals is permanent.

Urticarial eruptions or plaques which break out over various parts of the body are a frequent symptom seen in animals of either sex. These are sharply defined and edematous swellings of the skin about the size of a half dollar or may be even larger. The usual locations of these plaques are the croup, belly, and neck.

The intensity of the symptoms mentioned which are significant of the early stage of the disease may vary to a wide extent and in many instances be so mild as to escape the attention of any but the most careful observer. They commonly disappear after a brief period. The apparent recovery, however, is not permanent, for such animals after a period of variable length manifest constitutional or nervous symptoms. These may not appear for several months or even years. They consist of a general nervous disorder with staggering, swaying gait, especially in the hind limbs. The animal generally becomes emaciated, the abdomen assuming a tucked-up appearance. The first indication of paralysis will be noted in traveling, when the animal fails to pick up one of the hind feet as freely as the other, or both may become affected at the same time, at which time knuckling is a common symptom. Labored breathing is occasionally noted. When the paralysis of the hind limbs starts to appear the disease usually progresses rapidly. The horse goes down, is unable to rise, and dies in a short time from nervous exhaustion. The appetite usually remains good up to the last.

Although a case of dourine may now and then recover, as a rule the disease is present in the latent stage. Bad weather, exposure, insufficient feed, and complicating diseases like influenza, distemper, or in fact any condition which tends to lower the vitality of the animal, may hasten the termination of the disease.

Diagnosis.—The complement-fixation test furnishes by far the most reliable means of diagnosis and is especially valuable in a chronic affection of this character, when the symptoms manifested are variable and frequently so obscure as to escape observation. This is a laboratory test requiring special facilities and the services of a trained bacteriologist.

Treatment.—Little benefit can be obtained from medicinal treatment, nor is such treatment desirable in this country, where the disease has existed only in restricted areas, and where sanitary considerations demand its prompt eradication.

INFECTIOUS ABORTION IN MARES.

Infectious abortion (also known as contagious abortion, epizootic abortion, enzootic abortion, slinking of colts) is a disease of mares which from a specific cause results in the premature expulsion of the fetus and its membranes from the uterus. It is characterized by an inflammatory condition of the female reproductive organs.

The contagious nature of the disease had not been recognized until recently, the disease being principally attributed to various conditions, such as traumatic influences, various infectious diseases, spoiled feed, drugs, and other factors. Ostertag was the first to study premature births in mares, attributing as the cause of the same a streptococcus, which he was supposed to have been able to use successfully in artificially producing abortion, either by inoculations or feeding. His findings could not be substantiated by other investigators.

The earliest appearance of the disease in this country was in 1886, at which time it caused considerable damage to the horse-breeding industry in the Mississippi Valley. Smith and Kilbourne investigated an outbreak in Pennsylvania in 1893, at which time they incriminated another germ belonging to the paratyphus B group as the causative factor of the disease. These findings have been subsequently substantiated by many investigators abroad, as well as in this country, notably so by De Jong, Dassonville, and Rivière, and by Good and Meyer. More recently very valuable information was contributed to our knowledge on this disease by Schofield, of Canada, especially with regard to the biological tests for diagnosis. Good suggested *"Bacillus abortivus equinus"* as the name for the specific organism.

The causative agent of this disease is not identical with the germ causing abortion in cattle. It exerts its action, however, in a similar manner, and appears to have, under certain conditions, a predilection for the genital organs of the mare, where it induces certain morbid changes whereby a premature expulsion of the fetus is the result. The germ is usually present in the fetal membranes and also in the aborted fetus. Mares may harbor the infection without disclosing any apparent ill effects. It appears to exert its influence mainly upon the female genital organs, where it may induce an inflammatory condition of the uterus.

The infected animals may carry the fetus through the normal period of pregnancy, giving birth to either a normal or a weak colt, or again abortion may take place at any time during pregnancy, mostly, however, from the sixth to the ninth month.

Symptoms.—The symptoms suggestive of abortion are frequently entirely absent. At times the abortion may be ushered in by symptoms of colicky pains, restlessness, and periodical straining; these, however, are by no means constant, especially if the abortion takes place in the early months of pregnancy. The genital organs are usually swollen, showing a mucous discharge. Immediately before abortion the symptoms are more aggravated. Following abortion the discharge is more characteristic, being of a dark-brown color, sometimes even bloody, and contains streaky or flaky pus. The fetal membranes in all cases are not expelled with the aborted fetus, but there is a tendency toward retention of these membranes, which frequently has serious consequences upon the health of the animal. At times it becomes necessary to resort to manual removal of the afterbirth, and the inflammation of the uterus and a chronic discharge usually follow such conditions. The expelled fetuses, as a rule, die soon after the abortion, and if the expulsion has taken place at a time close to its full term the fetuses are usually poorly developed and subject to various kinds of digestive and septic disorders. The fetuses do not disclose any particular abnormal appearance on external examination; in many cases, however, the post-mortem examination reveals inflammatory changes of various organs.

The method of infection has not yet been satisfactorily established; nevertheless it is essential that we consider as the principal mode of infection the ways which have been proved for the contagious abortion in cattle. These are especially by ingestion; that is, by taking up the germs with the feed, water, or other means, which have become contaminated with the germs. The infection through the genital organs is probably not so frequent, but in this regard the stallion no doubt plays an important rôle in the spreading of the disease. Schofield considers this method of infection as the principal source of spreading the disease.

It must be considered that in infected stables the germs may be present throughout the premises, and by keeping animals which have aborted in such stables a contamination of feed and utensils may continually take place, since the aborted mares usually discharge a considerable quantity of material which is often heavily charged with the germs. The germ is taken up by the body with the feed or water, passing from the intestines into the blood, and from there is carried to the genital organs, where it finds suitable conditions for its development. Milk from an infected mare may also contain the germ, and colts may become infected by sucking the milk of infected mothers. In such instances the infection may remain dormant until the colt develops and becomes pregnant, when the organism, finding a condition suitable for its development, produces the disease.

On the other hand, stallions used in covering infected mares may be carriers of the germs, and when used for the breeding of healthy animals may in this manner readily transmit the disease to them.

Diagnosis.—Contagious abortion may be diagnosed by the changes which occur in the fetal membranes, and also in the expelled fetus. In order, however, to substantiate a diagnosis with certainty, demonstration of the germ by miscroscopical examination is necessary. The occurrence of frequent abortions among the mares in a stable is also an additional evidence of the contagious character of the malady. It must be considered that at times infected mares may carry the fetus to full maturity, in which case the diagnosis is possible only by blood examinations in a laboratory.

Infected animals usually abort only once; however, in a certain proportion of cases they may abort even two, three, or four times in succession.

Animals which establish a tolerance for the infection, and carry the fetus to full maturity, may nevertheless remain a source of danger for spreading the disease.

The tests used in laboratories for the diagnosis are the agglutination and complement-fixation tests, by which the disease may be diagnosed from a sample of blood from a suspected animal. Such tests, however, have to be confined to the laboratories, which are equipped for such work.

Treatment and prevention.—Medicinal treatment is usually of no avail, and all efforts should be directed toward the prevention of the disease. Various medicinal agents have been recommended and are being exploited for the treatment, but to the present time no satisfactory evidence has been established as to their merits. Bacterial vaccines prepared from the specific organism have been given limited trials, but to date they can not be considered as entirely satisfactory, since it will require considerable experience with them before their usefulness can be definitely established.

The prevention should consist largely in sanitary measures directed toward the disinfection of premises and animals. (For a method for disinfection of premises see article under that heading.)

The following procedure is advised for the disinfection of animals: To prevent a stallion from carrying the infection from a diseased mare to a healthy one the sheath and the penis should be disinfected with a solution of $\frac{1}{2}$ per cent of compound cresol solution, lysol, or trikresol, or a 1 per cent carbolic acid or 1 to 1,000 potassium permanganate solution in warm water. For this purpose it is advisable to use a soft-rubber tube with a large funnel attached to one end, or an ordinary syringe and tube would serve the purpose. The tube should be inserted into the sheath, and the foreskin held with the hand to prevent the immediate escape of the fluid. In addition to this the hair of the belly and inner side of the thighs should be sponged with an antiseptic. This disinfection should invariably precede and follow every service.

With regard to the mares, a period of three months should elapse between abortion and a subsequent breeding, and especially if there is any evidence of a discharge the breeding of the animal should not be undertaken. The mare showing signs of abortion should be immediately isolated and the fetus and membranes should be burned. The fetus should never be dragged across a barnyard or stable, but should be removed by other means by which the contamination of the premises may be prevented. The stall in which the animal aborted should be thoroughly disinfected and the genital organs of the mare washed daily with a disinfectant. The antiseptic washing recommended for the treatment of the stallions prior to and after breeding should be also used for the irrigation of the uterus of mares which have aborted. This treatment should be continued daily until all evidence of discharge has ceased. The isolation of the animal should be carried out for at least one month after the evidence of a discharge has ceased.

By carefully and persistently carrying out the sanitary measures it may be possible to control and finally eradicate the disease.

NAVEL ILL OF COLTS.

Navel ill of colts is also known as joint ill, omphalophlebitis, septic arthritis of sucklings, and pyosepticemia of the newly born.

The unfavorable outlook after the appearance of the disease, together with the fact that the disease when present requires the attention of a veterinarian, demands that the breeder concern himself with its prevention.

The disease is caused by a microorganism and several bacteria have been suspected of being responsible. Every one of the suspected organisms is found abundantly in manure and objects contaminated with manure. The infective material gains entrance into the colt through the open umbilical cord as a result of its coming into contact with litter, floors, or discharges from its dam contaminated by one of the organisms which cause the trouble. There are cases on record in which the infection has taken place before birth, and while some investigators assert that this method is the principal mode of infection still, in a large number of cases, the prophylactic measures adopted to guard against the infection through the navel cord have given good results. Since infection before birth can not be controlled satisfactorily, we are justified, for all practical purposes, in preventing navel ill by guarding against the infection through the cord at birth or soon afterwards.

Cleanliness of stables where pregnant mares are kept must be insisted upon. This is especially necessary where outbreaks of navel ill have been known to exist. Mares in the last stages of gestation should be placed in a box stall which has previously been cleaned and disinfected. The bedding should be frequently renewed and the external genitals and neighboring tissues should be kept clean and disinfected with a 2 per cent solution of carbolic acid or 1 per cent liquor cresolis compositus, or any other reliable disinfecting agent. Operations for opening abscesses and removal of afterbirths from cows should not be executed in the immediate vicinity of mares in an advanced stage of pregnancy.

The foal when dropped should be placed on clean bedding. In any event the cord of the foal should be washed in a disinfectant solution and tied at about 1½ inches from the navel with a band or string which has previously been soaked in a disinfectant solution. With a sharp pair of scissors the navel cord is then severed about one-half inch below the band and again disinfected. The ligature should not be tightened, however, until pulsation of the vessels in the cord has ceased. The stump of the cord is then painted with strong carbolic-acid solution, tincture of iodin, or a mixture of equal parts of tincture of iodin and glycerin. The stump should be washed daily with a disinfectant and either painted with iodin mixture or carbolic acid or dusted with some reliable antiseptic healing powder. After five days the parchmentlike dried stump may be cut off and the navel wound washed with a disinfectant solution and dusted with powder until healed.

The cases of navel ill resulting from infection before birth can not well be guarded against. By keeping mares, advanced in pregnancy, in good physical condition, the fetus will be expelled immediately upon the opening of the uterine cavity.

Once the infection of the navel cord has set in, the cord should not be ligated but should be washed in a disinfectant solution and a veterinarian called for the subsequent treatment.

INFECTIOUS ANEMIA OR SWAMP FEVER.

By JOHN R. MOHLER, V. M. D., *Chief, Bureau of Animal Industry.*

Infectious anemia of horses, known also by a number of other names, as swamp fever, American surra, malarial fever, typhoid fever of horses, the unknown disease, no-name disease, plains paralysis, and pernicious anemia, has recently been the subject of much investigation. The cause of the disease has now been definitely determined as an invisible virus, which is capable of passing through the pores of the finest porcelain filters, like the infection of foot-and-mouth disease, rinderpest, hog cholera, and similar diseases. The disease is most prevalent in low-lying and badly drained sections of the country, although it has been found on marshy pastures during wet seasons in altitudes as high as 7,500 feet. Therefore proper drainage of infected pastures is indicated as a preventive. It is also more prevalent during wet years than in dry seasons. It usually makes its appearance in June and increases in frequency until October, although the chronic cases may be seen in the winter, having been contracted during the warm season.

Cause.—It has been conclusively proved that infectious anemia is produced by an invisible filterable organism which is transmissible to horses, mules, and asses by subcutaneous inoculation of blood serum. The virus which is present in the blood may be transmitted to a number of equines in a series of inoculations by injecting either the whole blood, the defibrinated blood, or the blood serum which has been passed through a fine Pasteur filter, thus eliminating all the visible forms of organismal life, including bacteria, trypanosoma, piroplasma, etc. This virus has also been found to be active in the carcass of an affected animal 24 hours after death.

Following the injection of the infectious principle there is a period of incubation which may extend from ten days to one and one-half months, at the end of which time the onset of the disease is manifested by a rise of temperature. If uncomplicated, the infection runs a chronic course, terminating in death in from two months to one and one-half years, or even longer. The probability of the virus being spread by an intermediate host, such as flies, mosquitoes, internal parasites, etc., is now receiving careful investigation.

From experiments already conducted it appears that this disease, formerly supposed to be confined to Manitoba and Minnesota, is more or less prevalent in Kansas, Nebraska, Colorado, Wyoming, Montana, North Dakota, Virginia, Texas, and New York. It also occurs in Europe, having been reported in Germany under the name of infectious anemia and in France as infectious typho-anemia.

Symptoms.—The disease is characterized by a progressive pernicious anemia, remittent fever, polyuria, and gradual emaciation in spite of a voracious appetite. It begins to manifest itself by a dull, listless appearance and by general weakness, the animal tiring very easily. This stage is followed closely by a staggering, swaying, uncertain gait, the hind legs being mostly affected. There is also noted a weakness and tenderness in the region of the loins, and at the same time the pulse, though weak, stringy, and intermittent, increases in rapidity and may run as high as 70. The temperature may rise to 103° F. or higher, remaining high for several days, and then dropping to rise again irregularly. Toward the end of the disease the temperature occasionally remains persistently high. The horse may improve for a time, but usually this improvement is followed by a more severe attack than the first. Venous regurgitation is sometimes noticed in the jugular before death. The quantity of urine passed is enormous in some cases. Death finally occurs from exhaustion or syncope.

The blood shows a slight decrease in the number of white blood cells, while there is a gradual but marked diminution of red corpuscles, the count running as low as 2,000,000 per cubic millimeter, the normal count being 7,000,000. If the blood is drawn from such an animal, the resulting red clot will be about one-fifth of the amount drawn. Occasionally a slow dripping of blood-tinged serum from the nostrils is observed as a result of this very thin blood oozing from the mucuous membranes. Petechiæ, or small hemorrhagic points, are sometimes noticed on the nictitating membrane and conjunctiva, while paleness of the visible mucous membranes of the nose and mouth is usually in evidence, although they may have a yellow or mahogany tinge. Often a fluctuating, pendulous swelling may appear on the lower lip, point of elbow, sheath, legs, under the belly, or on some other pendent portion, especially late in the disease, which is indicative of poor circulation, thinning of the blood, and consequent loss of capillary action.

Lesions.—After death the carcass is found to be very much emaciated and anemic, the visible mucosa being very pale. This marked absence of adipose tissue makes the skinning of the animal a difficult task. Subcutaneous and intermuscular edema and hemorrhages are frequently observed, although in many cases it is remarkable to see how few macroscopic lesions may be present. The predominating and most constant lesion is probably the petechiæ, so often observed in the muscle or on the serous membranes of the heart. The heart is generally enlarged and may be the only organ to show evidence of disease. In other cases the lungs may be studded with petechiæ, with a serous exudate present in the thoracic cavity. In addition to the petechiæ already noted, the pericardial sac generally contains an increased quantity of fluid. The abdominal cavity may show peritonitis and a hemorrhagic condition of the intestines, which probably result from overfeeding in consequence of the ravenous appetite. The liver, although usually normal, sometimes presents a few areas of degeneration. The spleen is at times found to be enlarged and covered with petechiæ. The kidneys may appear normal or anemic and flaccid, but microscopically they usually show a chronic parenchymatous degeneration. The lymph glands may be enlarged and hemorrhagic.

Diagnosis.—The diagnosis of the disease is not difficult, especially in advanced stages. The insidious onset, remittent fever, progressive emaciation and anemia, unimpaired or ravenous appetite, staggering gait and polyuria are a train of symptoms which make the disease sufficiently characteristic to differentiate it from other diseases affecting horses in this country. The peculiar relapsing type of fever, the great reduction in the number of red blood cells, and the absence of eosinophila are sufficient to differentiate it from the anemias produced by internal parasites, while it may be readily distinguished from surra by the nonsusceptibility of cattle and by the great ease with which the trypanosoma may be found in the latter affection.

Prognosis.—The prognosis of the disease is very unfavorable. Veterinarians in different sections of the country where it is prevalent report a mortality of 75 per cent or even higher. Recovery takes place only when treatment is begun early or when the animal has a long convalescent period.

Treatment.—The treatment of the disease has so far been far from satisfactory. The iodid, permanganate, and carbonate of potash have been used. Arsenic, axytol, quinin, and silver preparations have been suggested, but all have been uniformly without success. Intestinal antiseptics have been resorted to, and the results are encouraging but not altogether satisfactory. Symptomatic treatment seems to be the most dependable. For instance, Davison, of this bureau, was able to reduce greatly the mortality from this affection by giving an antipyretic of 40 grains of quinin, 2 drams of acetanilid, and 30 grains of powdered nux vomica four times daily. In the late stages, with weak heart action, alcohol should be substituted for acetanilid. Cold-water sponge baths may be given, and in addition frequent copious injections of cold water per rectum, which has a beneficial effect in reducing the temperature and in stimulating peristalsis of the bowels, which, as a result of the disease, show a tendency to become torpid during the fever. Purgatives, on account of their debilitating effect, should not be given unless absolutely necessary, but laxatives and easily digested feeds should be given instead. Not infrequently a dirty yellowish tinge of the visible mucous membranes has been observed, in which cases 20 grains of calomel in from 2 to 4 drams of aloes in a ball, or 2-dram doses of fluid extract of podophyllin, may be given. Following the subsidence of the fever, a tonic should be administered, composed of the following drugs in combination:

Arsenious acid	grams	2
Powdered nux vomica	do	28
Powdered cinchona bark	do	85
Powdered gentian root	do	110

These should be well mixed and one-half teaspoonful given to the affected animal at each feed.

As in the case of all other infectious diseases, the healthy should be separated from the sick horses and thorough disinfection of the infected stables, stalls, litter, and stable utensils should be carried out in order to prevent the recurrence of the disease. As a disinfectant the compound solution of cresol, carbolic acid, or chlorid of lime may be used, by mixing 6 ounces of any one of these chemicals with 1 gallon of water. One of the approved coal-tar sheep dips may also be used to advantage in a 5 per cent solution (6 ounces of dip to 1 gallon of water). The disinfectant solution should be applied liberally to all parts of the stable, and sufficient lime may be added to the solution to make the disinfected area conspicious.

Investigations are now in progress with a view of producing a vaccine or serum that will protect horses that have been exposed to the disease.

SURRA.

By CH. WARDELL STILES, PH. D.

Professor of Zoology, United States Public Health Service.

Surra is not known to occur in the United States, but it is more or less common in the Philippine Islands and India. It is caused by a microscopic, flagellate animal parasite, known as *Trypanosoma evansi*, 20 to 34 μ long by 1 to 2 μ broad, which lives in the blood and destroys the red blood corpuscles. In general the disease is very similar to and belongs in the same general class with tsetse-fly disease, or nagana, of Africa and mal de caderas, of South America.

Surra is a wet-weather disease, occurring chiefly during or immediately after heavy rainfalls, floods, or inundations.

Surra attacks especially horses, asses, and mules, but it may occur in carabao, camels, elephants, cats, and dogs, and has been transmitted to cattle, buffaloes, sheep, goats, rabbits, guinea pigs, rats, and monkeys. No birds, reptiles, amphibia (frogs, etc.), or fish are known to suffer from it. It attacks both male and female animals, young and old. Australian breeds of horses and white and gray mules are said to be more susceptible than animals of other breeds and color.

Surra in equines and camels is said to be an invariably fatal disease, but cattle occasionally recover from it. There is no history of a definite onset of the disease, and the condition is progressive, usually with a number of relapses. The period of incubation may vary somewhat; in experimental cases it is from 2 to 75 (usually 6 to 8) days, according to conditions. The duration varies with the species of animal attacked, their age, and general condition. The average duration in the horse is reported at less than two months, though some cases may terminate fatally in less than one to two weeks.

Method of infection.—All evidence now available seems to indicate that surra is strictly a wound disease, namely, that the parasite may enter the body only through a wound of some kind. Apparently by far the most common method is through wounds produced by biting flies whose mouth parts are moist with the infected blood of some animal bitten by the same flies immediately before biting the healthy animal. Crows may also transmit the infection by pecking at sores on a diseased animal, soiling their beaks with blood, and transferring this infected blood to a healthy animal. Likewise, if a scratch is made on a horse and then infected blood is rubbed on the scratch, the horse will become diseased. If, in experiment, infected blood is fed to a healthy animal, the latter may contract surra in case it has an abraded or wounded spot in the mouth; but if no part of the lining of the alimentary canal is wounded, infection does not take place. Thus dogs and cats may contract the disease by wounding the lining of the mouth (as with splinters of bone) while feeding on the carcasses of surra subjects. All available evidence indicates that under normal conditions of pregnancy the disease is not transmitted from mother to fetus.

There is a popular view that surra may be contracted by drinking stagnant water and by eating grass and other vegetation grown upon land subject to inundation, but there is no good experimental evidence to support this view. Probably the correct interpretation of the facts cited in support of this theory is that biting flies are numerous around stagnant water and in inundated pastures; hence, that a great number of possible transmitters of the disease are present in these places.

Symptoms.[1]—The invasion of this disease when contracted naturally is usually marked by symptoms of a trivial character; the skin feels hot, and there may be more or less fever; there is also slight loss of appetite, and the animal appears dull and stumbles during action; early a symptom sometimes appears which may be the first intimation of the animal's indisposition, and which, as a guide to diagnosis, is of great importance; it is the presence of a general or localized urticarial eruption. If the blood is examined microscopically, it may be found to present a normal appearance; but in the majority of cases a few small, rapidly moving organisms will be observed, giving to the blood, as it passes among the corpuscles, a peculiar, vibrating movement, which if once observed will not easily be forgotten. If the parasite has not been discovered in the blood for several days, the symptoms mentioned above may be the only ones noticed, and, as a rule, when treated with febrifuges, the horse quickly improves in health and the appetite returns. This condition does not last for more than a few days, when the animal is again observed to present a dull and dejected appearance, and on examination well-marked symptoms are found; the skin is hot, the temperature more or less elevated—101.7° to 104° F.; the pulse full and frequent—56 to 64 beats a minute; the visible mucous membranes may appear clean, but the conjunctival membranes, especially those covering the membrana nictitans, are usually the seat of dark-red patches of ecchymosis, varying in size in different animals. There is more or less thirst and slight loss of appetite; the animal eats its grain and green grass, but leaves all or a portion of the hay with which it has been supplied. At the same time there are slight catarrhal symptoms present, including lacrimation and a little mucous discharge from the nostrils. Occasionally at this period of the disease the submaxillary glands may be found enlarged and perhaps somewhat tender on manipulation. One symptom is markedly absent, namely, the presence of rigors or the objective sign of chilliness. In addition, it will be noted that there is some swelling and edema of the legs, generally between the fetlock and the hock, which pits but is not painful on pressure, and in case of horses there may be also some swelling of the sheath at this stage of the disease. When the fever and concomitant symptoms have declared themselves for a short period, one thing becomes especially noticeable in every animal attacked, namely, the rapidity with which it loses flesh. If the blood has been examined microscopically during the second period of fever, at first a few parasites will have been observed in it, which day by day increase in number and reach a maximum, where they remain for a varying period, or at once suddenly or

---

[1] This summary of symptoms is based upon work by Lingard.

gradually disappear during the period of apyrexia. After the fever and the accompanying symptoms have for the second time been present for a few days—the period varying from one to six—the animal is found to have lost the dull, dejected appearance and to look bright. The temperature has fallen and, in some cases, has attained normal or even subnormal limits. The visible mucous membranes are clean, and the conjunctival petechiæ begin to fade; the pulse, however, will be found to be weak and thready in character, but the appetite excellent, and, in fact, if it were not for the loss of flesh and slight edema of the legs, there would be little to show that the animal was sick. Unfortunately, however, this condition does not continue for any great length of time, for again the temperature is elevated; in the course of a few hours the thermometer registers a still higher degree, the animal is dull and dejected, and by the following day the visible mucous membranes present a yellow tinge; large ecchymoses, dark in color, appear on the conjunctival membranes, the action of the heart is irritable, the pulse full and quick, or at times intermittent, and regurgitation may be observed in the jugulars, the breathing is quickened, and the individual respirations are shallow. On watching an animal in this condition it may be noticed that it takes seven or eight very short inspirations, followed by a much more prolonged and sonorous one; at the same time the breathing is more abdominal than thoracic in character. On examination of the legs it will be found that the swelling and edema have increased considerably, and that on the under surface of the abdomen, where previously it was confined to the sheath, it has now commenced to spread forward along the subcutaneous tissue between the skin and the muscles. During the whole of this time the appetite will have varied little, and the evacuations will be only slightly, if at all, altered in character. In the blood a repetition of the previous events takes place, the parasites make their appearance and increase to a maximum and again suddenly or gradually disappear, according to the length of the fever period. These periods, alternating with and without fever, may go on for a considerable time. The progress of the disease is variable and greatly depends upon the condition of the animal attacked, the weak one succumbing very rapidly, but each return of the fever brings with it, as a rule, an increase in the severity of the symptoms. There is increased yellowness of the membranes, fresh crops of petechiæ on the conjunctiva, a collection of gelatinous material at the inner angle, which at times becomes red in color from an admixture of blood, and which on microscopic examination is found to contain a varying number of the surra parasites; increased swelling and edema of the extremities and abdomen, which now extends between the fore limbs and up the chest. During this time the wasting has been steadily progressive, especially of the muscles of the back and those surrounding the hip joint and the glutei.

Toward the termination of the disease it will be noticed that an animal is disinclined to move, and when made to do so there is manifest loss of power over the hind quarters, somewhat simulating a slight partial paralysis, and the hind quarters of the animal reel from side to side. In connection with this it may be noted that frequently there is paralysis of the sphincter ani and a dilated condition of the anus. These symptoms taken together point to some interference with the normal functions of the spinal cord in the lower dorsal and lumbar regions, and are probably owing to pressure caused by an exudation within the spinal membranes. In many cases shortly before death the heart's action becomes exceedingly violent, shaking the whole frame at each beat, so that the sound can be heard at some distance from the animal. In some of these cases the animal may suddenly drop dead; in others the emaciation and weakness become so pronounced that it falls to the ground, and, after a short struggle, succumbs to the disease. In other cases, again, the animal falls to the ground and appears to be suffering from acute pain, struggles violently, sweat covers the body, and respiration is very hurried. The struggles soon exhaust the patient's strength, and for a time it lies quiet; soon, however, the struggles commence again, continuing until death occurs. In some cases the appetite is voracious.

The symptoms of the disease as observed in experimentally inoculated animals are as follows: Twenty-four hours after the subcutaneous injection of a small quantity of surra blood, in the great majority of cases, a small circumscribed and somewhat raised swelling is noticed at the seat of the inoculation. After forty-eight hours the tumor has increased in size and is accompanied with some edema; it presents a certain amount of tension of the parts involved, and is generally tender on manipulation. These conditions continue to increase, until by the fourth day the tumor may measure 3 or 4 inches in one direction by 2 or 3 in the other, and raised to the extent of an inch or an inch and a half above the surrounding tissues, or in some cases the tumor presents an almost circular form throughout. It will be also found that, if the tumor is firmly grasped, it is not fixed, but can be lifted up from the subcutaneous tissue. According to the nature and quantity of the inoculated blood, these symptoms rapidly present themselves, and either attain a maximum or are retarded until, varying from the fourth to the thirteenth day, the tumor at the seat of inoculation will be found to have lost a certain amount of its tension and tenderness. From this date the swelling and edema gradually begin to grow less, until finally, after a period of

10 to 14 days, the only sign left of the former swelling is a slight thickening of the skin over the point of the injection; but at the moment when the tension and tenderness of the parts at the seat of inoculation become suddenly decreased a symptom of the utmost clinical importance takes place, namely, at that moment the parasite of surra enters the blood of the general circulation.

The temperature on the day of inoculation, and, in fact, for several days afterwards, may remain normal in character, there being only a few degrees difference between the morning and evening observations. In other cases there may be a slight rise from the first evening, and a gradual progressive rise until the swelling at the seat of inoculation shows signs of reduction in size, when the temperature generally takes a decided rise again, and may attain 104° or 105.8° F. This elevation will last a varying period of from two to six days, and on the day following its onset the ordinary symptoms of fever will be noticed, and in addition there will be petechiæ on the conjunctival membranes, lacrimation, a slight mucous discharge from the nose, and in severe cases some edema of the lower portion of the legs, and perhaps of the sheath in horses. At the termination of the period of fever the temperature will be found to have fallen to normal or nearly so; the animal will present a brighter aspect, and there is every appearance of its return to health; in a few days, however, the animal again appears dull and half asleep; the temperature is elevated, a relapse takes place, and a repetition of all the symptoms in the primary paroxysm, including the reappearance of the parasite, is observed.

Diagnosis.—A diagnosis may also be established by the complement-fixation or agglutination tests with the sera from suspected animals. This, however, can be carried out only in laboratories and requires special facilities for its execution.

Treatment.—No satisfactory treatment is known. Intravenous injections of Fowler's solution of arsenic give temporary relief, but relapses occur. In view of the great economic importance of this disease, it would not be advisable to attempt to treat any sporadic cases should they occur in this country. On the contrary, the animals should be slaughtered immediately and their carcasses promptly burned.

54763°—23——37

OSTEOPOROSIS OR BIGHEAD.

By JOHN R. MOHLER, V. M. D., *Chief, Bureau of Animal Industry.*

Osteoporosis is a general disease of the bones which develops slowly and progressively and is characterized by the absorption of the calcareous or compact bony substance and the formation of enlarged, softened, and porous bone. It is particularly manifest in the bones of the head, causing enlargement and bulging of the face and jaws, thereby giving rise to the terms "bighead" and "swelled head," which are applied to it. The disease affects horses, mules, and asses of all ages, classes, and breeds, and of both sexes, and is found under all soil, dietetic, and climatic conditions. It may occur in sporadic form, but in certain regions, such as South Africa, Australia, Madagascar, India, Hawaii, and in this country it seems to be enzootic, several cases usually appearing in the same stable or on the same farm, and numerous animals being affected in the same district. In the United States the disease has been found in all the States bordering the Delaware River and Chesapeake Bay, in some of the New England States, and in many of the Southern States, especially in low regions along the coast. In Europe the disease appears to be quite rare, and is usually described as a form of osteomalacia, a disease which is not uncommon among cattle of that continent. The opinion that bighead is only a form of osteomalacia, however, can not be accepted, nor can the infrequency of the former among European horses and the frequency of the latter among other live stock be conceded on the argument which has been presented, namely, that the better care which horses receive prevents them from becoming affected. In the Southwest, where osteomalacia, or creeps, has not infrequently been observed among range cattle by the writer, no case of osteoporosis of the horses using the same range has been noted, although the latter animals are given no more attention than the cattle.

The appropriate treatment of osteomalacia in cattle is so effective that if osteoporosis were a similar manifestation of disease a similar line of treatment should prove equally efficacious. However, this is not the fact. On the other hand, the occurrence of osteomalacia on old, worn-out soil, or on land deficient in lime salts, or from eating feed lacking in these bone-forming substances, or drinking water with a lime deficiency, is in perfect accord with our knowledge of the disease. But osteoporosis may occur on rich, fertile soil, in the most hygienic stables, and in animals receiving the best of care and of bone-forming feeds with a proper amount of mineral salts in the drinking water.

Cause.—The cause of this disease still remains obscure, although various theories have been advanced, some entirely erroneous, others more or less plausible; but none of them has been established. Thus the idea that feeding fodder and cereals poor in mineral salts and grazing in pastures where the soil is poor in lime and phosphates will cause the disease has been entirely disproved in many instances. Others have considered that the disease starts as a muscular rheumatism which is followed by an inflammatory condition of the bones, terminating in osteoporosis. The idea that the disease is contagious has been advanced by many writers, although no causative agent has been isolated. Numerous experiments have been made by inoculating the blood of an affected horse into normal horses without results. A piece of bone taken by Pearson from the diseased lower jaw of a colt was transplantetd into a cavity made for it in the jaw of a normal horse, but without reproducing the disease. Pétrone believes that the *Micrococcus nitrificans* causes osteomalacia in man as a result of its producing nitrous acid, which dissolves the calcareous tissues, and when injected into dogs in pure culture a similar disease is produced. It is probable that if this work is confirmed a somewhat similar causative factor will be discovered for osteoporosis.

Elliott considers the latter disease to be of microbic origin, the result of climatic conditions, and divides the island of Hawaii into two districts, in one of which the rainfall is 150 inches annually, where bighead is very prevalent, and the second of which is dry and rarely visited by rain, where the disease is unknown. Removal of animals from the wet to the dry district is followed by immediate improvement and frequently by recovery. In the wet district horses in both good and bad stables take the disease, but in the dry districts no unfavorable or unhygienic surroundings produce the affection. As both native and imported horses are equally susceptible, there is no indication of an acquired immunity to be observed.

Theiler has recently stated that his experiments in transfusing blood from diseased to normal horses were negative, and has suggested that the causative agent may be transmitted by an intermediate host only, as in the case of Texas fever. He draws attention to this method of spreading East African coast fever, although blood inoculations, as in osteoporosis, are always without result. We know that coast fever is infectious, and that it can not be transmitted by blood inoculations, but is conveyed with remarkable ease by ticks from diseased cattle. That the cause has not been observed may be accounted for by its being invisible even to the high magnification of the microscope.

On some farms and in some stables bighead is quite prevalent, a number of cases following one after another. On one farm of Thoroughbreds in Pennsylvania all the yearling colts and some of the aged horses were affected during one year, and on a similar farm in Virginia a large proportion of the horses for several years were diseased, although the cows and sheep of this farm remained unaffected.

Symptoms.—The commencement of the disease is usually unobserved by the owner, and those symptoms which do develop are generally not well marked or are misleading unless other cases have been noted in the vicinity. Until the bones become enlarged the symptoms remain so vague as not to be diagnosed readily. The disease may be present itself under a variety of symptoms. If the bones of the hock become affected, the animal will first show a hock lameness. If the long bones are involved, symptoms of rheumatism will be the first observed, while if the dorsal or lumbar vertebræ are affected indications of a strain of the lumbar region are in evidence. Probably the first symptom to be noticed is a loss of vitality combined with an irregular appetite or other digestive disturbance and with a tendency to stumble while in action. These earlier symptoms, however, may pass unobserved, and the appearance of an intermittent or migratory lameness without any visible cause may be the first sign to attract attention. This shifting and indefinite lameness, involving first one leg and then the other, is very suggestive, and is even more important when it is associated with a tendency to lie down frequently in the stall and the absence of a desire to get up, or the presence of evident pain and difficulty in arising.

About this time, or probably before, swelling of the bones of the face and jaw, which is almost constantly present in this disease, will be observed. The bones of the lower jaw are the most frequently involved, and this condition is readily detected with the fingers by the bulging ridge of the bone outside and along the lower edge of the molar teeth. A thickening of the lower jawbone may likewise be identified by feeling on both sides of each branch at the same time and comparing it with the thinness of this bone in a normal horse. As a result mastication becomes difficult or impossible and the teeth become loose and painful. The imperfect chewing which follows causes balls of feed to form which drop out of the mouth into the manger. Similar enlargements of the bones of the upper jaw may be seen, causing a widening of the face and a bulging of the bones about midway between the eyes and the nostrils. In some cases the nasal bones also become swollen and deformed, which, together with the bulging of the bones under the eyes, gives a good illustration of the reason for the application of the term bighead.

Other bones of the body will undergo similar changes, but these alterations are not so readily noted except by the symptoms they occasion. The alterations of the bones of the spinal column and the limbs, while difficult of observation, are nevertheless indicated by the reluctance of the animal to get up and the desire to remain lying for long periods of time. The animal easily tires, moves less rapidly, and if urged to go faster may sustain a fracture or have a ligament torn from its bony attachments, especially in the lower bones of the leg. An affected horse weighing 1,000 pounds was seen by the writer to fracture the large pastern bone from rearing during halter exercise.

The animal becomes poor in flesh, the coat is rough and lusterless, and the skin tight and harsh, producing a condition termed "hidebound," with considerable "tucking up" of the abdomen. The horse shows a short, stilted, choppy gait, which later becomes stiffer and more restricted, while on standing a position simulating that in founder is assumed, with a noticeable drop to the croup. The animal at this stage usually lies down and remains recumbent for several days at a time. Bed sores frequently arise and fractures are not uncommon in consequence of attempts to arise, which complications, in addition to emaciation, result in death.

The disease may exist in this manner for variable periods extending from two or three months to two years. The termination of the disease is uncertain at best, but is likely to be favorable if treatment and a change of feed, water, and location is adopted in the early stages of the malady.

Lesions.—As has been stated, the bones are the principal tissues involved. The nutrition of the bone is disturbed, as is indicated by the diminished density or rarefaction of the bony substances, the increase in the size or widening of the Haversian canal and the medullary cavity, and the enlargement of the network of spaces in the spongy tissue, the absorptive changes following the course of the Haversian system. In this process of absorption there are formed within the substance of the bone areas of erosion, indentations, or hollow spaces of irregular shape. These spaces increase in size and become confluent, causing an appearance resembling some varieties of coral. The affected bone may be readily incised with a knife, the cut surface appearing finely porous. This porous area is soft, pliable, and yields easily to the pressure of the finger. It has been shown by chemical analysis that the bone of an osteoporotic horse, when compared with that of a normal horse, shows a reduction in the amount of fat, phosphoric acid, lime, and soda, but a slight increase in organic matter and silicic acid. The bones lose their yellowish-white appearance, becoming gray and brittle. The affected bones may be those of any region or portion of the body. Besides the change already noted in the bones of the face, the ends of the long bones, such as the ribs, are involved, and may be sectioned, though not so readily as the facial bones. The bones of the vertebræ are also frequently involved, necessitating great care in casting a horse, as the writer has seen several cases of broken backs in casting such animals for other operations. The marrow and cancellated tissue of the long bones may contain hemorrhages and soft gelatinous material or coagulated fibrin. The internal organs are usually normal, but a catarrhal condition of the gastrointestinal tract may be noted as the result of the improper mastication, resulting from the enlargement of the jaws and soreness of the teeth.

Treatment.—The affected animal should be immediately placed under new conditions, both as to feed and surroundings. If the horse has been stable fed, it is advisable to turn it out on grass for two or three months, preferably in a higher altitude. If the disease has been contracted while running on pasture, place the animal in the stable or corral. In the early stages of the disease beneficial results have followed the supplemental use of lime given in the drinking water. One peck of lime slaked in a cask of water and additional water added from time to time is satisfactory and can be provided at slight expense. This treatment may be supplemented by giving a tablespoonful of powdered bone meal in each feed, with free access to a large piece of rock salt, or the bone meal may be given with four tablespoonfuls of molasses mixed with the feed. Feeds containing mineral salts, such as beans, cowpeas, oats, and cottonseed meal, may prove beneficial in replenishing the bony substance that is being absorbed. Cottonseed meal is one of the best feeds for this purpose, but it should be fed carefully. The animal should not be allowed to work at all during the active stage of the disease, nor should it be used for breeding purposes.

HORSESHOEING.

By John W. Adams, A. B., V. M. D.,

*Professor of Surgery and Lecturer on Shoeing, Veterinary Department,
University of Pennsylvania.*

Bad and indifferent shoeing so frequently leads to diseases of the feet and in irregularities of gait, which may render a horse unserviceable, that it has been thought appropriate to conclude this book with a brief chapter on the principles involved in shoeing healthy hoofs.

In unfolding this subject in the limited space at my disposal, I can only hope to give the intelligent horse owner a sufficient number of facts, based on experience and upon the anatomy and physiology of the foot and leg, to enable him to avoid the more serious consequences of improper shoeing.

Let us first examine this vital mechanism, the foot, and learn something of its structure and of the natural movements of its component parts, that we may be prepared to recognize deviations from the normal and to apply the proper corrective.

GROSS ANATOMY OF THE FOOT.

(Pls. XXXII–XXXIV.)

The bones of the foot are four in number, three of which—the long pastern, short pastern, and coffin bone, placed end to end—form a continuous straight column passing downward and forward from the fetlock joint to the ground. A small accessory bone, the navicular, or "shuttle," bone, lies crosswise in the foot between the wings of the coffin bone and forms a part of the joint surface of the latter. The short pastern projects about 1½ inches above the hoof and extends about an equal distance into it.   (See also page 395.)

The pastern and the coffin bone are held together by strong fibrous cords passing between each two bones and placed at the sides so as not to interfere with the forward and backward movement of the bones. The joints are therefore hinge joints, though imperfect, because, while the chief movements are those of extension and flexion in a single plane, some slight rotation and lateral movements are possible.

583

The bones are still further bound together and supported by three long fibrous cords, or tendons. One, the extensor tendon of the toe, passes down the front of the pasterns and attaches to the coffin bone just below the edge of the hair; when pulled upon by its muscle this tendon draws the toe forward and enables the horse to place the hoof flat upon the ground. The other two tendons are placed behind the pasterns and are called flexors, because they flex, or bend, the pasterns and coffin bone backward. One of the tendons is attached to the upper end of the short pastern, while the other passes down between the heels, glides over the under surface of the navicular bone, and attaches itself to the under surface of the coffin bone. These two tendons not only flex, or fold up, the foot as the latter leaves the ground during motion, but at rest assist the suspensory ligament in supporting the fetlock joint.

The foot-axis is an imaginary line passing from the fetlock joint through the long axes of the two pasterns and coffin bone. This imaginary line, which shows the direction of the pasterns and coffin bone, should always be straight—that is, never broken, either forward or backward when viewed from the side, or inward or outward when observed from in front. Viewed from one side, the long axis of the long pastern, when prolonged to the ground, should be parallel to the line of the toe. Viewed from in front, the long axis of the long pastern, when prolonged to the ground, should cut the hoof exactly at the middle of the toe.

Raising the heel or shortening the toe not only tilts the coffin bone forward and makes the hoof stand steeper at the toe, but slackens the tendon that attaches to the under surface of the coffin bone (perforans tendon), and therefore allows the fetlock joint to sink downward and backward and the long pastern to assume a more nearly horizontal position. The foot-axis, viewed from one side, is now broken forward; that is, the long pastern is less steep than the toe, and the heels are either too long or the toe is too short. On the other hand, raising the toe or lowering the heels of a foot with a straight foot-axis not only tilts the coffin bone backward and renders the toe more nearly horizontal, but tenses the perforans tendon, which then forces the fetlock joint forward, causing the long pastern to stand steeper. The foot-axis, seen from one side, is now broken backward—an indication that the toe is relatively too long or that the heels are relatively too low.

The elastic tissues of the foot are preeminently the lateral cartilages and the plantar cushion. The lateral cartilages are two irregularly four-sided plates of gristle, one on either side of the foot, extending from the wings of the coffin bone backward to the heels and upward to a distance of an inch or more above the edge of the hair, where they may be felt by the fingers. When sound, these plates are elastic and yield readily to moderate finger pressure, but from various causes may undergo ossification, in which condition they are hard and unyielding. The plantar cushion is a wedge-shaped mass of tough, elastic, fibro-fatty tissue filling all the space between the lateral cartilages, forming the fleshy heels and the fleshy frog, and serving as a buffer to disperse shock when the foot is set to the ground. It extends forward underneath the navicular bone and perforans tendon, and protects these structures from injurious pressure from below. Instantaneous photographs show that at speed the horse sets the heels to the ground before other parts of the foot—conclusive proof that the function of this tough, elastic structure is to dissipate and render harmless violent impact of the foot with the ground.

The horn-producing membrane, or "quick," as it is commonly termed, is merely a downward prolongation of the "derm," or true skin, and may be conveniently called the pododerm (foot skin). The pododerm closely invests the coffin bone, lateral cartilages, and plantar cushion, much as a sock covers the human foot, and is itself covered by the horny capsule, or hoof. It differs from the external skin, or hair skin, in having no sweat or oil glands, but, like it, is richly supplied with blood vessels and sensitive nerves. And, just as the derm of the hair skin produces upon its outer surface layer upon layer of horny cells (epiderm), which protect the sensitive and vascular derm, so, likewise, in the foot the pododerm produces over its entire surface soft cells, which, pushed away by more recent cells forming beneath, lose moisture by evaporation and are rapidly transformed into the corneous material which we call the hoof. It is proper to regard the hoof as a greatly thickened epiderm having many of the qualities possessed by such epidermal structures as hair, feathers, nails, claws, etc.

The functions of the pododerm are to produce the hoof and to unite it firmly to the foot.

There are five parts of the pododern, easily distinguishable when the hoof has been removed, namely: (1) The perioplic band, a narrow ridge from one-sixteenth to one-eighth of an inch wide, running along the edge of the hair from one heel around the toe to the other. This band produces the perioplic horn, the thin varnishlike layer of glistening horn, which forms the surface of the wall or "crust," and whose purpose seems to be to retard evaporation of moisture from the wall. (2) The coronary band, a prominent fleshy cornice encircling the foot just below and parallel to the perioplic band. At the heels it is reflected forward along the sides of the fleshy frog, to become lost near the apex of this latter structure. The coronet produces the middle layer of the wall, and the reflexed portions produce the "bars," which are, therefore, to be regarded merely as a turning forward of the wall. (3) The fleshy leaves, 500 to 600 in number, parallel to one another, running downward and forward from the lower edge of the coronary band to the margin of the fleshy sole. They produce the soft, light-colored horny leaves which form the deepest layer of the wall, and serve as a strong bond of union between the middle layer of the wall and the fleshy leaves with which they dovetail. (4) The fleshy sole, which covers the entire under surface of the foot, excepting the fleshy frog and bars. The horny sole is produced by the fleshy sole. (5) The fleshy frog, which covers the under surface of the plantar cushion and produces the horny frog.

The horny box or hoof consists of wall and bars, sole and frog. The wall is all that part of the hoof which is visible when the foot is on the ground (see fig. 8). As already stated, it consists of three layers—the periople, the middle layer, and the leafy layer.

The bars (see fig. 1c) are forward prolongations of the wall, and are gradually lost near the point of the frog. The angle between the wall and a bar is called the "buttress." Each bar lies against the horny frog on one side and incloses a wing of the sole on the other, so that the least expansion or contraction of the horny frog separates or approximates the bars, and through them the lateral cartilages and the walls of the quarters. The lower border of the wall is called the "bearing edge," and is the surface against which the shoe bears. By dividing the entire lower circumference of the wall into five equal part, a toe, two side walls, and two quarters will be exhibited. The "heels," strictly speaking, are the two rounded soft prominences of the plantar cushion, lying one above each quarter. The outer wall is usually more slanting than the inner, and *the more slanting half of a hoof is always the thicker.* In front hoofs the wall is thickest at the toe and gradually thins out toward the quarters, where in some horses it may not exceed one-fourth of an inch. In hind hoofs there is much less difference in thickness between the toe, side walls, and quarters. The horny sole, from which the flakes of old horn have been removed, is concave and about as thick as the wall at the toe. It is rough, uneven and often covered by flakes of dead horn in process of being loosened and cast off. Behind the sole presents an opening into which are received the bars and horny frog. This opening divides the sole into a body and two wings.

The periphery of the sole unites with the lower border of the wall and bars through the medium of the white line, which is the cross section of the leafy horn layer of the wall and of short plugs of horn which grow down from the lower ends of the fleshy leaves. This white line is of much importance to the shoer, since its distance from the outer border of the hoof is the thickness of the wall, and in the white line all nails should be driven.

The frog, secreted by the pododerm covering the plantar cushion or fatty frog, and presenting almost the same form as the latter, lies as a soft and very elastic wedge between the bars and between the edges of the sole just in front of the bars. A broad and shallow depression in its center divides it into two branches, which diverge as they pass backward into the horny bulbs of the heel. In front of the middle cleft the two branches unite to form the body of the frog, which ends in the point of the frog. The bar of a bar shoe should rest on the branches of the frog. In unshod hoofs the bearing edge of the wall, the sole, frog, and bars are all on a level; that is, the under surface of the hoof is perfectly flat, and each of these structures assists in bearing the body weight.

With respect to solidity, the different parts of the hoof vary widely. The middle layer of the wall is harder and more tenacious than the sole, for the latter crumbles away or passes off in larger or smaller flakes on its under surface, while no such spontaneous shortening of the wall occurs. The white line and the frog are soft-horn structures, and differ from hard horn in that their horn cells do not under natural conditions become hard and hornlike. They are very elastic, absorb moisture rapidly, and as readily dry out and become hard, brittle, and easily fissured. Horn of good quality is fine grained and tough, while bad horn is coarse grained and either mellow and friable or hard and brittle. All horn is a poor conductor of heat, and the harder (drier) the horn the more slowly does it transmit extremes of temperature.

THE PHYSIOLOGICAL MOVEMENTS OF THE HOOF.

A hoof while supporting the body weight has a different form, and the structures inclosed within the hoof have a different position than when not bearing weight. Since the amount of weight borne by a foot is continually changing, and the relations of internal pressure are continuously varying, a foot is, from a physiological viewpoint, never at rest. The most marked changes of form of the hoof occur when the foot bears the greatest weight, namely, at the time of the greatest descent of the fetlock. Briefly, these changes of form are: (1) An expansion or widening of the whole back half of the foot from the coronet to the lower edge of the quarters. This expansion varies between one-fiftieth and one-twelfth of an inch. (2) A narrowing of the front half of the foot, measured at the coronet. (3) A sinking of the heels and a flattening of the wings of the sole. These changes are more marked in the half of the foot that bears the greater weight.

The changes of form occur in the following order. When the foot is set to the ground the body weight is transmitted through the bones and sensitive and horny leaves to the wall. The coffin bone and navicular bone sink a little and rotate backward. At the same time the short pastern sinks backward and downward between the lateral cartilages and presses the perforans tendon upon the plantar cushion. This cushion being compressed from above and being unable to expand downward by reason of the resistance of the ground acting against the horny frog, acts like any other elastic mass and expands toward the sides, pushing before it the yielding lateral cartilages and the wall of the quarters. This expansion of the heels is assisted and increased by the simultaneous flattening and lateral expansion of the resilient horny frog, which crowds the bars apart. Of course, when the lateral cartilages are ossified, not only is no expansion of the quarters possible, but frog pressure often leads to painful compression of the plantar cushion and to increase of lameness. Frog pressure is therefore contraindicated in lameness due to sidebones (ossified cartilages). Under the descent of the coffin bone the horny sole sinks a little; that is, the arch of the sole around the point of the frog and the wings of the sole become somewhat flattened. All these changes of form are most marked in sound unshod hoofs, because in them ground pressure on the frog and sole is pronounced; they are more marked in fore hoofs than in hind hoofs.

The movement of the different structures within the foot and the changes of form that occur at every step are indispensable to the health of the hoof, so that these elastic tissues must be kept active by regular exercise, with protection against drying out of the hoof. Long-continued rest in the stable, drying out of the hoof, and shoeing decrease or alter the physiological movements of the hoof and sometimes lead to foot diseases. Since these movements are complete and spontaneous only in unshod feet, shoeing must be regarded as an evil, albeit a necessary one, and indispensable if we wish to keep horses continuously serviceable on hard, artificial roads. However, if in shoeing we bear in mind the structure and functions of the hoof and apply a shoe whose branches have a wide and level bearing surface, so as to interfere as little as may be with the expansion and contraction of the quarters, in so far as this is not hindered by the nails, we need not be apprehensive of trouble, provided the horse has reasonable work and his hoofs proper care.

GROWTH OF THE HOOF.

All parts of the hoof grow downward and forward with equal rapidity, the rate of growth being largely dependent upon the amount of blood supplied to the pododerm, or "quick." Abundant and regular exercise, good grooming, moistness and suppleness of the hoof, going barefoot, plenty of good feed, and at proper intervals removing the overgrowth of hoof and regulating the bearing surface. by increasing the volume and improving the quality of the blood flowing into the pododerm, favor the rapid growth of horn of good quality; while lack of exercise, dryness of the horn, and excessive length of the hoof hinder growth.

The average rate of growth is about one-third of an inch a month. Hind hoofs grow faster than fore hoofs and unshod ones faster than shod ones. The time required for the horn to grow from the coronet to the ground, though influenced to a slight degree by the precited conditions, varies in proportion to the distance of the coronet from the ground. At the toe, depending on its height, the horn grows down in 11 to 13 months, at the side wall in 6 to 8 months, and at the heels in 3 to 5 months. We can thus estimate with tolerable accuracy the time required for the disappearance of such defects in the hoof as cracks, clefts, etc.

Irregular growth is not infrequent. The almost invariable cause of this is an improper distribution of the body weight over the hoof—that is, an unbalanced foot. Colts running in soft pasture or confined for long periods in the stable are frequently allowed to grow hoofs of excessive length. The long toe becomes " dished "—that is, concave from the coronet to the ground—the long quarters curl forward and inward and often completely cover the frog and lead to contraction of the heels, or the whole hoof bends outward or inward, and a crooked foot, or, even worse, a crooked leg, is the result if the long hoof be allowed to exert its powerful and abnormally directed leverage for but a few months upon young plastic bones and tender and lax articular ligaments. All colts are not foaled with straight legs, but failure to regulate the length and bearing of the hoof may make a straight leg crooked and a crooked leg worse, just as intelligent care during the growing period can greatly improve a congenitally crooked limb. If breeders were more generally cognizant of the power of overgrown and unbalanced hoofs to divert the lower bones of young legs from their proper direction, and, therefore, to cause them to be moved improperly, with loss of speed and often with injury to the limbs, we might hope to see fewer knock-kneed, bowlegged, " splay-footed," " pigeon-toed," cow-hocked, interfering, and paddling horses.

If in shortening the hoof one side wall is, from ignorance, left too long or cut down too low with relation to the other, the foot will be unbalanced, and in traveling the long section will touch the ground first and will continue to do so till it has been reduced to its proper level (length) by the increased wear which will take place at this point. While this occurs rapidly in unshod hoofs, the shoe prevents wear of the hoof, though it is itself more rapidly worn away beneath the high (long) side than elsewhere, so that by the time the shoe is worn out the tread of the shoe may be flat. If this mistake be repeated from month to month, the part of the wall left too high will grow more rapidly than the low side whose pododerm is relatively anemic as a result of the greater weight falling into this half of the hoof, and the ultimate result will be a " wry," or crooked foot.

THE CARE OF UNSHOD HOOFS.

The colt should have abundant exercise on dry ground. The hoofs will then wear gradually, and it will only be necessary from time to time to regulate any uneven wear with the rasp and to round off the sharp edge about the toe in order to prevent breaking away of the wall.

Colts in the stable can not wear down their hoofs, so that every four to six weeks they should be rasped down and the lower edge of the wall well rounded to prevent chipping. The soles and clefts of the frog should be picked out every few days and the entire hoof washed clean. Plenty of clean straw litter should be provided. Hoofs that are becoming " awry " should have the wall shortened in such a manner as to straighten the foot-axis. This will ultimately produce a good hoof and will improve the position of the limb.

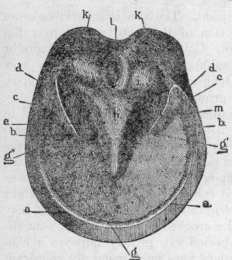

Fig. 1.—Ground surface of a right fore hoof of the regular form: *a, a,* wall; *a-a,* the toe; *a-b,* the side walls; *b-d,* the quarters; *c, c,* the bars; *d, d,* the buttress; *e,* lateral cleft of the frog; *f,* body of the sole; *g, g', g'',* leafy layer (white line) of the toe and bars; *h,* body of the frog; *i, i,* branches of the frog; *k, k,* horny bulbs of the heels; *l,* middle cleft of the frog.

CHARACTERISTICS OF A HEALTHY HOOF.

A healthy hoof (figs. 1 and 8) is equally warm at all parts, and is not tender under pressure with the hands or moderate compression with pincers. The coronet is soft and elastic at all points and does not project beyond the surface of the wall. The wall (fig. 8) is straight from coronet to ground, so that a straightedge laid against the wall from coronet to ground parallel to the direction of the horn tubes will touch at every point. The wall should be covered with the outer varnishlike layer (periople) and should show no cracks or clefts. Every hoof shows " ring formation," but the rings should not be strongly marked and should always run parallel to the coronary band. Strongly marked ring-formation over the entire wall is an evidence of a weak hoof, but when limited to a part of the wall is evidence of previous local inflammation. The bulbs of the heels should be full, rounded, and of equal height. The sole (fig. 1) should be well hollowed out, the white line solid, the frog well developed, the middle cleft of the frog broad and shallow, the spaces between the bars and the frog wide and shallow, the bars straight from the buttress toward the point of the frog, and the buttresses themselves so far apart as not to press against the branches of the frog. A hoof can not be considered healthy if it presents reddish discolored horn, cracks in the wall, white line, bars, or frog, thrush of the frog, contrac-

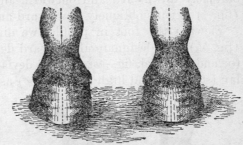

FIG. 2.—Pair of fore feet of regular form in regular standing position.

tion or displacement of the heels. The lateral cartilages should yield readily to finger pressure.

VARIOUS FORMS OF HOOFS.

As among a thousand human faces no two are alike, so among an equal number of horses no two have hoofs exactly alike. A little study of different forms soon shows us, however, that the form of every hoof is dependent in great measure on the direction of the two pastern bones as viewed from in front or behind, or from one side; and that all hoofs fall into three classes when we view them from in front and three classes when we observe them in profile. Inasmuch as the form of every foot determines the peculiarities of the shoe that is best adapted to it, no one who is ignorant of, or who disregards the natural form of, a hoof can hope to understand physiological shoeing.

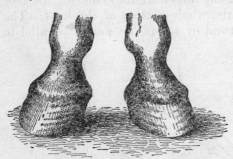

FIG. 3.—Pair of fore feet of base-wide form in toe-wide standing position.

FORMS OF FEET VIEWED FROM IN FRONT AND IN PROFILE.

Whether a horse's feet be observed from in front or from behind, their form corresponds to, or at least resembles, either that of the regular position (fig. 2), the base-wide or toe-wide position (fig. 3), or the base-narrow position (fig. 4).

By the direction of the imaginary line passing through the long axes of the two pasterns (figs. 2, 4, 5) we determine whether or not the hoof and pasterns stand in proper mutual relation.

In the regular standing position (fig. 2) the foot-axis runs straight downward and forward; in the base-wide position (fig. 3) it runs obliquely downward and outward, and in the base-narrow position (fig. 4) it runs obliquely downward and inward.

Viewing the foot in profile, we distinguish the regular position (fig. 5b) and designate all forward deviations as acute-angled (long toe and low heel, fig. 5a), and all deviations backward from the regular (steep toe and high heel, fig. 5c) as steep-toed, or stumpy. When

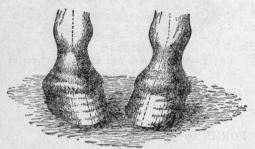

the body weight is evenly distributed over all four limbs, the foot-axis should be straight; the long pastern, short pastern, and wall at the toe should have the same slant.

A front hoof of the regular standing position.— The outer wall is a little more slanting and some-

FIG. 4.—Pair of fore feet of base-narrow form in toe-narrow standing position.

what thicker than the inner. The lower border of the outer quarter describes the arc of a smaller circle—that is, is more sharply bent than the inner quarter. The weight falls near the center of the foot and is evenly distributed over the whole bottom of the hoof. The toe forms an angle with the ground of 45° to 50° and is parallel to

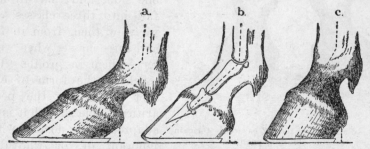

FIG. 5.—*a,* Side view of an acute-angled fore foot (shod) ; *b,* side view of a regular fore foot, showing the most desirable degree of obliquity (34°) ; *c.* side view of a stumpy, or "upright," fore foot ; obliquity above 50°. In *a, b, c,* note particularly the relation between the length of the shoe and the overhanging of the heels. Note also the toe roll of the shoes.

the direction of the long pastern. The toe points straight ahead, and when the horse is moving forward in a straight line the hoofs are picked up and carried forward in a line parallel to the middle line of the body, and are set down flat. Coming straight toward the observer the hoofs seem to rise and fall perpendicularly.

A *hoof of the base-wide position* is always awry. The outer wall is more slanting, longer, and thicker than the inner, the outer quarter more curved than the inner, and the outer half of the sole wider than the inner. The weight falls largely into the inner half of the hoof. In motion the hoof is moved in a circle. From its position on the ground it breaks over the inner toe, is carried forward and inward close to the supporting leg, thence forward and outward to the ground, which the hoof meets first with the outer toe. Horses that are toe-wide ("splay-footed"—toes turned outward) show all these peculiarities of hoof-form and hoof-flight to a still more marked degree and are therefore more prone to "interfere" when in motion.

A *hoof of the base-narrow position* is awry, but not to so marked a degree as the base-wide hoof. The inner wall is usually a little more slanting than the outer, the inner half of the sole wider than the outer, and the inner quarter more curved than the outer. The outer quarter is often flattened and drawn in at the bottom. The weight falls largely into the outer half of the hoof. In motion the hoof breaks over the outer toe, is carried forward and outward at some distance from the supporting leg, thence forward and inward to the ground, which it generally meets with the outer toe. The foot thus moves in a circle, whose convexity is outward, a manner of flight called "paddling." A base-narrow horse, whose toes point straight ahead, frequently "interferes," while a toe-narrow (pigeon-toed) animal seldom does.

A *regular hoof* (fig. 5b), viewed from one side, has a straight foot-axis inclined to the horizon at an angle of 45° to 50°. The weight falls near the center of the foot and there is moderate expansion of the quarters.

An *acute-angled hoof* (fig. 5a) has a straight foot-axis inclined at an angle less than 45° to the horizon. The weight falls more largely in the back half of the hoof and there is greater length of hoof in contact with the ground and greater expansion of the heels than in the regular hoof.

Upright or stumpy hoof.—In the upright or stumpy hoof (fig. 5c) the foot-axis is straight and more than 55° steep. The hoof is relatively short from toe to heel, the weight falls farther forward, and there is less expansion of the heels than in the regular hoof.

Wide and narrow hoofs.—Finally, there are wide hoofs and narrow hoofs, dependent solely upon race and breeding. The wide hoof is almost circular on the ground surface, the sole but little concave, the frog large, and the quality of the horn coarse. The narrow hoof has a strongly "cupped" sole, a small frog, nearly perpendicular side walls, and fine-grained, tough horn.

54763°—23——38

Hind hoofs are influenced in shape by different directions of their pasterns much as front feet are. A hind hoof is not round at the toe as a front hoof is, but is more pointed. Its greatest width is two-thirds of the way back from toe to heel, the sole is more concave, the heels relatively wider, and the toe about 10° steeper than in front hoofs.

EXAMINATION PRELIMINARY TO SHOEING.

The object of the examination is to ascertain the direction and position of the limbs, the shape, character, and quality of the hoofs, the form, length, position, and wear of the shoe, the number, distribution, and direction of the nails, the manner in which the hoof leaves the ground, its line of flight, the manner in which it is set to the ground, and all other peculiarities, that at the next and subsequent shoeings proper allowances may be made and observed faults corrected. The animal must, therefore, be observed both at rest and in motion.

At rest, the observer should stand in front and note the slant of the long pasterns. Do they drop perpendicularly, or slant downward and outward (base-wide foot), or downward and inward (base-narrow foot)? Whatever be the direction to the long pastern, an imaginary line passing through its long axis, when prolonged to the ground, should apparently pass through the middle of the toe. But if such line cuts through the inner toe the foot-axis is not straight, as it should be, but is broken inward at the coronet, an indication that either the outer wall of the hoof is too long (high) or that the inner wall is too short (low). On the contrary, if the center line of the long pastern falls through the outer toe the foot-axis is broken outward at the coronet, an indication that either the inner wall is too long or the outer wall too short.

The observer should now place himself at one side, two or three paces distant, in order to view the limb and hoof in profile. Note the size of the hoof in relation to the height and weight of the animal, and the obliquity of the hoof. Is the foot-axis straight—that is, does the long pastern have the same slant as the toe, or does the toe of the hoof stand steeper than the long pastern (fig. 6c)? In which case the foot-axis is broken forward at the coronet, an indication, usually, that the quarters are either too high or that the toe is too short.

If the long pastern stands steeper than the toe (fig. 6a) the foot-axis is broken backward, in which case the toe is too long or the quarters are too low (short). In figures 6a and 6c the dotted lines passing from toe to quarters indicate the amount of horn which must be removed in order to straighten the foot-axis, as shown in figure 6b. Note also the length of the shoe.

Next, the feet should be raised and the examiner should note the outline of the foot, the conformation of the sole, form and quality of the frog, form of the shoe, wear of the shoe, and the number and distribution of the nails. Does the shoe fully cover the entire lower border of the wall? or is it too narrow, or fitted so full on the inside that it has given rise to interfering? or has the shoe been nailed on crooked? or has it become loose and shifted? is it too short, or so wide at the ends of the branches as not to support the buttresses of the hoof? Does the shoe correspond with the form of the hoof? Are the nails distributed so as to interfere as little as possible with the expansion of the quarters? are there too many? are they too large? driven too "fine" or too high? These are questions which the observer should put to himself.

Note carefully the wear of the old shoe. It is the unimpeachable evidence of the manner in which the hoof has been set to the ground since the shoe was nailed to it, and gives valuable "pointers" in leveling the hoof. Wear is the effect of friction between the shoe and the

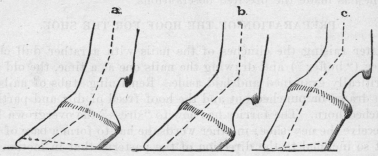

FIG. 6.—*a*, Side view of foot with the foot-axis broken backward as a result of too long a toe. The amount of horn to be removed from the toe in order to straighten the foot-axis is denoted by a dotted line; *b*, side view of a properly balanced foot, with a straight foot-axis of desirable slant; *c*, side view of stumpy foot with foot-axis broken forward, as a result of overgrowth of the quarters. The amount of horn to be removed in order to straighten the foot-axis is shown by a dotted line.

ground at the moment of contact. Since the properly leveled hoof is set flat to the ground, the "grounding wear" of a shoe should be uniform at every point, though the toe will always show wear due to scouring at the moment of "breaking over." Everything which tends to lengthen the stride tends also to make the "grounding wear" more pronounced in the heels of the shoe, while all causes which shorten the stride—as stiffening of the limbs through age, overwork, or disease—bring the grounding wear nearer the toe.

An exception should be noted, however, in founder, in which the grounding wear is most pronounced at the heels.

If one branch of the shoe is found to be worn much thinner than the other, the thinner branch has either been set too near the middle line of the foot (fitted too close), where it has been bearing greater weight while rubbing against the ground, or, what is much more often the case, the section of wall above the thinner branch has been too long (too high), or the opposite-section of wall has been too short (too low). "One-sided wear, uneven setting down of the feet, and an unnatural course of the wall are often found together." How much an old shoe can tell us, if we take time and pains to decipher its scars!

The horse should next be observed at a walk and at a trot or pace, from in front, from behind, and from the side, and the "breaking over," the carriage of the feet, and the manner of setting them to the ground carefully noted and remembered. A horse does not always move just as his standing position would seem to imply. Often there is so great a difference in the form and slant of two fore hoofs or two hind hoofs that we are in doubt as to their normal shape, when a few steps at a trot will usually solve the problem instantly by showing us the line of flight of the hoofs and referring them to the regular, base-wide, or base-narrow form.

No man is competent either to shoe a horse or to direct the work till he has made the precited observations.

PREPARATION OF THE HOOF FOR THE SHOE.

After raising the clinches of the nails with a rather dull clinch cutter ("buffer") and drawing the nails one at a time, the old shoe is critically examined and laid aside. Remaining stubs of nails are then drawn or punched out and the hoof freed of dirt and partially detached horn. The farrier has now to "dress" the overgrown hoof to receive the new shoe; in other words, he has to form a base of support so inclined to the direction of the pasterns that in motion this surface shall be set flat upon the ground. He must not rob the hoof nor leave too much horn; either mistake may lead to injury. If he has made a careful preliminary examination he knows what part of the wall requires removal and what part must be left, for he already knows the direction of the foot axis and the wear of the old shoe and has made up his mind just where and how much horn must be removed to leave the hoof of proper length and the foot axis straight.

A greatly overgrown hoof may be quickly shortened with sharp nippers and the sole freed of semidetached flakes of horn. The concave sole of a thick-walled, strong hoof may be pared out around the point of the frog, but not so much as to remove all evidences of exfoliation. The wall should be leveled with the rasp till its full thickness, the white line, and an eighth of an inch of the margin of the sole are in one horizontal plane, called the "bearing surface of the hoof." The bars, if long, may be shortened, but *never pared on the side.* The branches of the sole in the angle between the bars and the wall of the quarters should be left a little lower than the wall, so as not to be pressed upon by the inner web of the shoe. "Corns," or bruises of the pododerm, are usually a result of leaving a thick mass of dry, unyielding horn at this point. The frog should not be touched further than to remove tags or layers that are so loose as to form no protection. A soft frog will shorten itself spontaneously by the exfoliation of superficial layers of horn, while if the frog is dry, hard, and too prominent it is better to soften it by applying moisture in some form, and to allow it to wear away naturally than to pare it down. It is of advantage to have the frog project below the level of the wall an amount equal to the thickness of a plain shoe, though we rarely see frogs of such size except in draft horses. The sharp lower border of the wall should be rounded with the rasp to prevent its being bent outward and broken away. Finally, the foot is set to the ground and again observed from all sides to make sure that the lines bounding the hoof correspond with the direction of the long pastern.

THE SHOE.

The shoe is an artificial base of support, by no means ideal, because it interferes to a greater or less degree with the physiology of the foot, but indispensable except for horses at slow work on soft ground. Since a proper surface of support is of the greatest importance in preserving the health of the feet and legs, it is necessary to consider the various forms of shoes best adapted to the different forms of hoofs. Certain properties are common to all shoes and may be considered first. They are form, width, thickness, length, surfaces, borders, " fullering," nail holes, and clips.

Form.—Every shoe should have the form of the hoof for which it is intended, provided the hoof retains its proper shape; but for every hoof that has undergone change of form we must endeavor to give the shoe that form which the hoof originally possessed. Front shoes and hind shoes, rights and lefts, should be distinctly different and easily distinguishable.

Width.—All shoes should be wider at the toe than at the ends of the branches. The average width should be about double the thickness of the wall at the toe.

Thickness.—The thickness should be sufficient to make the shoe last about four weeks and should be uniform except in special cases.

Length.—This will depend upon the obliquity of the hoof viewed in profile. The acute-angled hoof (fig. 5a) has long overhanging heels, and a considerable proportion of the weight borne by the leg falls in the posterior half of the hoof. For such a hoof the branches of the shoe should extend back of the buttresses to a distance nearly double the thickness of the shoe. For a hoof of the regular form (figs. 5b and 8) the branches should project an amount equal to the thickness of the shoe. In a stumpy hoof (fig. 5c) the shoe need not project more than one-eighth of an inch. In all cases the shoe should cover the entire " bearing surface " of the wall.

Surfaces.—The surface that is turned toward the hoof is known as the " upper," or " hoof surface," of the shoe. That part of the hoof surface which is in actual contact with the horn is called the " bearing surface " of the shoe. The " bearing surface " should be perfectly horizontal from side to side, and wide enough to support the full thickness of the wall, the white line, and about an eighth of an inch of the margin of the sole. The bearing surface should also be perfectly flat, except that it may be turned up at the toe ("rolling-motion " shoe, fig. 5 *a*, *b*, *c*.) The surface between the bearing surface and the inner edge of the shoe is often beaten down or concaved to prevent pressure too far inward upon the sole. This " concaving," or " seating," should be deeper or shallower as the horny sole is less or more concave. As a rule, strongly " cupped " soles require no concaving (hind hoofs, narrow fore hoofs).

Borders.—The entire outer border should be beveled under the foot. Such a shoe is not so readily loosened, nor is it so apt to lead to interfering.

Fullering.—This is a groove in the ground surface of the shoe. It should pass through two-thirds of the thickness of the shoe, be clean, and of uniform width. It is of advantage in that it makes the shoe lighter in proportion to its width and, by making the ground surface somewhat rough, tends to prevent slipping.

Nail holes.—The shoe must be so " punched " that the nail holes will fall directly on the white line. They should be confined to the fore half of front shoes, but may occupy the anterior two-thirds of hind shoes. For a medium-weight shoe three nail holes in each branch are sufficient, but for heavier shoes, especially those provided with long calks, eight holes are about right, though three on the inside and four on the outside may do.

Clips.—These are half-circular ears drawn up from the outer edge of the shoe either at the toe or opposite the side wall. The height of a clip should equal the thickness of the shoe, though they should be even higher on hind shoes and when a leather sole is interposed between the shoe and hoof. Clips secure the shoe against shifting. A side clip should always be drawn up on that branch of the shoe that first meets the ground in locomotion.

SPECIAL FEATURES AND FITTING THE SHOES.

A shoe for a regular hoof (figs. 7 and 8) fits when its outer border follows the wall closely in the region of the nail holes and from the last nail to the end of the branch gradually projects beyond the surface of the wall to an eighth of an inch and extends back of the buttresses an amount equal to the thickness of the shoe. The shoe must be straight, firm, air-tight, its nail holes directly over the white line, and its branches far enough from the branches of the frog to permit the passage of a foot pick. Branches of the shoe must be of equal length.

In fitting a shoe to a hoof of regular form we follow the form of the hoof, but in base-wide and base-narrow hoofs, which are of irregular form, we must pay attention not only to the form of the hoof but also to the direction of the pasterns and the consequent distribution of weight in the hoof, because where the most weight falls the surface of support of the foot must be widened, and where the least weight falls (opposite side of the hoof) the surface of support should be narrowed. In this way the improper distribution of weight within the hoof is evenly distributed over the surface of support.

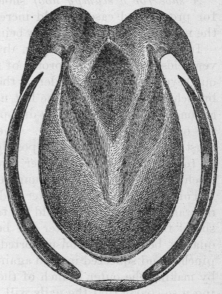

FIG. 7.—Left fore hoof of regular form, shod with a plain "fullered" shoe. Note the distribution of the nails, length of the fuller (crease), and the closeness of the ends of the shoe to the branches of the frog.

A *shoe for a base-wide hoof* should be fitted full on the inner side of the foot and fitted close on the outer side, because the inner side bears the most weight. The nails in the outer branch are placed well back, but in the inner branch are crowded forward toward the toe.

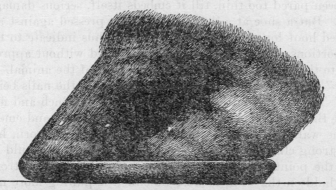

FIG. 8.—Side view of hoof and shoe shown in fig. 7. Note the straight toe, weak ring formation running parallel to the coronet, clinches low down and on a level, length of the shoe, and the under-bevel at the toe and heel.

A *shoe for a base-narrow hoof* should be just the reverse of the preceding. The outer branch should be somewhat longer than the inner.

A shoe for an acute-angled hoof should be long in the branches, because most of the weight falls in the posterior half of the foot. The support in front should be diminished either by turning the shoe up at the toe or by beveling it under the toe (fig. 5a).

A shoe for a stumpy hoof should be short in the branches, and for pronounced cases should increase the support of the toe, where the most of the weight falls, by being beveled downward and forward.

In many cases, especially in draft horses, where the hoofs stand very close together, the coronet of the outer quarter is found to stand out beyond the lower border of the quarter. In such cases the outer branch of the shoe from the last nail back must be fitted so full that an imaginary perpendicular dropped from the coronet will just meet the outer border of the shoe. The inner branch, on the other hand, must be fitted as " close " as possible. The principal thought should be to set the new shoe farther toward the more strongly worn side. Such a practice will render unnecessary the widespread and popular fad of giving the outer quarter and heel calk of hind shoes an extreme outward bend. Care should be taken, however, that in fitting the shoe " full " at the quarter the bearing surface of the hoof at the quarter be not left unsupported or incompletely covered, to be pinched and squeezed inward against the frog. This will be obviated by making the outer branch of the shoe sufficiently wide and punching it so coarse that the nails will fall upon the white line.

Hot fitting.—Few farriers have either the time or the skill necessary to adjust a cold shoe to the hoof so that it will fit, as we say, " air-tight." Though the opponents of hot fitting draw a lurid picture of the direful consequences of applying a hot shoe to the hoof, it is only the abuse of the practice that is to be condemned. If a heavy shoe at a yellow heat be held tightly pressed against a hoof which has been pared too thin, till it embeds itself, serious damage may be done. But a shoe at a dark heat may be pressed against a properly dressed hoof long enough to scorch, and thus indicate to the farrier the portions of horn that should be lowered without appreciable injury to the hoof and to the ultimate benefit of the animal.

Nailing.—The horse owner should insist on the nails being driven low. They should pierce the wall not above an inch and five-eighths above the shoe. A nail penetrating the white line and emerging low on the wall destroys the least possible amount of horn, has a wide and strong clinch, rather than a narrow one, which would be formed near the point of the nail, and, furthermore, has the strongest possible hold on the wall, because its clinch is pulling more nearly at a right angle to the grain (horn tubes) of the wall than if driven high. Finally, do not allow the rasp to touch the wall above the clinches.

THE BAR SHOE.

The bar shoe (fig. 9) has a variety of uses. It enables us to give the frog pressure, to restore it to its original state of activity and development when, by reason of disuse, it has become atrophied. It gives the hoof an increased surface of support and enables us to relieve one or both quarters of undue pressure that may have induced inflammation and soreness. The bar of the shoe should equal the average width of the remainder of the shoe and should press but lightly on the branches of the frog. The addition of a leather sole

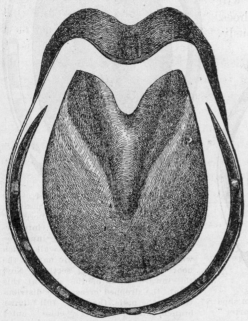 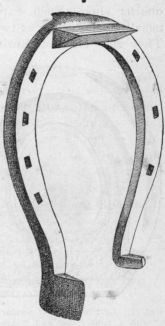

FIG. 9.—An acute-angled left fore hoof shod with a bar shoe. Note the width and position of the bar and the fact that the nails are placed well toward the toe, so as not to interfere with the expansion of the quarters.

FIG. 10.—A fairly formed right fore ice shoe for a roadster. The toe and outer-heel calks cut at right angles, and the inner-heel calk is slender and blunt. The back surface of the toe calk should be perpendicular.

with tar and oakum sole-packing allows us to distribute the weight of the body over the entire ground surface of the hoof.

THE RUBBER PAD.

Various forms of rubber pads, rubber shoes, rope shoes, fiber shoes, and other contrivances to diminish shock and prevent slipping on the hard and slippery pavements of our large cities are in use in different parts of the world. In Germany the rope shoe (a malleable-iron shoe with a groove in its ground surface in which lies a piece of tarred rope) is extensively used with most gratifying results. It is cheap, durable, easily applied, and effective.

In the large cities of England and the United States rubber pads are extensively used. They are rather expensive, but are quite efficient in preventing slipping on polished and gummy pavements, though not so effective on ice. Figure 11 is an illustration of one of the best of many rubber pads. The rubber is stitched and cemented to a leather sole and is secured by the nails of a three-quarter shoe. Such a pad will usually last as long as two shoes. They may be used continuously,

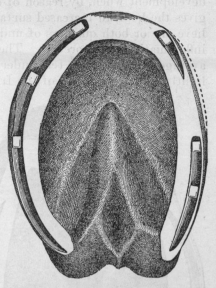

FIG. 12.—A narrow right fore hoof of the base-wide (toe-wide) standing position, shod with a plain "dropped-crease" shoe to prevent the toe cutting (interfering). The dotted line at the inner toe indicates the edge of the wall which was rasped away in order to narrow the hoof along the striking section. Note the inward bevel of the shoe at this point, the dropped crease, the distribution of the nails, the long "full" inner branch, and the short "close" outer branch.

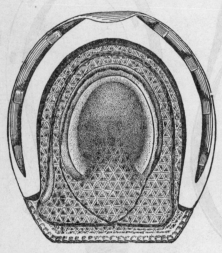

FIG. 11.—Left fore hoof of regular form shod with a rubber pad and "three-quarter" shoe. (Ground surface.)

not only without injury to the hoof, but to its great benefit. The belief, unsupported by evidence, that rubber pads "draw the feet" keeps many from using them. A human foot encased in a rubber boot may eventually be blistered by the sweat poured upon the surface of the skin and held there by the impervious rubber till decomposition takes place with the formation of irritating fatty acids; but there is no basis for an analogy in the hoof of a horse.

OTHER SPECIAL FORMS.

Some drawings, designed to illustrate shoeing in connection with "interfering" and "forging," and other special conditions, are shown in figures 13 to 18.

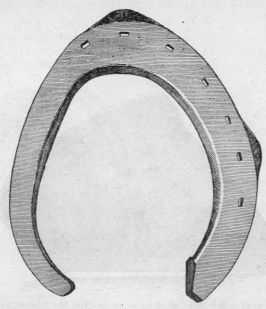

FIG. 13.—Hoof surface of a right hind shoe to prevent interfering. The inner branch has no nail holes and is fitted and beveled under the hoof. Note the number and position of the nail holes, the clip on the outer side wall, and the narrowness and bend of the inner branch.

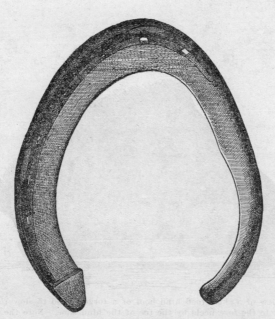

FIG. 14.—Ground surface of shoe shown in the previous figure. The inner, nailless branch has the thickness of the outer branch plus its calk. so that the inner and outer quarters of the hoof are equidistant from the ground.

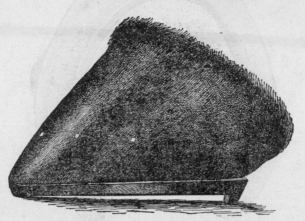

Fig. 15.—Side view of a fore hoof shod so as to quicken the "breaking over" (quicken the action) in a "forger." Note the short shoe, heel calks inclined forward, and the rolled toe.

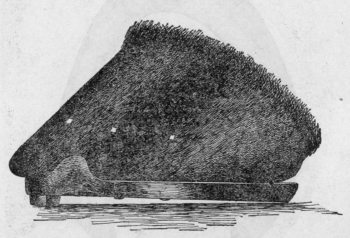

Fig. 16.—Side view of a short-toed hind hoof of a forger, shod to slow the action and to prevent injury to the fore heels by the toe of the hind shoe. Note the elevation of the short toe by means of a toe calk and the projection of the toe beyond the shoe. When such a hoof has grown more toe, the toe calk can be dispensed with and the shoe set farther forward.

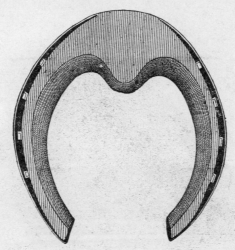

FIG. 17.—A toe-weight shoe to increase the length of stride of fore feet. The nails are placed too far back, and the shoe has no characteristic form but the weight is properly placed.

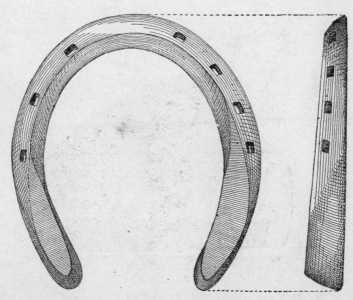

FIG. 18.—Most common form of punched heel-weight shoe to induce high action in fore feet. The profile of the shoe shows a " roll " at the toe and " swelled " heels. The weight is well placed, but " rolling " the toe and raising the heels lower action. The shoe would be much more effective if of uniform thickness and with no roll at the toe.

INDEX.